S0-AFC-533

GEORGE H. MULLER, D.V.M.

Clinical Associate Professor of Dermatology
Stanford University School of Medicine
Palo Alto, California

ROBERT W. KIRK, D.V.M.

Professor of Small Animal Medicine
New York State Veterinary College
Cornell University, Ithaca, New York

**With a foreword by:**

EUGENE M. FARBER, M.D.

Professor and Executive Head,
Department of Dermatology,
Stanford University School of Medicine, Palo Alto, California

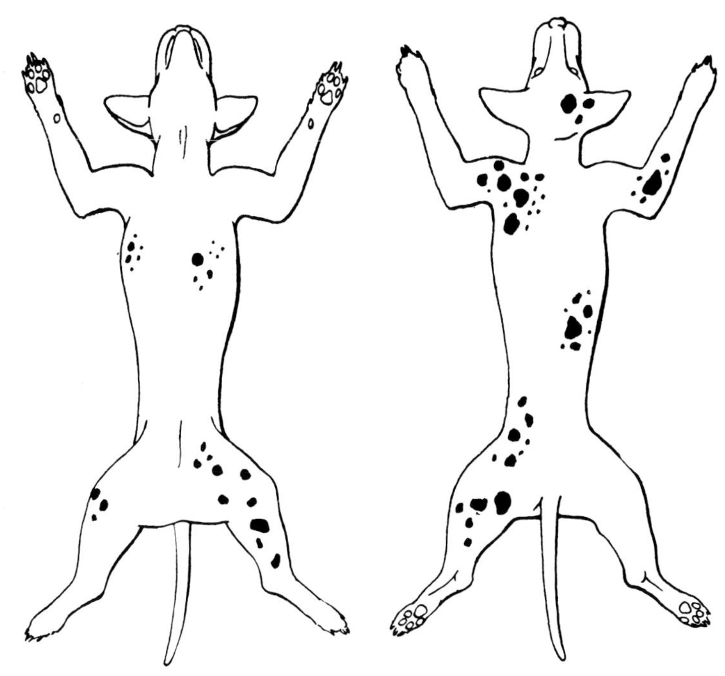

# SMALL ANIMAL DERMATOLOGY

W. B. SAUNDERS COMPANY · PHILADELPHIA · LONDON · TORONTO

W. B. Saunders Company: West Washington Square
Philadelphia, Pa. 19105

12 Dyott Street
London W.C.1

1835 Yonge Street
Toronto 7, Ontario

Reprinted October, 1969

Small Animal Dermatology

# PREFACE

This textbook of small animal dermatology is designed for students and clinicians. The authors have attempted to present a complete discussion of the entire subject in one volume. The book covers basic science, clinical aspects and therapeutic methods in a manner designed primarily for those who struggle daily with clinical dermatologic problems.

Although one fifth of a small animal practice deals with skin problems, this is the first complete text directed exclusively to that subject. Because of the broad scope of the book, some areas have not been developed in depth. In these cases, general principles are outlined, and the reader is advised to consult the lists of suggested reading which follow each chapter.

Dermatology is unique in that pathology of the lesions can be observed directly. The color illustrations provide an accurate method of teaching skin disease characteristics, and are arranged with an outline-form discussion of each disease for easy reading by busy clinicians.

The dermograms are original line drawings which illustrate the various steps in the pathogenesis of a dermatosis. The symbolic interpretations which are used are standardized in all the diagrams for ease in comparing tissue reactions in each disease. Most of the drawings and charts in the text were prepared especially for this volume.

Original too, and presented for the first time in veterinary dermatology, are the distribution patterns of skin lesions in typical canine and feline dermatoses.

Throughout the text, key principles and clinical guides are outlined in gray blocks for emphasis as "pearls" of knowledge.

The book can be used as a textbook for a complete course in small animal dermatology if one studies the chapters in consecutive order. However, the busy clinician can go directly to Section Five on specific dermatoses for concise information. The cross reference system will enable him to study any one skin disease in more detail if necessary. Terminology has been kept forthright, with use of as many English names as possible.

A brief survey of comparative dermatology stresses similar diseases in man and animals. The authors hope that mutual understanding and increased interest in diseases of the skin in several species may be fostered to the advantage of all.

The authors dedicate this book to clinicians who deal daily with small animal dermatoses, and to those who for years have requested that it be written. We hope they will find encouragement in it and answers to many of their questions.

GEORGE H. MULLER

ROBERT W. KIRK

*Palo Alto, California*

# ACKNOWLEDGMENTS

We particularly appreciate the enthusiastic encouragement of Dr. E. M. Farber, who wrote the foreword and made the facilities of the Dermatology Department, Stanford University School of Medicine, available to us.

Many authorities have read sections of the text pertaining to their specialties and offered constructive criticism. These include R. M. Adams, M.D., Faye Arundell, M.D., D. W. Baker, D.V.M., B. E. Belshaw, D.V.M., M. S. Blois, M.D., A. J. Cox, M.D., J. F. Cummings, D.V.M., H. E. Evans, Ph.D., W. Kaplan, D.V.M., S. R. Roberts, D.V.M., and Mrs. Jean Miller Mahoney.

Sketches and drawings were skillfully depicted by members of the Stanford Medical Illustrations Department: Louise Follett, Jill Leland, and Doreen Davies Masterson. We are especially pleased with the illustrations of Jill Leland, whose artistry clearly interpreted dermatologic processes.

Expert photographic advice was provided by Leonard Winograd and Daniel Zimm; both also helped with the production of some of the black and white photographs.

Most of the arduous task of typing the manuscript was ably completed by Helen Brown. The secretarial assistance and language translations of Christa Frisch were most helpful.

The E. R. Squibb Company and Eaton Laboratories have partially defrayed the cost of illustrations and color photographs. This help is acknowledged gratefully.

The National Science Foundation partially supported one of the authors (R. W. K.) with a Science Faculty Fellowship during the preparation of a portion of the manuscript.

We are grateful to Opal and Helen for their patience, understanding and help during the long preparation of the book.

The staff of W. B. Saunders Company has been most understanding, and a source of strength as we toiled together to produce this text.

G. H. M.

R. W. K.

# FOREWORD

EUGENE M. FARBER, M.D.

The multitude and variety of cutaneous diseases of animals have occupied the time and efforts of many veterinarians and have presented an area as complex as human skin disease.

Drs. Muller and Kirk have combined their talents and energies to publish a scholarly and practical book, the first of its kind.

Dr. George H. Muller has had over twenty-five years of experience in small animal practice. Since 1958 he has been on the Clinical Faculty of the Department of Dermatology at the Stanford University School of Medicine, where he has lectured to residents and medical students and carried out original studies on the biology of animal skin. He is a well-known lecturer at many schools of veterinary medicine and has participated actively in national meetings of veterinary and medical societies. Among his more recent publications is *Canine Skin Lesions.* He has a comprehensive and considerable knowledge of dermatology, both animal and human.

Dr. Robert W. Kirk is a Professor of Veterinary Medicine at Cornell University, where he has had seventeen years of experience in teaching small animal medicine. He is a well-known lecturer, the author of two books, *Current Veterinary Therapy* and *A Manual of Veterinary Procedures and Emergency Treatment.* He is also the author of articles and chapters in numerous other texts.

Dr. Kirk has been on sabbatical leave from Cornell University to carry out investigative studies in the Department of Dermatology at Stanford University and to work with Dr. Muller in the writing of this book. Both authors have expanded existing knowledge of veterinary dermatology through close contact with the basic scientists and clinicians in the Department of Dermatology at Stanford. They have with ingenuity adapted therapeutic methods in human care to animal dermatoses.

The color photography deserves a special comment. Dr. Muller is a nationally known amateur photographer. Most of the color photographs came from his collection of over 2000 Kodachromes of canine and feline dermatoses.

The section on "Comparative Dermatology" reminds us that the diseases of skin in animals and man have much in common. This outstanding contribution to the medical literature will serve to stimulate an increased interest in the study of animal and human skin diseases as they relate to one another.

# CONTENTS

## SECTION THREE—ETIOLOGIC FACTORS



## SECTION FOUR—DERMATOLOGIC THERAPY



## SECTION FIVE—CANINE AND FELINE DERMATOSES

# SMALL ANIMAL DERMATOLOGY

# FUNDAMENTALS OF DERMATOLOGY

---

*Section One*

# ONE

# *Anatomy of the Skin*

The skin serves as an anatomic and physiologic barrier between the animal body and its environment. It provides protection from physical, chemical and microbiologic injury, and its sensory components enable the animal to perceive heat, cold, pain, touch and pressure. Although the skin and hair coat of dogs and cats serve a heat-regulating function, they do not function in the same manner as in animals which do not pant. The skin may help in the synthesis of vitamin D, and its deeper layers have important fat storage and insulating qualities.

The skin, hair and subcutaneous tissue of a newborn puppy represent 24 per cent of its body weight (Lovell and Getty, 1964). By the time of maturity these structures only compose 12 per cent of body weight. Skin is made up of the epidermis and dermis which are closely associated with the hypodermis. It is difficult to dissect these layers from underlying structures, since subcutaneous tissue and superficial muscles are attached closely. Some areas of skin are specially modified in thickness and structure to adapt to specific function. The structure of skin is determined embryologically, and thick areas transplanted to other skin areas retain their characteristic anatomy in the new site (Pillsbury, Shelley and Kligman, 1961).

Skin is continuous at each body opening with the mucous membrane located there (digestive, respiratory, ocular and urogenital portals). The thickness of various layers of the skin varies greatly from one area to another. In general the skin is thickest over the dorsum and neck and thinnest on the abdomen, sternum and in the axillary and inguinal regions. The hair covering also varies in density in each individual. Usually the coat is heavy and thick over the back and sides of the body, but the inside of the ears and flanks and the under side of the tail often are practically hairless. Adnexal structures (hair, glands and claws) of dogs and cats have special variations of structure which will be discussed in detail later.

Four areas typify the variations found in canine integument—nasal, footpad, scrotal and hairy skin (Muller and Schneidman, 1967). Since hairy skin is abundant and important in disease processes it is discussed in detail; the other areas are mentioned for comparative purposes.

## HAIRY SKIN

Canine skin is composed of two layers which function as a unit: an outer layer, the epidermis, and an inner layer, the dermis (Fig. 1:1*A* and *B*).

***Cutaneous Anatomy***

I. Skin (cutis)
  A. Epidermis
    1. Horny layer (stratum corneum)
    2. Clear layer (stratum lucidum)
    3. Granular layer (stratum granulosum)
    4. Prickle layer (stratum spinosum)
    5. Basal layer (stratum basale)
  B. Epidermal appendages (adnexa)
    1. Glands of the skin
      a. Sebaceous glands
      b. Apocrine sweat glands
      c. Eccrine sweat glands
    2. Claw (ungues)
    3. Hair (pili)
  C. Dermis (corium)
II. Hypodermis (subcutis)

### Epidermis

The outer layer or epidermis is composed of multiple layers of cells, ranging from cuboid to flat. These are of two distinct types, keratinocytes and melanocytes. In addition, specialized appendages of the epidermis project into the underlying dermis.

The keratinocytes are the most important and abundant cells. They produce the dead fibrous protein, keratin, which is the main constituent of the outermost horny layer of the skin.

Production of the horny layer (the body's "miracle wrap") is the most important function of the epidermis.

For purposes of identification, certain areas of the epidermis are classified as "layers" and named, from within outward, as follows:

#### BASAL LAYER

The *basal layer* (stratum basale) is a single row of columnar cells resting on the basement membrane and separating the epidermis from the dermis. Most of

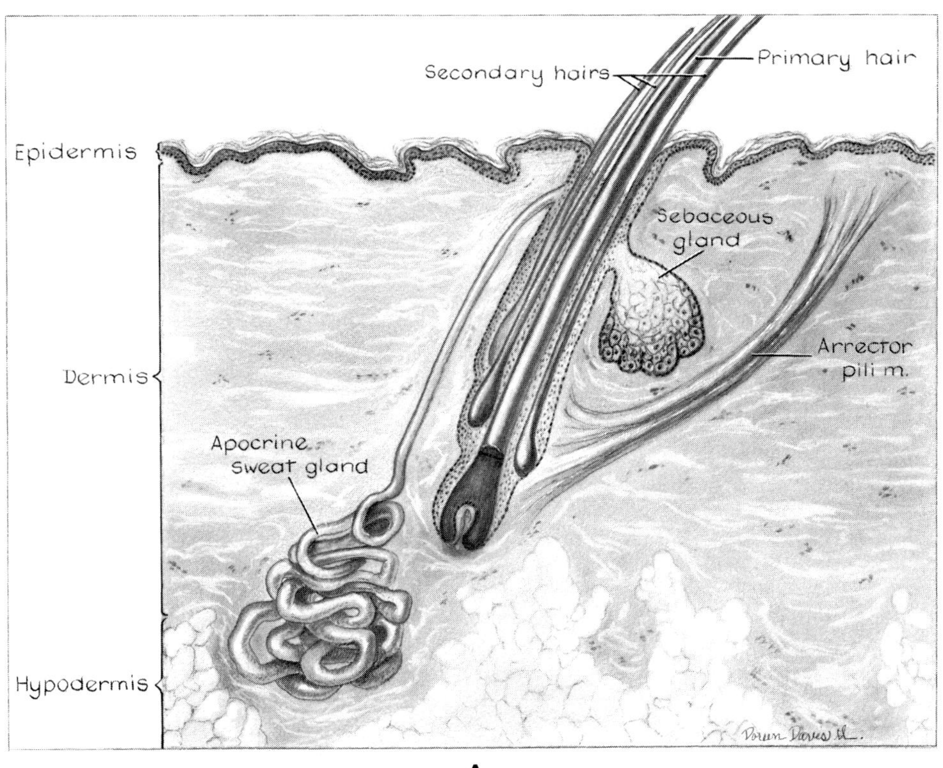


A

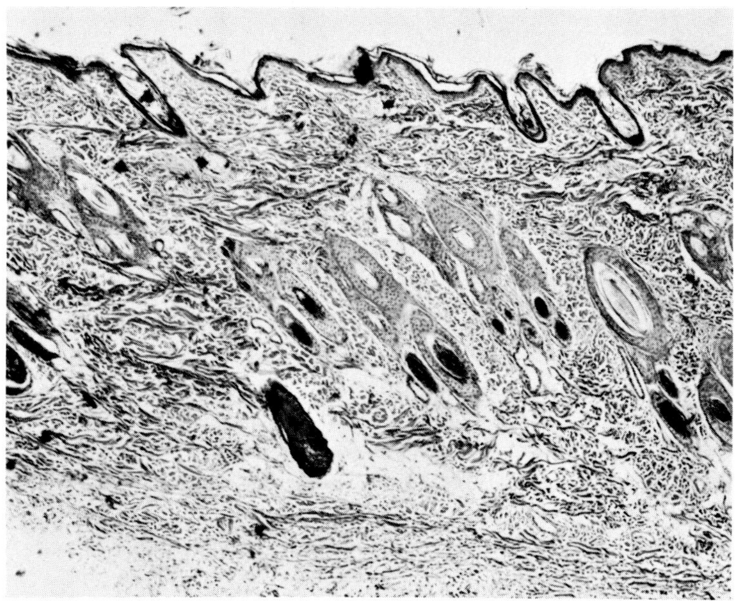

B

**Figure 1:1.** *A*, Normal canine skin (diagrammatic). *B*, Normal canine skin (Low power).

these cells are keratinocytes but a few are melanocytes (clear cells). The keratinocytes are constantly reproducing and pushing upward to replenish the epidermal cells above. The daughter cells move into the outer layers of the epidermis and are ultimately shed as dead horny cells.

#### PRICKLE CELL LAYER

The *prickle cell layer* (stratum spinosum or stratum malpighii) is composed of the daughter cells of the basal layer. This layer in hairy skin is two to three cells thick and comprised of flattened cuboid cells. In skin from the footpad and planum nasale they appear to be connected by fine spines or intercellular bridges, which are tonofibrils radiating from desmosomes in the cell wall (Lovell and Getty, 1964). These cells are not active mitotically except when the surface layers above are stripped off. However, they are viable, nucleated cells which are actively synthesizing keratin (Figs. 1:2 and 1:3).

#### GRANULAR LAYER

The *granular layer* (stratum granulosum) may not be present, but if observed it is only one cell thick. Cells in this layer are distinctly flattened (parallel to the surface) and contain shrunken nuclei and large basophilic staining keratohyaline granules (Fig. 1:3). These cells are dying.

#### CLEAR LAYER

The *clear layer* (stratum lucidum) is a fully keratinized, compact thin layer of non-nucleated dead cells. In dogs and cats it is found *only* in the footpads.

#### HORNY LAYER

The *horny layer* (stratum corneum) is the thin outer layer of completely keratinized tissue which is constantly being shed (Fig. 1:3). Its gradual desquamation normally is balanced by proliferation of the basal cells to maintain a constant epidermal thickness.

It must be stressed again that these layers are only various stages in a continuing process in the production of keratin. The horny layer is the body's "miracle wrap." Together with the granular layer it forms the barrier zone which prevents outward loss of moisture and other elements, and inward diffusion of chemicals, bacteria and other noxious agents. Diseases which interfere with the function of the barrier zone allow rapid passage of substances through the skin and upset the internal milieu. One therapeutic example of the clinical use of the outward growth of keratinocytes concerns griseofulvin. This drug is taken orally and absorbed. Subsequently it is deposited in the basal cells of the epidermis and moves with them outward until it is present in the horny layer. There it produces its inhibiting effect on dermatophytes which affect the skin. Since it takes several weeks to reach the horny layer, griseofulvin must be administered for a long time.

The melanocytes are the second type of cell found in the basal layer of the epidermis. Since they do not stain readily in H & E preparations, they appear as "clear" cells (Fig. 1:4). They are derived from the neural crest and migrate into

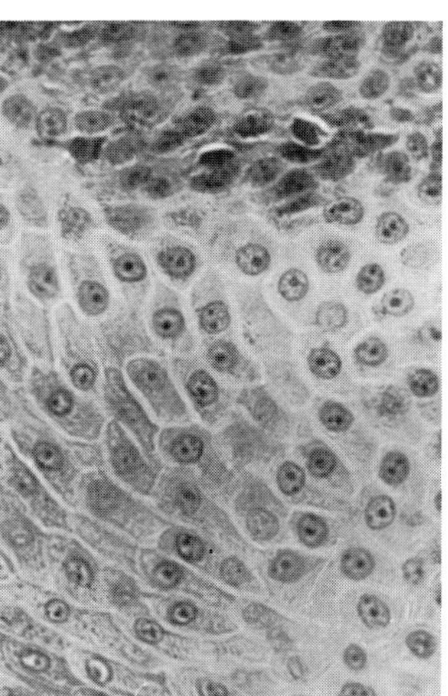

**Figure 1:2.** Prickle cells from footpad showing intercellular bridges (High power).

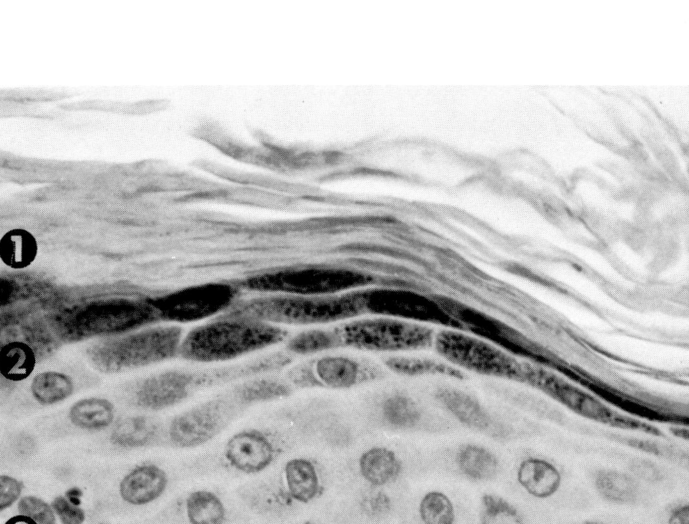


**Figure 1:3.** *1*, Horny layer; *2*, granular layer; and *3*, prickle cell layer from the planum nasale (High power).

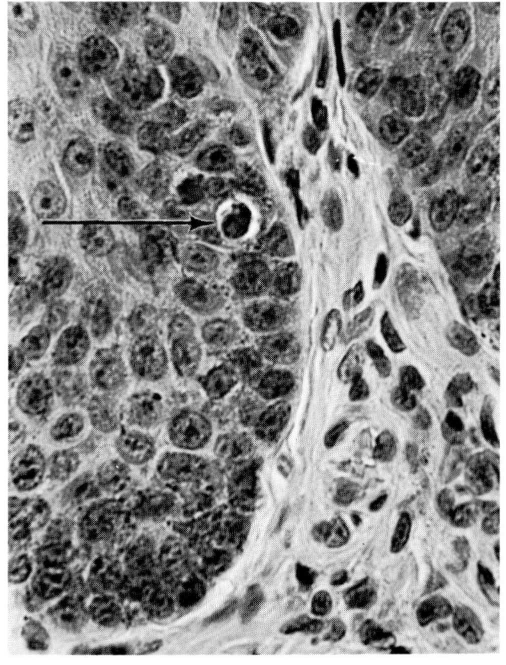

**Figure 1:4.** Melanocyte or "clear cell" in the basal layer of the planum nasale (High power, H & E stain).

the epidermis early in fetal life. Although they are of nondescript appearance, with special stains they can be shown to have long cytoplasmic extensions that weave among the epidermal cells, even extending into the upper layers of the epidermis. These dendritic processes are thought to inject pigment into the neighboring keratinocytes. Melanocytes contain tyrosinase, and are cells capable of producing the pigment melanin from the amino acid tyrosine. On exposure to sunlight or inflammation, melanocytes are stimulated to produce increased numbers of melanin granules. White and dark skin do not differ in the number of melanocytes they contain. Dark skin, however, contains more melanin—a reflection of greater activity of the melanocytes. Most of the pigment in skin is located in the basal layers of the epidermis. The horny layer is usually nonpigmented.

## Dermis (Corium)

The major function of the dermis is to support and nourish the epidermis and its appendages.

It is an integral part of the body's connective tissue system, and is of mesodermal origin. It may be affected by diffuse systemic collagen diseases and thus reflects their effect on the skin. In areas of thick hairy skin, the dermis accounts for most of the depth, whereas the epidermis is especially thin. In very thin skin, such as on the scrotum, the decreased thickness results from the thinness of the dermis. The dermis is composed of fibers, ground substance and cells. It also contains the epidermal appendages, arrector pili muscles, blood and lymph vessels and nerves.

The dermal fibers are collagenous, reticular and elastic. Collagenous fibers have great tensile strength and are the largest and most numerous. They are thick bands composed of multiple protein fibrils. The reticular fibers (precollagen) are fine branching structures that become closely approximated to collagen fibers with age. They can be detected only by special silver stains. Elastic fibers are composed of single fine branches which possess great elasticity. They are well visualized by the elastic van Gieson stain (Fig. 1:5).

The main component of the dermis is the ground substance. It is a mucoid gel-sol composed of mucopolysaccharides (hyaluronic acid and chondroitin sulfuric acid). It fills the spaces and surrounds other structures of the dermis, but allows electrolytes, nutrients and cells to traverse it freely in passing from the dermal vessels to the avascular epidermis. As animals age the ground substance decreases in amount.

There are three types of dermal cells—fibroblasts, mast cells and histiocytes (Fig. 1:6). Fibroblasts are immature cells with indistinct cytoplasm but spindle-shaped nuclei that have a fine vesicular appearance. They produce collagenous fibers and are often found adjacent to the surface of collagen bundles. Mast cells are histiocytic cells that are spindle-shaped, but with a round or oval nucleus. They characteristically have numerous large, intracytoplasmic,

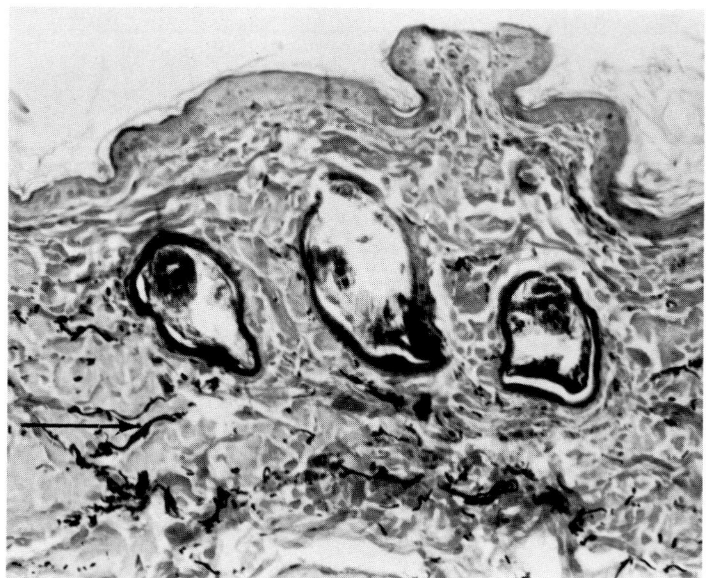

**Figure 1:5.** Elastic fibers from section of skin stained with elastic van Gieson (note epidermal papilla at surface of skin) (Low power).

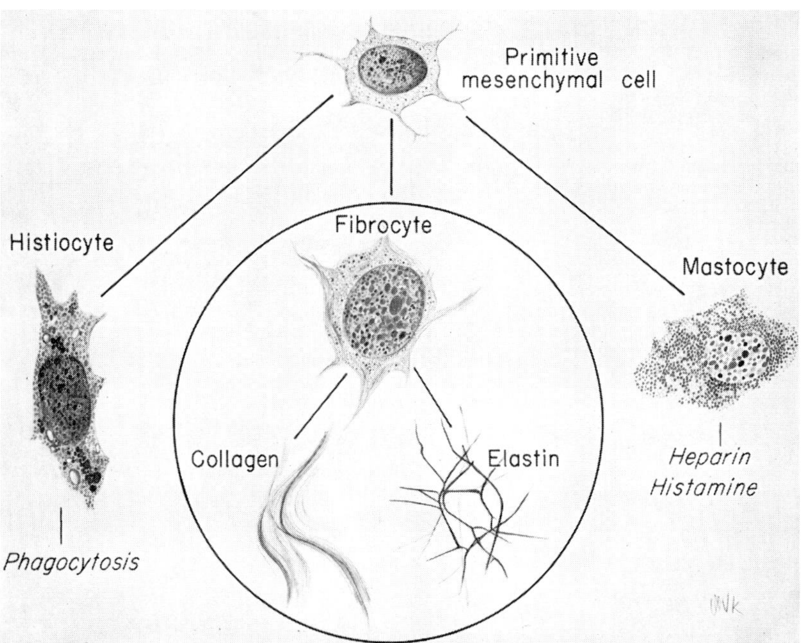


**Figure 1:6.** Schematic representation of the "cellular morphogenesis" in normal skin. (From Pillsbury, Shelley and Kligman: *Cutaneous Medicine.* W. B. Saunders Co., Philadelphia, 1966.)

basophilic, metachromatic granules which contain heparin and histamine. These granules are not evident with H & E stain but do show nicely with Giemsa stain, methylene blue or toluidine blue. Mast cells occur in all areas of connective tissue but especially around blood vessels.

Histiocytes are mature lymphoid type cells which are also called "wandering or tissue monocytes." They have round or bean-shaped nuclei that stain slightly paler than fibroblasts. Histiocytes form abundant reticular fibers and possess the ability to phagocytize bacteria and particulate material. Histiocytes may migrate to areas where material digestible to them is present. Those cells containing phagocytized material are called macrophages. If the material is melanin they are called melanophages; if it is lipid they become "foam cells." When individual macrophages are unable to deal with large particles, the cells fuse together to form multinucleated foreign-body giant cells.

### Hypodermis (Subcutis)

The hypodermis is predominantly fat which is mesodermal in origin. This region is composed of lipocytes, blood vessels, nerves and connective tissue. Some areas of the body (eyelids, ears, scrotum) have very little subcutaneous fat, whereas other areas have abundant amounts. There is a hormonal influence which results in female fat distribution. The shock-absorbing effect of fat depots in the footpads of dogs and cats is extremely important.

In general, the hypodermis functions to store fat, acts as a heat insulator and supports the overlying dermis and epidermis to give body contour.

## EPIDERMAL APPENDAGES

### Glands of the Skin

Epidermal appendages include sebaceous glands, apocrine and eccrine sweat glands, the nail matrix and hair follicles. They all develop embryologically as specialized groups of epidermal cells which proliferate into the underlying dermis.

#### *SEBACEOUS GLANDS*

Sebaceous glands are simple alveolar holocrine glands which appear as evaginations of the hair follicle. In a few places they are not associated with hairs. This is the case, for example, in the anus, external ear canal and the meibomian (tarsal) glands of the eyelid. The glands of Zeis are special sebaceous glands associated with the cilia of the upper eyelid. Sebaceous glands are located in the superficial layers of the dermis, and where hair is dense they tend to be long and narrow (squeezed). Where hair is sparse the glands are larger. There are no glands in the planum nasale; large sebaceous glands tend to associate with small hairs, and the largest of all are found at the mucocutaneous borders. In the cat they are present only on the hairy skin, but are especially large on the dorsal tail (supracaudal organ), on the lip and beneath the lip—the submental organ (Strickland and Calhoun, 1963). Sebaceous glands are often multilobular, club shaped and coiled. Several glands may enter into the single opening of the hair follicle complex. A ring of sebaceous glands opens into the follicle of the tactile hairs.

Each sebaceous gland is connected to the upper part of the hair follicle (or to the epidermal surface) by a short duct. The gland has a peripheral germinative layer of basal cells which surround a central mass of large foamy lipid-filled cells (Fig. 1:7). Excretion is produced by complete disruption of the foamy cells, and this effect may be actuated by contraction of the arrector pili muscle of the pilosebaceous-arrector muscle complex. While there is no neural control of secretion, there is evidence of hormonal control. Testosterone causes hypertrophy and estrogen causes involution of the glands.

Sebum production is increased by androgens and decreased by estrogens.

The oily secretion produced by sebaceous glands contains cholesterol, cholesterol esters, squalene, waxes, and esterified fatty acids. It tends to keep the skin

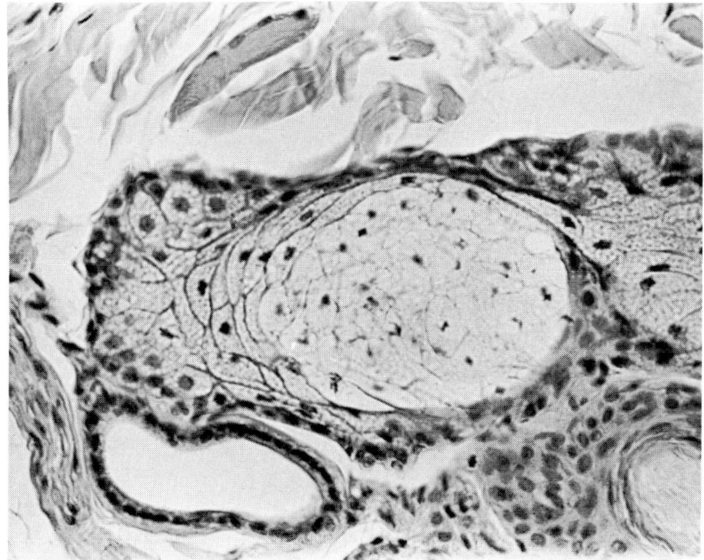

**Figure 1:7.** Canine sebaceous gland (apocrine duct in lower left corner, hair follicle and hair in lower right corner). (High power.)

soft and pliable by forming a surface emulsion which spreads over the surface of the horny layer to retain moisture and thus maintain proper hydration. The oily film also spreads over the hair shafts and gives them a glossy sheen. During periods of illness or malnutrition, the hair coat may become dull and dry as a result of inadequate functioning of the skin glands (both sebaceous and apocrine).

#### APOCRINE SWEAT GLANDS

Apocrine sweat glands are located deep in the dermis. They are serpentine in the dog and glomiform in the cat. One gland is associated with each hair follicle complex and its duct enters the follicle just above the entrance of the sebaceous duct (Fig. 1:1*A*). The body of the gland is composed of widely dilated secretory tubules surrounded by a layer of stellate myoepithelial cells (Fig. 1:8). The secretory epithelium is a single layer of columnar cells with budlike apical projections, finely basophilic cytoplasm containing pigment granules, and a spheroid nucleus (Fig. 1:9). At the completion of secretion the glands have a wider lumen and the secretory cells have become low cuboid in shape with a flattened nucleus. Apocrine glands are located throughout the body of the dog (except planum nasale). Specialized apocrine glands are present in the external ear canal and in the eyelids associated with the cilia (glands of Moll). Saccular coiled apocrine glands of the cat are present in all the general body skin but are prominent in the scrotum (Strickland and Calhoun, 1963).

Apocrine sweat is a proteinaceous, white odorless milky fluid which is formed slowly and continuously. It is stored in the lumen of the secretory tubule and expelled by myoepithelial contraction under sympathetic (adrenergic) stimulation (Iwabuchi, 1967).

Bacteria on the skin surface act on apocrine secretions to produce characteristic odors.

Mammary glands are specialized apocrine skin glands.

#### ECCRINE SWEAT GLANDS

Eccrine sweat glands in the dog and cat (Fig. 1:10) are found only in the footpads. The glands are located deep in the dermis at its junction with the hypodermis. A long duct connects the secretory tubule with a pore on the surface of the pad (Fig. 1:11). These glands have no thermoregulatory function in the dog or cat.

### Specialized Glandular Structures

#### CIRCUMANAL GLANDS

Circumanal glands are closely allied with the skin of the anus. They are composed of a sebaceous component which is associated superficially with the

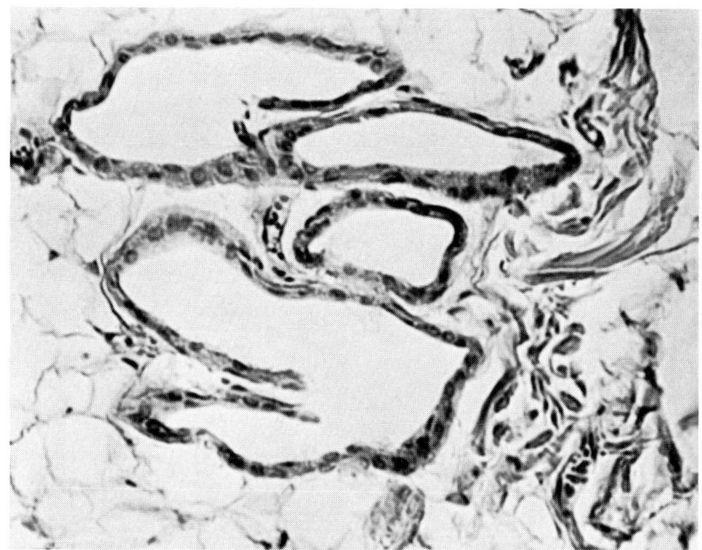

**Figure 1:8.** Section through coiled portion of apocrine sweat gland. (High power.)

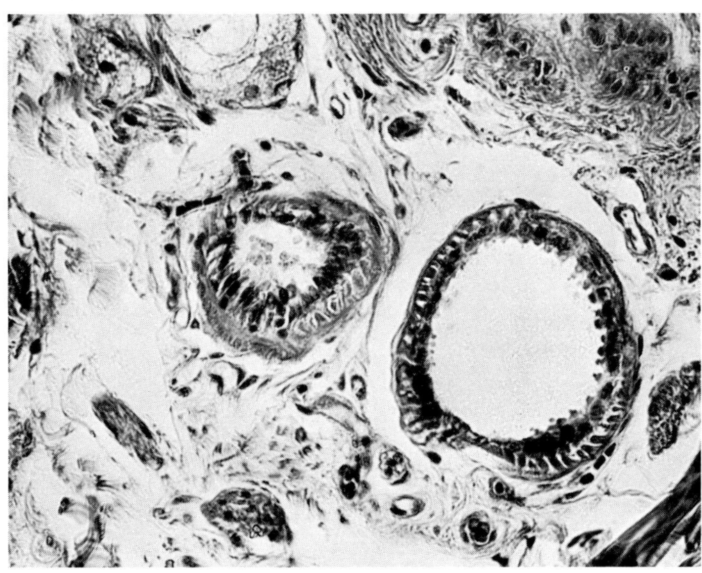

**Figure 1:9.** Apocrine gland showing secretory epithelium. (High power.)

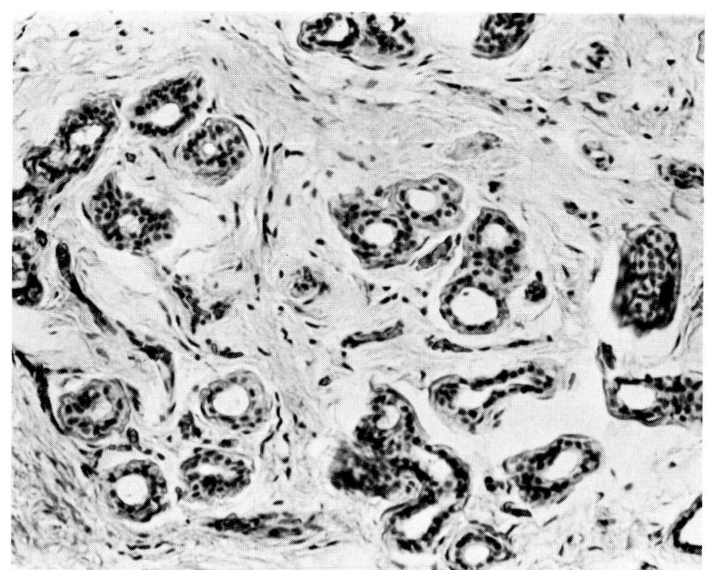

**Figure 1:10.** Eccrine sweat glands from canine footpad. (High power.)

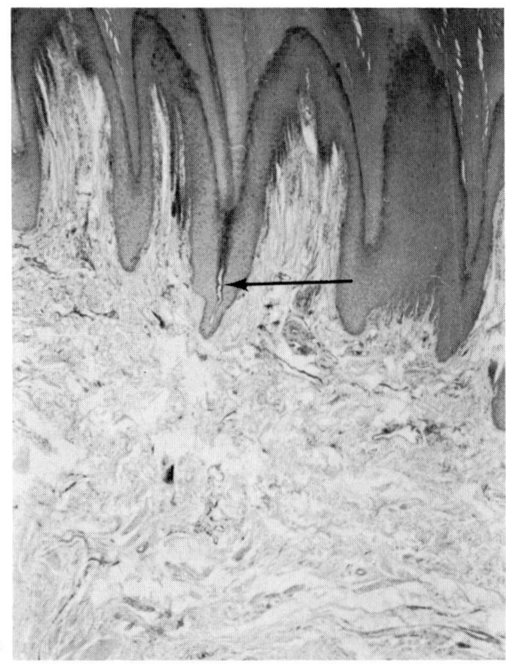

**Figure 1:11.** Eccrine duct traversing the epidermis of the footpad. (High power.)

hair follicles of the region. The deeper component consists of solid masses of large polygonal cells that are not sebaceous in nature and have no secretory activity (Parks, 1950).

### *TAIL GLAND*

The tail gland is located on the dorsal surface of the tail about two inches distal to the anus. It is an oval area of skin which is unique (Fig. 1:12). The hair coat of the region is characterized by stiff, coarse hairs, each emerging singly from its follicle. The surface of the skin may be yellow and waxy from the abundant secretion of the numerous large sebaceous and apocrine glands of the

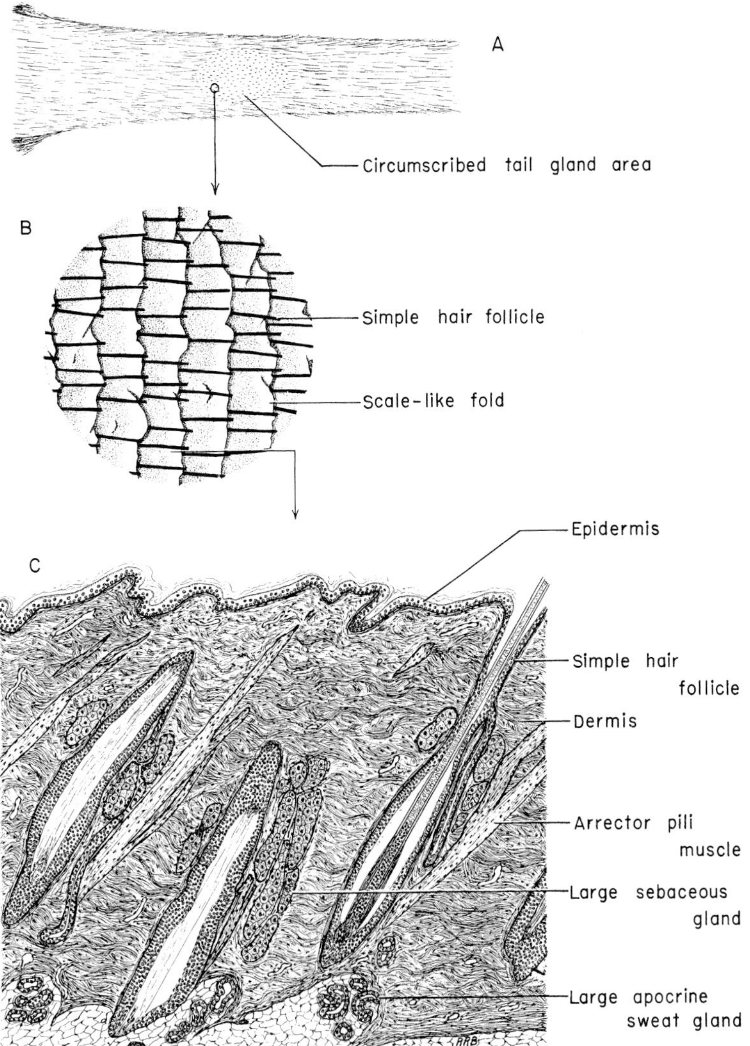


**Figure 1:12.** Surface contour, hair arrangement and histology of the tail gland area. (From Miller, Christensen and Evans: *Anatomy of the Dog.* W. B. Saunders Co., Philadelphia, 1964. After Lovell and Getty, 1957.)

area. Hildebrand (1952) believes this secretion aids in olfactory recognition of the species. This area of the tail may be severely affected in clinical cases of seborrhea. Strickland and Calhoun (1963) comment on the numerous large sebaceous glands which are present in the cat on the dorsal surface of the tail for its entire length. They are not localized to a circumscribed area as in the dog. This region of sebaceous glands in the cat has been named the "supracaudal organ." Excess accumulation of its secretion causes a condition called "stud tail."

#### GLANDS OF THE EXTERNAL AUDITORY CANAL

The skin lining of the external ear canal is stratified squamous epithelium with sebaceous and apocrine glands and hair follicles. Just under the epithelium the sebaceous glands are abundant. The tubular (apocrine) glands are located deeper in the dermis. Normal ear wax is thought to be a mixture of the secretions of both types of glands (Nielsen, 1953). In inflammation, the apocrine glands become cystic and their secretion increases markedly (Kirk and Spreull, 1968).

#### ANAL SACS

Anal sacs are paired structures located between the internal and external sphincter muscles on each side of the anus. Each is really a pocket of skin which opens into the anal canal by a single duct. Sebaceous glands are more abundant in the skin lining the duct, whereas apocrine glands are concentrated in the skin of the fundus (Fig. 1:13). The oily, disagreeable-smelling fluid which accumulates in the sacs is a product of both types of glands (Montagna and Parks, 1948). In contrast to this arrangement in the dog, the cat has large numbers of seba-

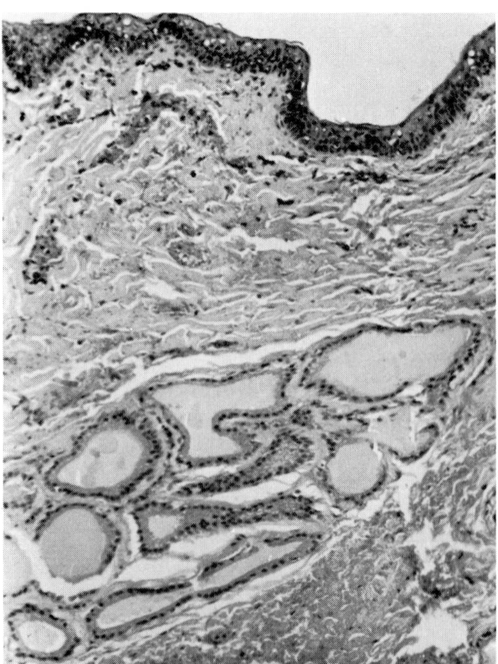

**Figure 1:13.** Section through wall of the anal sac showing apocrine type glands in the dermis.

ceous glands comprising much of the fundic wall of its anal sacs (Strickland and Calhoun, 1963).

## CLAWS

The claw (nail) is a direct continuation of the dermis and epidermis with specialized structure (Fig. 1:14*A*). The distal phalanx of each toe has a crescent-shaped dorsal process called the ungual crest. The dermis of adjacent skin is continuous with and extends distally from this bony process as the periosteum of the phalanx. It has a rich blood supply and is the source of the profuse hemorrhage which occurs if the claw is trimmed too short. The structures making up the claw are compressed laterally, and the dermis can thus be divided into the sole (ventral), the dorsal ridge of the coronary band, and the lateral and medial walls. Most of the claw is formed from the coronary band and the dorsal ridge. In many areas the dermis has fine papillae which project distally and interdigitate with soft epidermal lamellae.

The epidermis of adjacent skin also is continuous with that of the claw. The basal layer of the epidermis, supported by the dermis, is most active in the coronary and dorsal ridge areas and so causes the claw to grow in a circular fashion and produces a curved claw. This is why the claw may grow around into the volar surface of the footpad. The horny walls grow over the sole of the claw for the same reason. The epidermis of the claw sole has distinct granular and clear layers as well as the usual structures. However, the epidermis of the rest of the claw is largely composed of a thick horny layer which consists of flat cornified epidermal cells fused into a horny plate. On the ventral surface the claw is separated from the footpad by a distinct furrow. A fold of modified skin hides the dorsal junction of hairy skin and claw. This claw fold is free of hair on its inner surface and produces the thin stratum tectorium which is the outer layer of the proximal claw.

## HAIR

The skin of dogs and cats is completely covered with hairs except for the nose, footpads and mucocutaneous junctions. Hairs are flexible, elastic, horny threads. They are divided into the free part (the hair shaft) and the proximal part (the root).

The hair shaft which extends above the surface of the skin is a dead structure with three parts, the cuticle, the cortex and the medulla. The medulla of dog and cat hair is moderately wide. In the cat the profile of the hair is distinctly serrated. The cortex is made up of tightly packed keratin cells. Primary hairs have a cortex and medulla but secondary hairs have only a cortex. The cuticle is a thin layer of cells which overlap much like shingles. However, they are tightly pressed to the surface of the cortex. Each hair root has a knob-like, hollow proximal end (like the bottom of a champagne bottle) which is called the hair bulb. This bulb attaches the hair to its underlying dermal papilla. The hair roots arise from epithelial pits called hair follicles. The epithelial part of the hair follicle is divided into an outer root sheath, which is continuous with the basal layer of the skin, and an inner root sheath, which grows upward from the dermal

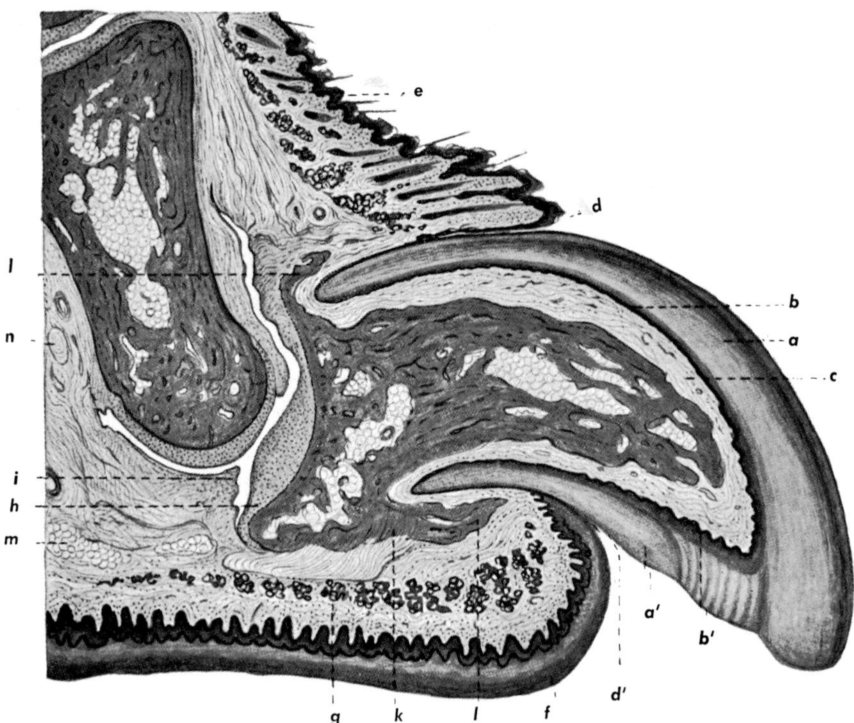


**Figure 1:14***A*. Midsagittal section through the claw of the dog. *a*, Stratum corneum of the epidermis of the claw; *a'*, stratum corneum of the epidermis of the sole; *b,b'*, deep, noncornified epidermal layers of the dorsum and sole of the claw; *c*, corium (papillated in the area of the sole); *d*, claw fold; *d'*, limiting furrow separating the sole from the digital pad; *e*, skin with hair and glands; *f*, epidermis of the digital pad with stratum granulosum and lucidum; *g*, tubular glands in the digital pad; *h*, articular cartilage of the third phalanx; *i*, meniscus; *k*, Sharpey's fibers from a tendon insertion; *l*, ungual crest; *m*, fat cushion within the digital pad; *n*, lamellar corpuscle. (Reprinted from A. Trautmann and J. Fiebiger: FUNDAMENTALS OF THE HISTOLOGY OF DOMESTIC ANIMALS. Copyright 1952 by Cornell University. Used by permission of Cornell University Press.)

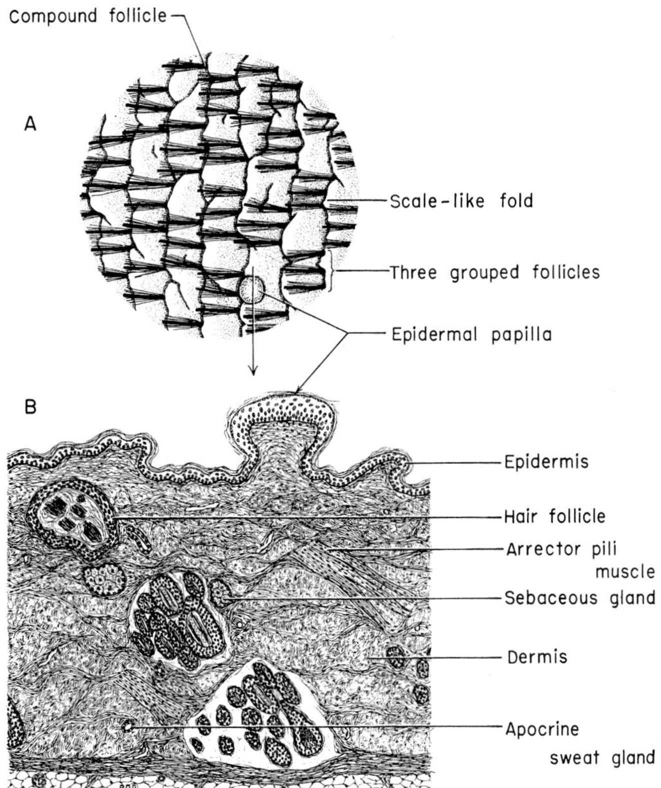


**Figure 1:14***B*. Surface contour, hair arrangement and histology of the hairy skin. *A*, View of scalelike folds and arrangement of hair follicles; *B*, histological section of hairy skin. (From Miller, Christensen and Evans: *Anatomy of the Dog*. W. B. Saunders Co., Philadelphia, 1964. After Lovell and Getty, 1957.)

papilla to the level of the sebaceous gland. Hairs are set into the skin at an oblique angle with bundles of hair sharing common openings on the surface. These bundles usually are arranged in groups of three and these in turn are aligned in irregular rows. The skin surface is thrown into scale-like folds which form compound hair follicle depressions from which the hair bundles emerge. Knob-like projections called epidermal papillae are seen occasionally (Fig. 1:14*B*).

Hair shafts that share a common skin opening have a single follicle down to the level of the sebaceous glands, but here they separate and each hair has its own follicle. A typical bundle may have seven to 15 hairs—one large, long, stiff cover hair, which has a deeper follicle, and many fine lanugo or under hairs with superficially located follicles. Within a group of three hair bundles, the guard hair of the central bundle is coarser than those in the lateral bundles (Fig. 1:15*A*).

The hair follicle unit consists of the hair follicle and its arrector pili muscle together with apocrine and sebaceous glands.

Certain structures are always associated with hairs and form the "hair follicle unit" or apopilosebaceous complex (Fig. 1:15*B*). Sebaceous glands from each hair follicle are bunched into clusters and sometimes fuse. All empty into the common hair follicle. Each hair's arrector pili muscle joins with others of the same follicle unit and together they insert into the dense layer of dermis immediately beneath the epidermis. When these muscles contract the follicle complex is elevated and sebum is expressed into the common canal. Each follicle unit also possesses one apocrine gland which empties into the common follicle distal to the sebaceous duct.

Dogs and cats have three general kinds of hairs: tactile or sinus hair, coarse or guard hair, and fine or lanugo hair.

## Tactile Hairs

Tactile hairs are also called whiskers (Fig. 1:16*A*). They are most numerous on the sides of the muzzle where some of the longest grow from two tubercles, one on either side of the face. A tuft of such hairs grows from the submental region of the lower jaw and several grow from above each eye. The eyelashes (cilia) are large hairs but they are not sinus hairs. The typical tactile hair of carnivores has a well-developed connective tissue sheath around the hair follicle which is rich in elastic fibers. A blood sinus lined with endothelium is interposed between the inner and outer layers of the dermal portion of the follicle (Fig. 1:16*B*). This thin-walled blood sinus (of tactile hairs of the face) is abundantly supplied with branches of the trigeminal nerve. The entire complex assists in improving the acuity of sensory perception and may help animals orient themselves in poor light. The tactile hairs probably help demonstrate emotional feeling, as cats show supreme adoration by rubbing their face (and whiskers) against the object of their affection.

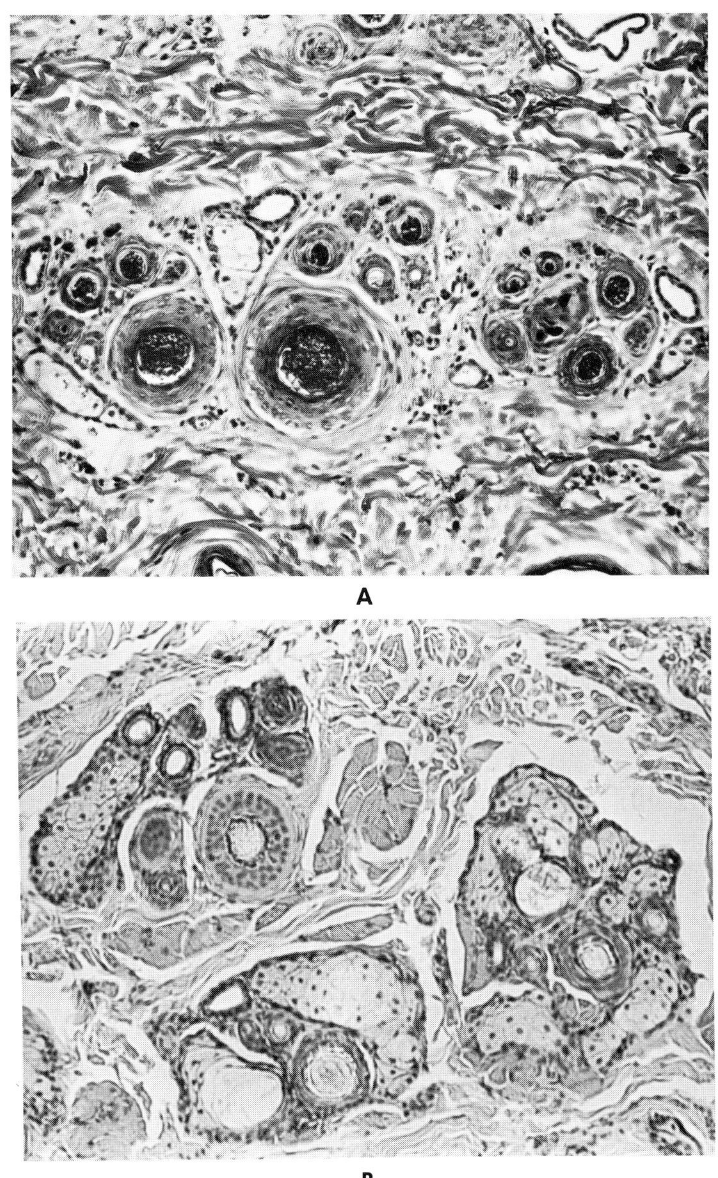


**Figure 1:15***A*. Three multiple hair follicle units. (High power.)

**Figure 1:15***B*. Three apopilosebaceous complexes, each showing primary and secondary hairs, sebaceous and apocrine glands and arrector pili muscles. (High power.)

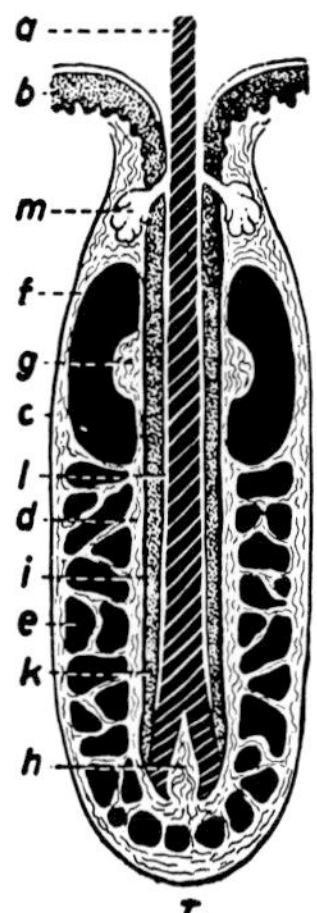


**Figure 1:16***A*. Hair follicle of sinus hair of cat in longitudinal section, semidiagrammatic (150×). *a*, Hair; *b*, epidermis; *c*, outer, *d*, inner, layer of the dermal follicle; *e*, the blood sinus (this sinus has been differentiated into a nontrabecular annular sinus *f*, into which projects the sinus pad *g*); *h*, hair papilla; *i*, glassy membrane of the follicle; *k*, outer root sheath; *l*, inner root sheath; *m*, sebaceous glands. (Reprinted from A. Trautmann and J. Fiebiger: FUNDAMENTALS OF THE HISTOLOGY OF DOMESTIC ANIMALS. Copyright 1952 by Cornell University. Used by permission of Cornell University Press.)

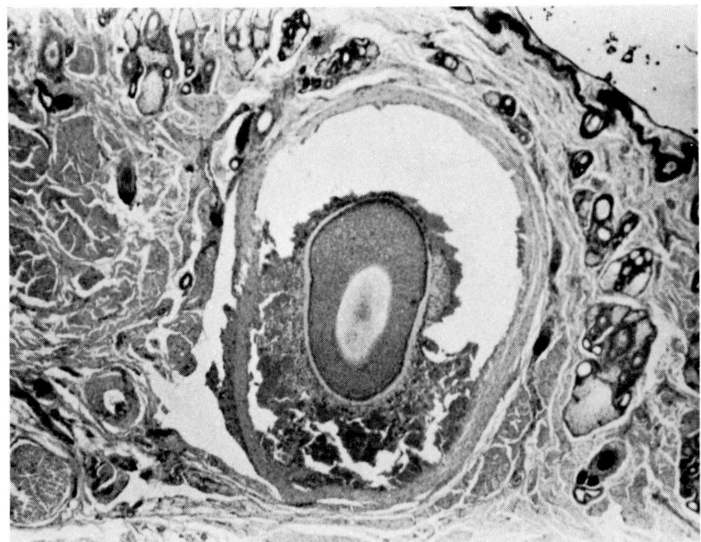

**Figure 1:16***B*. Tactile hair from upper lip of dog showing blood sinus. (High power.)

## Hair Types

Although hair types of dogs are extremely diverse, various authors have attempted to classify them on the basis of color, length, type of bristle and characteristics of the medulla and cortex. Although Lovell and Getty (1964) have summarized these classifications, we have attempted to further simplify the classification presented by Gair. Hair types of dogs can be divided into normal (intermediate length), short and long coats.

### *NORMAL COAT*

The normal coat is typified by that seen in the German shepherd, the Corgi and wild dogs such as wolves and coyotes. It is composed of primary hairs (coarse guard hairs or bristles) and secondary hairs (fine lanugo hairs or undercoat). A high proportion of the hairs, by number but not by weight, are lanugo hairs.

The next two classes of hair coats also are made up basically of primary and secondary hairs, but the relative sizes of hairs and their numbers vary markedly from the normal coat.

### *SHORT COAT*

The short coat can be divided into coarse and fine subdivisions. The coarse short hair is typified by the Rottweiler and many of the terriers. This type of coat has a strong growth of primary hairs and a much lesser growth of secondary hairs. The total weight of hair is less, and the secondary hairs especially are less in weight and numbers than in the normal coat. The fine short coat is exemplified by boxers, dachshunds and miniature pinschers. This type of coat has the largest number of hairs per unit area. The secondary hairs are numerous and well developed and the primary hairs are reduced in size as compared to the normal coat.

### *LONG COAT*

The long coat also can be arranged into two subdivisions—the fine long coat and the woolly or coarse long coat. The fine long coat is found in the cocker spaniel, the Pomeranian and the chow. This coat has greater weight of hair per unit area than does the normal coat, except in the toy breeds where the weight may be less because the hair is finer. The woolly or coarse long coat is found in the poodle, and perhaps also in the Bedlington terrier and the Kerry blue terrier. Lanugo hairs (secondary hairs) make up 70 per cent of the total weight of these coats and 80 per cent of the number of hairs (Rook and Walton, 1965). For secondary-type hairs these are relatively coarse and nonmedullated and the three breeds mentioned have little tendency to shed hair.

The hair coat of cats is of two types, longhair or Persian, and shorthair or "domestic." The shorthair is the natural and dominant gene. Long-haired cats, which were probably mutations, are severely handicapped by matted hair when forced to live in a wild state. The hairs of cats project as groups of hairs from a common follicular canal at the skin surface, but the bundles are farther apart in the cat than in the dog (Creed, 1958). Strickland and Calhoun (1963) state that the bundles of hair are arranged in clusters of two, three, four and five with clusters of two and three bundles being common on the dorsal body and clusters of four and five being found ventrally. Each bundle or group contains three primary hairs surrounded by six to 12 secondary hairs.

## Hair Color

Coat color in cats is complex but a few generalizations are possible. White is dominant over all colors. It is followed in order of dominance by black, tabby and red. In the Siamese breed seal point is the dominant gene while blue point is its recessive. Chocolate point is a diluent of seal point, and lilac point is a diluent of blue point.

The genetic aspects of coat color in dogs also is a complex subject which has been documented by Little (1957). Pigmentation in individual hairs may be uniform throughout the length of the shaft or it may vary. In the agouti-type hair (German shepherd, Norwegian elkhound) the tip is white or light, the heavy body is pigmented brown or black and the base is a light yellow or red-brown. Pigment cells in the bulb of the hair deposit pigment in or between the cortical and medullary hair cells. The amount of pigment deposited in the hair and its location there produce different optical effects. However, there are only two types of pigment. The black-brown pigment is designated tyrosine-melanin; and the yellow-red pigment is called pheo-melanin (Lovell and Getty, 1964).

## Hair Cycle

Hairs do not grow continuously as claws do, but grow in cycles (Fig. 1:17). Each cycle consists of a growing period (anagen) when the follicle is actively producing the hair and a resting period (telogen) when the hair is retained in the follicle as a dead or "club" hair which is subsequently lost. There is also at least one transitional period (catagen) between these two stages. Chase (1965) has outlined a detailed classification of the steps of hair growth. This is also discussed by Ebling (1965). During anagen, or active growth, hair is produced by mitotic division of cells in the matrix surrounding the dermal papilla. At the end of active growth the middle region of the hair bulb starts to become constricted. Above this area the hair root becomes expanded and keratinized to form a "club." At this transitional stage (catagen) the connective tissue sheath of the follicle thickens and becomes corrugated just below the newly formed "club" and this cord of cells pushes the "club" hair up the hair canal. The distal portion of the hair follicle left in the canal below the club shortens to form a little nipple called the secondary germ. This is telogen or the resting stage. When the next period of activity starts, often weeks or months later, the secondary germ elongates, grows down to enclose the dermal papilla and gives rise to the new hair bulb. Mitosis begins and a new hair pushes upward and emerges alongside the old club, which is then lost. The metabolic activity engendered during anagen is tremendous. Hair is practically solid protein (keratin) and, although each hair grows only 0.04 to 0.18 mm. daily (Comben, 1951), when several hundred thousand hairs are growing it means 60 to 70 feet of hair is produced daily.

Hair growth in dogs and cats follows definite cycles, but hair replacement is in a mosaic pattern so there is no synchronized wave pattern of shedding.

The knowledge of normal patterns of hair growth in domestic animals is fragmentary. Little is known about hair growth of the dog and cat. Many rodents shed their hair coats in definite, synchronized wave-patterns. This means that many hairs in adjacent follicles are in the same period of their cycle. Waves of replacement start at the midline of the abdomen and move laterally and dorsally. Man, the guinea pig, the dog and the cat have hair follicle growth which is not synchronized and therefore hair replacement is said to have a mosaic pattern. Adjacent hairs may be in any stage of the hair cycle – telogen, anagen or catagen. No critical studies of hair growth in the dog have been done. With over 300 recognized breeds and innumerable coat patterns in mongrels this would be a supreme task. Not only do coat types vary from breed to breed but they may even vary on individuals. Breeds such as the collie, chow and other similar types have long hair on the body but short hair on the face and feet. These variations can be explained if there is a different rate of hair growth on each part of the body or a different length of hair cycle on each part or a combination of both variables.

It seems reasonable to assume that a major portion of this difference in dogs may be due to a different length of hair cycle in different breeds or on

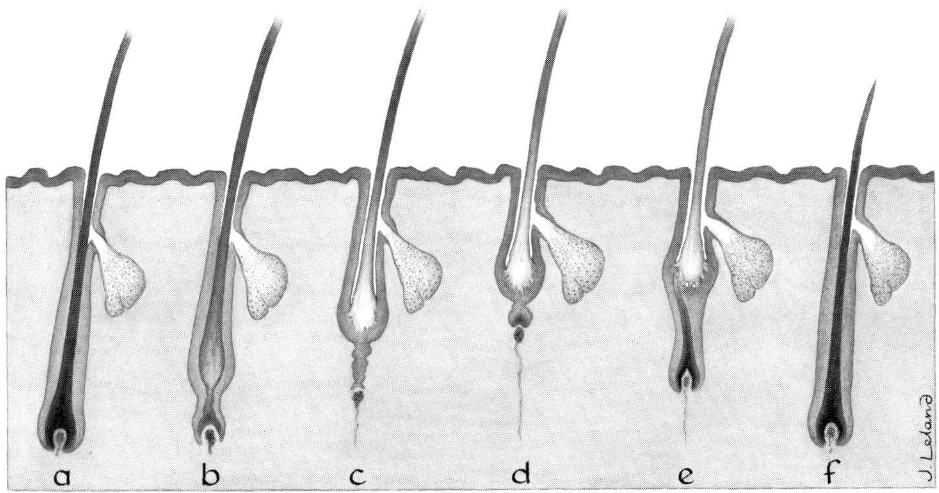


**Figure 1:17.** The hair cycle. *a,* Anagen: During anagen, the growing stage, hair is produced by mitosis in cells of the dermal papilla. *b,* Early catagen: In early catagen, the transitional stage, a constriction occurs at the hair bulb. The hair above this will become a "club." *c,* Catagen: The distal follicle becomes thick and corrugated and pushes the hair outward. *d,* Telogen: This is the resting stage. The dermal papilla separates and an epithelial strand shortens to form a secondary germ. *e,* Early anagen: The secondary germ grows down to enclose the dermal papilla and a new hair bulb forms. The old "club" is lost. *f,* Anagen: The hair elongates as growth continues.

various body areas, just as such differences occur in man. Scalp hair (man) may grow in anagen for up to 25 years without resting and attain lengths of several feet. Eyebrows or hair of the body, on the other hand, grow only about six months before going into telogen, which lasts an equal time (Pillsbury, Shelley and Kligman, 1961). The hair is shed and a new cycle begins.

Under conditions of ill health or generalized disease, the growing stage (anagen) may be considerably shortened. Accordingly, a large percentage of body hairs may be in telogen (resting) at one time. Telogen hairs are more easily lost because they are less firmly anchored and so the animal may "shed" excessively. Actually the removal of "club" hair may stimulate the growth cycle (anagen).

Disease states also may lead to faulty formation of hair cuticle. In some cases the cuticle cells are not pressed tightly against the cortex, and light striking the hair surface is reflected abnormally. Thus the hair looks dull and lusterless. Severe illness or systemic stress, such as the burden of pregnancy or parturition, may cause many body hairs to enter telogen prematurely but in synchronization. Later, shedding of these hairs occurs simultaneously. This postpartum or telogen effluvium is found in several species, including the dog (Bosse, 1965).

A hair that falls out at the end of a growth cycle is a club hair. The club consists of a tiny dry white ball at the root end. Root sheaths are not present but the club may be surrounded by an epithelial sac. Hair plucked in anagen shows a larger expanded root, which is moist and glistening, often pigmented at the end and surrounded by a root sheath (Fig. 1:18*A*). Hair plucked at telogen shows a club root with root sheaths and a keratinized sac (Fig. 1:18*B*). Hair affected by mild disease or poisonings may have abruptly tapered shafts or local constric-

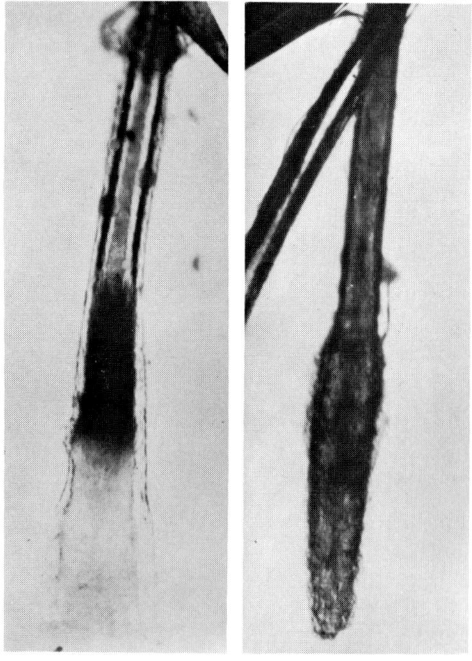


**Figure 1:18***A*. Anagen hair plucked from hair follicle. (Low power.) *B*, Telogen hair plucked from hair follicle. (Low power.) (Courtesy of Drs. E. J. Van Scott and P. Frost, National Institutes of Health, Bethesda, Maryland.)

tions at the distal end. Severe hair damage causes the hair to break off and fall out. In these cases the root of the hair looks like a spear (Lewis and Wheeler, 1967). Hair with the most rapid growth and the longest growth cycle is apt to be affected the most, so body hair often will be lost before that of the extremities. It is interesting to note that guinea pigs and mice experimentally infected with *T. mentagrophytes* show fungal invasion of hairs only in the anagen period of growth.

Telogen-anagen ratios may be helpful in studying abnormal coat conditions in the future. At least 100 hairs must be carefully and firmly plucked and classified.

Little has been documented concerning normal canine shedding, but certain wild dogs shed rather generally in the spring and again in the fall. Ebling (1965) has shown that the photoperiod is more important to shedding than environmental temperature. In some species, as the hours of light per day increase, rate of shedding increases, the coat becomes coarser and the hair density decreases.

The photoperiod is more important to shedding than the environmental temperature.

Sebaceous secretion increases. All these effects seem to be designed to allow air to circulate through the coat. As the daily photoperiod is decreased the coat sheds profusely, there is a stimulation of new hair growth, an increase in coat thickness and a decrease in sebum production. These effects produce a dense coat with improved insulating qualities.

Steroid hormones of the testis, ovary or adrenal cortex all may prolong the telogen (resting) stage. Thyroid hormone may shorten telogen. The pituitary gland may have an effect on hair growth through the action of thyrotropic hormone or gonadotropic hormones. Hormones also influence the type of hair produced—i.e., hypophysectomy or natural disease of the pituitary (German shepherd pups) results in retention of "puppy" hair (Ebling, 1965). However, general hormonal effects are without a solid basis of fact in all species and the preceding statements should be accepted as actions that were noted only in certain cases.

Hair growth is a confusing subject which needs much research. It is well to remember that the hair coat of pet animals is a cosmetic or ornamental object in addition to its other functions. Every effort should be made to minimize or prevent procedures (clipping and shaving) which may affect the animal's appearance for many weeks. Although generalizations may be misleading, normal or short coats usually take about 130 days to regrow after shaving, while long coats such as found in the Afghan may take as long as 18 months.

## MUSCLES OF THE SKIN

Arrector pili muscles, which attach to general body hair follicles, are involuntary (smooth muscle) and are more abundant in the dorsal line of the neck, back and tail. Tactile hairs are attached to striated muscle fibers extending from the cutaneous muscle to their follicles and can be moved voluntarily.

## BLOOD SUPPLY OF THE SKIN

Blood is supplied to the region of the skin by two types of arteries, simple cutaneous arteries whose main purpose is to feed the skin, and mixed cutaneous arteries which initially supply muscles but terminate in the skin. Both types of vessels are involved in the formation of the three vascular plexuses which make up the microscopic arterial system of the skin (Fig. 1:19).

The subcutaneous plexus forms a network of vessels in the hypodermis. Branches from this network form a middle plexus which is located at the level of the hair follicles and skin glands. The most superficial plexus arises from the middle plexus and supplies the epidermal papillae. Arteriovenous anastomoses are seen in the deeper layers of the skin and in the ear flap and the tip of the tail. These may have a function in thermoregulation, but they are less significant than in man. In the dog the papillary body is poorly developed or absent where hair abounds, and the capillary loops projecting into these papillae from the superficial plexus are not prominent. This would be a real detriment to effective heat loss. In hairless areas a superficial plexus is found which does send capillary loops to the fairly well defined papillary body in these regions (Hughes and Dransfield, 1959).

## NERVES OF THE SKIN

The region of the skin is supplied with adrenergic sympathetic motor nerves to blood vessels, to arrector pili muscles, and to myoepithelial cells around the apocrine glands. There appear to be no motor nerves to the apocrine or sebaceous glands themselves or to hairs or other epidermal appendages (tactile hairs excepted).

There is a rich supply of sensory nerves to the epidermis and dermis. Sensations of touch, temperature, pain and itching are probably mediated by both specialized and nonspecialized nerve endings and by both myelinated (sheathed) and nonmyelinated nerves. Nerve fibers from cells of the dorsal root ganglia come together in the skin where they form fine networks. These fibers become finer as they approach their final destination. They end as terminal twigs in the skin and mucous membrane. These twigs form the principal end-organ called the dermal network. Winkelmann (1960) has suggested that sensory nerve fibers are modified into three types of terminal receptors: the dermal nerve network, the hair follicle network and the specialized end-organs (Fig. 1:20).

The dermal network, the fundamental receptor in mammalian skin, is the same type of end-organ found in mucous membrane. In the skin the density of dermal network endings per unit surface area varies inversely with the pelage. Thus in glabrous skin the network is extensive but in hairy skin it is rather sparse.

In regions of hairy skin the sensory nerve fibers form a double network around each primary hair called the hair follicle network. The outer series of

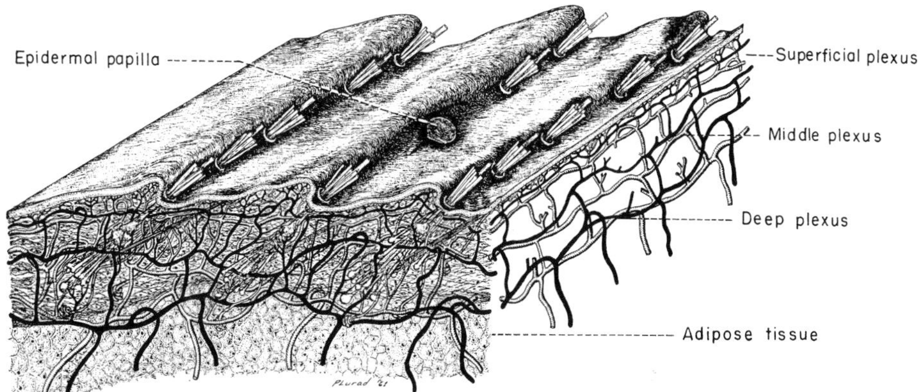


**Figure 1:19.** Schematic section of the skin of the dog, showing epidermal papilla and blood vessels (veins in black). (From Miller, Christensen and Evans: *Anatomy of the Dog.* W. B. Saunders Co., Philadelphia, 1964.)

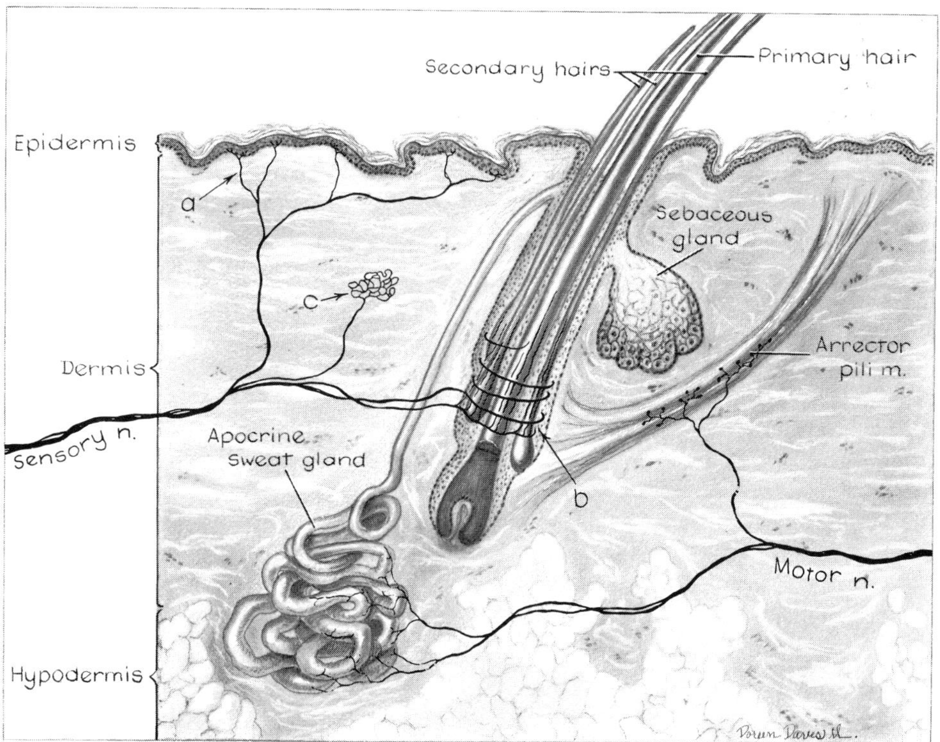


**Figure 1:20.** Nerve supply of the canine skin. *a,* Dermal nerve network. *b,* Hair follicle network. *c,* Specialized end organs.

fibers is coarse and encircles the hair follicle in the cells of the middle layer of the dermal coat; the inner series lies among the cells of the outer root sheath parallel to the hair shaft (Weddell, 1956).

Although glabrous skin contains fibrils of the dermal nerve network, it also contains a great many encapsulated nerve endings which are formed into specialized receptors. These special end-organs are particularly prominent in the mucocutaneous function, and in the footpads. Actually the special end-organs are somewhat similar to the hair follicle network except that the final axon filaments are rolled into a coil or a ball instead of being wrapped around the hair follicle. The bulb-type corpuscle so formed is encapsulated but not as heavily as similar receptors in human skin.

Present evidence has shown that there is no morphologic basis to the old theory that specific receptors perceive specific sensation (Sinclair et al., 1952). In mammals the principal organ for perception, especially for touch, is the hair follicle network. This mechanism is further refined in the sinus or tactile hairs of dogs and cats where engorgement of the vascular sinus surrounding the base of the hair follicle seems to enhance sensory acuity. Other nerve endings, the dermal network and the mucocutaneous end-organ, also may serve as touch receptors. The dermal network is active in the perception of pain and in temperature variation. Weddell suggests that thermal sensations are distinguished from those related to pain, not on the basis that different terminals served by different axons have been stimulated but on the basis that different patterns of spike potentials reach the central nervous system along one and the same set of nerve fibers. Thus sensory differentiation may be a function of central interpretation.

## The Sensation of Pruritus

Itching is an unpleasant sensation which provokes the desire to scratch. It may be a distinct sensation although it could be a specialized type of pain (Lewis and Wheeler, 1967). It can be elicited only from the epidermis, the upper dermis and the palpebral conjunctiva. There are no specialized itch receptors, although there are "itch points" in the skin where nerve endings are especially numerous. The number of "itch points" vary from site to site and from animal to animal. After skin damage the number of functioning itch points may increase. Changes in skin temperature, dryness, and diseases of the skin and internal organs are associated with pruritus. Application of certain mechanical, chemical, electrical and thermal stimuli to the skin surface and the systemic administration of certain drugs and allergens result in itching.

It is not known what actually triggers the nerve ending to produce the itch impulse and, although protein enzymes have produced the sensation experimentally, a number of mechanisms probably are involved.

The action potential for itching is conducted chiefly over unmyelinated fibers at a slow rate. There probably are two types of itch:

1. A slowly conducted, poorly localized, dull form conducted over C fibers. These are small fibers which conduct at two to three meters per second and have a high electrical threshold. They are easily blocked by a local anesthetic but are hard to block with pressure.

2. A rapidly conducted, well-localized, bright form conducted over delta

fibers of the A group. These are larger, faster, myelinated fibers which have a lower threshold to electrical stimulation. They are easily blocked by pressure but slowly depressed by anesthetics.

The neuron pathway of itch perception is probably complex but is thought to proceed through the lateral spinothalamic tract to the posterior lateral ventral nucleus of the thalamus and finally to the sensory area of the cortex (Lewis and Wheeler, 1967).

## SPECIALIZED AREAS OF THE SKIN

### Footpads

The skin covering the footpads is modified to absorb shock and to resist abrasion. The outer layers are tough, thick and heavily pigmented, and the surface is covered with numerous conical papillae which may be worn smooth with wear. Histologically the most striking feature is an exceptionally thick horny layer. This is the upper layer of the thick epidermis (1800 microns), which is acanthotic and arranged in a jagged, sawtooth or papillary manner (Fig. 1:21). A clear layer may be seen between the horny layer and the prominent granular layer. The prickle cell layer is many cells thick. There is usually an abundant amount of pigment present in the basal layer and adjacent tissues. Collagen tissue in the upper dermis is fine and fibrillar. It is denser in the deeper layer of the dermis. Eccrine sweat glands, which are present in dogs and cats only in the footpads, are numerous in the lower dermis. Ducts from these glands pass through the upper dermis and enter the epidermis at the very depths of the epidermal pegs (Fig. 1:11). These ducts spiral through epidermal structure to

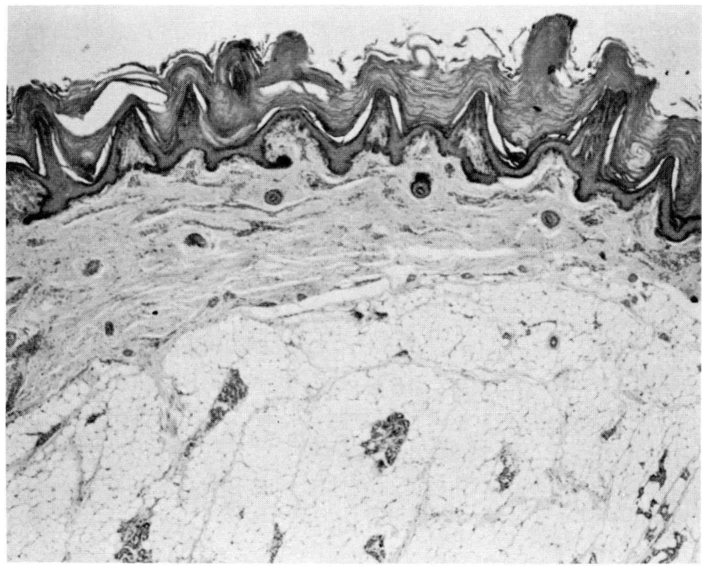

**Figure 1:21.** Histologic section of canine footpad. (Low power.)

discharge the glandular secretion at the surface. The hypodermis is substantial and consists of abundant layers of adipose tissue which serves as a cushion.

### Planum Nasale

The nasal skin is heavily pigmented, tough and moist. The surface has an irregular appearance caused by shallow grooves which divide the surface into polygonal, plaque-like areas. The epidermis is thick (630 microns) but composed of only three layers, the horny layer, the prickle cell layer, and the basal layer (Fig. 1:22). There are many pigment granules in the lower layers of the epidermis but the granular layer of the upper epidermis is slight because the keratinocytes in this type of skin do not undergo typical keratinization. A complete absence of appendages such as hairs and glands is a significant feature of nasal skin. Blood vessels and nerves are larger in the deeper layers of the dermis than in the more superficial layers.

### Scrotal Skin

The scrotal skin is very thin. Histologically the horny layer is thin but the epidermis as a whole is thick and has numerous prominent epidermal ridges (Fig. 1:23). The basal layer contains large numbers of melanin pigment granules. Hair follicles are exceedingly sparse. The dermis is particularly thin, and this is the reason the skin appears to be fine and delicate. Capillaries are abundant in the dermis and there are numerous smooth muscle fibers.

## EMBRYOLOGY

Complete, accurate information about the embryologic development of the skin of the dog and cat and its adnexa is not available. Basic facts pertaining to mammals certainly would seem to be valid for the dog, and some information is available on development of the hair follicles in this species (Balinsky, 1960).

Keratinocytes, or basal epidermal cells, are derived from ectoderm. Melanocytes, the other cell type in the epidermis, migrate from the neural crest (of the ectoderm) to the skin in early fetal life. In the first weeks of intrauterine life the skin is present as a single layer of both types of cells. It is called the stratum germinativum. During fetal development second, third and fourth layers appear in the epidermis; prickle cells, cornification and finally true keratinization develop before birth. The deeper section of the skin, the dermis, is derived from the dermatomes of the mesoderm. It is first apparent as loose mesenchymal tissue with abundant ground substance. As development progresses collagen appears and finally elastic fibers arise. Many of the latter are formed postnatally. Subcutaneous fat may be found prenatally.

The first hairs to appear on the fetus are vibrissae and sinus or tactile hairs which develop on the chin, eyebrows and upper lip. The general body hair appears first on the head and gradually spreads posteriorly. Hair follicles develop as solid cords of epidermal cells which grow obliquely downward into the dermis. As the peg of epidermis advances it becomes bulbous and partially enve-

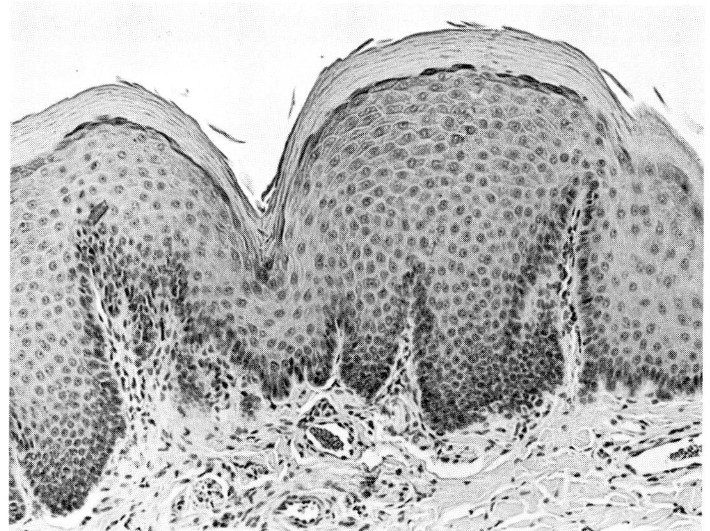

**Figure 1:22.** Histologic section of the planum nasale.

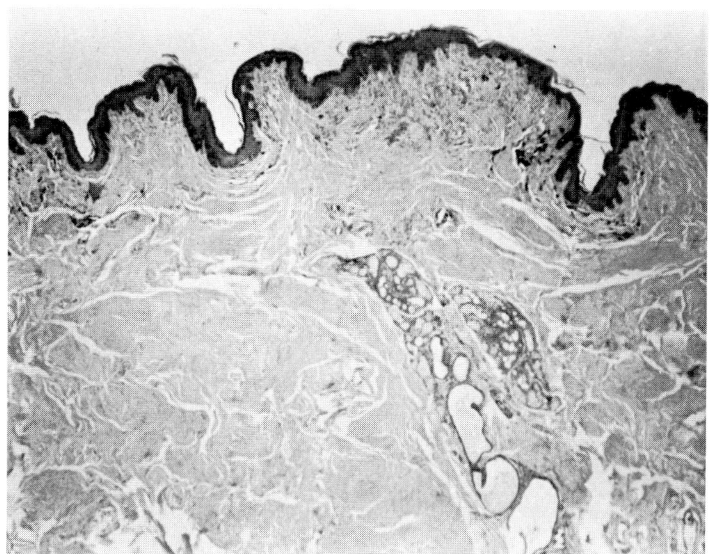

**Figure 1:23.** Histologic section of scrotal skin showing rete ridges.

lops a bit of mesenchymal tissue. This structure differentiates into the hair bulb (from epidermis) and dermal papilla (from mesenchyme). These primary hair follicles develop at regular intervals in the skin and, as the fetus enlarges, new follicles appear among the older ones. At birth, primary hair follicles are present in groups of two, three or four, but each follicle has only a single hair. It takes as long as six months for the secondary follicles to develop and for the accessory hairs to emerge from the follicular orifice (Fig. 1:24). Follicles from short-haired animals tend to be straight and long whereas those from long-haired breeds tend to be curved. The primary hair of puppies is often fluffy or fine and as maturity is reached it is replaced by coarser adult fibers.

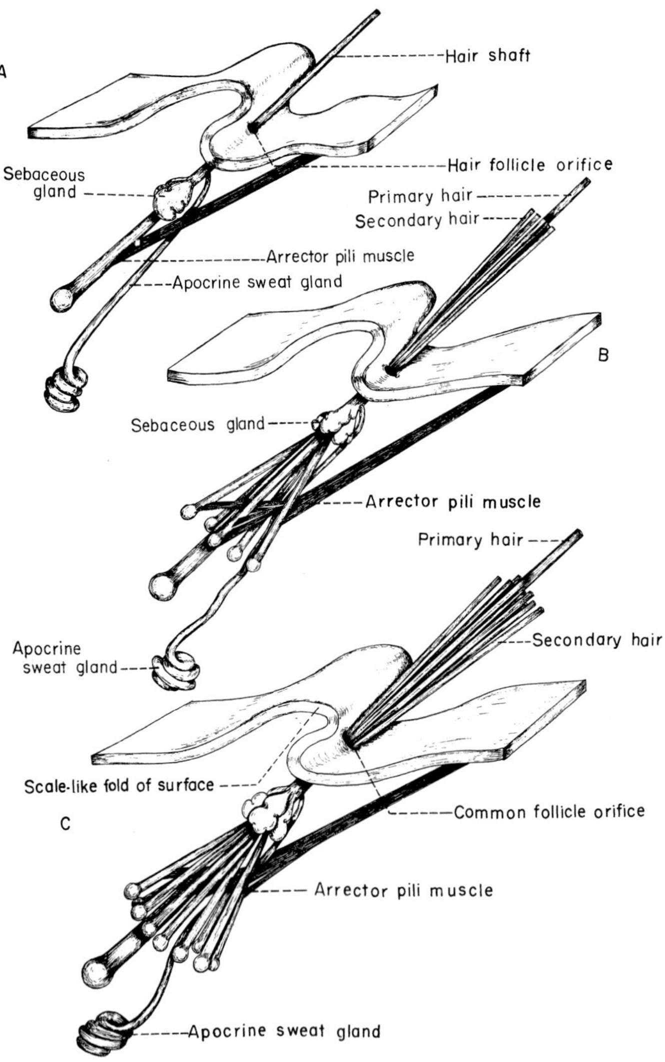


**Figure 1:24.** Development of postnatal canine hair follicle, schematic. *A*, Simple hair follicle during the first week of life; *B*, compound hair follicle during the twelfth week of life; *C*, more elaborate compound hair follicle during the twenty-eighth week of life. (From Miller, Christensen and Evans: *Anatomy of the Dog*. W. B. Saunders Co., Philadelphia, 1964.)

Sebaceous glands develop with the hair as solid outgrowths from the upper part of each follicle. The central cells in each cord accumulate lipid and then disintegrate to form alveoli and ducts. These glands are probably functional before birth.

Apocrine sweat glands appear as buds from the hair follicle above the level of the sebaceous glands. They grow downward in a spiral manner and form coils deep in the dermis or subcutis. In man these glands have limited distribution and do not function until seven to eight years of age. Delay in their function in animals may be the reason for the absence of telltale body scent in fawns and some other newborns during the neonatal period. Roy states that apocrine function in the dog is not completely developed until seven to 10 months of age (puberty).

Eccrine sweat glands are found only in the footpads. They develop as solid cords growing downward from the epidermis and progress deeply into the dermis and subcutis.

Claws of puppies and kittens are well developed at birth.

## References


Aoki, T., and Woda, M.: Functional Activity of the Sweat Glands of the Hairy Skin of the Dog. Science *114*:123, 1951.

Balinsky, B. I.: *An Introduction to Embryology*. W. B. Saunders Co., Philadelphia, 1960.

Bosse, K.: Prospects for Comparative Dermatology. *In* Rook, A. J., and Walton, G. S.: *Comparative Physiology and Pathology of Skin*. F. A. Davis Co., Philadelphia, 1965.

Chase, H. B.: Cycles and Waves of Hair Growth. *In* Lyne, A. G., and Short, B. F. (ed.): *Biology of the Skin and Hair Growth*. American Elsevier Publishing Co., New York, 1965.

Comben, N.: Observations on the Mode of Growth of the Hair of the Dog. Brit. Vet. J. *107*:231-235, 1951.

Creed, R. F. S.: The Histology of the Mammalian Skin with Special Reference to the Dog and Cat. Vet. Rec. *70*:736-743, 1958.

Ebling, F. J.: Comparative and Evolutionary Aspects of Hair Replacement. *In* Rook, A. J., and Walton, G. S.: *Comparative Physiology and Pathology of Skin*. F. A. Davis Co., Philadelphia, 1965.

Farber, E. M.: *Cutaneous Medicine; Diagnosis and Management*. Handbook, Dept. of Dermatology, Stanford University School of Medicine, Oct., 1966.

Gair, R.: Die Wuchstormen des Haarkleides bei Haustieren nach Untersuchungen beim Hunde. Z. Tiersucht. u. Zuchtungsbiol. *11*(1):57-88, 1928.

Hildebrand, M.: The integument in canidae. J. Mammal. *33*:419-428, 1952.

Hughes, H. V., and Dransfield, J. W.: Blood Supply to the Skin of the Dog. Brit. Vet. J. *115*:299-310, 1959.

Iwabuchi, T.: General Sweating on the Hairy Skin of the Dog and its Mechanisms. J. Invest. Derm. *49*:61-69, 1967.

Kirk, R. W.: *Otitis Externa in the Dog*. Veterinary Scope, The Upjohn Co., 1957.

Kligman, A. M.: Pathophysiology of Ringworm Infections in Animals with Skin Cycles. J. Invest. Derm. *27*:171, 1956.

Lewis, G. M., and Wheeler, C. E.: *Practical Dermatology*. W. B. Saunders Co., Philadelphia, 1967.

Little, C. C.: *The Inheritance of Coat Color in Dogs*. Comstock Publishing Assoc., Ithaca, N.Y., 1957.

*Lovell, J. E., and Getty, R.: The Integument. *In*: Miller, M. E., Christensen, G. C., and Evans, H. E.: *Anatomy of the Dog*. W. B. Saunders Co., Philadelphia, 1964.

Lyne, A. G., and Short, B. F.: *Biology of the Skin and Hair Growth.* American Elsevier Publishing Co., New York, 1965.

Montagna, W., and Parks, H. E.: A Histochemical Study of the Glands of the Anal Sac of the Dog. Anat. Rec. *100*:297-318, 1948.

Montagna, W.: *The Structure and Function of Skin.* Academic Press, New York, 1956.

Montagna, W., and Ellis, R. A.: *The Biology of Hair Growth.* Academic Press, New York, 1958.

Nielsen, S. W.: *Glands of the Canine Skin.* A.J. Vet. Res. *14*:448-454, 1953.

Parks, H.: Morphological Cytochemical Observations on the Circumanal Glands of the Dog.: Ph.D. thesis, Cornell University, Ithaca, N.Y. 1950.

*Pillsbury, D. M., Shelley, W. B., and Kligman, A. M.: *Dermatology.* W. B. Saunders Co., Philadelphia, 1956.

Pillsbury, D. M., Shelley, W. B., and Kligman, A. M.: *Cutaneous Medicine.* W. B. Saunders Co., Philadelphia, 1961.

Rook, A. J., and Walton, G. S.: *Comparative Physiology and Pathology of the Skin.* F. A. Davis Co., Philadelphia, 1965.

Roy, W. E.: Role of the Sweat Gland in Eczema in Dogs. A.V.M.A.J. *124*:51-54, 1954.

Schneidman, H.: Personal communication, 1967.

Schwartzman, R. M., and Orkin, M.: *A Comparative Study of Skin Diseases of Dog and Man.* Charles C Thomas, Springfield, Ill., 1962.

Sinclair, D. C., Weddell, G., and Zander, E.: Relationship of Cutaneous Sensibility to Neurohistology in Human Pinna. J. Anat. *86*:402-411, 1952.

Spreull, J. S. A.: Otitis Externa. *In* Kirk, R. W. (ed.): *Current Veterinary Therapy III.* W. B. Saunders, Philadelphia, 1968.

Stewart, W. D., Danto, J. L., and Maddin, S.: *Synopsis of Dermatology*: C. V. Mosby Co., St. Louis, Mo., 1966.

Strickland, J. H., and Calhoun, M. L.: The Integumentary System of the Cat. Amer. J. Vet. Res. *24*:1018-1029, 1963.

*Trautman, A., and Fiebiger, J.: *Fundamentals of the Histology of Domestic Animals*: Revised and edited by Habel and Biberstein, Comstock Publishing Assoc., Ithaca, N.Y.

Van Scott, E. J., Reinertson, R. P., and Steinmuller, R.: The Growing Hairroots of the Human Scalp and the Morphologic Changes following Amethopterin Therapy. J. Inv. Derm. *29*:197, Sept. 1957.

Weddell, G.: Studies Related to the Mechanism of Common Sensibility in Cutaneous Innervation: a Brown Univ. Symposium. *In* Montagna, W. (ed.): *Advances in Biology of the Skin,* Vol. I. Pergamon Press, London, 1960.

Weddell, G., Palmer, E., and Pallie, W.: Nerve Endings in the Mammalian Skin. Biol. Rev. *30*:159-195, 1956.

Winkelmann, R. K.: Similarities of Cutaneous Nerve End-Organs in Cutaneous Innervation: a Brown Univ. Symposium. *In* Montagna, W. (ed.): *Advances in Biology of the Skin.* Vol. I. Pergamon Press, London, 1960.

---

*Suggested supplemental reading.

# TWO

# *Physiology of the Skin*

## GENERAL FUNCTIONS OF THE SKIN

Skin is an indispensable organ which is especially adapted for animal life and activity. Lewis and Wheeler (1967) listed the general functions of skin and these have been modified to apply to animal skin as follows:

1. *Enclosing barrier.* Perhaps the most important function of skin is to make possible an internal environment for all other organs by maintaining an effective barrier to the loss of water, electrolytes and macromolecules.
2. *Environmental protection.* A corollary function is the exclusion of external injurious agents—chemical, physical and microbiological—from entrance into the internal environment.
3. *Temperature regulation.* Skin plays a role in the regulation of body temperature through its support of the hair coat and through regulation of the cutaneous blood supply.
4. *Sensory perception.* Skin is a prime sense organ for touch, temperature, pain and itch.
5. *Motion and shape.* The flexibility, elasticity and toughness of the skin allow motion and provide shape and form.
6. *Antimicrobial.* The skin surface has antibacterial and antifungal properties.
7. *Blood pressure control.* Changes in the peripheral vascular bed affect blood pressure.
8. *Secretion.* Skin is a secretory organ by virtue of its apocrine and sebaceous glands.
9. *Adnexa production.* Skin produces keratinized structures such as hair, nails and the horny layer of the epidermis.
10. *Storage.* The skin is a reservoir of electrolytes, water, vitamins, fat, carbohydrates, protein and other materials.
11. *Pigmentation.* Processes in the skin (melanin formation, vascularity and keratinization) help determine the coat and skin color.
12. *Excretion.* The skin functions in some species in a limited way as an excretory organ.
13. *Vitamin D production.* Vitamin D is produced in or on the skin.
14. *Indicator.* The skin may be an important indicator of internal disease.

Many of the items in the preceding list have been discussed previously, and several will be covered later in the text. There are some facets of skin function, however, which deserve more discussion.

The most important function of the skin is to act as a barrier. Epidermis, particularly the horny layer, limits permeability.

## Skin Permeability

The most important function of the skin is to produce a tough, flexible barrier, without which life is impossible. Skin permeability thus is important in limiting the loss of critical substances, as well as in controlling absorption of medications and noxious agents. In animals with a dense hair coat the hair itself has an excellent protective function. It insulates the skin from its external environment and not only serves a heat-conserving function but also physically protects the skin from contact with toxic or noxious agents. This forms the first line of external defense.

Although the skin as a whole has a barrier function, certain areas have more activity than others, and different levels of skin offer resistance to different agents. Chemical groups of keratin, amino acid and other materials at all levels of the skin probably bind or react chemically with some agents to prevent further penetration. The surface film of lipids exerts a repelling force on water and electrolytes.

The horny layer of dried keratinized cells appears loose and ineffective as a barrier when observed histologically. However, present opinion is that in life the horny layer is a thin but tough, effective barrier. It is the most important deterrent to penetration of the skin. The fact that blisters form indicates that the horny layer is inhibiting passage of fluid, but also indicates that the dermal-epidermal junction has a membrane effect too. Percutaneous absorption and resistance to absorption are thought to be passive processes. In the past it was felt that absorption through the pilosebaceous apparatus was important. At present this route may be functional for absorption in certain circumstances, but most of the time absorption through the epidermis between these structures is the major route. Absorption through the skin can be enhanced by increasing temperature and moisture content and by increasing the concentration of the material applied. These effects are additive and form the basis for the use of occlusive dressings such as "Saran wrap" in dermatologic therapy. Vehicles of medications have a minor effect on absorption unless they traumatize or modify the horny layer. Agents such as salicylic acid, DMSO, alcohol or chloroform may damage the skin or remove lipid and so enhance absorption. Vehicles which bind the drug or release it easily or which change viscosity markedly may increase or decrease the contact of the active agent with the skin surface and thus modify absorption. The horny layer may be removed by "stripping," a process of peeling which employs application and removal of "Scotch" tape. This process is a strong stimulus to mitosis in the region of cells below the stripped area so that new horny material is formed rapidly. In the interim, however, part of the barrier function of that section has been breached.

Some generalizations can be made regarding percutaneous absorption. Usually small molecules pass through the skin more easily than large, molecules penetrate better than ions, volatile agents pass better than nonvolatile, and substances which are soluble in organic solvents pass better than those soluble in water alone. Solubility in both water and lipid solvents at a ratio of one to one may be associated with maximum penetration of some agents.

Occasionally tables are presented showing drugs which are well absorbed through the skin. These lists may be misleading, however, as the absorption is measured by systemic effect, and some drugs produce profound effects with minute dosage while others have little effect with huge dosage. Water is well absorbed into the skin and produces a marked softening effect on keratin. Drugs which are well absorbed from the skin may have serious toxic consequences. These include anticholinesterases, alkaloid bases such as nicotine and strychnine, certain insecticides, gases, volatile oils, phenol and tetraethyl lead. Lipid soluble materials, fat soluble vitamins, and steroid hormones may also be absorbed reasonably well.

Water absorbed into the skin markedly softens keratin.

## Skin pH

In man the pH of the skin has been extensively studied and reported by Marples (1965) and others. Children with seborrheic dermatitis were found to have a significantly higher pH on the abnormal areas of skin as compared with children with normal skin. The acid pH of normal human skin presents an unattractive environment for many organisms and may account for the limited normal bacterial flora. Draize (1942) studied the pH of different skin regions in many mammalian species. The dog was the most alkaline of all species tested. Samples were made from six areas of each dog's skin. The pH range was 5.18 to 9.18. Ninety-five per cent of the samples fell within the range 6.2 to 8.6 and the average of all readings was 7.52. It is not clear whether pH has an influence on skin disease in the dog.

## Pigmentation

Melanin is a dark pigment that is responsible for the color of hair (along with pheomelanin), and for naturally occurring general and local pigmentation of the skin. It is produced by a special cell, the melanocyte, which is derived from the neural crest and migrates to the basal cell layer of the epidermis. The melanocyte is a mature melanin-producing and melanin-containing cell that in its embryonic form is called a melanoblast. Within this cell are small organelles or saccules whose sole task is the manufacture of pigment. These organelles are called melanosomes. They possess tyrosinase activity, and this enzyme catalyzes tyrosine to melanin. The melanosomes, seen by electron microscope, are clear at first, but soon develop fibrous strands which become granular as the synthesis of melanin proceeds and nodules form on the fibers (Blois, 1968). When melanin formation is fairly complete the melanosomes are dense black. Conglomerations of melanosomes (five to eight) are surrounded by a "cell membrane" and form the melanin granules seen with a light microscope. Melanin granules vary in size, but their number and also their disposition within the melanocyte cause the variation in skin color. Melanin granules are transferred to adjacent keratinocytes to increase pigmentation of these epithelial cells. The exact method of transfer is not known, but the dendritic processes of the melanocyte may be engulfed by the epithelial cells, or the pigment granules may be extruded into the intercellular spaces where they are engulfed by the epithelial cells (keratinocytes).

The actual formation of melanin is a complex polymerization, which occurs in the melanocyte. Tyrosine is the amino acid substrate. The enzyme tyrosinase, when photochemically oxidized by ultraviolet light in the presence of a copper protein, converts tyrosine to dopa (dihydroxyphenylalanine). This is then oxidized through a complex series of steps to melanin. Sulfhydryl (—SH) groups and copper in the cupric form will suppress tyrosinase activity.

Engstrom (1966) has reported a rare condition in chow puppies characterized by rapid depigmentation of the buccal mucosa, the tongue and the hair. The condition was shown to be caused by a lack of active tyrosinase.

Melanin formation is under the control of melanin-stimulating hormone (MSH) produced in the intermediary lobe of the pituitary gland. Melanin production is thus influenced by diseases of the pituitary gland and, through the pituitary, by other endocrine glands. It appears that adrenal cortical hormones inhibit stimulation of melanin production by the pituitary gland.

## Excretory Function

The skin is not a completely impermeable membrane and so certain amounts of water are lost insensibly. In animals with numerous eccrine sweat glands, the excretory function of the skin may eliminate small amounts of urea, creatinine, ammonia and lactate ion. In addition large amounts of water and certain electrolytes may be excreted. Since dogs and cats have eccrine sweat glands only on the footpads, it is doubtful that the excretory function of these glands is of much consequence.

## Temperature Regulation

Dog and cat skin does not possess the extensive superficial arteriovenous shunts of man and pigs which are designed to disseminate heat in hot weather. Therefore their heat regulatory mechanisms and their response to thermal burns vary markedly (Ham, 1944). In addition, carnivores lack eccrine sweat glands in the hairy skin, so the relative importance of this thermoregulatory mechanism differs from that of mammals that do sweat. Aoki and Wada (1951) have shown that the abundant apocrine sweat glands of the dog do not participate in central heat regulation. Apocrine glands do respond to local heat stimulation, however, and probably serve locally in a minor way to protect the skin from an excessive rise in temperature.

### MECHANISMS TO CONSERVE HEAT

When the environmental temperature falls, the body attempts to reduce heat loss by vasoconstriction in the skin and erection of the hairs to improve the insulating qualities of the skin and coat. The external temperature at which the heat-retaining mechanisms are no longer able to maintain a constant body temperature and at which heat production has to be increased is known as the *critical temperature.* Normal dogs with intact pelage had a critical temperature of 57° F. but when their coats were shaved off they produced a critical temperature of 77° F. Thick subcutaneous fat also acts as efficient insulating material. Animals that are nonfasting have a lower critical temperature than fasting individuals, and thus the former are better able to stand a low environmental temperature. When the aforementioned mechanisms of heat conservation are no longer effective in preventing a fall in body temperature, an increase in heat production begins. A rapid increase in heat production is accomplished mainly by shivering. In normal dogs shivering begins when the rectal temperature falls about 2° F.

### MECHANISMS TO DISSIPATE HEAT

Heat is regularly lost from the body by radiation, conduction and convection, by vaporization of water from the skin and respiratory passages, and by the excretion of urine and feces. The excretory losses are relatively unimportant in heat dissipation. Ordinarily 75 per cent of the heat loss is accomplished by radiation, conduction and convection. The efficiency of these mechanisms varies with the external temperature and humidity, and is modified further by the animals' vasomotor and pilomotor responses. These become quite ineffective at higher temperatures and heat loss by vaporization of water from the skin and lungs becomes more influential. Since they cannot "sweat," dogs and cats have developed the ability to vaporize large volumes of water from their respiratory passages. In dogs as the environmental temperature rises above 80 to 85° F. the rate of breathing also rises, but the depth of breathing (tidal volume) is markedly reduced. This helps to prevent excess carbon dioxide blow-off and severe blood-gas changes. At a rectal temperature of 105° F. the dog is in danger of thermal imbalance, and at 109° F. collapse is imminent.

The rectal temperature of the cat begins to rise at an environmental temperature of 90° F., but as the respiratory rate increases the tidal volume is only slightly reduced, so the cat is more susceptible to a lowering of its blood carbon dioxide level (respiratory acidosis). However, the cat possesses an additional compensatory mechanism. A hot environment, or sympathetic stimulation, produces a copious flow of watery saliva from the submaxillary gland. The cat spreads this on its coat for additional water vaporization, and cooling results. Similar stimulation in dogs produces only a scanty secretion of thick saliva which can not help the cooling process (Dukes, 1955).

The problem of temperature regulation in dogs and cats is often complicated by the physical condition of the coat, and by the environmental temperature. Breeds with heavy coats intended for cold climes are often moved to regions of high temperatures where they may suffer. The problem is greatly accentuated by a matted, unkempt coat which stifles air circulation through the hair. Proper grooming will greatly increase the comfort of these animals. (See Chapter 19, Care of the Skin and Hair Coat.)

## References

Aoki, T., and Wada, M.: Functional Activity of the Sweat Glands of the Hairy Skin of the Dog. Science *114*:123, 1951.

Blois, A. S. Personal communication, 1968.

Draize, J. H.: The Determination of the pH of the Skin of Man and Common Laboratory Animals. J. Invest. Derm. *5*:77-85, 1942.

*Dukes, H. H.: *Physiology of Domestic Animals.* Comstock Publishing Assoc., Ithaca, N.Y., 1955.

Engstrom, D.: Tyrosinase Deficiency in the Chow Chow. *In* Kirk, R. W. (ed.) Current Veterinary Therapy, 1966-67. W. B. Saunders Co., Philadelphia, 1966.

Ham, A. M.: Histopathology of Burns. Ann. Surg. *120*:689-697, 1944.

*Lewis, G. M., and Wheeler, C. M.: *Practical Dermatology.* W. B. Saunders Co., Philadelphia, 1967.

*Marples, M. J.: *The Ecology of Human Skin.* Charles C Thomas, Springfield, Ill., 1965.

*Pillsbury, D. M., Shelley, W. B., and Kligman, A. M.: *A Manual of Cutaneous Medicine.* W. B. Saunders Co., Philadelphia, 1961.

---

*Suggested supplemental reading.

# THREE

# *Dermatohistopathology*

Study of the skin in daily practice actually involves a study of its gross pathology. Skin is one of the few organs in which such observation is possible. Since this entire book is in a sense a study of dermatopathology, this section will emphasize cutaneous histopathology. Physicians have developed this aspect of diagnostic dermatology to a high degree—veterinary clinicians have not. It is our hope that this chapter will stimulate interest in exploring the potential of veterinary dermatohistopathology.

## LABORATORY METHODS

Although the basic principles of histopathology apply to skin, we will summarize here the aspects of fixation, processing and staining which are most pertinent.

Biopsy specimens should be blotted to remove excess blood and placed in 10 per cent formalin, the fixative of choice. This preserves the specimen indefinitely. It is best to prepare the formalin dilution just prior to use by adding 1 ml. of formalin to 9 ml. of tap water. However, if a buffered formalin is used it may be prepared in larger amounts beforehand.

Almost all laboratories use the Autotechnicon for processing specimens. This ensures automatic control of fixation, dehydration and embedding. Part of the process involves alcohol and xylene treatment, which removes fat, so if lipid studies and stains are necessary, the laboratory should be forewarned. Part of the specimen will then be prepared as a formalin-fixed frozen section.

All routine specimens are cut on a rotary microtome into sections 5 to 8 microns thick and stained with hematoxylin and eosin. Table 3:1 lists several useful stains which are employed commonly in cutaneous histopathology.

## DEFINITION OF TERMS

The following list is an attempt to explain briefly those words used to describe the histopathologic changes noted in the section on diseases of the skin. Some of these terms have not been described in small animal dermatoses but they are fundamental pathologic changes which the reader should recognize.

TABLE 3:1. Useful Staining Methods

A. Fixation in Formalin, Processed by Autotechnicon

| *Stain* | *Results* |
|---|---|
| H & E (Hematoxylin and Eosin) | *For routine:* Nuclei, blue. Muscle, nerve, collagen, red. |
| EVG (Elastic Van Gieson, Verhoeff) | *For elastic and collagen:* Collagen, red. Elastic tissue, nuclei, black or gray. Muscles, nerves, yellow. |
| PAS (Periodic-Acid Schiff Reaction) | *For polysaccharides, fungi, basement membrane, hyalin:* Fungi, magenta or purple-red. Nuclei, blue if counterstained with hematoxylin. Basement membrane and some kinds of hyaline, pink-red. |
| Giemsa | *For mast cells, eosinophils and organisms:* Mast cell granules, purple. Nuclei, epidermis, bacteria, blue, collagen, pink. Granules of eosinophils, histoplasma, red. |
| Gram | *For bacteria:* Gram-positive bacteria, blue. Gram-negative bacteria, red. |
| Von Kossa | *For calcium:* Calcium, black. |
| Masson Trichrome | *For collagen:* Collagen, green. Nuclei, nerves, muscle, dark red. |

B. Fixation in Formalin, Frozen Section

| *Stain* | *Results* |
|---|---|
| Scarlet Red | *For lipids:* Neutral fat, orange. Cholesterol and fatty acids do not stain. |

C. Fresh Tissue, Frozen Section

| *Stain* | *Results* |
|---|---|
| Dopa | *For melanocytes*: Melanocytes, dark brown granules. |

D. Histochemical staining usually requires complex research techniques, but some are of practical importance. The PAS stain (Hotchkiss-McManus) is listed above. The Alcian Blue reaction demonstrates acid mucopolysaccharides, and the Feulgen reaction stains desoxyribonucleic acid (DNA) red. The latter is present in many viral inclusion bodies. All three stains can be applied to formalin-fixed, paraffin-embedded tissues. Further information on histochemical reactions is described by Winkelmann in Montgomery's Dermatopathology.

## Epidermal Changes

*Atrophy* of the epidermis may result from neoplastic or inflammatory changes in the dermis. Normal thinning occurs in some patients with senility. In man, and in skin which characteristically shows epidermal rete projections, the disappearance of these ridges is a useful sign of atrophy. One layer or all layers of the epidermis may be atrophied.

*Acanthosis* means an increase in thickness of the prickle cell layer. In areas with rete ridges they may be elongated and prominent.

*Hyperkeratosis* is an increased or thickened horny layer. The thickening may be increased proportionately more than other epidermal layers.

*Parakeratosis* is a retention of epidermal nuclei in the horny layer. It is a result of abnormal keratinization and may be associated with deposits of amorphous material that is PAS-positive.

*Edema* may be seen between prickle cells and makes them appear to be distinctly separated. This intercellular edema is also called spongiosis. Intracellular edema appears as hydropic or vacuolar degeneration.

*Liquefaction degeneration* is a loss of the sharp outline of the basal cell layer. It results from underlying edema and a cellular infiltrate from the dermis, but loss of basal cell orientation may also be caused by dystrophy or anaplasia.

*Bullae and vesicles* are fluid (lymph) filled spaces. Subcorneal, spongiotic and acantholytic vesicles (and bullae) are sometimes first found microscopically. They are not commonly observed in animals. When observed, it is important to note whether the accumulation is subcorneal (separates the horny layer from the prickle cell layer) or subepidermal (separates the epidermis from the dermis).

*Dyskeratosis* refers to abnormal keratinization of individual cells in the epidermis. As a result, normal and abnormal cells may be adjacent to each other in a patchy pattern.

*Acantholysis* is a condition associated with lysed or dying cells which lose their intercellular bridges and become detached from surrounding cells. Their cytoplasm may condense into a halo at the cell periphery. The nucleus chromatin may become homogeneous and intensely stained.

*Papillomatosis* is an upward proliferation of papillae so that the surface of the epidermis is thrown into irregular waves.

*Anaplasia* refers to a loss of normal cell differentiation, organization and function. Anaplastic cells are variable in size, with deep-staining, irregular-shaped nuclei.

*Metaplasia* is a change in the type of adult cells in a tissue to a form which is not normal for that tissue.

## Dermal Changes

#### FIBROUS STRUCTURE

The fibrous tissue of the dermis is composed of elastic, collagenous and reticulum fibers embedded in a homogeneous ground substance. The proportion of each structure varies in different areas of the body and in different disease processes. Smooth muscle also is present in vessels and as arrector pili muscles. These structures can best be delineated by the special stains described previously.

#### CELLULAR STRUCTURE

The cellular elements of the dermis include the various blood cells and fixed tissue cells that participate in dermal reactions. These mesodermal cells are divided into three groups: the myeloid group, the lymphoid group and the reticulohistiocytic group, which includes fibroblasts and endothelial cells.

Certain types of cells invade the skin in inflammatory dermatoses and in granulomas and lymphomas.

**Myeloid Group.** This group includes the polymorphonuclear leukocyte (neutrophil) and the eosinophilic leukocyte. The neutrophil has a lobated nucleus and a cytoplasm that contains neutrophilic granules. It has phagocytic capabilities for bacteria and consequently is called a microphage. (The macrophage is a large histiocyte which can engulf hemosiderin, lipids and melanin, in addition to bacteria.) Neutrophils invade the skin in response to bacterial infections and other agents that cause dermatitis. The eosinophil appears much like the neutrophil, except that its cytoplasmic granules are a brilliant red when stained with eosin. They are especially prominent in Giemsa-stained sections. Although eosinophils can phagocytize bacteria, they are most commonly found in tissues undergoing anaphylactic and allergic reactions. According to Litt (1964), they act as part of the defense against certain immune complexes.

**Lymphoid Group.** This group includes stem cells and lymphoblasts which are seen only in malignant lymphomas, and lymphocytes which also are found invading the skin in acute and chronic inflammation and granulomas. Lymphocytes have very dark-staining, spherical nuclei and sparse cytoplasm. Large lymphocytes may be easily confused with macrophages.

**Reticulohistiocytic Group.** This group is comprised of phagocytic cells which also have the ability to phagocytize and to form reticulum and collagen fibers. Some of these cells derive from the same stem cell as the lymphocyte, while others are formed from adventitious tissue cells. Reticulum cells are immature cells with oval, pale-staining nuclei and abundant cytoplasm. These irregular cells form reticulum cell tumors. Histiocytes look like reticulum cells except that they may be smaller. They may produce reticulum fibers and phagocytize bacteria and particulate matter. Those cells which have ingested such material are called macrophages. If the engulfed material was fat they are called foam cells; if it was melanin, they are called melanophores. When individual macrophages are unable to deal with particles, several cells may fuse together to form multinucleated foreign-body giant cells. There are several arrangements. Giant cells may be associated with reactions from tuberculosis, sarcoidosis, granulomas and deep mycotic infections.

Under special influences histiocytes may change into epithelioid cells. These are large cells with an ill-defined eosinophilic cytoplasm and large pale, oval nuclei. They often group together into the Langhans type of giant cell, which has a semihorseshoe-shaped arrangement of nuclei. These cells often grow together in tubercles.

Fibroblasts can be derived from histiocytes or from adventitious cells or possibly from histiocytes. Fibroblasts form collagen fibers and are often found adjacent to these bundles. Fibroblast nuclei are pale staining and have a vesicular appearance. The cytoplasm gives the cell an elongated spindle shape.

Mast cells are histiocytic cells with metachromatic granules containing histamine and heparin. They are found everywhere in the connective tissue, but especially near the walls of blood vessels and capillaries. In aggregate they form mast cell tumors, which are common in boxer dogs. They may also be abundant in granulomas and near healing wounds. Mast cells tend to be spindle-shaped with round nuclei. The intracytoplasmic granules stain best with Giemsa, methylene blue or toluidine blue stains.

The origin of plasma cells is uncertain. They may arise from reticulum or lymphocytic cells. Plasma cells have abundant basophilic cytoplasm and a round, eccentrically placed nucleus. Deeply basophilic chromatin particles are arranged in the periphery of the nucleus and give it a cartwheel appearance. Plasma cells are found in chronic inflammations and granulomas.

## INTERPRETATION

The evaluation of histologic specimens has not been well developed in small animal dermatology. The reader is referred to Lever (1967) and to Montgomery (1967) for helpful descriptions of human lesions. The following list enumerates the lesions which at present we feel will show significant histologic changes. Further details of many of the conditions will be found in the sections on diseases of the skin (pp. 225 to 392).

Acanthosis nigricans
Acral lick dermatitis
Allergic reaction
Calcinosis circumscripta
Calcinosis cutis
Deep mycotic infection
Demodectic mange
Dermatitis, acute
Dermatitis, chronic
Dermatomycosis
Epidermal cyst
Hypothyroidism
Insect bite
Lentigo
Sarcoptic mange
Tumors
  Basal cell carcinoma
  Esoinophilic granuloma

Tumors *(Continued)*
  Fibroma
  Fibrosarcoma
  Granuloma
  Hemangioma
  Histiocytoma
  Lipoma
  Lymphosarcoma
  Mast-cell tumor
  Melanoma
    Benign
    Malignant
  Neurofibroma
  Papilloma
  Perianal adenoma
  Sebaceous gland tumor
  Squamous cell carcinoma
  Sweat gland (apocrine) tumor
  Transmissible venereal tumor

## References

Jubb, K. V. F., and Kennedy, P. C.: *Pathology of Domestic Animals.* Academic Press, New York, 1963.

*Lever, W. F.: *Histopathology of the Skin*; 4th Edit. J. B. Lippincott Co., Philadelphia, 1967.

Litt, Mortimer, Studies in Experimental Eosinophilia. J. Cell Biol. *23*:355-361, 1964.

*Montgomery, Hamilton: *Dermatopathology.* Harper and Row (Hoeber Medical Div.), New York, 1967.

Moulton, J. E.: *Tumors in Domestic Animals.* University of California Press, Berkeley, 1961.

Mulligan, R. M.: *Neoplasms of the Dog.* Williams & Wilkins, 1949.

*Suggested supplemental reading.

# DIAGNOSTIC METHODS

*Section Two*

# FOUR

## *Clinical Examination*

In making a diagnosis of a skin disease it is most important to treat the skin like any other major system and carefully evaluate the case with a thorough examination and appropriate diagnostic procedures. Ideally, this should be accomplished the first time the patient is seen and before any masking treatments have been initiated. A complete unbiased history should be obtained and a careful physical examination of the skin completed.

History, examination and laboratory procedures should precede dermatologic therapy.

The clinician should obtain a complete medical history and perform a thorough physical examination in all cases. The morphology of the skin lesion and its distribution pattern may be the only aids to diagnosis, although clinical impressions often may be substantiated with appropriate laboratory tests.

### HISTORY

Some dermatologists prefer to examine the skin quickly at first, so that pertinent questions can be emphasized in taking the history, while inappropriate items can be omitted. However, it is vital to use a systematic, detailed method of examination and history-taking so that important information is not overlooked. At times the history can be confined to the dermatologic aspects of the case, but usually a general medical history is an obvious and desirable necessity.

#### Age

Age is important dermatologically as some disorders are age-related. For example, demodectic mange usually begins in young dogs before sexual maturity. Allergies tend to appear in more mature individuals, probably because repeated exposure to the antigen must occur before clinical signs develop. Hormonal disorders tend to occur in animals between six and ten years of age.

## Sex

Sex obviously limits certain problems, but is especially important in sex hormonal imbalances. Perianal adenomas are seen almost exclusively in male dogs. One should determine whether the patient is sexually intact, and if so whether the skin problem bears any relationship to the estral cycle.

## Breed

Breed predilection determines the incidence of some skin disorders. Seborrhea is common in cocker spaniels; acanthosis nigricans usually occurs in dachshunds; anal adenomas are often found in male wire-haired fox terriers; and many of the wiry-coated terrier breeds (Scotties, cairns, Sealyhams, West Highland whites, Irish terriers and Welsh terriers) seem to be particularly cursed by a predisposition to allergic skin disease.

## Owner's Complaint

The owner's complaint or chief cause of concern is often the major sign used in compiling a differential diagnosis. The clinician who can "draw out" a complete history in unbiased form has indeed a valuable skill. It is important that the questions presented to the client do not suggest answers, or tend to shut off discussion. A friendly "Let's help this patient together" attitude often stimulates the client to reveal more information. Some owners purposely or unconsciously withhold pertinent facts, especially about neglect, diets, previous medication or other procedures they feel may not be well received by the examining veterinarian. The skillful clinician is ever tuned to listen for side comments by the client or by the children. These may be veritable "pearls" of information in a mass of extraneous trivia.

Next, obtain the following information from the owner: Chief complaint, date of onset, original locations of the lesions, description of the initial lesions, tendency to progression or regression, factors affecting the course and previous treatment (home, proprietary or pet shop remedies used as well as veterinary treatment).

Almost all animals with skin disorders have been bathed, dipped, sprayed or larded with one or more medications, and the owner may be reluctant to disclose a complete and honest list of previous treatments. It is important that the types of medication and dates of application be completely divulged, as modification of pertinent signs may have resulted.

Although the patient cannot relate subjective findings (symptoms) it is possible to determine the degree of hyperesthesia, pruritus and pain reasonably well. The owner's idea of intensity of itching, however, may vary considerably from the veterinarian's. Consequently, it is helpful to phrase the questions:

"How many times daily do you see your dog scratch?" "Does he itch in many sites, or just a few?" "Does he shake his head?"

The same type of specific question is helpful when discussing diets, as the owner often remembers the atypical feedings. A more representative answer is often secured if one asks, "What did your pet eat yesterday (or over the last 48 hours)?"

Since contact irritants or allergens are important it is necessary to inquire about the dog's external environment. "Does he live in an apartment or is he outdoors in the fields and forests? Does he sleep in a dog house or in the owner's bed? Is the bedding straw, shavings, wool blankets or silk sheets?"

In determining contagion one should inquire about the skin health of other animals on the premises. The presence of skin disease in the people associated with the patient also may be highly significant in some disorders (scabies and ringworm).

At this point the clinician has usually acquired a general idea of the problem and is ready to proceed with a careful physical examination. In some cases he may want to come back to the general medical history if further developments indicate more serious or underlying systemic disease.

## PHYSICAL EXAMINATION

In dermatology the clinician can observe the pathologic lesions directly. He need not rely on vague shadows or referred sounds to determine abnormality, as skin lesions are clearly visible. By careful, systematic inspection alone the diagnosis of many dermatoses becomes apparent.

---

Good lighting is of paramount importance.

---

Normal daylight without glare is best, but any artificial light of adequate candle power is sufficient if it produces bright uniform lighting. The lamp should be adjustable to illuminate all body areas. A combination loupe and light (Fig. 4:1) provides magnification of the field as well as good illumination.

Before concentrating on the individual lesions always observe the entire animal from a distance of several feet for a general impression of abnormalities.

Does he appear to be in good health? Is he fat or thin, unkempt or well groomed? Is the problem generalized or localized? What is the distribution of the lesions? Are they bilaterally symmetrical or unilaterally irregular?

To answer some of these questions examine the patient more closely. Inspect the dorsal aspect of the body (Fig. 4:2) and then carefully observe the lateral surfaces. Next turn the patient over for a careful examination of the ventral region (Fig. 4:1).

Report the findings in detail on the patient's chart. The initial documentation of a skin case and its progress during treatment can be easily visualized by using the rubber stamps illustrated in Figure 4:3. The extent of the lesions can be sketched on the stamped outline of the dog or cat, and the descriptive terms listed can be circled where they are pertinent (Fig. 4:4). This system saves much time, and insures that no important information is omitted (see also p. 75).

A large rubber stamp has been designed which fits exactly into the lines of a 5 × 8-inch. Histaccount hospital record card. The stamp is used as follows:

1. For new cases, the receptionist fills out the regular hospital record card with routine information of the owner's name, address, breed, age, sex and so

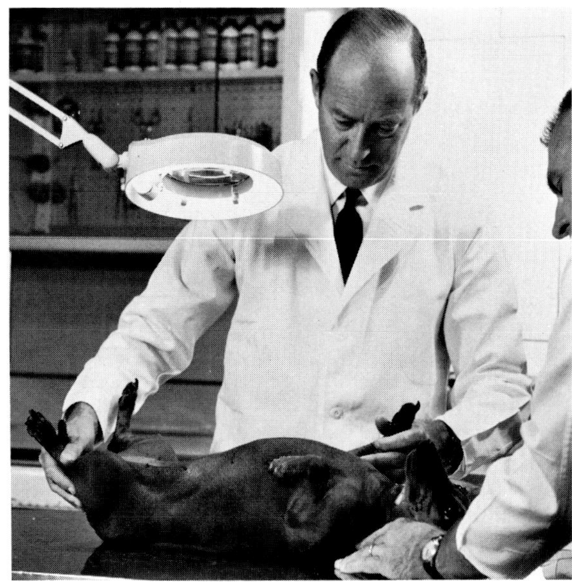

**Figure 4:1.** Examining the ventral surface of the patient. Combination lens and light provides illumination and magnification for close examination.

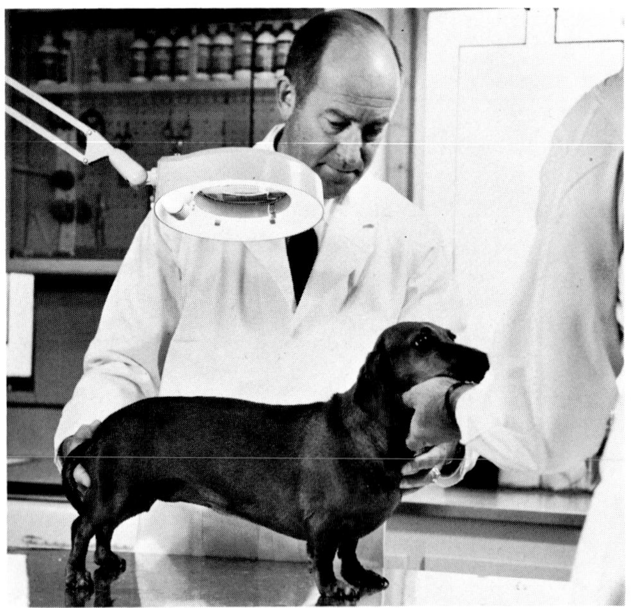

**Figure 4:2.** Examining the dorsal surface of the patient.

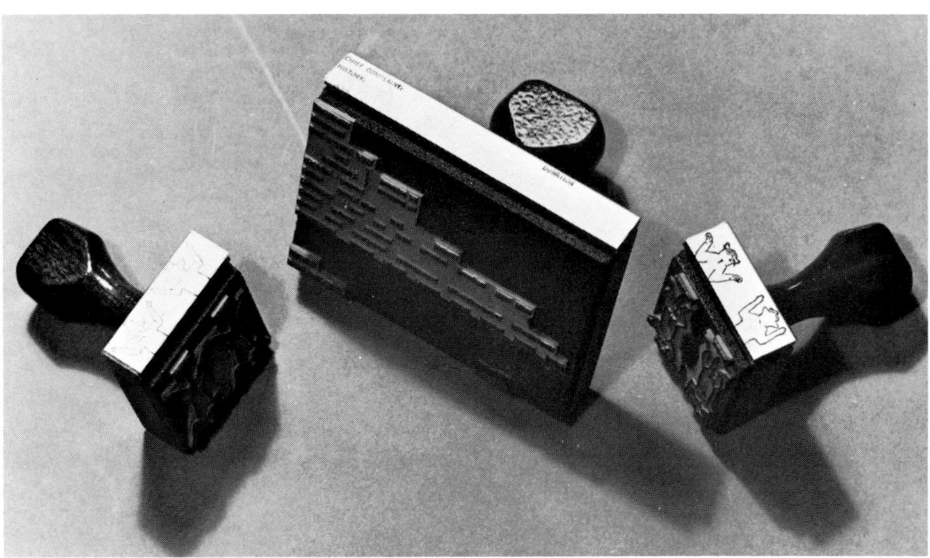

**Figure 4:3.** Rubber stamps used for easy, complete recording of facts about dermatologic cases. (See p. 468, San Francisco Rubber Stamp Co.)

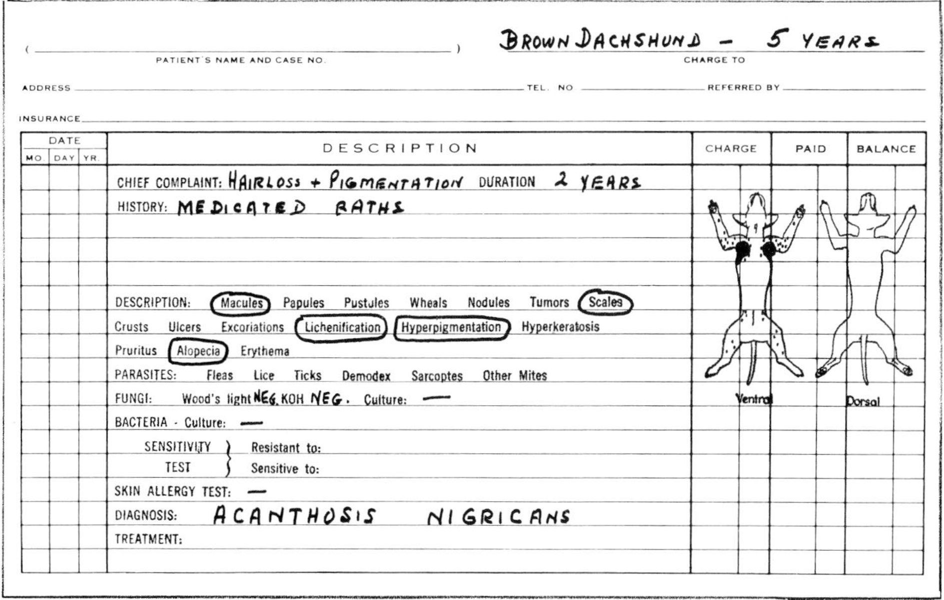

( ______________________ ) BROWN DACHSHUND – 5 YEARS

PATIENT'S NAME AND CASE NO. CHARGE TO

ADDRESS ______ TEL. NO ______ REFERRED BY ______

INSURANCE ______

| DATE MO | DATE DAY | DATE YR | DESCRIPTION | CHARGE | PAID | BALANCE |
|---|---|---|---|---|---|---|
| | | | CHIEF COMPLAINT: HAIRLOSS + PIGMENTATION DURATION 2 YEARS | | | |
| | | | HISTORY: MEDICATED BATHS | | | |
| | | | DESCRIPTION: (Macules) Papules Pustules Wheals Nodules Tumors (Scales) | | | |
| | | | Crusts Ulcers Excoriations (Lichenification) (Hyperpigmentation) Hyperkeratosis | | | |
| | | | Pruritus (Alopecia) Erythema | | | |
| | | | PARASITES: Fleas Lice Ticks Demodex Sarcoptes Other Mites | | | |
| | | | FUNGI: Wood's light NEG. KOH NEG. Culture: — | Ventral | Dorsal | |
| | | | BACTERIA - Culture: — | | | |
| | | | SENSITIVITY TEST } Resistant to: | | | |
| | | | Sensitive to: | | | |
| | | | SKIN ALLERGY TEST: — | | | |
| | | | DIAGNOSIS: ACANTHOSIS NIGRICANS | | | |
| | | | TREATMENT: | | | |

**Figure 4:4.** Circled items record clinical findings on the history and physical examination form. Note shading on animal outline to indicate lesion distribution.

on. As soon as she realizes she is dealing with a skin case, she can imprint the stamp on the first available line. Under the heading "Chief Complaint" she fills in the owner's reason for bringing the animal to the clinic.

2. During the office visit, a few pertinent questions by the clinician will give the "Duration" and "History" of the present and former dermatoses. This includes home remedies and treatment by other veterinarians.

3. In precise and dermatologically descriptive terms the description of the lesions is noted by circling the appropriate words. Parasites are noted and recorded. An exclamation mark (!) is placed within the circle to emphasize the most significant facts.

4. The lesions are marked on the outline of the dog's or cat's dorsal and ventral aspect.

5. Results of mycotic and bacterial cultures are marked in their appropriate spaces. There is a space for the results of antibiotic sensitivity tests and skin allergy testing.

6. If a "Diagnosis" has been made by this time, the proper term can be placed in this column. If in doubt, it can be left blank or a "Tentative Diagnosis" can be filled in and so designated.

7. Under "Treatment" the therapeutic agents used and dispensed can be listed. This will be very valuable if another veterinarian on the staff has to see the patient next time.

For the busy small animal practitioner the rubber stamp form has these advantages:

1. *Compactness.* Since the material needs to become part of the permanent hospital records, it should take up as little space as possible.

2. *Uniformity.* One form is used for all dermatoses. Dermatologic descriptions and laboratory results are standardized automatically.

3. *Timesaving.* The "fill in" spaces and preprinted dermatologic terms reduce the time needed to record information.

After an impression is obtained from a distance the skin should be examined more closely. Palpation now becomes important too. What is the texture of the hair? Is it coarse or fine, dry or oily, and does it epilate easily? The texture, elasticity and thickness of the skin should be determined and impressions of heat or coolness recorded. It is important to examine every inch of skin and mucous membranes. It is easier to find important skin lesions in some breeds than in others, depending on the thickness of the coat. There is a variation in density of an individual's coat in different body areas. Lesions can be discerned easier in sparsely-haired regions. However, the clinician must part the hair in many areas to observe and palpate lesions which are partially covered. When abnormalities are discovered it is important to establish their general distribution as well as their configuration within an area. Are they single, multiple, discrete, diffuse, grouped or confluent? With sharp observation linear or annular configuration of the lesions may be noted (Table 4:1). At this point one should focus upon individual lesions and examine them minutely with good light and a hand lens or a head loupe with 4 to 6 power magnification (Fig. 4:5).

---

Examine individual lesions minutely with a magnifying head loupe.

---

TABLE 4:1. Dermatologic Description
(Other than Primary and Secondary Lesions)

| | |
|---|---|
| *Distribution* | *Consistency* |
| Generalized | Indurated |
| Localized | Soft |
| Bilaterally symmetrical | Rolled border |
| Asymmetrical | Fluctuent |
| Patchy | Atrophied |
| Scattered | *Quality* |
| *Arrangement* | Dry |
| Discrete | Moist |
| Confluent | Greasy |
| Grouped | Oozing |
| Well defined | Bleeding |
| Poorly defined | Secondarily infected |
| *Configuration* | Purulent |
| Annular | *Color* |
| Arciform | Erythematous |
| Polycyclic | Violaceous |
| Linear | Yellow |
| Serpiginous | Brown |
| Central healing | White |
| *Depth* | Gray |
| Elevated | Black |
| Surface | |
| Deep | |

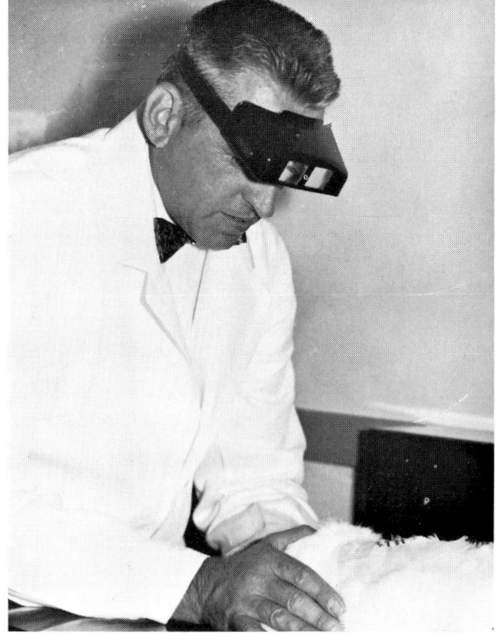

**Figure 4:5.** Close examination of lesions with a 4-power magnifying head lamp.

# FIVE

# *Morphology of Skin Lesions*

Search for individual skin lesions: scrutinize and identify.

Morphology of skin lesions is the essential feature of canine dermatologic diagnosis and sometimes the *only* guide if laboratory procedures yield no useful information. Learn to recognize primary and secondary lesions! Careful inspection of the diseased skin will frequently reveal a primary lesion pathognomonic of a specific dermatosis. In many cases, however, the significant lesion must be differentiated from the mass of secondary debris. The ability to discover a characteristic lesion and understand its significance is the first step toward mastering dermatologic diagnosis. Always remember that variations are common, since early as well as advanced stages exist in most skin diseases. In addition, the appearance of skin lesions may change with medication, self-inflicted trauma and secondary infection.

Most skin diseases, however, are characterized by a single type of lesion. This primary lesion varies slightly from its initial appearance to its full development. Later, through regression, degeneration or traumatization, it changes in appearance and in its new, altered form becomes a secondary lesion.

The diagrams and photographs of this chapter help, in a graphic way, to identify the primary and secondary lesions. The definitions and examples explain the importance and relationship of skin lesions to canine and feline dermatoses.

The skin lesions depicted in the diagrams that follow graphically demonstrate how the pathologic morphology varies from the normal.

*Primary Lesions*

| | | | |
|---|---|---|---|
| Macule | Nodule | Pustule | Vesicle |
| Papule | Tumor | Wheal | |

*Secondary Lesions*

| | | | |
|---|---|---|---|
| Scale | Scar | Excoriation | Hyperpigmentation |
| Crust | Ulcer | Lichenification | Hyperkeratosis |

# NORMAL CANINE SKIN

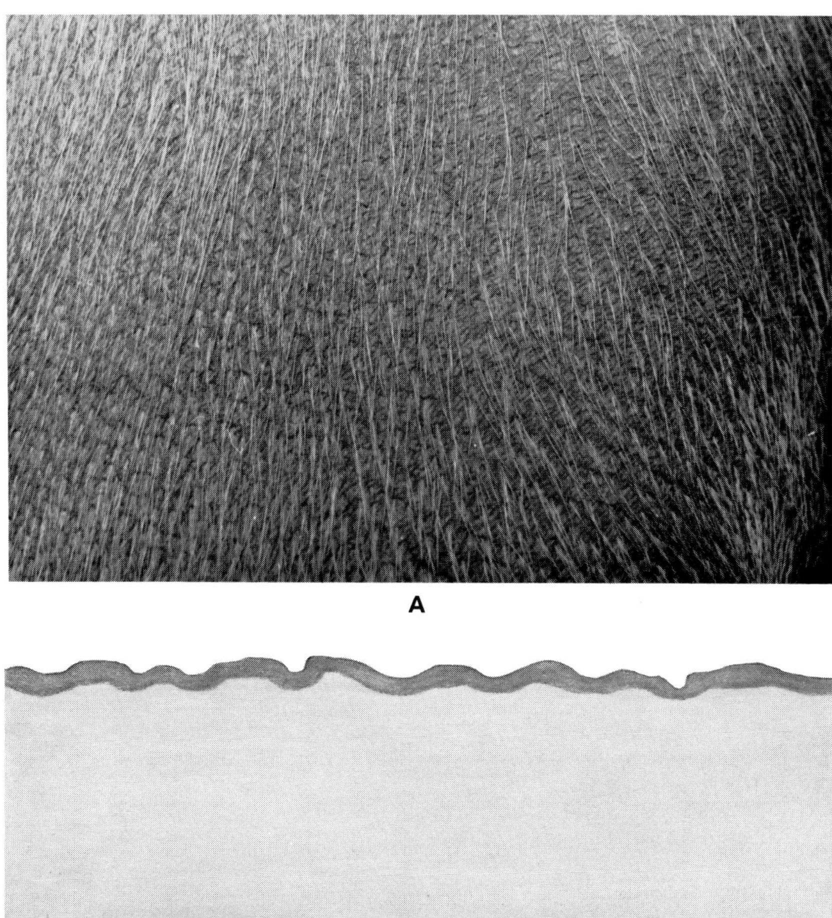

A

B

**Figure 5:1.** *A*, Normal canine skin. *B*, The skin is shown here diagramatically. The dark (upper) zone represents the epidermis, which in canine skin is thin and without prominent epidermal pegs. The light (lower) zone represents the dermis.

# *Primary Lesions*

## MACULE

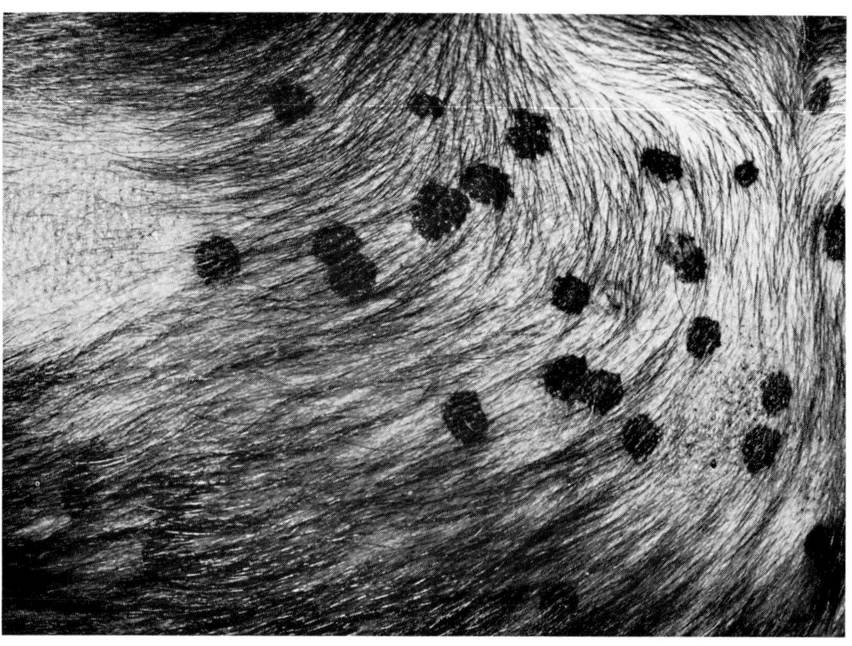

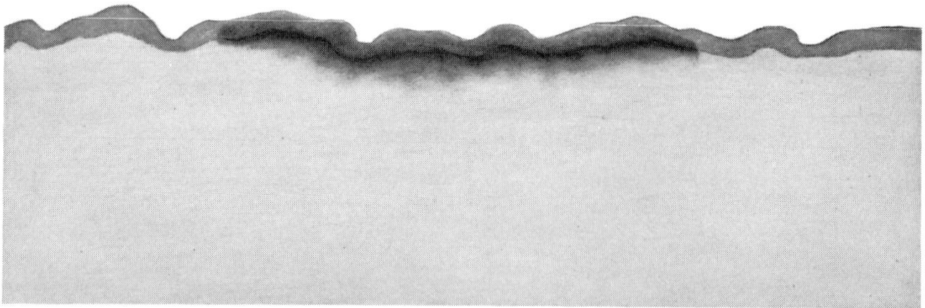

**Figure 5:2.** Macule – a circumscribed, flat spot characterized by change in color of the skin. A larger macule, over 1 cm. in size, is called a "patch." The discoloration can result from three processes: increase in melanin pigmentation, depigmentation and erythema. Examples are the hyperpigmentd patches in the axillae of dogs with acanthosis nigricans, erythematous macules in many types of acute dermatitis and pigmented nevi. (Photo illustrates lentigo.)

# PAPULE

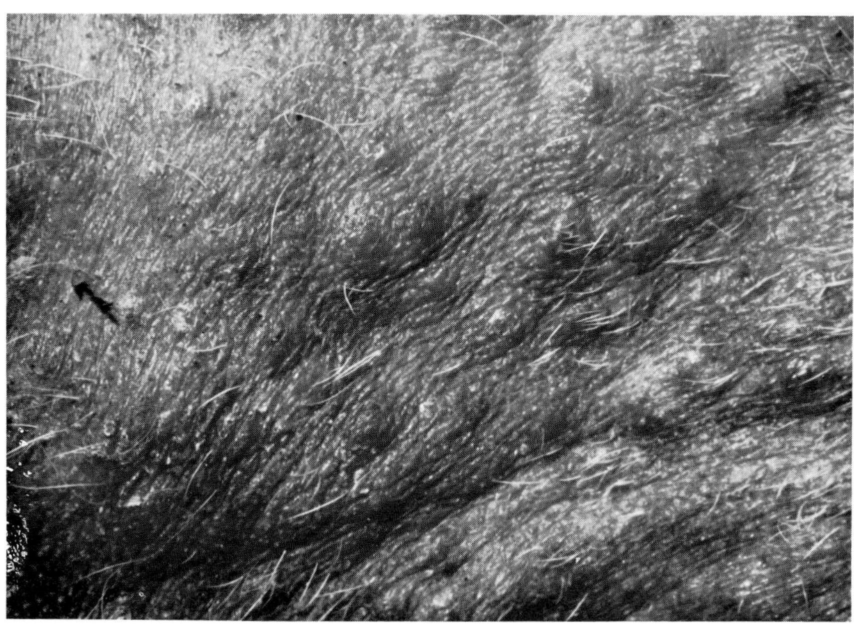

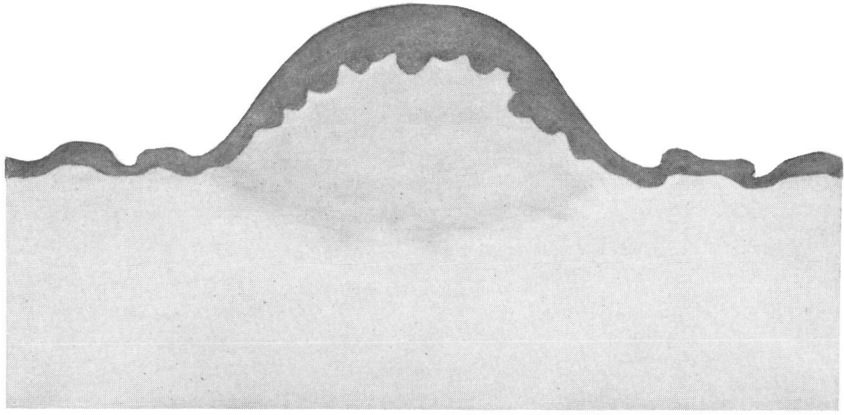

**Figure 5:3.** Papule—a small, solid elevation of the skin up to 1 cm. in diameter. A larger, flat-topped elevation is called a "plaque." A papule can always be palpated as a solid mass. Many papules are pink or red swellings produced by tissue infiltration of inflammatory cells, by intraepidermal and subepidermal edema or by epidermal hypertrophy. Examples are the erythematous papules seen in chronic allergic contact dermatitis of dogs after exposure to plants. (Photo illustrates allergic contact dermatitis.)

## NODULE

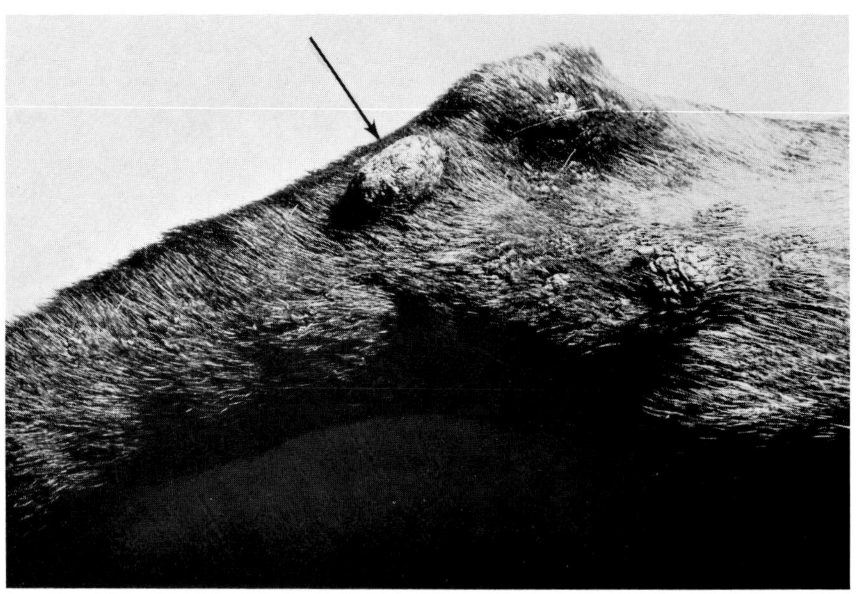

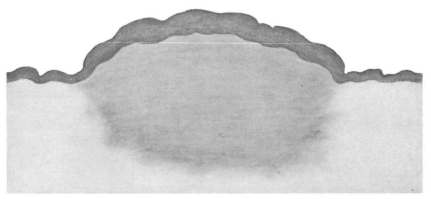

**Figure 5:4.** Nodule—a small, circumscribed, solid elevation that usually extends into the deeper layers of the skin. Nodules may be inflammatory or neoplastic. Examples are warts and small epidermal cysts. (Photo illustrates seborrheic keratosis.)

## TUMOR

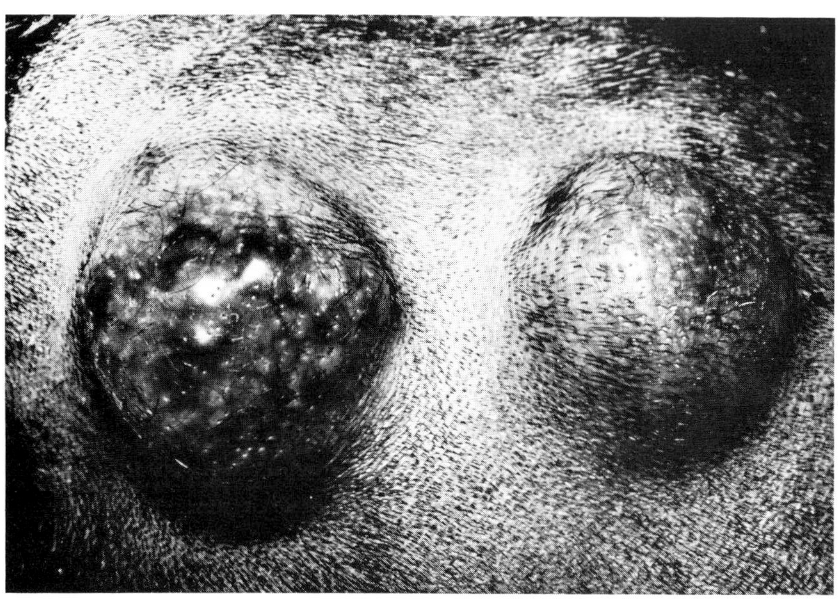

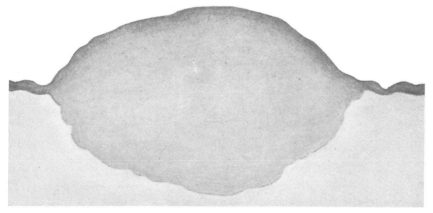

**Figure 5:5.** Tumor—a neoplastic enlargement of larger size that may be composed of any structure of the skin or subcutaneous tissue. Examples are fibromas, mastocytomas, melanomas and carcinomas. (Photo illustrates calcifying epitheliomas.)

# PUSTULE

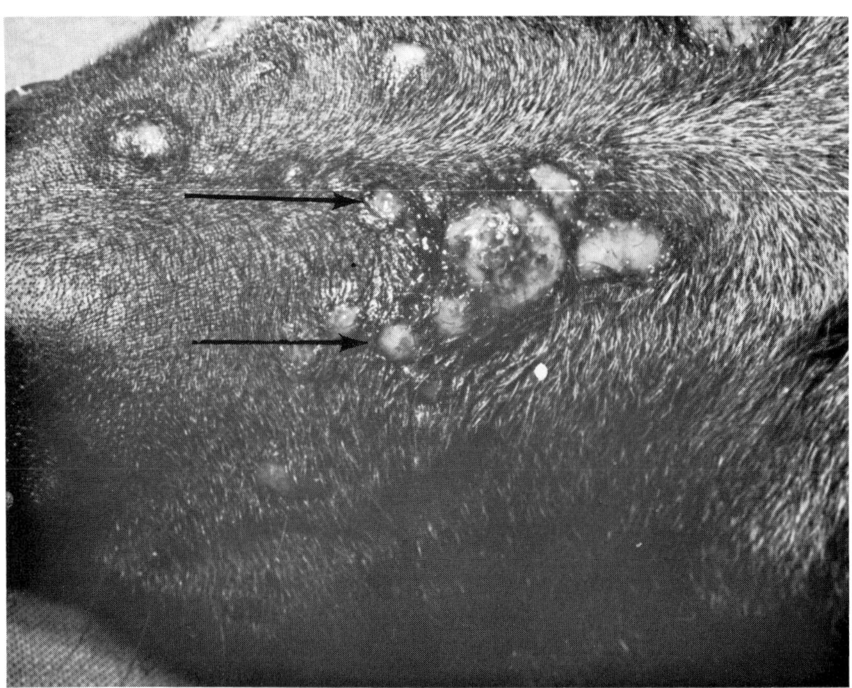

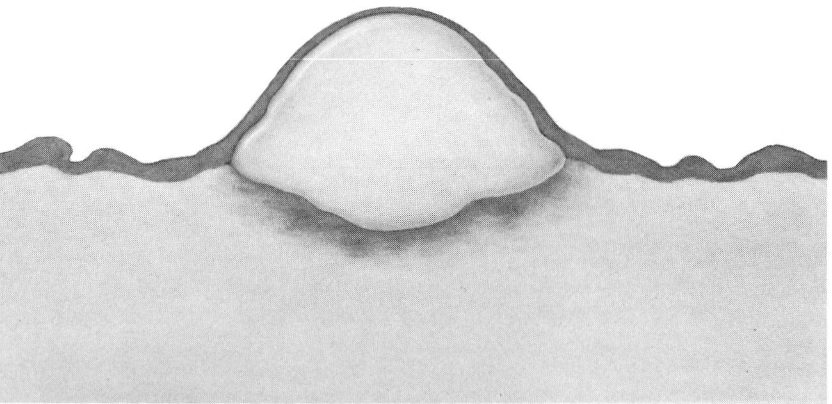

**Figure 5:6.** Pustule—a small circumscribed elevation of the skin filled with pus. It is technically a small abscess (occasionally sterile) of the superficial area of the skin. The color is usually yellow but may be pink or red. Examples are acne, folliculitis and the pustules seen on the abdomen of puppies with impetigo. (Photo illustrates nasal pyoderma.)

## WHEAL

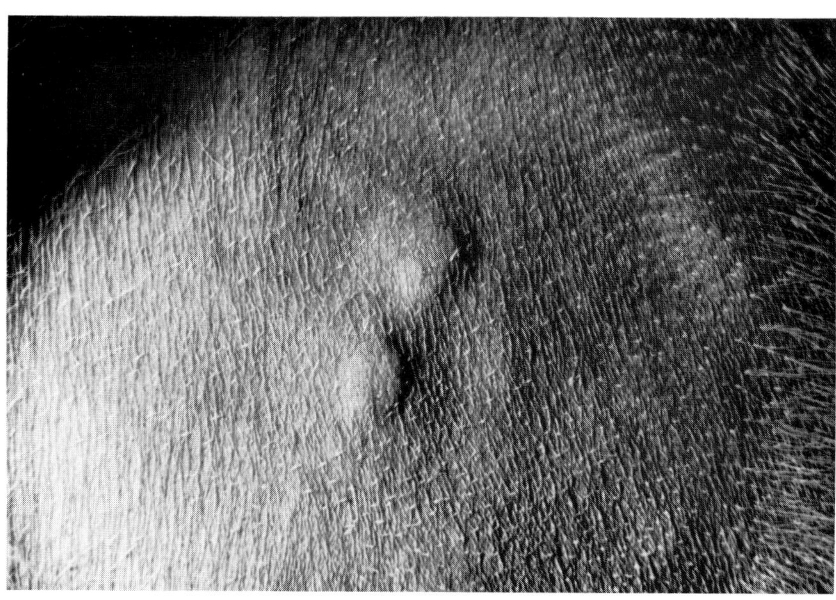

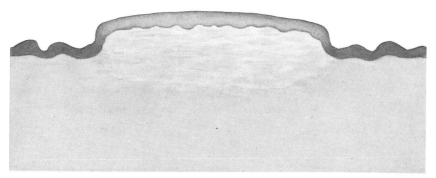

**Figure 5:7.** Wheal—a sharply circumscribed, raised lesion consisting of edema. Wheals are characteristically white or pink elevated ridges or round edematous swellings. In dogs they produce characteristic raised areas of the hair coat that are especially prominent on the back. Examples are urticaria, fleabites and positive reactions to allergy skin tests. (Photo illustrates urticaria.)

# VESICLE

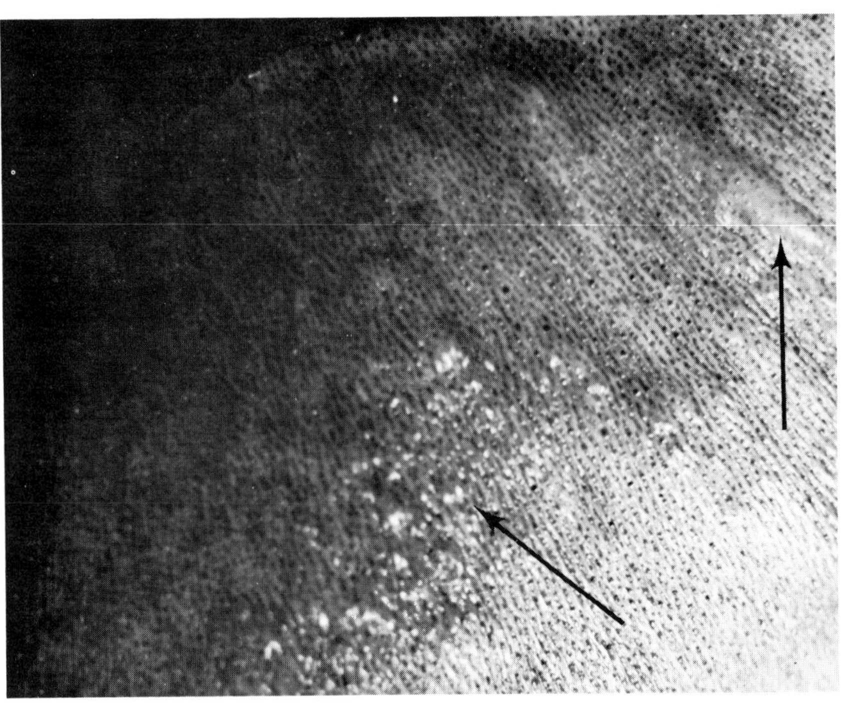

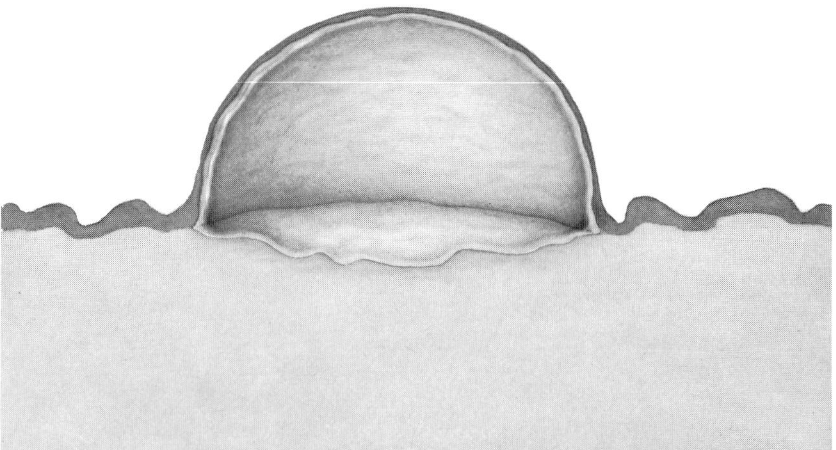

**Figure 5:8.** Vesicle—a sharply circumscribed elevation of the skin filled with clear, free fluid and up to 1 cm. in diameter. A large vesicular lesion is called a "bulla." Vesicles are seen rarely in dogs and cats. They occasionally occur with acute dermatitis caused by primary irritants. (Photo illustrates poison oak contact dermatitis.) (Courtesy R. M. Schwartzman.)

# *Secondary Lesions*

## SCALE

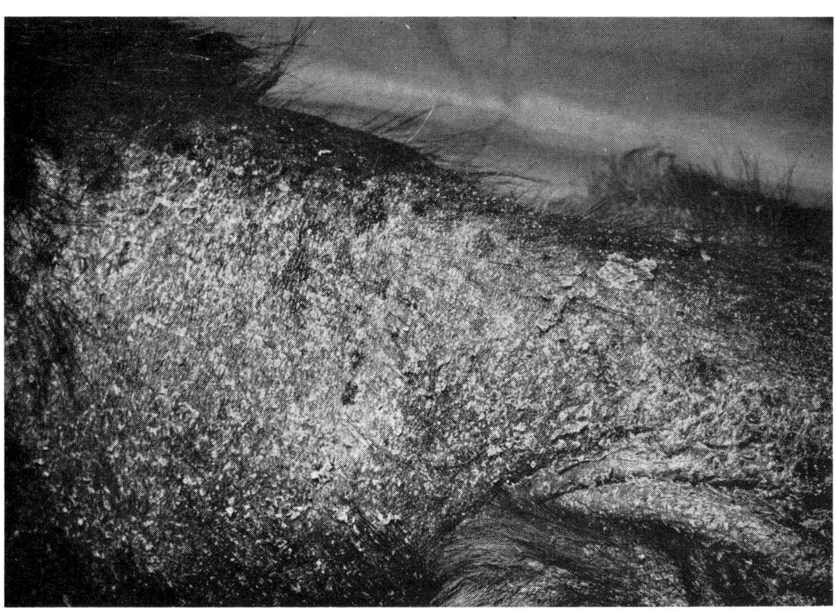

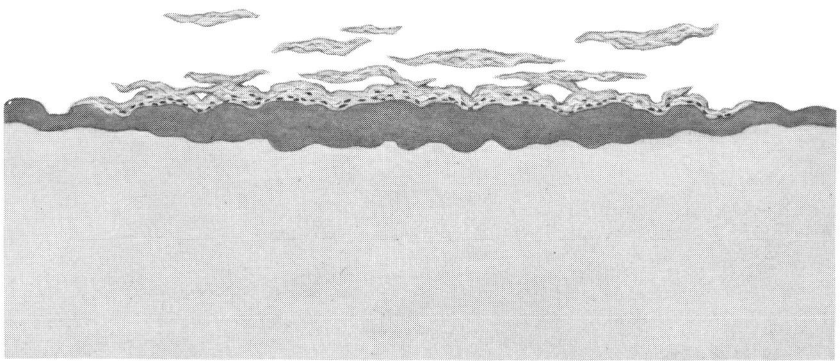

**Figure 5:9.** Scale—an accumulation of loose fragments of the horny layer of the skin. The scale is the final product of epidermal keratinization. In seborrhea, for example, scales are the result of an increased rate of keratinization. The consistency of flakes varies greatly and they can appear branny, fine, powdery, flaky, plate-like, greasy, dry, loose, adhering or "nit-like." The color varies from white, silver, yellow or brown to gray. Scales are seen in seborrhea, generalized demodectic mange and chronic allergic dermatitis. (Photo illustrates seborrhea sicca.)

## CRUST

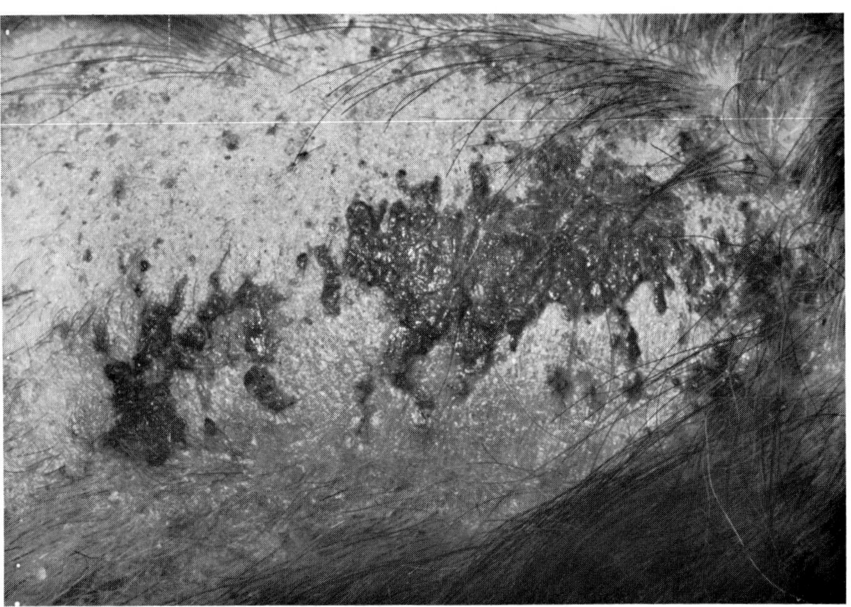

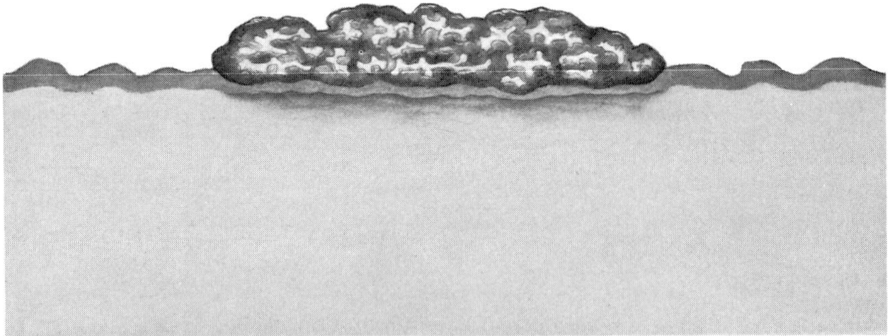

**Figure 5:10.** Crust—a dried exudate on the surface of a lesion. A crust is formed when dried exudate, serum, pus, blood, scales or medications adhere to the surface and often mingle with hair. Unusually thick crusts are found in hairy areas because the dried material tends to adhere more tightly than in glabrous skin. Hemorrhagic crusts in staphylodemodicosis are brown or dark red; yellowish-green crusts appear in some cases of pyoderma; tan, lightly adhering crusts are found in impetigo. For diagnosis it helps to remove a crust and examine the underlying lesions. (Photo illustrates superficial dermatitis.)

## SCAR

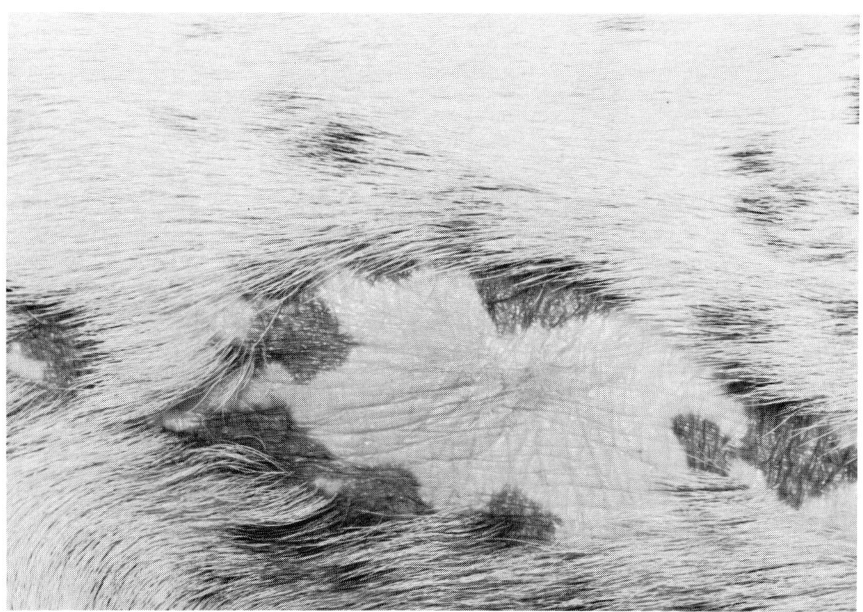

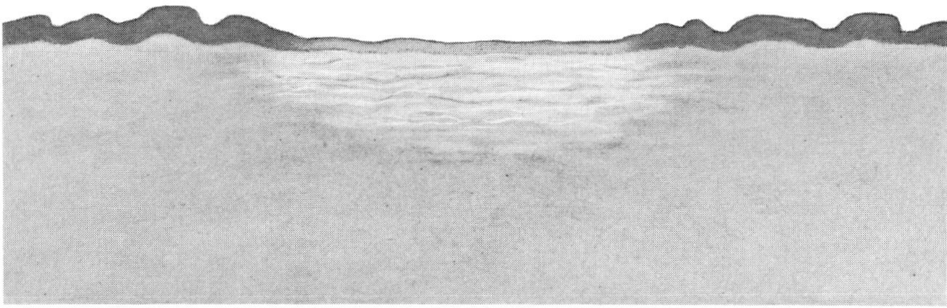

**Figure 5:11.** Scar—an area of fibrous tissue that has replaced the damaged dermis or subcutaneous tissue. Scars are the remnants of trauma or dermatologic lesions. Most scars in dogs and cats are atrophic and depigmented. Proliferative scars do occur and in dark-skinned dogs scars can be hyperpigmented. Scars are observed following severe burns and in deep pyoderma. (Photo illustrates burn scarring.)

## ULCER

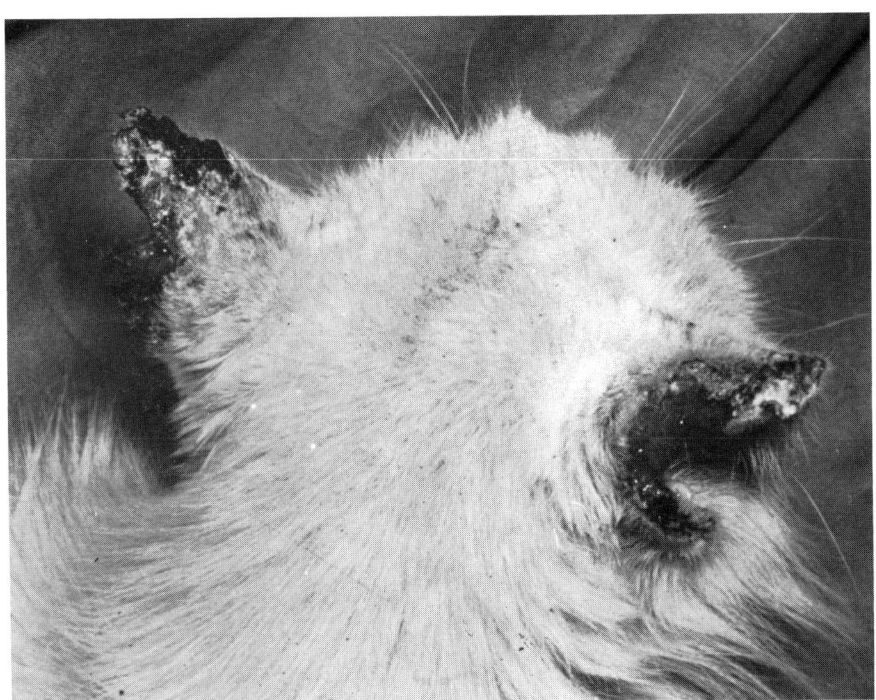

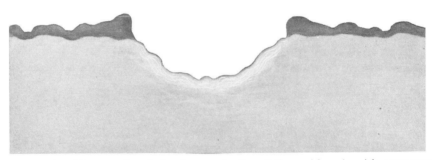

**Figure 5:12.** Ulcer—a break in the continuity of the epidermis with exposure of the underlying dermis. A severe pathologic process is required to form an ulcer; therefore, a search for the cause is always indicated. It is important to note the structure of the edge, the firmness of the ulcer and the type of exudate in the crater. A scar is always left after healing of ulcers. An *erosion* can be considered a shallow ulcer that does not penetrate the basal cell layer and consequently heals without scarring. Examples are feline rodent ulcers and chronic nasal solar dermatitis in collies. (Photo illustrates feline solar dermatitis.)

## EXCORIATION

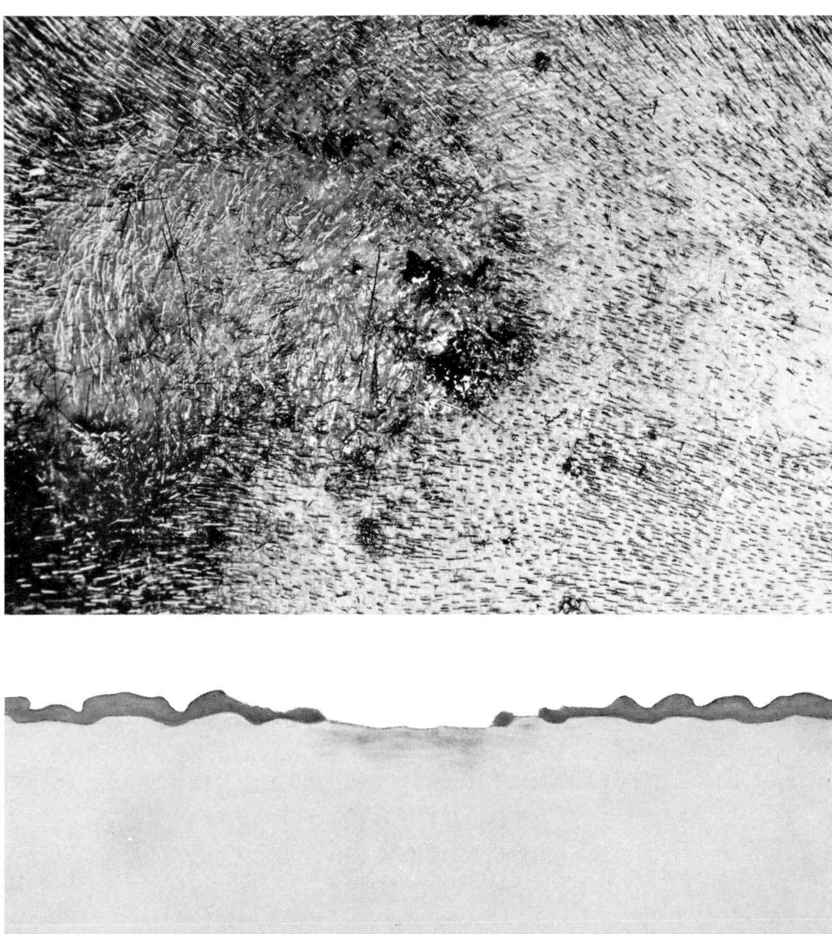

**Figure 5:13.** Excoriation—a superficial removal of epidermis caused by scratching, biting or rubbing. Most excoriations are self-produced, caused by pruritus, and they invite secondary bacterial infection. Acute moist dermatitis caused by self-inflicted trauma is such an example. (Photo illustrates acute moist dermatitis.)

## LICHENIFICATION

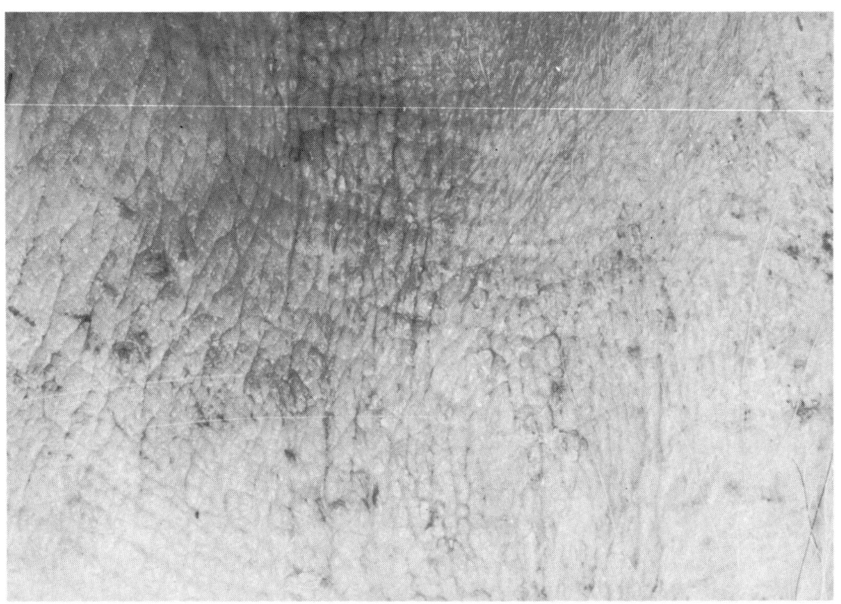

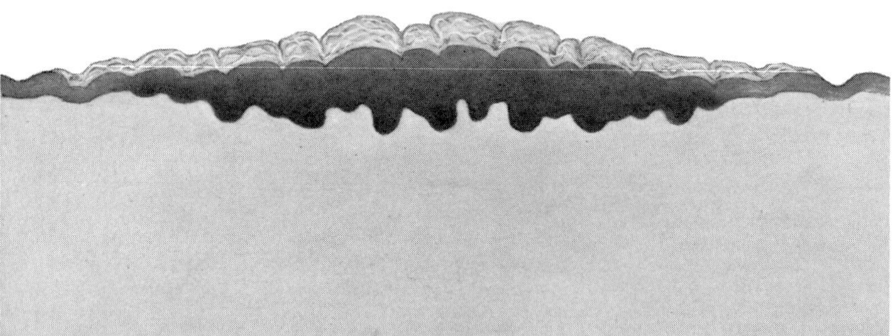

**Figure 5:14.** Lichenification—a thickening and hardening of the skin characterized by an exaggeration of the superficial skin markings. Lichenified areas frequently result from friction. They may be normally colored but more often are hyperpigmented. Examples are the hyperpigmented, lichenified flanks in the male feminizing syndrome and the axillae in acanthosis nigricans. (Photo illustrates chronic atopic dermatitis.)

# HYPERPIGMENTATION

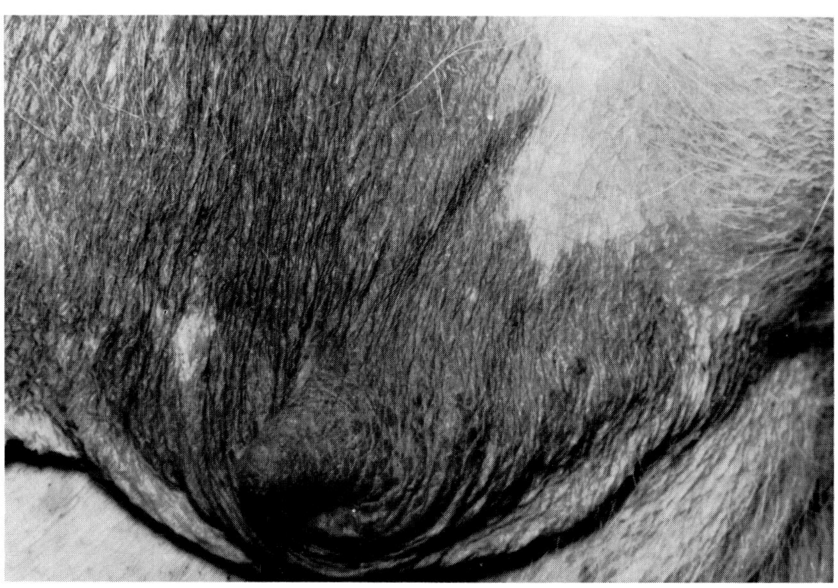

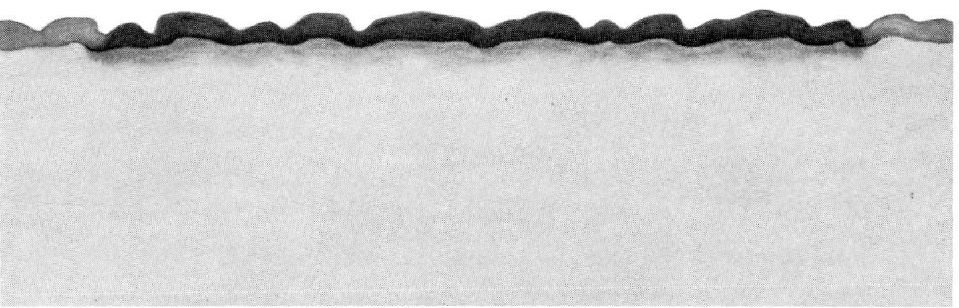

**Figure 5:15.** Hyperpigmentation—an excessive coloration of the skin caused by increased deposition of melanin. Increase in pigmentation varies from light gray to black. Examples are acanthosis nigricans, male feminizing syndrome, ovarian imbalances, chronic dermatitis and neurodermatitis. (Photo illustrates ovarian imbalance.)

## HYPERKERATOSIS

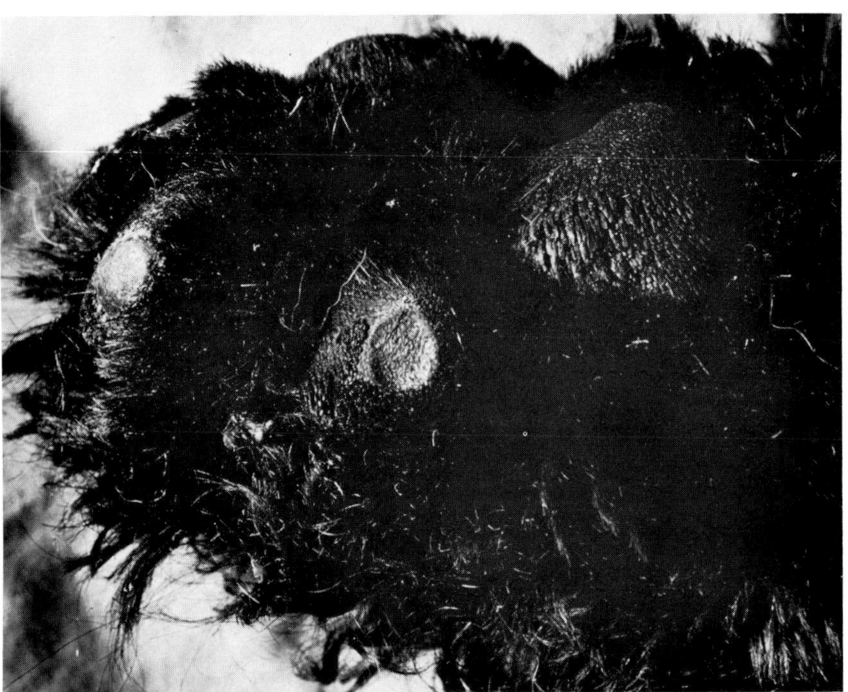

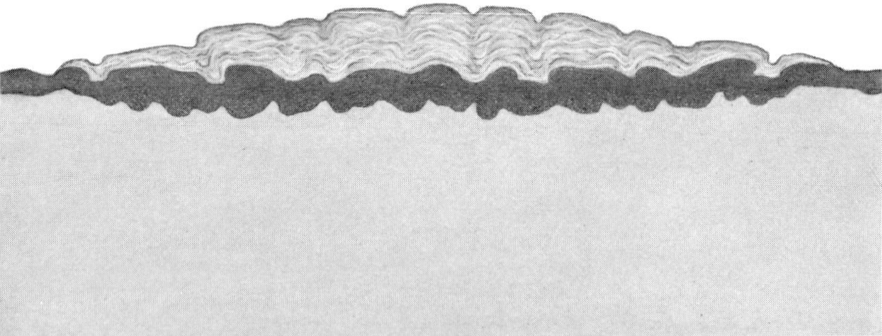

**Figure 5:16.** Hyperkeratosis—an increase in thickness of the horny layer of the skin. This condition occurs in normal skin and also on specialized areas such as the digital pads and planum nasale. Examples are callus formation and nasodigital hyperkeratosis (hardpad). The keratogenic hyperplasia can occur in plaques, ridges, circular areas or even "feathered" projections of digital pads. (Photo illustrates digital hyperkeratosis.)

# SIX

# *Distribution Patterns of Skin Lesions*

A dramatic change becomes apparent when a skin disorder affects an animal whose body is covered with a dense hair coat. Even the most casual observer is aware of the loss of hair in certain areas. The alopecic pattern—which is often sharply demarcated—assumes a new meaning when it is accurately interpreted. When alopecia and other hair changes are evaluated according to their distribution pattern over the entire body, significant diagnostic clues appear. Comparatively speaking, only on the human scalp is alopecia as striking and meaningful.

Recognizing the distribution pattern of skin lesions is a valuable diagnostic aid.

In animals the primary skin lesions are often hidden under the hair coat; in fact, it requires painstaking observation to see them. Only when the animal is clipped can the distribution pattern of such lesions be seen with ease. Consequently, in animals there are two distinctly different patterns that aid in diagnosis: Changes in external hair coat, and definition of primary and secondary skin lesions. These two factors do not necessarily have a reciprocal relationship.

Symmetry is of great importance! The dorsal and ventral views are significant, while the lateral aspect is of little value in this respect. When cutaneous lesions are bilaterally symmetrical, the skin may reflect an internal disease (for example, hyperadrenocorticism). Conversely, external (environmental) causes create a characteristically irregular lesional pattern (for example, fungal infections).

## DIFFERENT STAGES

As a skin disease progresses from its earliest appearance to its final, fully developed state, the pattern must necessarily change. A small patch of alopecia can enlarge into almost total hair loss in some cases. Obviously, if all intermediate stages of such a disease were drawn diagrammatically the result would be more confusing than helpful. It was necessary, therefore, to select for each skin disorder a single distribution pattern which is of greatest diagnostic value. It must be kept in mind at all times that different stages of each disease exist. The total impact of all diagrams should be interpreted with that fact constantly in mind.

In the description that accompanies each diagram other stages are referred to when necessary. Also, it is noted whether the distribution pattern represents alopecia or changes of the skin surface.

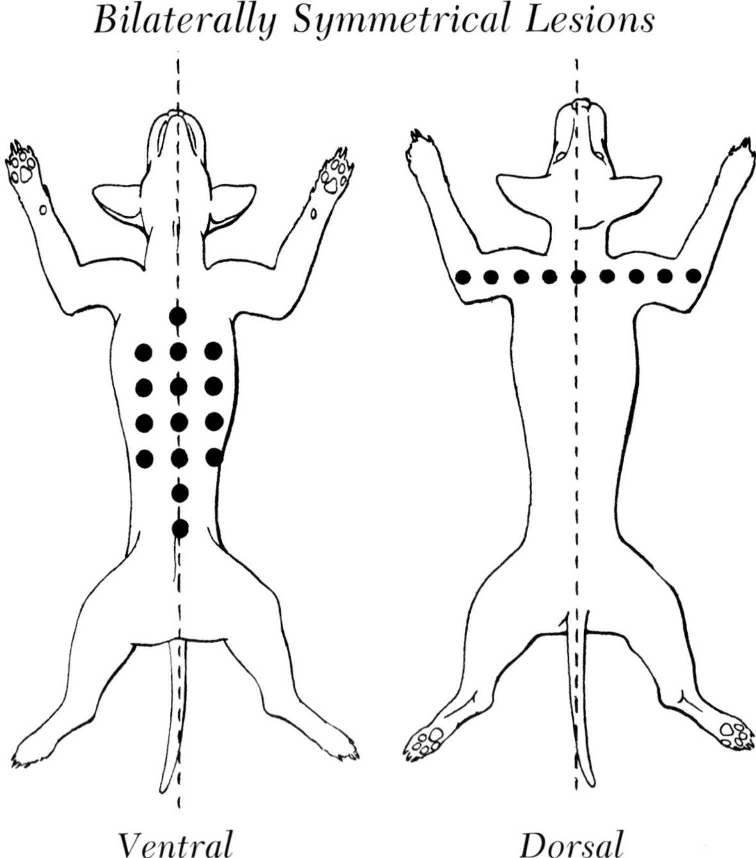


**Figure 6:1.** When a line is drawn from the tip of the nose to the end of the tail and the distribution of the lesions is the same on the right side as on the left side, the pattern is called bilaterally symmetrical. Most such skin disorders have an internal cause; frequently the skin becomes a reflection of internal disease. Examples are hypothyroidism, hyperadrenocorticism and Sertoli cell tumor.

*Asymmetric Distribution Pattern*

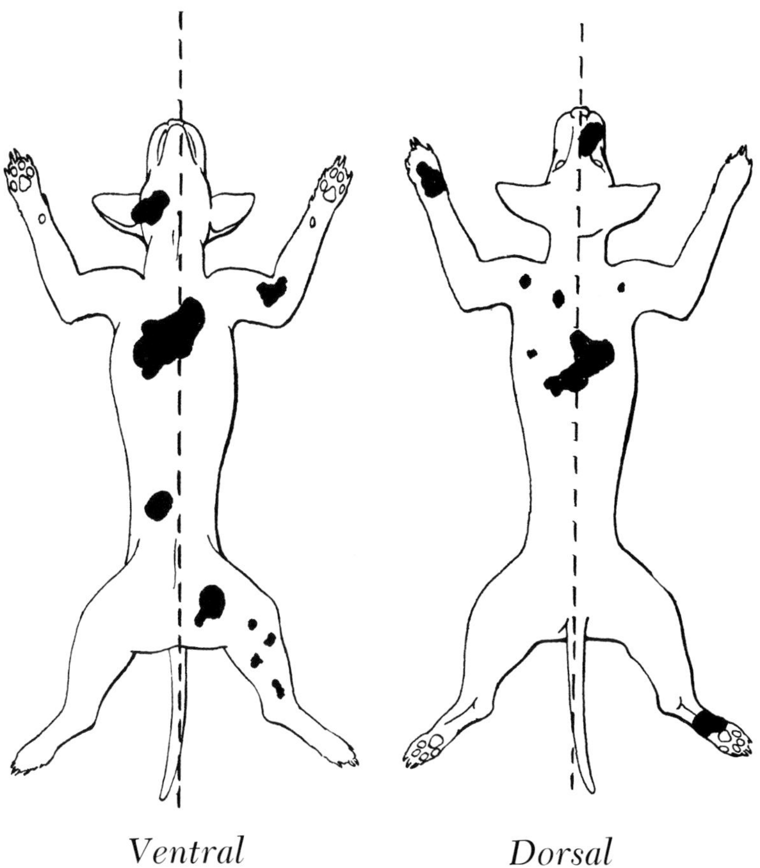

*Ventral* *Dorsal*

**Figure 6:2.** When a line is drawn from the tip of the nose to the end of the tail and the lesions on one side are not identical with those on the other side, the distribution pattern is asymmetric. External environmental causes, such as ectoparasites or contact allergens, usually cause such skin disorders.

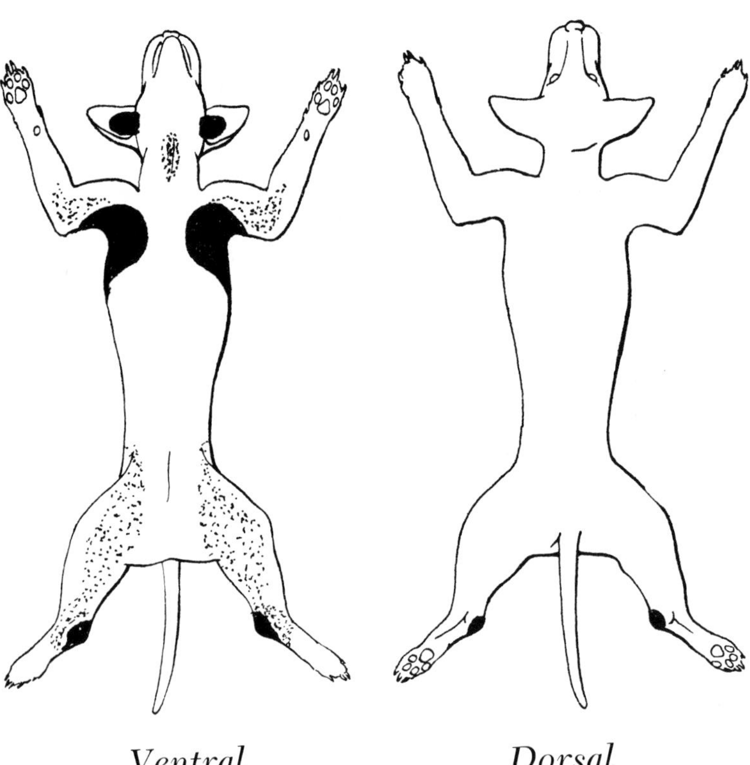


**Figure 6:3.** The lesions are bilaterally symmetrical areas of hyperpigmentation with alopecia, hyperkeratosis and lichenification. A greasy, seborrheic film covers the surface of many lesions. In the early stage, a hyperpigmented patch appears in each axilla. According to the present concept of acanthosis nigricans, the initial appearance of axillary lesions is the most important feature in the differential diagnosis of this disorder. As the disease progresses this patch becomes larger, the skin thickens and verrucous ridges appear. After the axillary lesions appear, other areas become affected in the following order: medial forelegs, medial hindlegs, hocks, inside of the ears, flanks and chest. Eventually the paws are affected, with secondary interdigital pyoderma occurring in some cases. The dorsal surface remains remarkedly unaffected except for seborrheic scaling.

*Sertoli Cell Tumor*

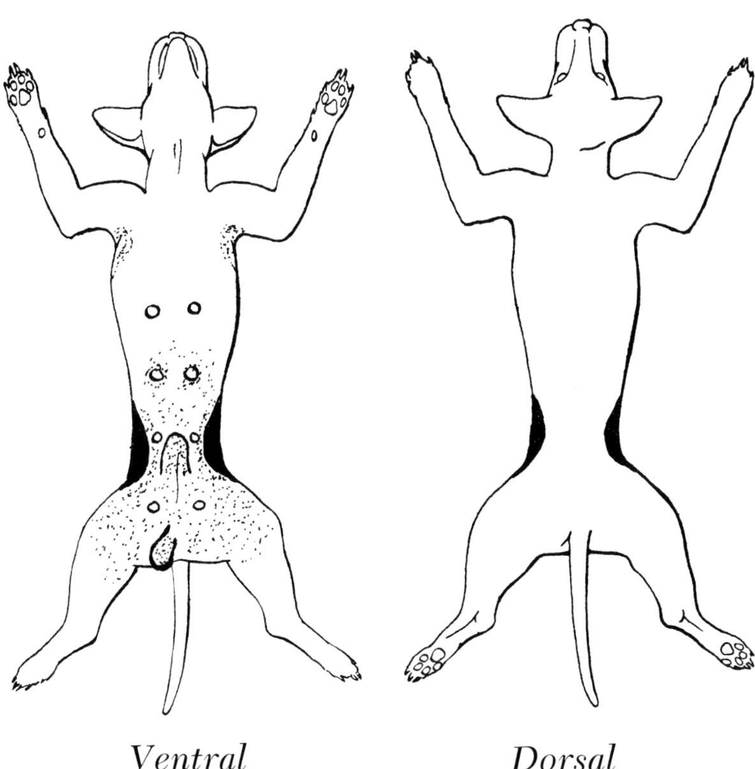

*Ventral* *Dorsal*

**Figure 6:4.** The diagram shows the characteristic distribution pattern. The area around the genital organs is characteristically affected with sharply circumscribed hyperpigmented patches. The normal skin between the lesions seems pale by comparison. There is slight involvement of the medial surfaces of the thigh and axillae. Hyperkeratosis and lichenification of the flanks are common and gynecomastia increases as the disease becomes chronic. In advanced cases alopecia affects most of the body, although only a narrow strip of hair may remain on the top of the head and dorsum of the back. In early cases of Sertoli cell tumor patients may not have skin lesions.

# *Feminizing Syndrome of Male Dogs (Hypoandrogenism)*

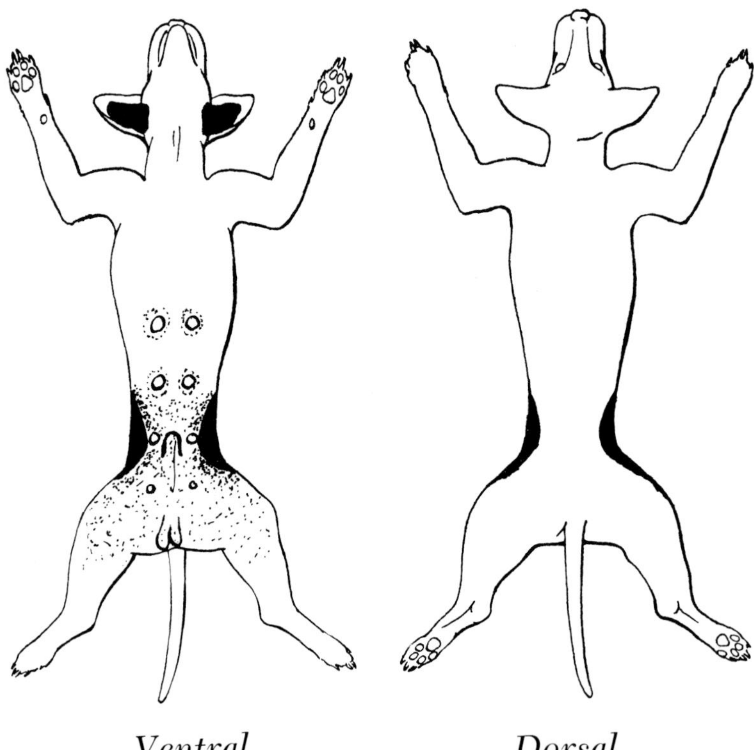


**Figure 6:5.** Hyperpigmentation and hyperkeratosis affect the flanks first and the area around the genital organs next, in a bilaterally symmetrical fashion. There are gynecomastia and ceruminous otitis. A severe secondary seborrhea afflicts the entire body. The diagram shows two normal testicles in the scrotum. In general, the distribution pattern of lesions is similar to that in Sertoli cell tumor cases, but there is no evidence of testicular neoplasia or widespread hair loss.

*Hypothyroidism*

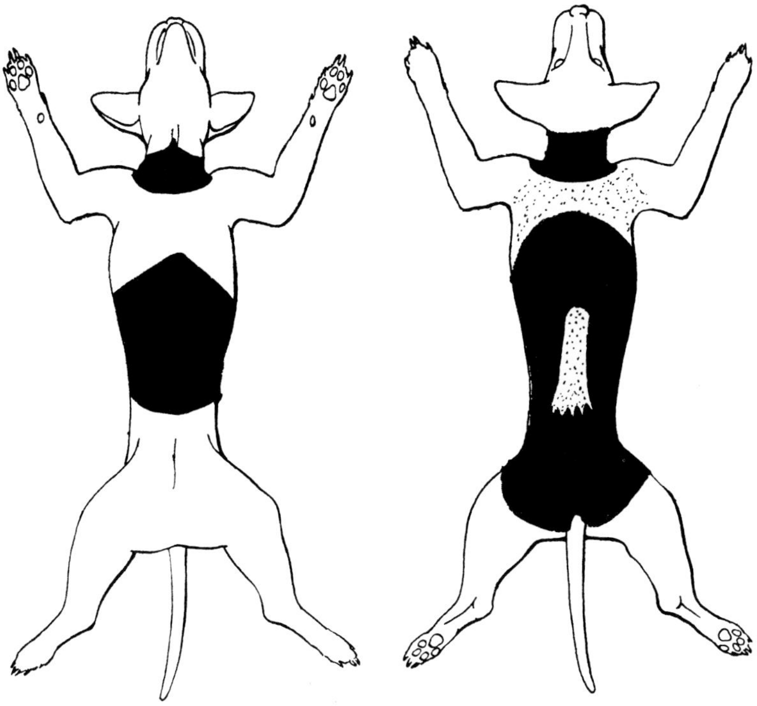

*Ventral* *Dorsal*

**Figure 6:6.** Alopecia occurs in a bilaterally symmetrical pattern as shown by shaded areas. The lateral trunk, dorsum and neck are the regions most commonly affected, and the head and legs are often spared. The skin of the affected areas is dry and cool to the touch; the entire hair coat is lusterless and brittle. The typical pattern may vary from one or two barely visible areas in short-haired dogs to spectacular sharply circumscribed alopecia in long-haired dogs.

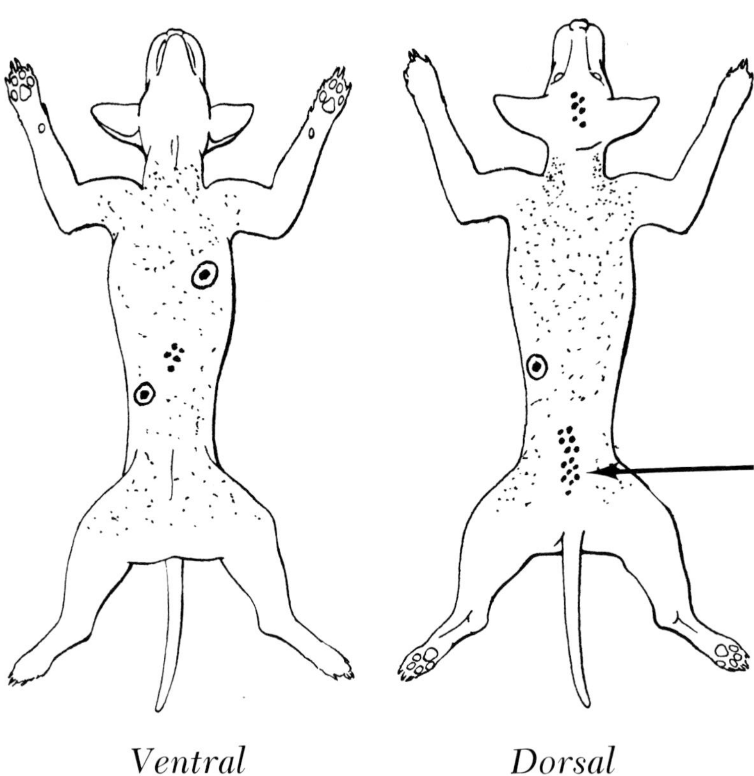


**Figure 6:7.** The distribution pattern of alopecia is not distinctly characteristic in the early stage. There is a "moth-eaten" pattern of hair loss, which in general is bilaterally symmetrical. The most noticeable lesions are found on the trunk and abdomen. Calcinosis cutis, if present, is most common on the posterior region of the back, the abdomen and the top of the head. Large blue veins can be seen on the distended abdomen and macules with a pigmented center and flaky margin are seen on the lateral side of the trunk. In advanced cases, most of the hair is lost except on the head and extremities. This pattern is very dramatic in long-haired dogs. The skin also becomes hyperpigmented on the alopecic areas. An arrow points to a common area of calcinosis cutis. The circled lesions represent the characteristic pigmented macules with their keratin rim.

## *Feline Endocrine Alopecia*

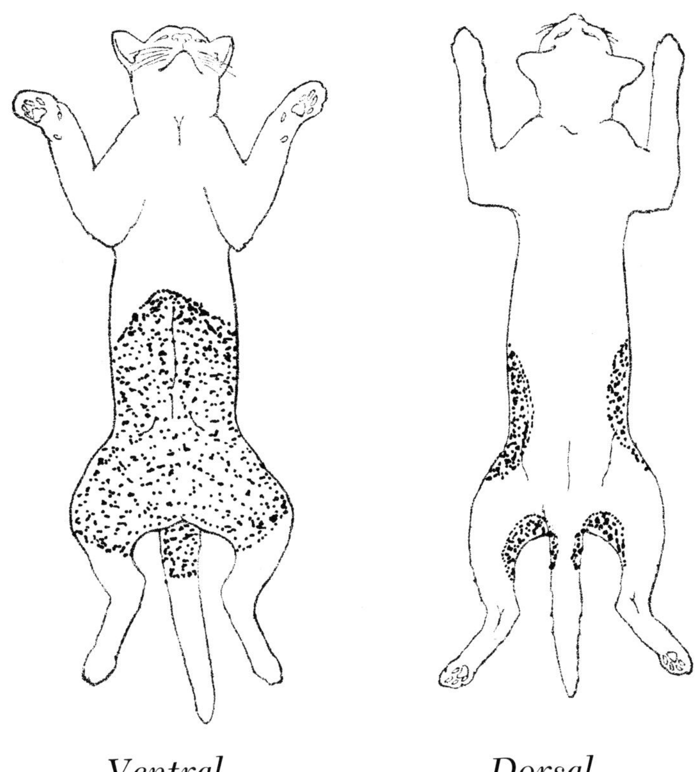


**Figure 6:8.** There is a partial or complete hair loss in the areas marked on the diagram. The distribution pattern of the alopecia is bilaterally symmetrical. The affected areas of skin are not pruritic, scaly or inflamed, but the hair in the region is dry, brittle and stubby.

*Flea Allergy Dermatitis*

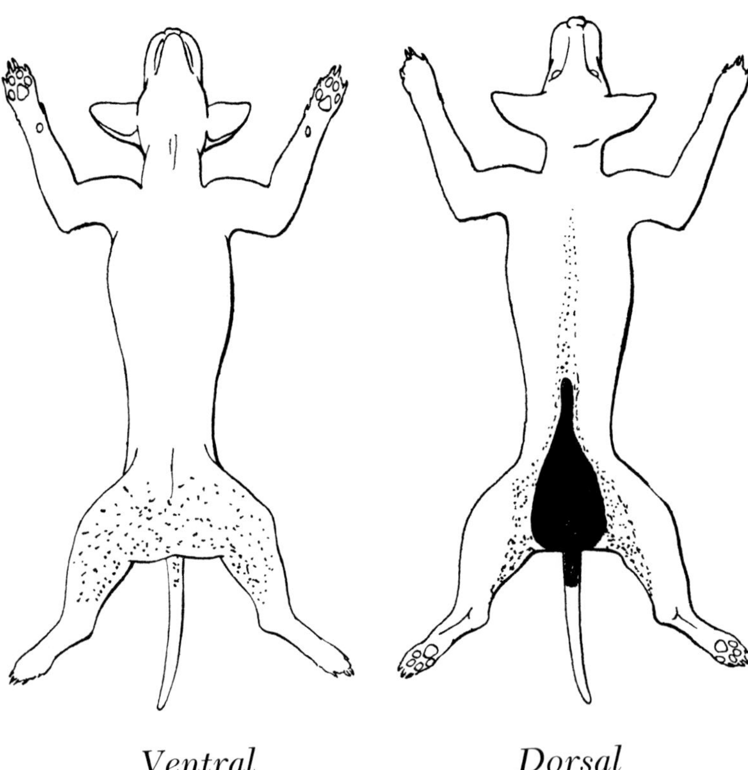


**Figure 6:9.** The shaded area of the sketch shows the location of the main erythematous and pruritic lesions. The posterior and medial surfaces of the thighs and posterior abdomen may be affected also. Fleas are commonly found on the affected areas and excoriations are caused by the dog's biting at his skin. Acute moist dermatitis may result from this self-inflicted trauma.

*Contact Dermatitis*

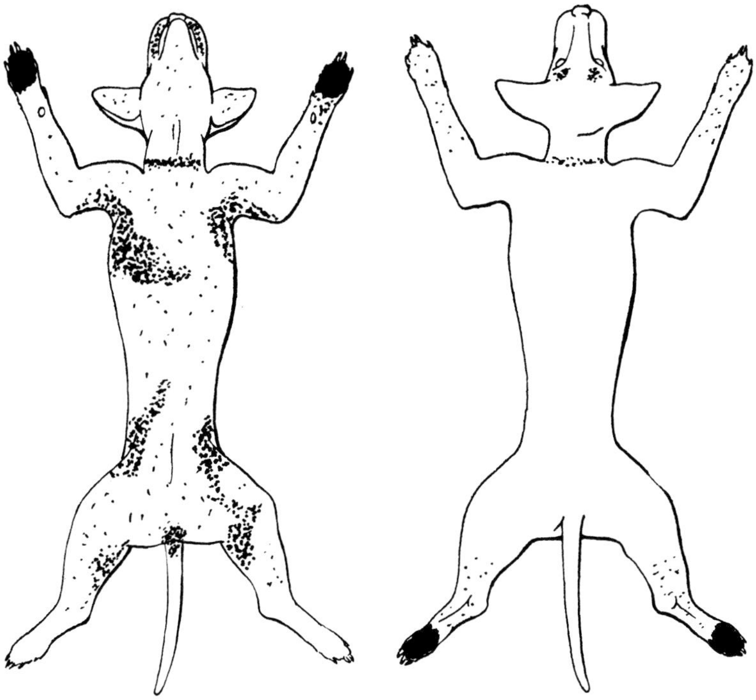

*Ventral* *Dorsal*

**Figure 6:10.** Lesions occur in areas that are sparsely covered with hair or that are hairless. Most lesions are on the ventral surface of the body. The abdomen, chest, axillae, flanks, interdigital spaces, legs, perianal area and eyelids are the most likely areas for an allergen to produce contact dermatitis. When the offending agent is a liquid the hairy regions may be involved.

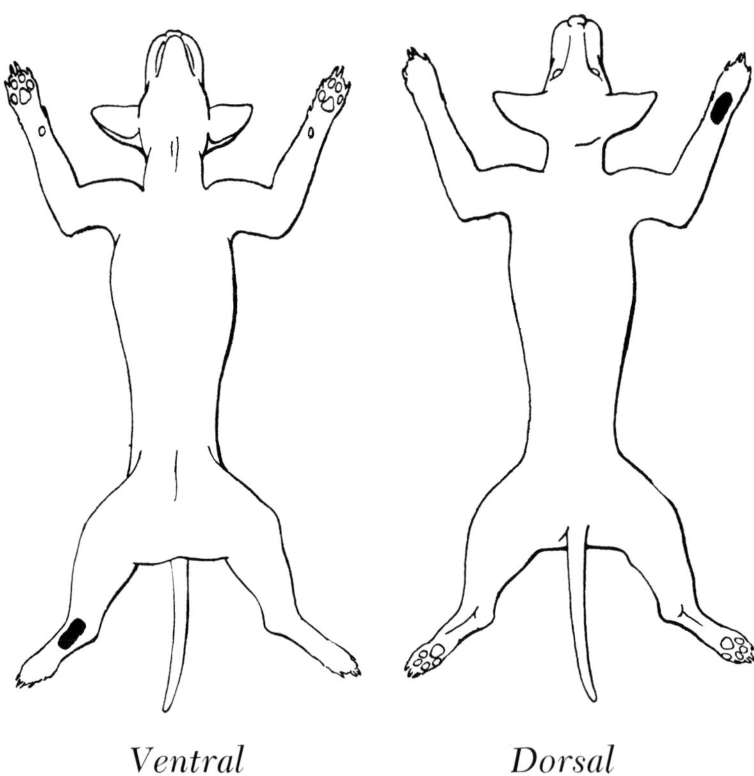


**Figure 6:11.** This is a unilateral, firm, hairless nodule with a moist, glistening surface. It occurs most commonly on the anterior surface of the carpus. In some cases it may be seen instead on the metacarpal or metatarsal surface and can be located laterally as well as anteriorly. The size varies from about 1 cm. to several centimeters in diameter. The shape is most frequently oval, but round and partially rectangular lesions have been observed. This condition is also known as lick granuloma and acral pruritic nodule.

## *Feline Neurodermatitis (Lick Granuloma)*

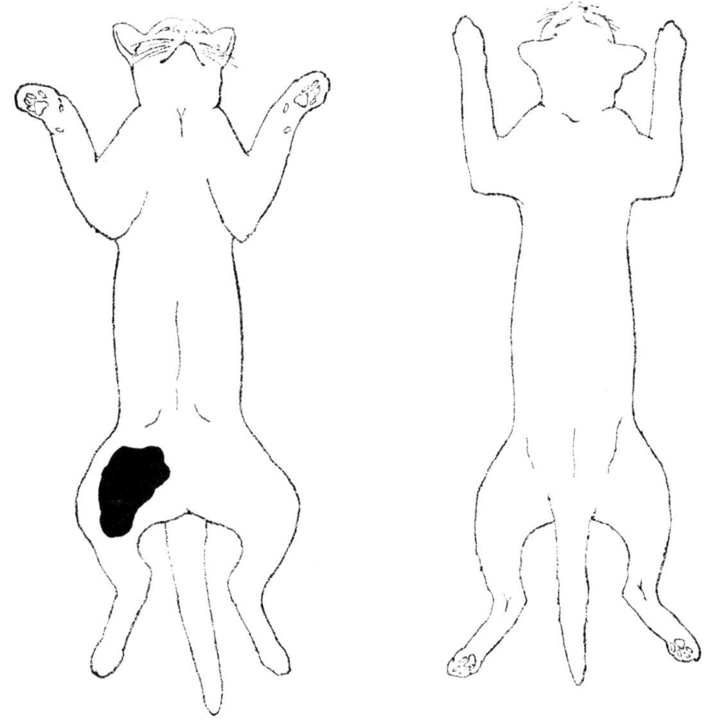


**Figure 6:12.** The shaded area represents a solitary hairless lesion with an ulcerated or eroded surface. It is produced by constant licking of the cat. Although the inside of the hindleg is the area most commonly affected, this lesion can also be found on other parts of the cat's body.

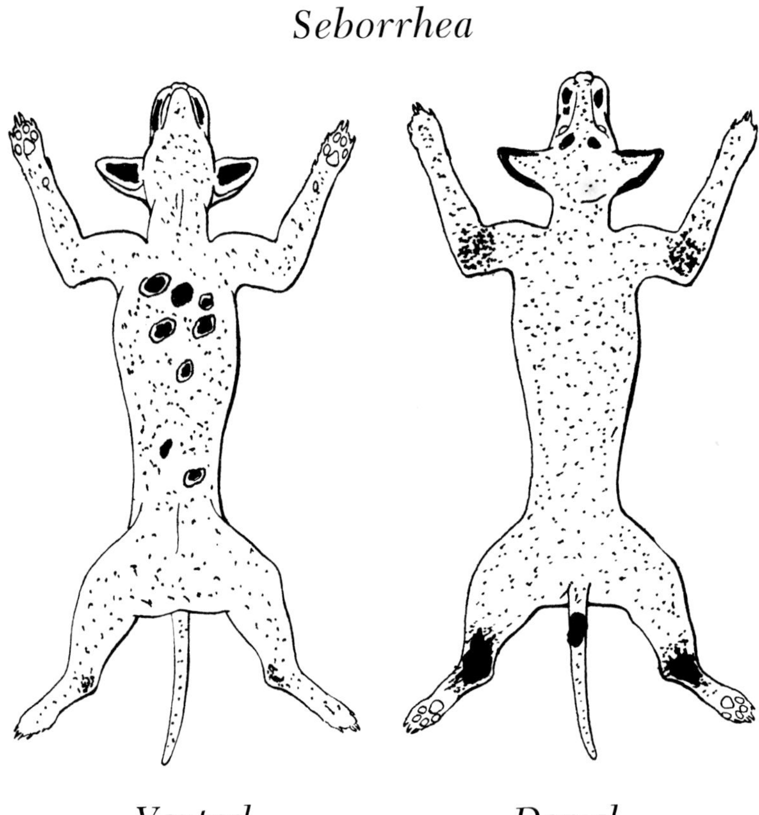


**Figure 6:13.** Although the shaded areas are the most consistently affected sites, seborrheic lesions can be found on any part of the body. The lesions consist of scaly crusted areas that often are somewhat circular. In chronic cases, as in cocker spaniels, the circular thoracic and abdominal lesions resemble fungal infections. The scales can be white, yellow, dry, greasy, branny, loose or adhering. In seborrheic dermatitis there is considerable erythema under the scaly surface. Ceruminous otitis is a common finding.

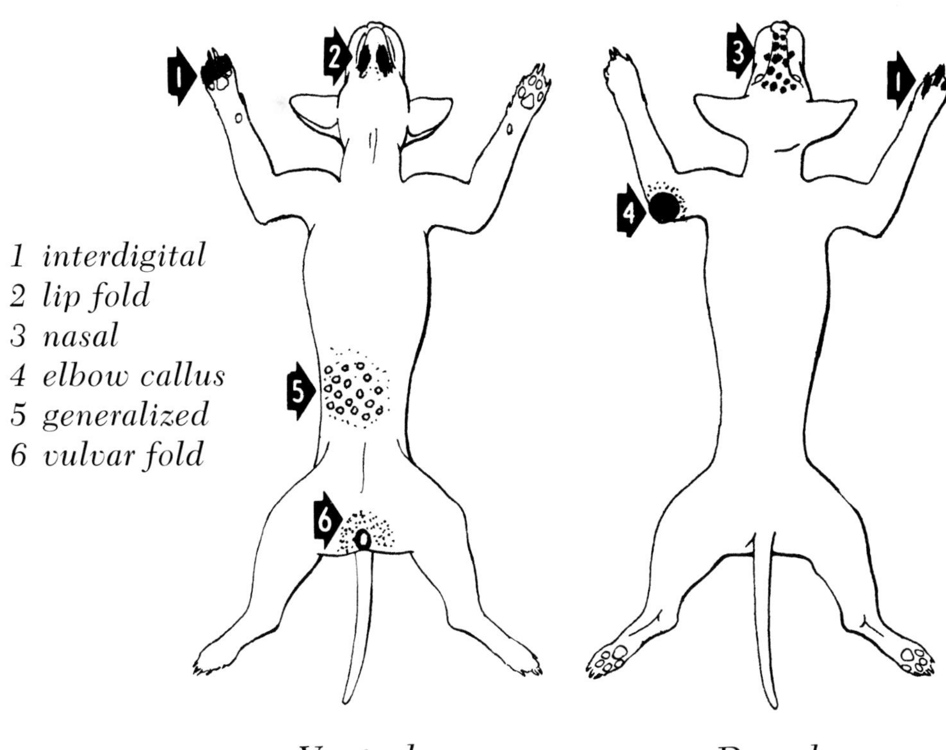


**Figure 6:14.** It is convenient to divide the pyodermas into regional groupings because of the tendency for bacterial infections to occur in certain sites. An anatomic defect can lead to pyoderma of the lip fold and vulvar fold, whereas the elbows and interdigital spaces are subject to environmental trauma. Generalized pyoderma may be confined to one of these areas, although in severe cases most of the cutaneous surface may be involved. The affected areas show pustules, furuncles and fistulas, and may be covered with hemorrhagic crusts.

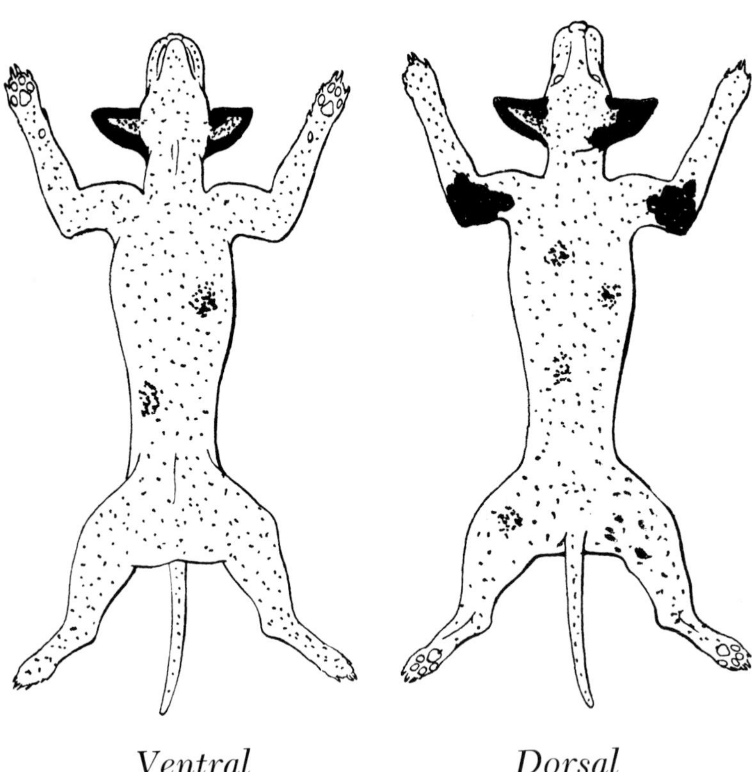


**Figure 6:15.** Sarcoptic mites *(Sarcoptes scabiei* var. *canis)* will parasitize all areas of the skin; however, the mites have a decided preference for certain regions. The external ears are definite sites of predilection and often show the greatest amount of trauma from the dog's scratching. The extremities, especially the elbows and hocks, also are involved frequently. Typically the affected areas show partial alopecia, erythema, excoriations and crusting.

*Localized Demodectic Mange*

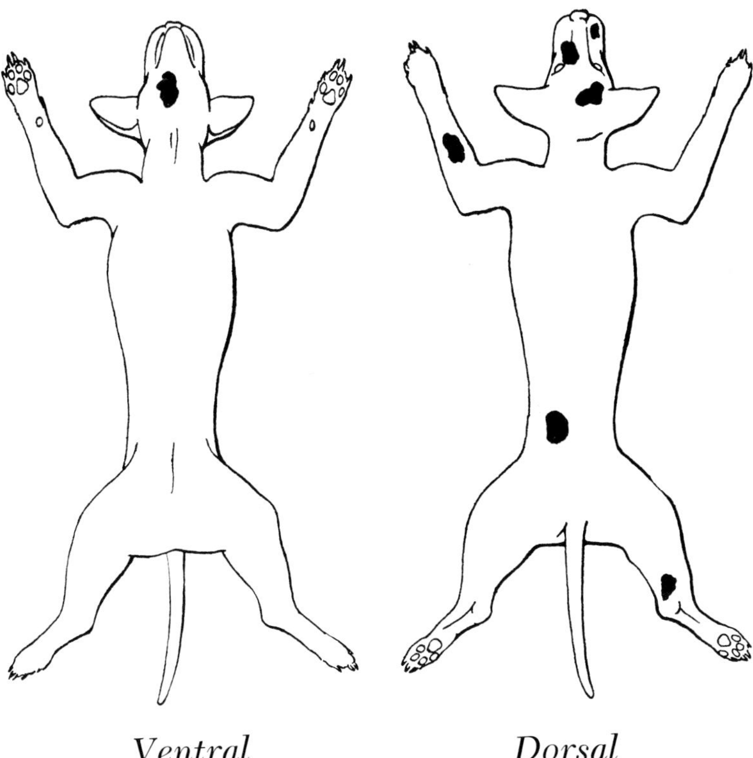

*Ventral* *Dorsal*

**Figure 6:16.** The head and forelegs are the most commonly affected areas. The average patient seldom has more than five lesions, each characterized by alopecia, erythema and scaling. The periocular area and the lips are frequently the sites of the first lesions. Next in order of occurrence are the face, neck and forelegs. A solitary lesion of demodectic mange can be found anywhere on the body.

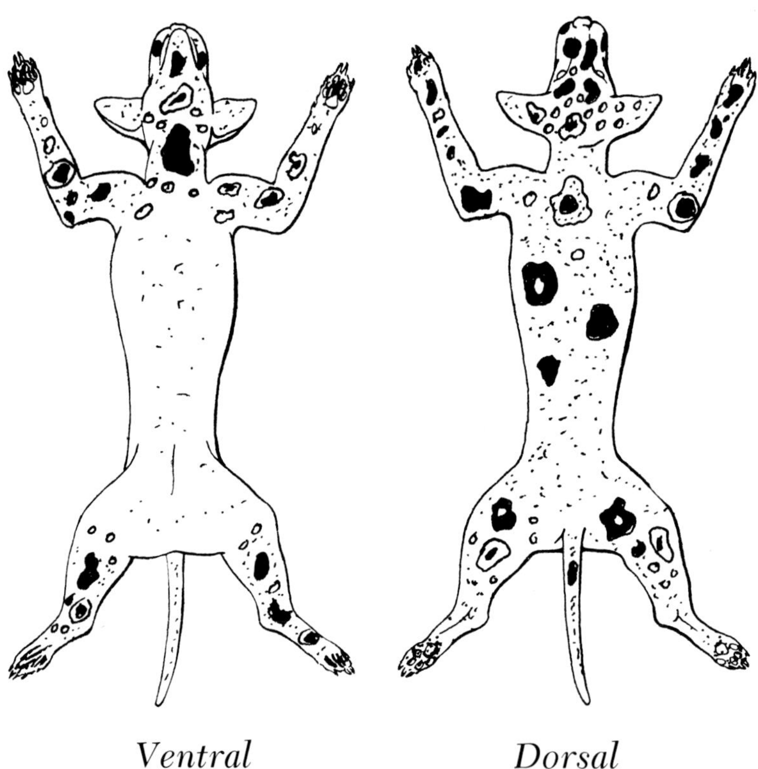


**Figure 6:17.** Although every part of the body can be involved, the face and legs usually become affected most severely. The chest and abdomen are sometimes spared. Most cases are complicated by pyoderma, which chronically affects the dorsum of the nose and the cheeks, throat, periorbital areas and legs. The involved areas show erythema, alopecia, pustules, furuncles, fistulas and hemorrhagic crusts.

# SEVEN

# *Laboratory Procedures*

Dermatologic laboratory procedures interpreted in the proper perspective can be useful diagnostic aids. In some cases laboratory procedures can establish the diagnosis accurately, help to confirm the clinical findings and provide a logical basis for successful therapeutic management. This discussion deals primarily with the equipment needed and the method used to perform each test. More detail about the test results and their significance will be found in other appropriate chapters of the text (i.e., Dermatohistopathology, Cutaneous Parasitology, and Cutaneous Bacteriology).

A routine laboratory procedure frequently will solve an undiagnosed dermatosis.

## EXAMINATIONS FOR PARASITES

### The Skin Scraping

This is one of the most frequently used tests in veterinary dermatology, and it should be performed whenever the diagnosis is not absolutely established. Its purpose is to enable the clinician to find and identify microscopic ectoparasites that inhabit the skin.

The equipment needed to perform a skin scraping (Fig. 7:1) is mineral oil or glycerine in a small dropper bottle, a scalpel handle and blade, microscope slides and coverslips, and a microscope. In addition, 10 per cent KOH solution, lactophenol cotton blue stain, tweezers and an alcohol lamp or other heat source are often useful.

It is essential to choose a "typical" or favorable area of skin on which to make the scraping to enhance the chances of finding parasites. Typical areas for each condition vary in location, so selection must be made on the basis of the probable diagnosis. In dermatomycosis it is best to select an area near the margin

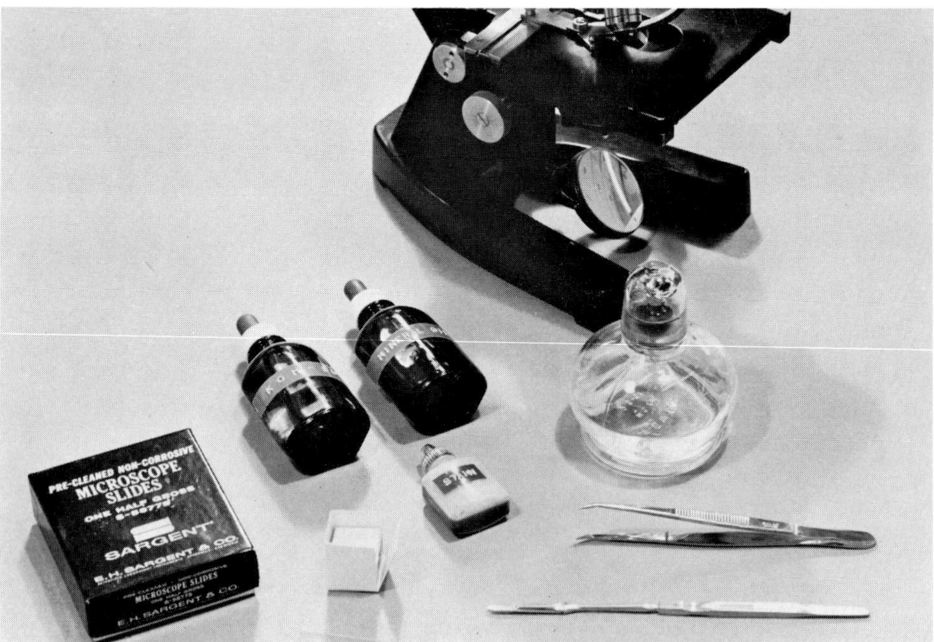


**Figure 7:1.** Equipment needed for making skin scrapings.

of a lesion which is growing rapidly. However, for other cases it is most desirable to choose a site which has not been disturbed by excoriations or other trauma and which has not been medicated.

---

Select undisturbed, unmedicated skin for a scraping site.

---

When attempting to find demodectic mites, a fold of skin should be pinched gently to express parasites. With sarcoptic mange this is not necessary. In either case, a drop of mineral oil or glycerine placed on the area to be scraped traps parasites, hair and scales and facilitates their adherence to the scalpel and thus their transfer to the slide. One should remember that parasites may be found on the surface, in the folds of epidermis, in the horny layer or the deeper epidermis, the hair follicle, or even in the dermis. Thus the scraping should be made gently, but deeply enough to draw blood, which indicates collection of material from the deeper layers.

The accumulated material is placed on a microscope slide and one or two drops of mineral oil are added. The mixture is stirred with a needle or applicator stick to spread it evenly. Always use a coverslip over material that is to be examined microscopically. With most parasitisms the preceding method is adequate to collect specimens for identification. If no parasites are found when looking for sarcoptic mites, it may be necessary to repeat the procedure on as many as eight to ten skin sites before diagnostic material is observed or the test is concluded as negative.

Occasional scrapings may be dense with much hair and debris. These can be "cleared" by adding a few drops of 10 per cent KOH to the slide and either allowing it to stand for 30 minutes, or heating it very gently (avoid boiling) for 15 to 20 seconds over a flame. High degrees of heat should be avoided.

Another technique for handling skin scrapings is especially useful when mites or their eggs are hard to find. This often occurs in cases of sarcoptic mange. In such instances an abundant amount of material is accumulated from several typical sites. All of the debris is placed in a small tube or beaker, 10 per cent KOH is added, stirred and the mixture heated gently. The KOH mixture is added to a saturated sugar solution in centrifuge tubes and spun until the mites and ova are floated to the surface. A drop or two of the surface solution is examined on a slide under a coverslip. This procedure is useful because it concentrates the eggs or parasites from the entire sample and the possibility of finding organisms is greatly enhanced.

Sarcoptic mange mites can often be graphically identified if the accumulated material from a scraping is placed in a plastic box, such as those in which tubes of ointment are packaged. The box is left at room temperature for 12 to 24 hours. The bottom of the box then can be examined with a powerful magnifying lens (9 ×) and the mites observed as slowly moving white specks.

#### *THE LARGER ECTOPARASITES*

Lice, ticks and fleas are large enough to be observed easily, although a hand lens is helpful, and a dissecting microscope (20 × to 40 ×) is needed for accurate identification of some specimens. These ectoparasites can be sprayed with alcohol or insecticide preparations and carefully picked off the surface of the skin with a forceps or by combing. The specimens should be placed in a vial of 70 per cent alcohol to insure death and to preserve them for identification. They can be mounted on slides in water, oil or glycerine for microscopic examination under several magnifications.

## EXAMINATIONS FOR DERMATOPHYTES

### The Potassium Hydroxide Preparation

This is a rapid method that can be meaningful only after one has considerable practice and experience in its use. The equipment necessary is 10 per cent KOH, microscope slides and coverslips, an alcohol or Bunsen burner, tweezers and a scalpel handle and blade. Material is collected as for a skin scraping, together with plucked hairs, and deposited on a slide. Several drops of 10 per cent KOH are applied, a coverslip added and the slide gently heated for 15 to 20 seconds. Alternately, it may merely be allowed to stand for 30 minutes at room temperature. An excellent result is obtained if the mount is placed on the microscope lamp for gentle heating. The preparation will be ready for examination in 15 to 20 minutes and the structures will be better preserved.

Identification of a mycotic infection, especially on glabrous skin, can be made by finding the branching mycelia. Hair shafts should be examined for spores. Ectothrix spores are found in *Microsporum* and *Trichophyton mentagrophytes* infections. Endothrix spores are found in some other dermatophytes.

Fungal cultures provide ultimate proof in diagnosis of dermatomycoses.

## Fungal Culture

The culture is the most reliable method for diagnosis and identification of dermatomycosis. It requires only a few minutes to inoculate media and most pathogens grow into distinctive colonies in one to three weeks at room temperature.

Equipment necessary includes disposable culture tubes or bottles (flat ½ ounce perfume bottles preferred) containing Sabouraud's dextrose agar with cyclohexamine and chloramphenicol, sterile Bard-Parker handle No. 7 with No. 15 blade, sterile forceps, sterile cotton and lactophenol cotton blue stain (Fig. 7:2).

The suspected lesion is cleansed with 70 per cent alcohol to reduce contamination. The sample for inoculation should be obtained from the periphery of a rapidly growing lesion. A small scraping of superficial keratin and hair should be obtained and deposited carefully on the center of the surface of culture medium (Fig. 7:3). The culture bottle should be closed, but the cap unscrewed a quarter turn to allow aerobic growth. The bottle ideally is placed on a cabinet shelf to incubate at room temperature. A pan containing water should be placed in the cabinet to insure relatively high humidity for growth and to prevent dehydration of the medium.

Because an adequate sample is vital, there are two additional techniques which may help assure a positive culture. If the case involves a dermatophyte which causes hair to fluoresce, the sample should be obtained from an area which is positive to this test. Often single hairs may be plucked from an area because of their brilliant fluorescence. This makes an ideal inoculum. Another technique has the advantage of accumulating much keratin debris as the inoculum. In this procedure a sterile toothbrush is rubbed vigorously over the suspected lesion. The bristles trap scaly material and hair which can be shaken out of the brush onto a sterile Petri dish for transfer to the culture bottle, or shaken directly onto the surface of the medium in a Petri dish. Alternately, a sterile scalpel blade can be used to scrape dry scales onto a piece of paper or the Petri dish.

Pluck hairs which fluoresce to the Wood's light for inoculating Sabouraud's agar.

Information on identification of cultures is given in the section on dermatophytes (p. 125).

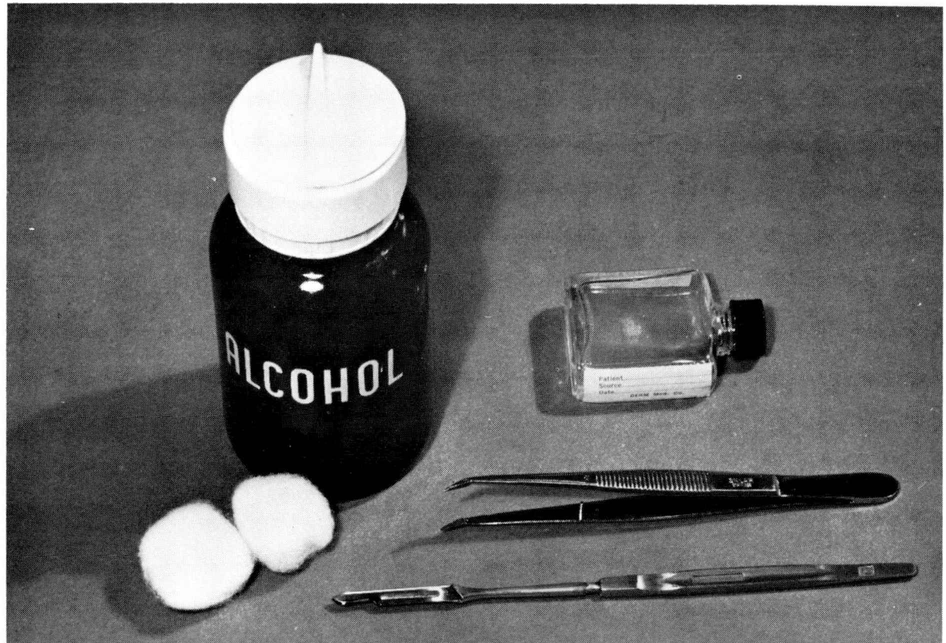


**Figure 7:2.** Equipment needed for making fungus cultures.

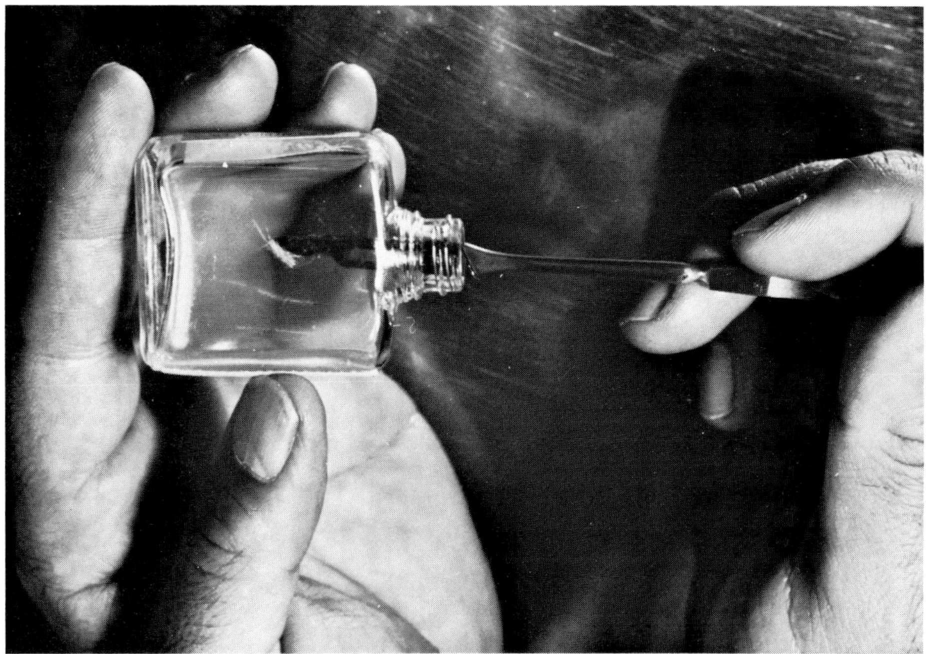

**Figure 7:3.** Depositing hair and keratin from skin scraping in a culture bottle containing Sabouraud's agar.

### Wood's Light

Ultraviolet light filtered through nickel oxide produces a beam called Wood's light. A useful unit has two light tubes, one on either side of a central magnifying glass and the entire complex is contained in a plastic rim with a comfortable handle (Fig. 7:4). In addition to its use in diagnosis, and to obtain infected material for culture, the Wood's light is helpful to follow the progress of therapy. However, it has several limitations.

All examinations must be made in a dark room. The only common dermatophyte of dogs and cats which causes hair to fluoresce is *Microsporum canis*, but even here less than half of the positive cultured cases also showed fluorescence. A positive response to Wood's light for this fungus is a bright yellow-green, not unlike that seen by shining the light on the numerals of a fluorescent watch face. Many other factors cause fluorescence (medications, dirt, petrolatum and scales) and these may give false positive reactions.

The usefulness of the Wood's light can be summarized—a positive response is highly suggestive, but a negative response is not conclusive, as the patient may be free of infection or affected by a nonfluorescing dermatophyte.

---

In Wood's light examination, positive fluorescence is a valuable clue; negative fluorescence is not conclusive.

---

### The Impression Smear

This test, described on page 100, is occasionally of limited use in identification of yeasts and fungi.

## EXAMINATIONS FOR BACTERIA

Much of the equipment used in a microbiology laboratory can now be purchased in disposable plastics. This has made office bacteriology feasible. For the simple tests described here, the following equipment is needed (Fig. 7:5): a microscope with light, condenser and appropriate objectives, 37° C. incubator, Bunsen burner or alcohol lamp, an inoculating loupe, an autoclave, an interval timer, staining rack, microscope slides and coverslips. Materials needed include: prepared sterile plastic Petri dishes with appropriate media, sterile swabs in culture tubes or plastic containers, appropriate antibiotic sensitivity discs, and appropriate stains and associated chemicals. Antibiotic discs should include penicillin, oxacillin, nafcillin, erythromycin, bacitracin, novobiocin, streptomycin, neomycin, polymyxin B, nitrofurazone, chloramphenicol and tetracycline. Staining equipment should be available for gram, new methylene blue, Giemsa, Wright's and lactophenol cotton blue stains.

While most of the simple media and culture tubes are received sterile and ready to use, the clinician should understand the three methods available for

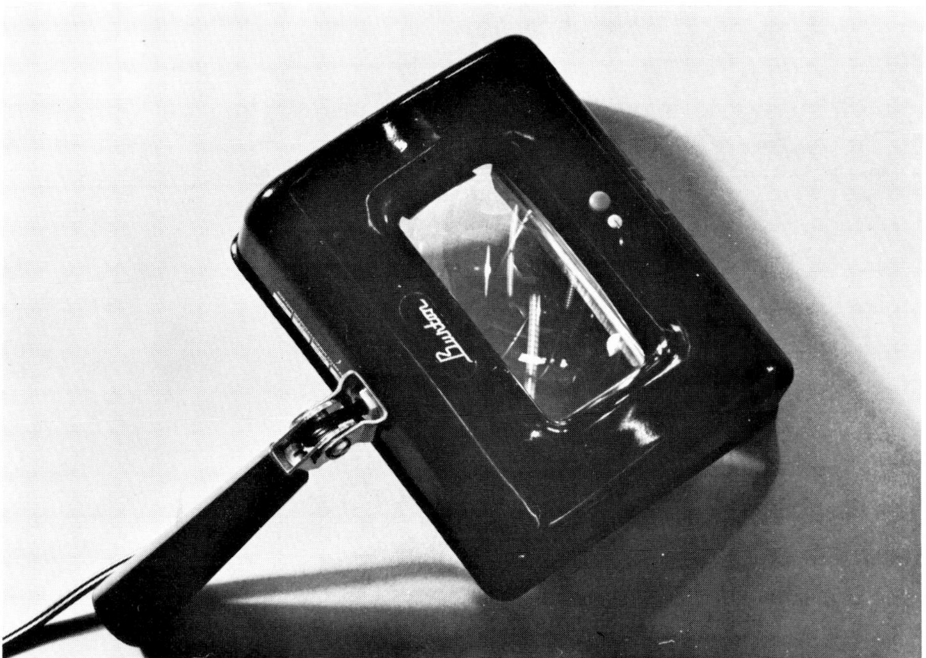


**Figure 7:4.** Wood's light with magnifying glass for examination of fungal materials for fluorescence.

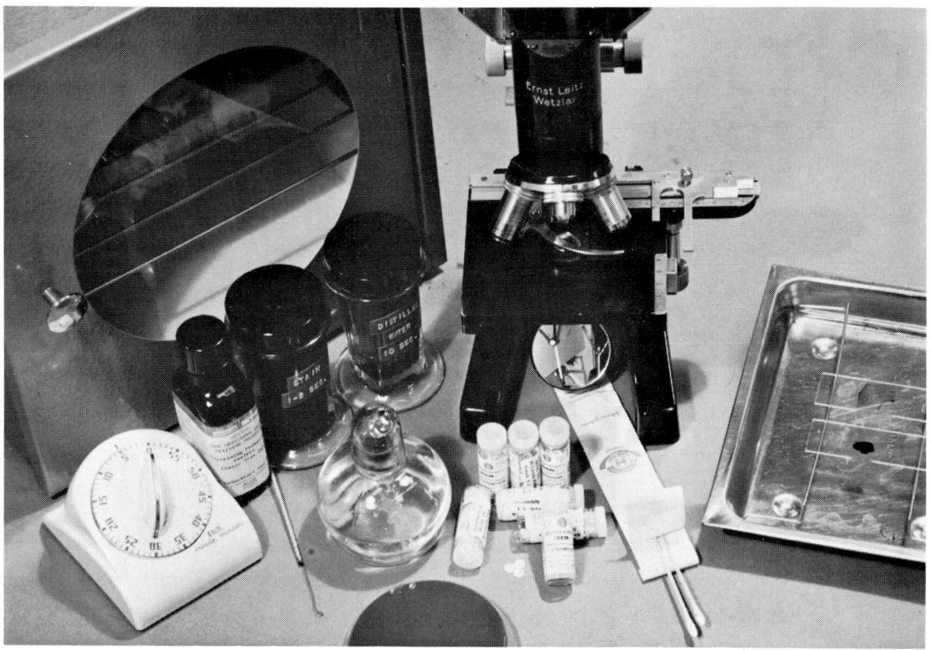


**Figure 7:5.** Equipment needed for diagnosis of bacterial diseases, and sensitivity testing.

sterilization. Glassware is ideally processed by heating in a hot air oven at 160° C. for at least one hour. This destroys all bacterial life including spores. Objects of rubber, metal, some glass, liquids, media and so on cannot be sterilized by dry heat. These items can be sterilized by exposure to steam under pressure of 15 pounds per square inch (121° C.) for 20 minutes. An open flame is needed to sterilize spatulas, forceps and inoculating loupes. They are first cleaned and then heated directly in the flame to ensure sterility.

## Direct Smears

A direct smear is a simple, inexpensive procedure that may reveal significant information rapidly. Variations of this test may be called touch or impression smears. To make the smear, a clean microscope slide can be pressed firmly against a raw or ulcerated lesion to transfer cellular material to the slide. Exudates may also be collected by sterile swab or aspirated into a sterile syringe. The swab can then be rolled gently across the slide, or a drop of the fluid in the syringe can be placed on the slide and carefully spread in a uniform film. Material from a block of tissue can be transferred to the slide by gently pressing the tissue onto the slide in several locations. In the latter case it is advisable to use only a freshly cut surface, and to blot it once with sterile gauze to remove excess blood before making the imprints.

Various stains can be utilized to identify different conditions.

For bacterial infections use Wright's stain and the gram stain. The presence of many bacteria and polymorphonuclear leukocytes is significant. Depending on the gram reaction one can often make a good guess at identification of the etiologic organism.

For fungal infections lactophenol cotton blue enables one to observe mycelia and spores.

Identification of the budding cells of *Candida albicans* is possible when the material is prepared in a wet mount stained with new methylene blue.

Some tumors may be diagnosed by impression smears. Mastocytoma, histiocytoma and malignant lymphoma may be identified occasionally. Giemsa stain is usually best.

## Bacterial Culture

Culture and identification of the organisms from superficial infections is usually reserved for refractory cases where special problems have developed. In these cases swabs from the infection are often inoculated into broth and then onto agar plates so that isolation and identification subcultures can be made. This is a procedure for a medical laboratory. In most instances of skin infection a gram stain of direct smear is made to identify the type of organism. A simultaneous heavy inoculation is made on an agar plate for antibiotic sensitivity tests (Fig. 7:6). These two procedures give the clinician adequate information to treat most infections properly.

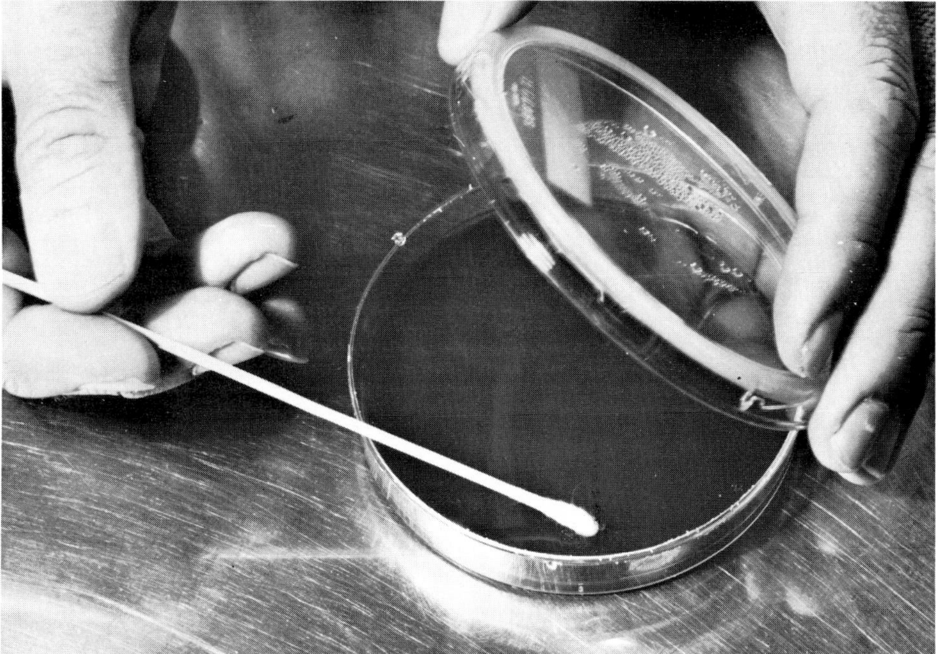

**Figure 7:6.** Inoculating blood agar directly from a culture swab.

## Antimicrobial Sensitivity Testing

This test is helpful in making a selection of effective antimicrobial agents. It is especially useful with staphylococcus, proteus and coliform infections where individual strains of the organisms may have different responses to antibiotics.

The test is only a guide — a positive test does not assure clinical success.

Conversely, a negative test does not always mean *no* clinical effect, but it usually would cause the veterinarian to look further for a more effective drug.

As with most tests, interpretation must be made in the proper perspective. Accuracy, of course, depends on obtaining a representative specimen. Pick an unopened lesion. Gently prepare the skin as for surgery and then open the lesion and swab its deep recess to obtain the sample. Inoculation on the blood agar plate must be heavy, so that dense growth is obtained. Usually ten or 12 discs are pressed onto the surface of the blood agar and incubation at 37° is continued for 12 to 24 hours before the test is read (Figs. 7:7 and 44:1*A*). The bacteria are either sensitive to or resistant to each disc and the results are only qualitative. They are reported as R (resistant) or S (sensitive). The size of the clear zone of inhibition around each disc is an indication of diffusibility of the drug, not sensitivity of the organism.

Common bacteria often associated with pyodermas are staphylococci, streptococci, corynebacteria, pseudomonas, proteus and *E coli.*

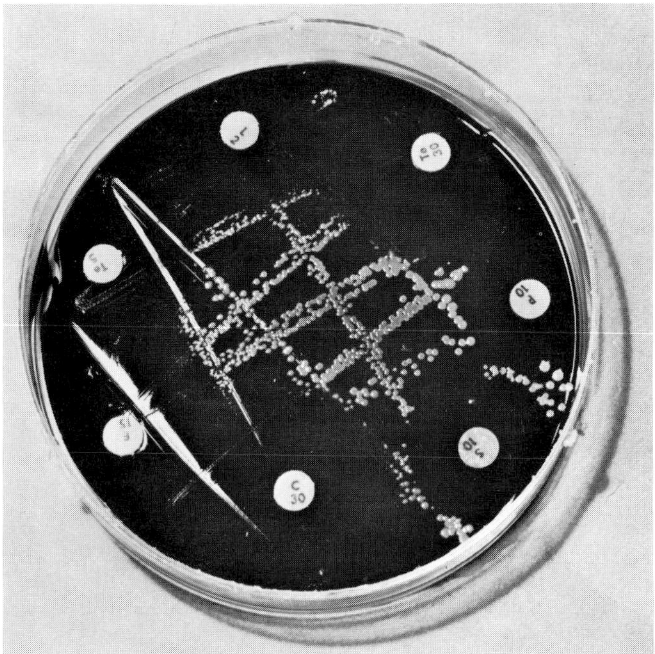

**Figure 7:7.** Antimicrobial sensitivity tests. This plate is not inoculated heavily enough. The color illustration in the section on pyoderma shows a better test result (Fig. 44:1, *A*).

## HISTOPATHOLOGICAL EXAMINATION

The practical value of biopsies in small animal practice is increasing as progress in histopathology of the skin develops new understanding of cutaneous lesions. A simple surgical tray for skin biopsies should include a Keyes cutaneous punch (4 mm. or 6 mm.), thumb forceps, mosquito hemostat, sharp scissors, scalpel, gauze sponges, 2 ml. and 5 ml. syringes and 25-gauge 1-inch needles (Fig. 7:8*A* and *B*). Ethyl chloride or Freon spray and 0.5 per cent lidocaine are needed for anesthesia. Ten per cent formalin (one part commercial formalin to nine parts of water) in wide-mouth 1-ounce jars and mailing tubes are needed for fixing and shipping the specimen. Many pathologists prefer formaldehyde that is buffered with dibasic sodium phosphate and monobasic potassium phosphate.

### Excision Biopsy

This is the preferred method of handling small nodules and tumors. It is both diagnostic and curative. An elliptical section of skin containing the lesion is removed and nylon or stainless steel sutures are used to repair the defect.

### Punch Biopsy

Proper selection of a typical area for biopsy is crucial. If possible, the specimen should contain normal and diseased tissue. The skin should be lightly

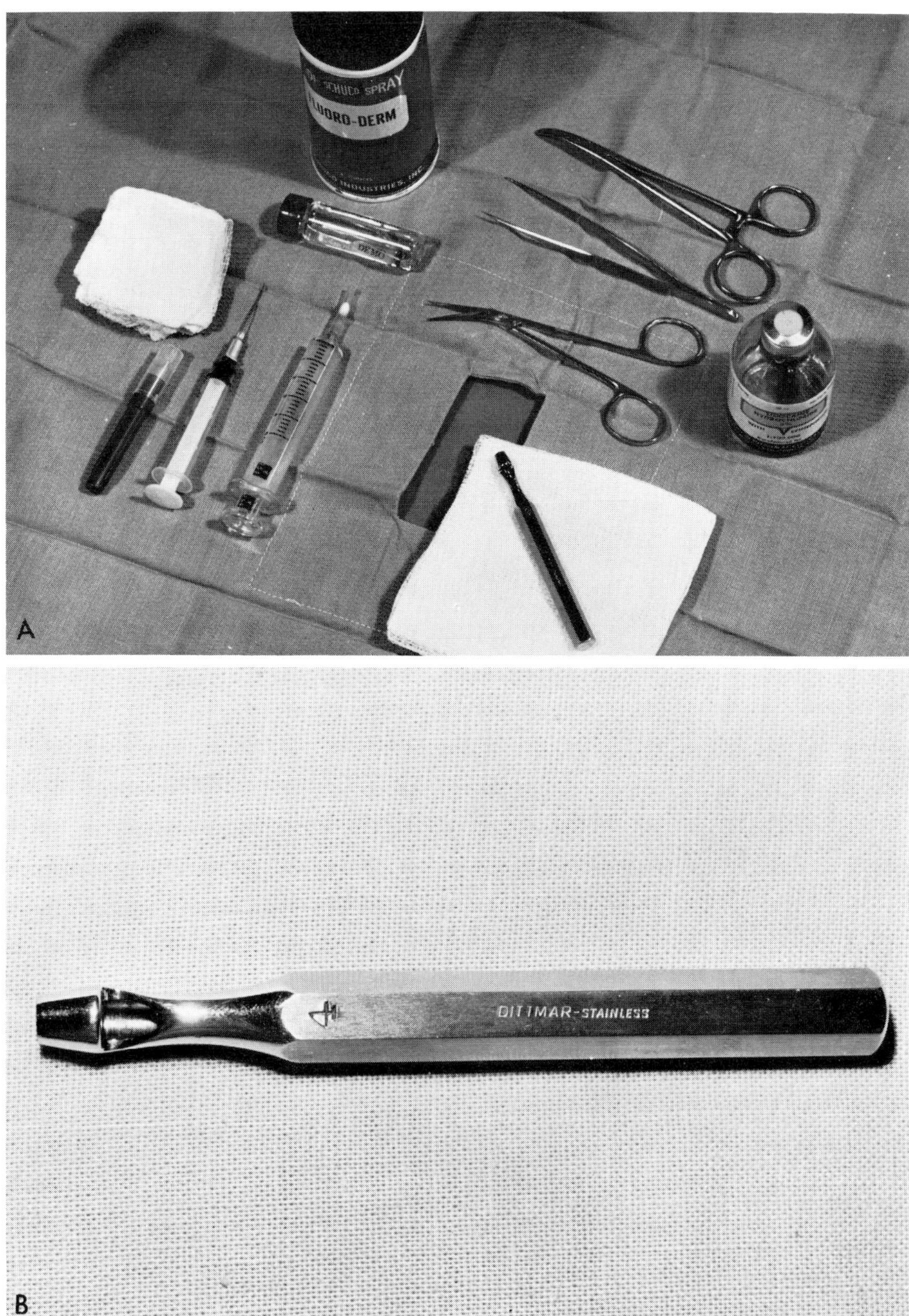


**Figure 7:8.** *A*, Equipment needed for skin biopsy procedure. Keyes 4 mm. cutaneous punch is in the foreground. *B*, Keyes 4 mm. cutaneous punch.

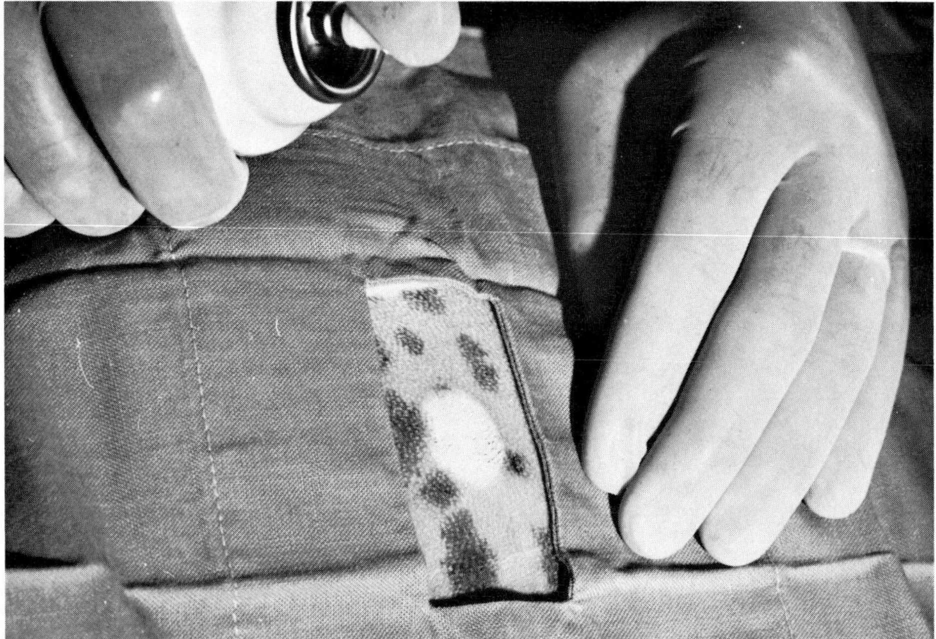

**Figure 7:9.** Spraying Freon on the skin.

sponged with 70 per cent alcohol. Trauma from a thorough surgical preparation may alter the appearance of the specimen, and should be avoided. A small bleb of 0.5 per cent lidocaine is injected subcutaneously for local anesthesia. This drug takes effect almost immediately. In order to make the skin firm so a sharp punch will remove a neat block of tissue, the skin is sprayed with a fine mist of ethyl chloride or Freon (Fig. 7:9). Gentle blowing or fanning of the skin will hasten the freezing process. When the skin is deep white with frost the Keyes biopsy punch is firmly pressed onto the skin and twisted rapidly back and forth until it has penetrated into the subcutaneous tissue (Fig. 7:10). The tissue plug is lifted from the crater with the thumb forceps (Fig. 7:11), the underlying tissue is severed with the scissors and the specimen placed on a piece of paper and smoothed out so it will not roll up. After about one minute it is placed in the jar of formalin fixative with the paper attached to it. Light pressure over the biopsy site will arrest any slight hemorrhage; however, a single suture can be taken to close the incision (Fig. 7:12*A* and *B*). It may be desirable to biopsy several sites, or to repeat biopsies at stated intervals.

Biopsy material is essential for diagnosis of neoplastic processes. It is useful in the following non-neoplastic dermatoses: demodectic and sarcoptic mange, dermatomycosis, acral pruritic granuloma, seborrhea, hypothyroidism, calcinosis circumscripta and calcinosis cutis.

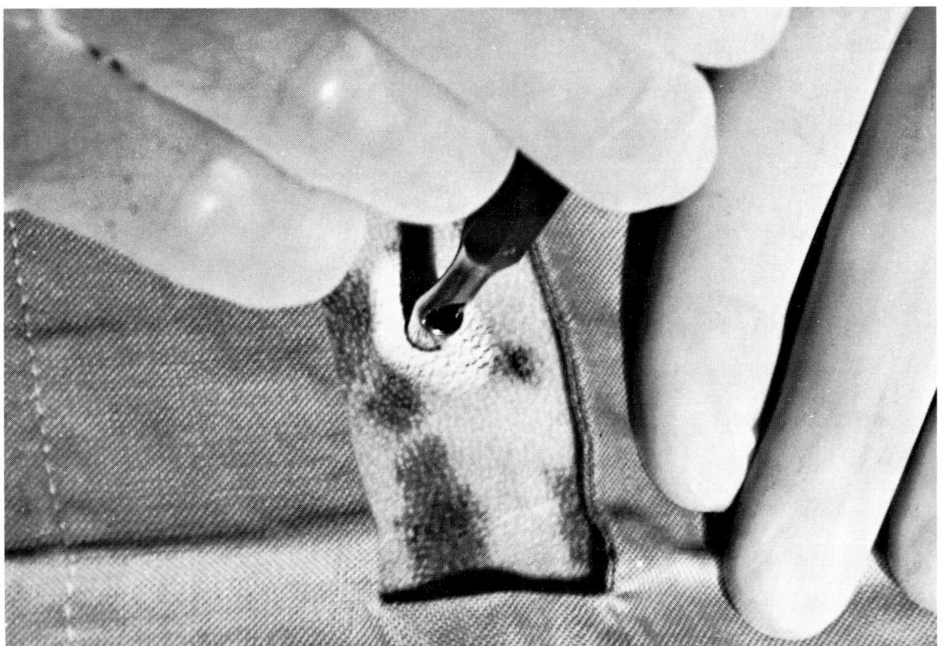

**Figure 7:10.** Rotation of the Keyes punch to obtain the biopsy specimen.

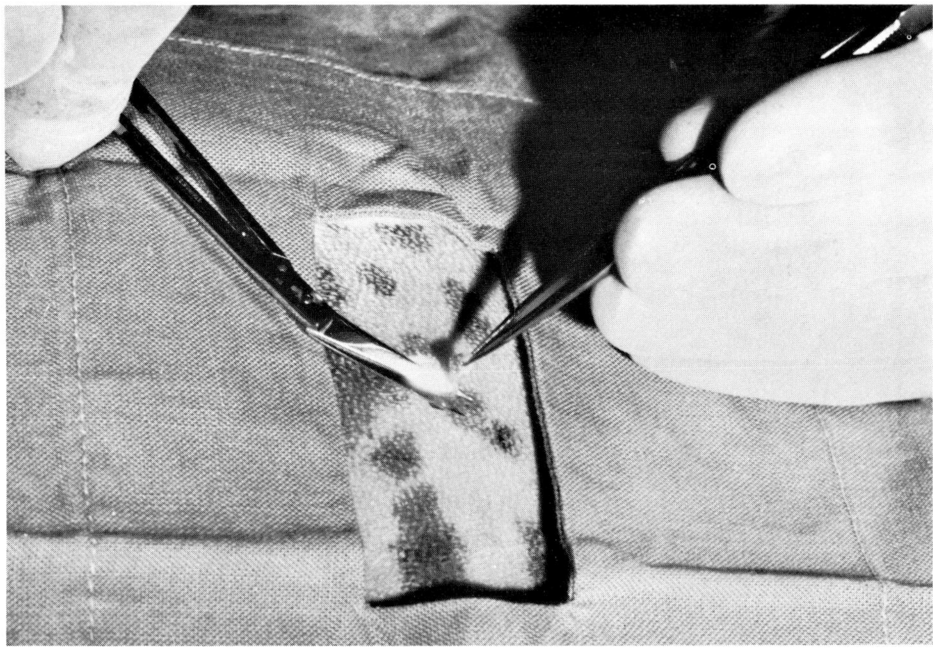

**Figure 7:11.** Removing the specimen with thumb forceps and scissors.

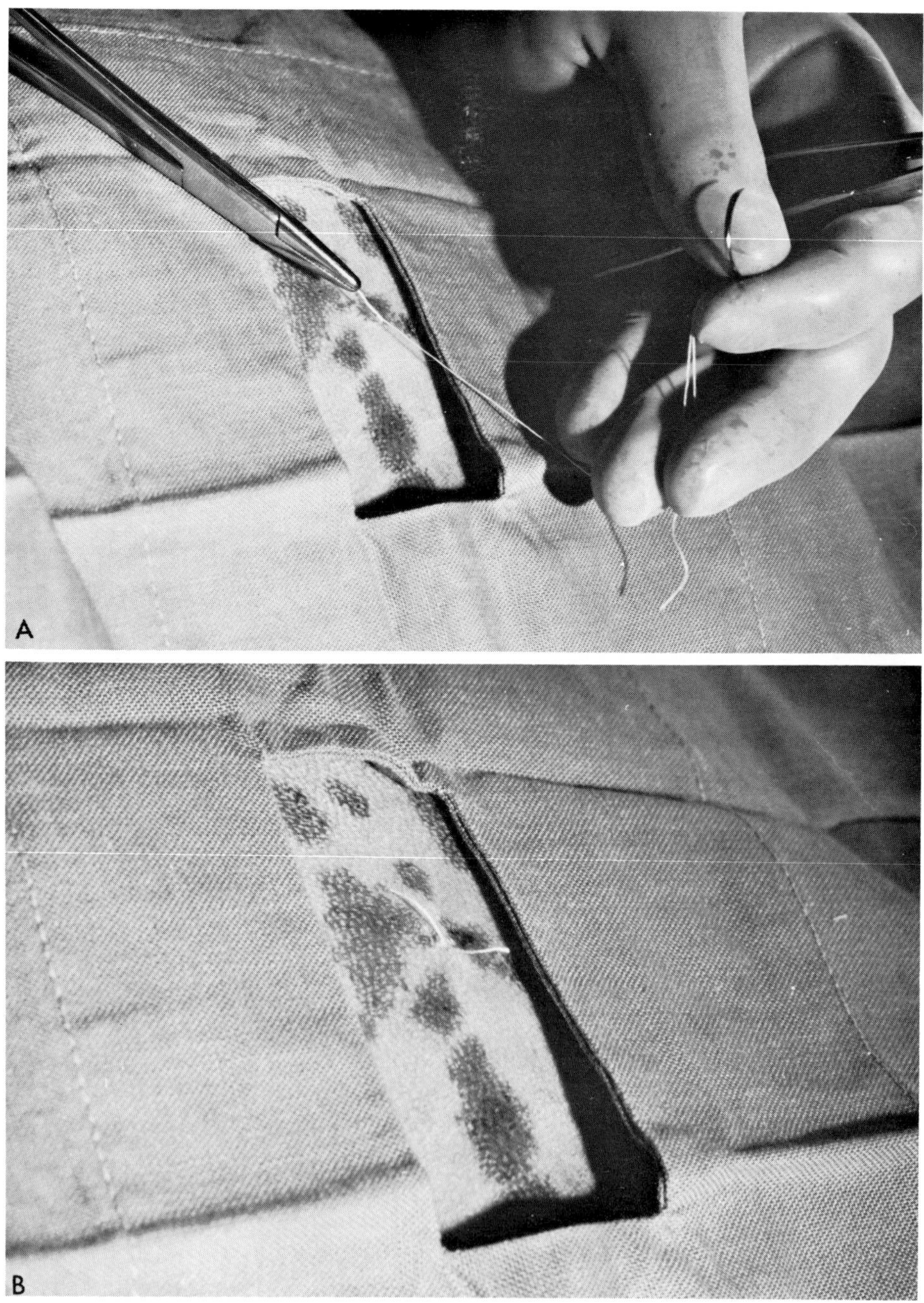

**Figure 7:12.** *A* and *B*, A single suture is optional in closing the wound.

## ALLERGY TESTING

There are three main methods of testing for cutaneous allergy: the patch test, the scratch test and the intradermal test. The patch test is not practical for dogs and cats at present since the patient may disturb the patch which holds the small amount of allergin in contact with the skin.

The scratch test is a simple, practical and safe method. It is made by scratching the skin with a needle and applying the test allergin to the excoriated area. A wheal and erythematous reaction at the site of the test denotes a positive test.

The intradermal test may be more accurate and has recently been made available in kits for the small animal clinician (see equipment list, p. 467). The rationale of this test kit seems reasonable but it has only started in field use and several years' trials will be necessary before final evaluation will be possible.

If the patient will not tolerate the procedure without sedation, a small amount of thiobarbiturate anesthesia may be used, and the test area on the lower abdomen or inguinal region is clipped carefully with a No. 40 blade. Each injection site should be premarked with a marking pen. A small amount of each allergin is injected intradermally to raise a small bleb. Several grouped allergins are used, each injected at a separate site. Prior to or during the test no corticosteroids, tranquilizers or antihistamine should be used. The test site is observed for a wheal or erythematous reaction at 2 minutes, 5 minutes, 10 minutes, 20 minutes, 40 minutes, one hour, 24 hours and 48 hours.

Proper utilization of this test is paramount to successful results. Careful selection of patients is essential and will affect the success or failure of its use. The test should be applied at the correct time in the fluctuating course of the disease and the results correlated with the case history.

# ETIOLOGIC FACTORS

*Section Three*

# EIGHT

## *General Discussion*

Section Three deals with the basic principles of the major causative factors of skin diseases. A knowledge of these principles is a prerequisite to the understanding of dermatology. In addition to six main causes, there are environmental factors and unknown factors to consider. Classification of skin diseases based on etiology is the best system for skin diseases of animals.

### CLASSIFICATION

In the past many attempts have been made to classify skin diseases, but none have been entirely satisfactory. Classification based on the morphology of lesions has been popular, grouping dermatoses into such categories as pustular eruptions, papular eruptions, alopecias and so on. Although the easy visualization of lesions may justify such a morphologic arrangement, many skin diseases can not be classified in that way. To fill this need, other classifications have been devised. The *anatomic* grouping allows discussion of such topics as diseases of the hair, diseases of the sebaceous glands and diseases of the nails. Along the same line, there have been discussions of skin diseases of the head, of the feet and of the abdomen. For certain purposes, the course has been used as a differentiating factor and the result has been grouping into chronic, acute and eczematous diseases. Unfortunately, this results in overlapping of entities and can lead to confusion. Another classification uses *functional disturbances,* stressing such factors as sebaceous secretion, sweating or altered sensory perception.

In human dermatology no classification so far devised has avoided criticism. In veterinary dermatology, devising a perfect classification is even more difficult because great gaps still exist in the knowledge of many dermatoses. The *etiologic* classification comes closest to perfection and will be used in this section. However, it is limited by the fact that the cause of many skin diseases is not clearly known.

#### Internal and External Factors

An interesting etiologic aspect of skin diseases can be pictured by grouping them arbitrarily into environmental factors that affect the skin from its

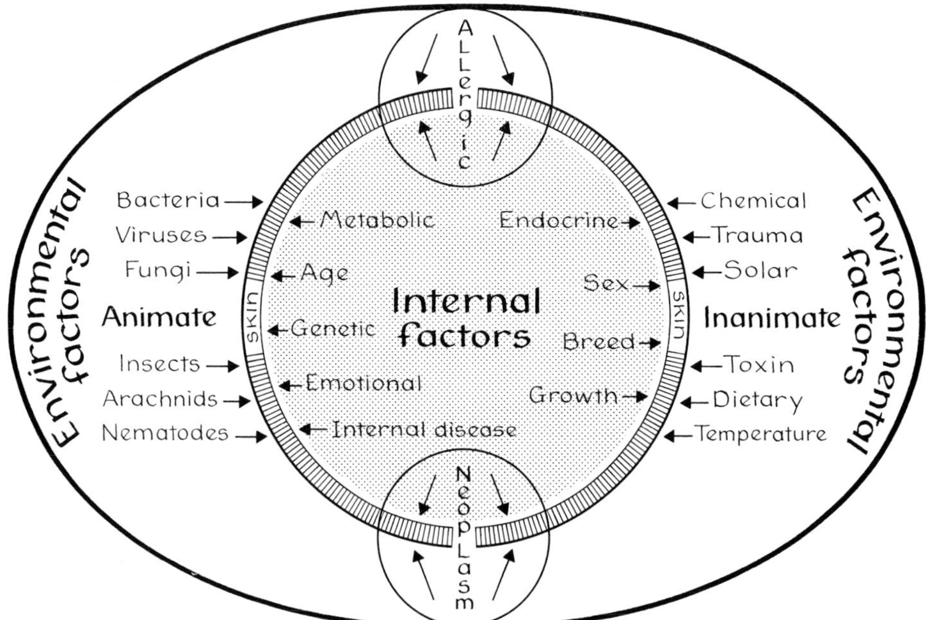


**Figure 8:1.** Etiology of skin diseases.

surface and internal factors that arise intrinsically. Figure 8:1 represents a simplified visualization of this idea. The clinician can coordinate information from the diagram with the bilateral symmetry of internally caused lesions and the asymmetry of externally caused lesions (Chapter Six). This should help him achieve greater accuracy in diagnosis.

Environmental factors are of two main types, animate and inanimate. The animate factors that plague the skin of animals are bacteria, viruses, fungi and ectoparasites. The inanimate factors are chemicals, solar radiation, trauma, toxins, heat, cold and diet.

Sometimes there is a simultaneous interaction of internal and external factors, such as in allergic or neoplastic disease. One example is atopic dermatitis, which requires an internal allergic predisposition and a corresponding external allergen (chemical). Another example is a carcinoma which may require an external factor such as solar radiation plus hypersensitivity to sunshine (feline solar dermatitis, p. 283, and nasal solar dermatitis, p. 305).

***ENVIRONMENTAL FACTORS***

The influence of environmental factors on the skin is less important in species that have dense hair coats to cover and protect the skin.

Exposure to sunlight causes many skin lesions in man. They occur on areas that are chronically irradiated. In dogs, a similar problem produces the photosensitization reactions of "collie nose" (p. 305). Chronic solar irritation of the ear tips can cause squamous cell carcinoma of white cats (p. 283).

Lack of hairy insulation of the ear tips may allow frostbite. This is common in cats and in small dogs exposed to the severe cold of northern climates. However, the heavy coat of many breeds also acts as insulation to protect the skin from burns caused by accidental contact with hot liquids, tar and caustic materials.

Primary irritants (chemicals, oil and fertilizers) and contact sensitizers (rhus, flea collars, leather, wool and fiber rugs) would be more common problems in animals if the pelage did not protect the skin from intimate contact. As it is, these substances often cause reactions on the glabrous areas of the flanks, the feet, and areas such as the rear of the legs, which frequently contact the ground. The reaction to local trauma is observed in the elbow callus of heavy breeds and in the so-called rodent ulcer of the feline lip.

Ringworm has a higher incidence in areas of the country like Florida where the climate and the presence of fungal elements in the soil and surroundings favor its growth. Conversely, the inhospitable environmental affects of high altitudes (above 5,000 feet) on the flea population is well known. Such areas cannot sustain flea colonies.

The skin is often injured by various plant particles, such as thorns, awns, foxtails, burrs and sharp seeds. When these particles penetrate the skin they set up a foreign body reaction. Foxtails have barbs that are pointed backward like small hooks and prevent "backing out." As a result the foxtail will travel under the skin and often produce troublesome fistulas. The feet of dogs are very likely to pick up such plant objects; however, they are also found in the ears, eyes, vulva, sheath and intertriginous areas.

Dogs occasionally ingest poisons such as thallium, which causes a typical dermatologic syndrome. However, they do not possess many of the foibles of their human companions, such as wearing cosmetics or exotic jewelry which may cause skin sensitivity. They have no occupational exposure to myriads of industrial allergens or irritants, and they do not experiment with exotic diet items. For all these reasons our animal pets are spared many of the environmental traumas which plague man.

### Unknown Factors

It is an unfortunate but realistic fact that the cause of many skin diseases is still unknown. Each year progress is made through research. When new entities are diagnosed, old and fallacious concepts are discarded. This is a sign of progress and hope for the future. In the meantime we must still diagnose and manage dermatoses of unknown etiology. Seborrhea is such a disease. Many theories exist about the cause of seborrhea but none have been proved. The very existence of the disease has been doubted by some. Paradoxically, the more causes postulated for a disease, the less is really known. Therfore, let us carefully learn what is known about etiologic factors today, and encourage research into the unknown causes of the other skin diseases.

# NINE

# *Cutaneous Bacteriology*

## NORMAL SKIN

In man a vast amount of research has been conducted to evaluate the normal skin flora, the host defense and other principles which have a bearing on the understanding of skin infections. In the dog and cat, there are almost no reports of investigations of bacteria on normal skin. Because the principles found in man may apply to dogs and cats, we will speculate here on the possible influence of these principles on skin health.

The skin provides a good culture medium for bacteria because it supplies water, carbohydrates, proteins, lipids, minerals and other nutrients. The normal flora of bacteria found on skin predominates because it is best adapted to that habitat. Organisms that do not persist are just not as well adapted and die out. It has been shown (Maibach, 1965) that the skin does not "kill" bacteria that are foreign or alien to it. Bacteria are found on the surface of the skin, in the superficial region of the horny layer, and abundantly in the outer area of the hair follicle to the depth of the sebaceous gland duct. Organisms occupy the hair follicle whether or not a hair is present. However, hair roots are sterile, and no bacteria can be cultured from apocrine or eccrine sweat gland secretions unless disease is present.

Bacteria cultured from the skin are classified as resident or transient, depending upon their ability to multiply in that habitat. The normal bacterial flora in human skin includes the following:

### Gram-Positive

1. Resident organisms (aerobic and anaerobic staphylococci, aerobic and anaerobic corynebacteria, and occasional hemolytic or nonhemolytic streptococci).
2. Transient organisms (sarcinae and aerobic spore-formers).

### Gram-Negative

1. Resident organisms (members of Mima-Herellea and aerobacter groups).

2. Transient organisms (*E. coli*, pseudomonas, proteus and alcaligenes). *Pityrosporon ovale* is a resident fungus.

Gram-negative organisms tend to flourish in moist, warm areas (i.e., axillae) and predominate when medications depress the gram-positive flora.

It is possible that some of the organisms listed may be present in the normal flora of dogs and cats, but documentation is lacking.

The numbers of resident bacteria on the skin tend to vary with individuals—some have many and others have few organisms. The number per individual may remain constant unless disturbed by antibacterial treatment or changes in climate. Moist, intertriginous areas tend to have large numbers, and individuals with oily skin have higher counts too. More bacteria are found on the skin in warm, wet weather than in cold, dry weather.

## Sterilization of the Skin

Total sterilization is a practical impossibility in spite of the superficial location of most bacteria. A two-minute scrub with soap and water followed by a two-minute soaking in 70 per cent alcohol usually is adequate for practical purposes. The resident organisms are soon back to their original levels, however, Maibach reports that 99.9 per cent of bacteria are removed by repeated application of a hexachlorophene cream (pHisoHex) followed by a final rinse of 0.5 per cent chlorhexidine in alcohol. In any method, the most important principle is mechanical removal with vigorous brushing.

The healthy, intact integument is remarkably resistant to bacterial infection even though potentially pathogenic bacteria continually threaten its integrity. Some of these defensive mechanisms are:

### DESICCATION

Organisms which fall on the dry, horny layer of the skin may be destroyed in the same way as those on a dry table top. Gram-negative organisms are especially sensitive to drying.

### MECHANICAL PROCESSES

The process of keratin exfoliation carries organisms away, and the dry keratin is a potent barrier to the penetration of bacteria. Washing and frictional rubbing remove huge numbers of bacteria.

### SURFACE FILMS

A number of fatty acids form a bacteriostatic or fungistatic film on the skin surface. The effect varies, however, as some organisms require fatty acids for growth and others are adversely affected by these lipid films. Beta-hemolytic streptococci may be destroyed by fatty acids on the skin surface, staphylococci are affected less, and gram-negative organisms may be quite resistant.

#### pH OF THE SKIN

Although human skin normally is more acid than dog skin, endocrine and infectious disease processes may alter the normal pH enough to markedly change the skin as a favorable habitat for some organisms.

#### ANTAGONISM OF ORGANISMS

One group of organisms may exert an inhibitory effect on others by elaborating antibiotic substances, competing for nutrients, changing the pH, or by the production of detrimental enzymes.

#### HOST DEFENSE

Leukocytes in the epidermis and macrophages and protein antibodies in the dermis may be a final and potent bulwark to the defense against invasion by microorganisms.

## SKIN INFECTIONS

The normal skin puts up a remarkable defense against pathogenic organisms, but damaged skin provides a much more favorable environment for their growth.

It can be accepted as a general rule that if skin infections are to be established some predisposition is necessary. The predisposing factors are almost always local, as constitutional influences such as anemia, malnutrition and so on are rarely important. The local factors are many, and include friction and trauma, excessive moisture (endogenous or exogenous), accumulated dirt and matted hair, chemical irritants, freezing and burns, irradiation and seborrhea. Bacterial infections may complicate dermatomycosis and insect and parasite infestations. In some instances the bacterial infection is of major importance and is the primary problem. In others, it is incidental. Thus skin infections may be classed as primary or secondary.

### Primary Infections

These occur in otherwise healthy skin, one species of organism is isolated, a characteristic disease pattern is evident, and the infection is cured by appropriate chemotherapeutic or antibacterial medication.

### Secondary Infections

These occur in diseased skin, more than one microorganism may be isolated, a less characteristic disease pattern is present, therapeutic agents are less effective, and treatment of the primary (or underlying) disease is vital to success.

The majority of nonspecific bacterial infections are caused by the pyogenic organisms, staphylococci and streptococci. These bacteria may be primarily invasive, and *S. aureus* infections are found more frequently. Other organisms may be prevalent in cultures from skin infections but they often are present as opportunists or secondary invaders. This may be the case with organisms such as *E. coli*, *P. aeruginosa* and *P. mirabilis*. Isolates of *S. faecalis*, *B. subtilis*, corynebacterium sp., nonhemolytic streptococci and diphtheroid organisms may be of even less significance.

It is important when dealing with skin infections to know what organisms are involved and to which antibiotics they are sensitive. The section on laboratory diagnosis details methods to use. We will discuss here the morphology and the cultural characteristics of the common skin pathogens.

## Staphylococci

*Staphylococcus albus* is rarely virulent, so *Staphylococcus aureus* is the major concern. Young cultures are always gram-positive and the organism is a uniform spherical coccus (0.8 micron) which is nonmotile and does not form spores. In pus the micrococci clump in irregular masses like a bunch of grapes. Colonies growing on solid blood agar media are porcelain white to yellowish orange in color (Fig. 44:1*A*). The darker colonies are thought to be more active biochemically and are usually more virulent. Some strains are strongly hemolytic; others are not.

Staphylococci are among the most resistant of the non-spore-forming organisms. They resist dehydration, are relatively heat-resistant and tolerate antiseptic medications better than the vegetative forms of most bacteria. Many strains produce one or several toxins. These may cause tissue necrosis at the point of infection, or on ingestion may cause "food poisoning."

Repeated injections of heat-killed staphylococci will protect rabbits against otherwise fatal doses of *S. aureus*. Bacterins, especially first-isolate, autogenous bacterins, are of real value in combating chronic infections in dogs and cats.

Chemotherapeutically, the staphylococci often present a dilemma, since they tend to become resistant to many antibiotics, especially penicillin. Sulfonamides usually are ineffective. Penicillin is the first choice if the organism is sensitive. With resistant strains methicillin, oxacillin, nafcillin, novobiocin, or lincomycin may be useful. Chloramphenicol or tetracycline will inhibit growth of some strains. The staphylococci are a group of organisms in which antibiotic sensitivity tests are essential to properly guide therapy.

## Streptococci

These cocci characteristically develop into chains of cells which are often quite pleomorphic and may be mistaken for short rods. In young cultures they are almost always gram-positive, non-spore-forming and nonmotile. Streptococci do not produce lush growth on culture media since they have delicate nutrient requirements. On blood agar they produce small (1 mm.) translucent colonies that are smooth, glistening and perfectly circular (Fig. 44:1*B*). With heavy inoculations the confluent growth is nearly transparent. Many strains are hemolytic; others are not. Although most streptococci are aerobic a few grow only under anaerobic conditions—a fact that the clinician should keep in mind before deciding that his culture is negative.

Streptococci exist primarily as animal parasites, they are found on mucous membranes and skin, and in milk of many species. Some strains are highly virulent and produce suppurative processes in their hosts, but others are relatively harmless organisms which assume a pathogenic role only when the host's resistance is markedly reduced. Most streptococci are easily killed by heat, drying or mildly antiseptic chemicals. This group of bacteria is divided into three groups *alpha* (viridans), *beta* (hemolytic) and *gamma* (anhemolytic). The beta group is further divided into the Lancefield serological types (A through P). Type A organisms are found only in man, and although types C and G have been reported in small animals, types L and M appear to be especially pathogenic to the dog.

Except for infections of *S. equi* in horses, one attack of a streptococcal infection does not cause immunity, so bacterins are generally of little use. Streptococcal infections are usually easily handled by chemotherapy. Penicillin is the drug of choice, but the sulfonamides are also effective. Other antibiotics such as bacitracin, erythromycin and tetracycline may be effective too.

## Pseudomonas Aeruginosa

This is seen as a secondary invader in skin infections. It is a highly motile, gram-negative rod. It grows well on simple media and the colonies are smooth, shiny, moist and spreading (Fig. 44:1*D*). An opalescent sheen appears on the surface of colonies, but this may be masked by the bright green pigment produced. There are really two water-soluble pigments, yellow green fluorescein and bluish green pyocyanin. This colony pigmentation and the characteristic, sweet odor reminiscent of beeswax are important aids to recognition of the organism.

*Pseudomonas aeruginosa* is prevalent in nature but has been isolated from ear and eye infections, from bladder and skin infections, and it is a major problem in severe burns. Most antibiotics are ineffective against this bacillus. It appears that gentamicin may be the first choice, with polymyxin B and neomycin as possible alternatives. Since it does not grow well at low pH, the use of 1 per cent acetic acid topically may be useful in the treatment of otitis externa caused by this organism.

## Escherichia Coli

This is a normal inhabitant of the lower bowel of all warm-blooded animals. It is a small rod-shaped gram-negative organism that may be motile. Spores are never formed. *E. coli* grows readily on all media as an aerobe or facultative anaerobe. The colonies are slightly raised, smooth, glistening, unpigmented and circular in outline. On EMB agar they have a green metallic sheen (Fig. 44:1*E*). Some strains are strongly hemolytic.

This enteric organism is fairly resistant to drying and antiseptic chemicals, and some strains are heat-resistant too. It is rarely highly pathogenic, being more of an opportunist. The most effective antibiotic must be determined by sensitivity testing of the specific strain but streptomycin (or dihydrostreptomycin), neomycin or chloramphenicol often work well. Injudicious use of antibiotics in primary skin infections caused by other organisms may have a profound effect on the emergence of resistant strains *E. coli* (or similar organisms).

## Proteus Mirabilis

This is another enteric organism that is widely distributed in nature. Under certain conditions it may become pathogenic, especially in infections involving the bladder, ear or skin. It is a motile, non-spore-forming, gram-negative rod which is highly pleomorphic. Its growth on solid media is profuse as it tends to swarm over the surface of the agar (Fig. 44:1*C*). The colonies are thin, transparent and confluent and, because the organism produces ammonia from urea, a typical ammoniacal odor may be associated with its growth.

Most of the basic information given in this chapter can be usefully applied to the superficial and deep pyodermas, which are covered separately in Chapter Forty-four (p. 321).

## *References*

*Bruner, D. W., and Gillespie, J. H.: *Hagan's Infectious Diseases of Domestic Animals.* Comstock Publishing Assoc., Ithaca, N.Y., 1966.
Coles, E. H.: *Veterinary Clinical Pathology.* W. B. Saunders Co., Philadelphia, 1967.
Jubb, K. V. F., and Kennedy, P. C.: *Pathology of Domestic Animals.* Academic Press, New York, 1963.
Lewis, G. M., and Wheeler, C. E.: *Practical Dermatology.* W. B. Saunders Co., Philadelphia, 1967.
*Maibach, H. I., and Hildick-Smith, G.: *Skin Bacteria and Their Role in Infection.* McGraw-Hill, New York, 1965.
Stewart, W. D., Danto, J. L., and Maddin, S.: *Synopsis of Dermatology.* C. V. Mosby Co., St. Louis, 1966.

*Suggested supplemental reading.

# TEN

# *Cutaneous Mycology*

Saprophytic fungi are omnipresent in our environment. Of the thousands of species, only a handful have acquired pathogenicity for animals. Fungi, however, are not nearly as common a cause of skin disease as supposed, and many nonspecific, pruritic dermatoses are diagnosed as dermatomycosis on inadequate evidence. Some clinicians use "grass fungus" as a catch-all term for these problems when in fact allergic contact dermatitis or factors other than fungi are involved.

Many dermatoses are erroneously called "fungus infections."

The host-parasite relationship in dermatomycosis is unusual. The fungi are efficient parasites which live on, not in the skin. Their growth takes place only in dead, keratinized structures and they avoid living tissue completely (Fig. 10:1).

Dermatomycosis can be transmitted from animals to man, from animals to other animals, and from man to animals. Zoophilic fungi prefer animals as hosts and often cause acute inflammatory reactions when they invade man. This inflammation is unfavorable to the invading fungus, thereby limiting the progress of the infection. Zoophilic fungus infections rarely cause an inflammatory reaction in animals, so that much of the time the dermatophyte is able to exist in a symbiotic relationship with its host.

Fungi are plants, and are typically parasites of plants, or saprophytes of plant products. Some fungi are also pathogenic for animals and man, although bacterial diseases usually capture a larger share of the clinician's attention.

## GENERAL CHARACTERISTICS OF FUNGI

Fungi, like bacteria, are heterotrophic organisms which have a nutritional requirement for some form of organic carbon. They are unable to utilize sunlight for energy and they thrive best in darkness. Some fungi are unicellular (yeasts), while others are multicellular. Some are dimorphic; that is, they grow as unicellular individuals under some circumstances and as multicellular organisms

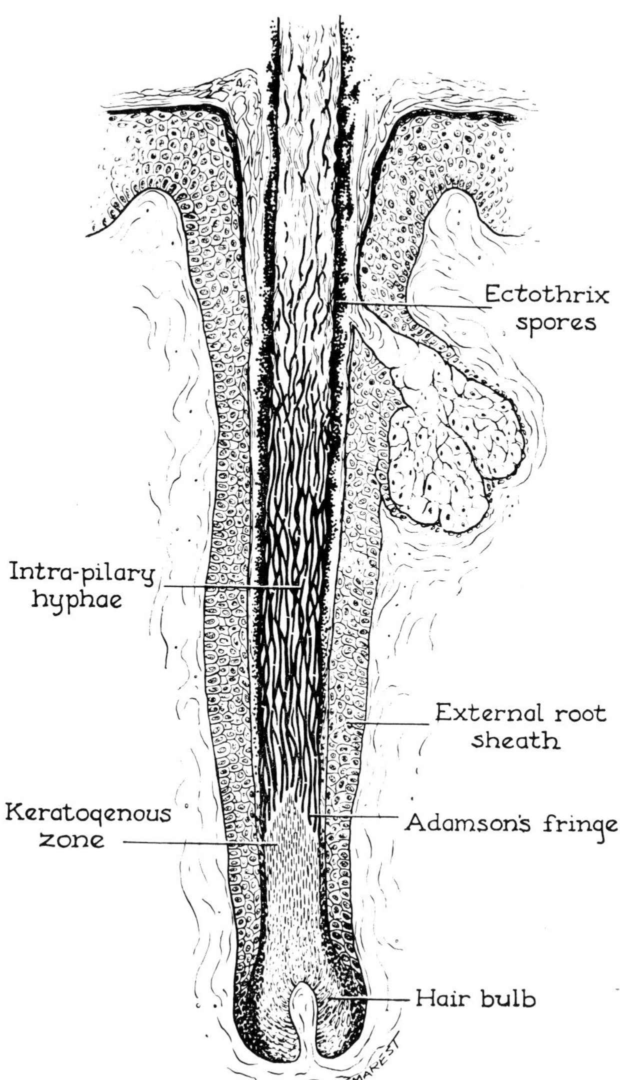


**Figure 10:1.** Diagrammatic representation of an infected hair illustrating the main features of the host-parasite relationship characteristic of dermatomycoses. The fungal filaments do not extend into the bulb of the hair but terminate abruptly in contact with hair matrix cells which still retain their nuclei. Only the *fully* keratinized portion of the hair shaft is invaded. (From Pillsbury, Shelley and Kligman: *Dermatology*. W. B. Saunders Co., Philadelphia, 1956.)

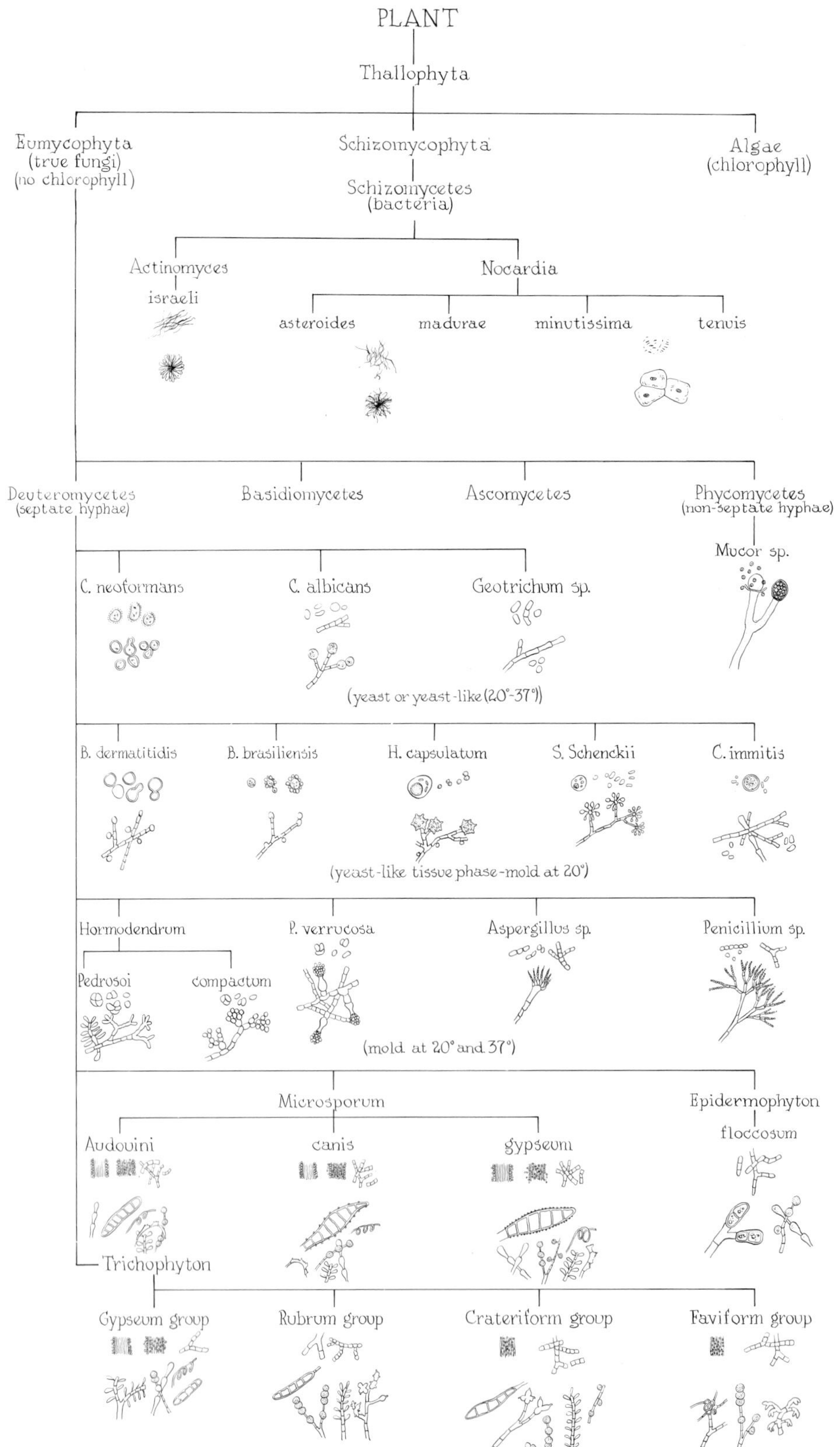


**Figure 10:2.** Classification—*Thallophyta.* (From Moss and McQuown: *Atlas of Medical Mycology.* 2nd Ed. Williams & Wilkins, Baltimore, 1969.)

under others. With some parasitic fungi the unicellular stage occurs in tissues and the multicellular stage occurs in cultures. Most pathogenic fungi are multicellular.

Multicellular fungi are made up of individual cells placed end to end to form filaments known as hyphae. The tangled mass of hyphae forming a single colony is known as the mycelium. Although the mycelial filaments of some molds are not divided by septa or cross walls but consist of single multinucleated cells, a greater number of species have septate hyphae. The species with septate hyphae (Fig. 10:2) belong to the classes Basidiomycetes, the Ascomycetes or Fungi Imperfecti. Basidiomycetes consist of mushrooms and bracket fungi. The Ascomycetes possess membranous sacs called asci (sing. ascus) which contain sexual spores, generally eight in number, called ascospores. The Fungi Imperfecti are forms for which no sexual spores have been observed, and the term imperfect refers to our knowledge of the organism, not to the fungus itself. As sexual phases for members of this group are found they are reclassified and transferred to the proper group.

The unit of fungus reproduction is the spore which may be formed by sexual fusion of nuclei – a "perfect" spore. Details of sexual spore formation are important in classification of fungi. Some fungi may develop asexual or "imperfect" spores, and some may produce alternation of perfect and imperfect states.

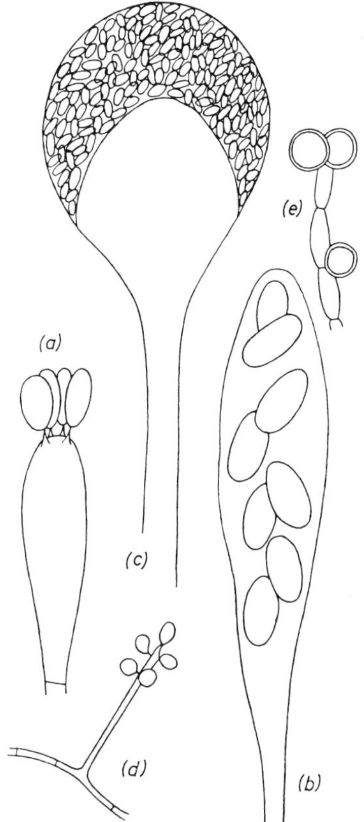


**Figure 10:3.** *a*, Basidium with four exogenous basidiospores. *b*, Ascus with eight endogenous ascospores. *c*, Sporangium of *Absidia ramosa* showing sporangiospores surrounding a central sterile columella. *d*, Conidia of *Sporotrichum schenkii* in culture. *e*, Pseudomycelium of *Candida albicans* bearing three chlamydospores. (All approximately × 500.) (From Stableforth and Galloway: *Infectious Diseases of Animals*. [Butterworth] Plenum, N.Y., 1959.)

There are four types of sexual spores, oospores, basidiospores, zygospores, and ascospores. However, since asexual spores are much more readily formed, more numerous and more conspicuous, they are more important in identifying most pathogenic fungi.

The simplest asexual spore is the arthrospore, which is a special portion of hypha that breaks off and is capable of reproducing the species. In many species of fungi, special spore-bearing hyphae develop which form spores by a process known as abjointing, i.e., by pinching and breaking off special elements. In some fungi, special cells appear at the end of a hypha which balloon into a sac-like structure in which spores are formed. This is called a sporangium. In other forms the spores are formed exogenously at the tip of special hyphae. This structure is called a conidiophore, and the spores are conidia. There are two types of conidia, multicelled macroconidia and small microconidia.

The number of cells, the characteristics of the cell wall of macroconidia, and the shape of the macroconidia are helpful in identification of species.

Chlamydospore is a general name used for thick-walled structures which are formed in the thallus and which apparently are resting forms, closely analogous in function to the spores of bacteria (Fig. 10:3).

## CHARACTERIZATION OF PATHOGENIC FUNGI

Fungi pathogenic to plants are distributed throughout all classes of the fungi, but those pathogenic for animals are found primarily in the Fungi Imperfecti and the Ascomycetes. Some plant pathogens are obligate parasites, while animal pathogens can usually be grown as saprophytes in vitro. Most fungi have less restrictive nutritive requirements than bacteria. They will grow on diverse media, over wide ranges of temperature and pH, and they are characteristically strongly aerobic. Pathogenic or saprophytic fungi may grow as mycelial or as yeast-like structures. Ringworm fungi are mycelial in culture and in the skin. *Cryptococcus neoformans*, a yeast, has budding cells both in culture and in animal tissue. *Histoplasma capsulatum*, on the other hand, grows as a mycelial fungus with large tuberculate chlamydospores on media, but as a small-celled yeast in vivo. This dimorphism is not uncommon with fungi pathogenic for animals and may be a function of environmental variation. In cultures it is often possible to affect the mycelium-yeast transformation by manipulation of the environment, and the unicellular state may be a result of growth under unfavorable conditions. A third type of growth in living tissues is the development of mycelial fungi as small grains or granules, similar to those of actinomycosis and maduromycosis, which are known as mycetomas. Here again the growth form of the pathogen probably results from an interaction between the host tissues and the fungus.

## CULTURE AND EXAMINATION OF FUNGI*

For proper identification of fungi it is mandatory that cultures be grown.

These ordinarily are made on Sabouraud's dextrose agar, but certain strains develop special cultural characteristics on special media such as polished rice grain, potato dextrose agar and corn meal agar. These cultures may be placed in the dark at a temperature of 25° to 30° C. for good growth, and the lower temperature allows fungi to develop while bacterial growth is suppressed. Many commercial agar preparations contain antibiotics such as streptomycin or chloramphenicol to inhibit bacterial growth. In addition cycloheximide is added for its inhibitory effect on many saprophytic molds. After one to three weeks the growth may be sufficient to make a tentative diagnosis on macroscopic appearance. Microscopic examination is usually necessary, however, to identify typical macroconidia. Preparations for this purpose are easily made with pressure-sensitive tape from stationery stores. No. 800 acetate-backed tape (Minnesota Mining and Mfg. Co.) preserves the preparation longer, but other tapes are adequate for most purposes. To make the preparation, a "flag of tape" ½″ × ½″ is fastened to the end of a wooden applicator stick (Fig. 10:4*A*) or grasped in forceps, and the sticky surface of the flag is touched to the surface of the colony just proximal to the advancing periphery. The tape is then pressed, sticky side down, on a slide with a drop of lactophenol cotton blue stain (Fig. 10:4*B*) and examined under the microscope. The tape selectively removes branches of hyphae-bearing conidia and avoids the taxonomically valueless vegetative mycelium.

Growth characteristics and the detailed structure of many fungi can be observed well in a "hanging drop" preparation or by making "block cultures." The latter are made by cutting 5 × 5 mm. blocks of agar from a 2 mm. deep layer in a Petri dish, transferring the block to a sterile microscope slide where it is inoculated, usually on two opposite sides, with a small amount of inoculum, covered with a sterile coverslip and incubated in a moist chamber. A moist chamber can be made by resting the slide on glass rods placed in the bottom of a covered Petri dish containing water (Fig. 10:5). When appropriate growth has taken place the coverslip with adhering mycelium may be removed and placed on a drop of lactophenol cotton blue stain on another slide. They are then ready for microscopic inspection.

Fungi in tissues are often satisfactorily stained by the usual hematoxylin-eosin method (H & E), but the periodic acid-Schiff stain (PAS) is superior. With this preparation the hyphae stain bright red and are recognized easily.

Examination of hairs and scales taken from skin scrapings and prepared with KOH offer an opportunity to obtain further information.

---

*See also Chapter Seven, Laboratory Procedures.

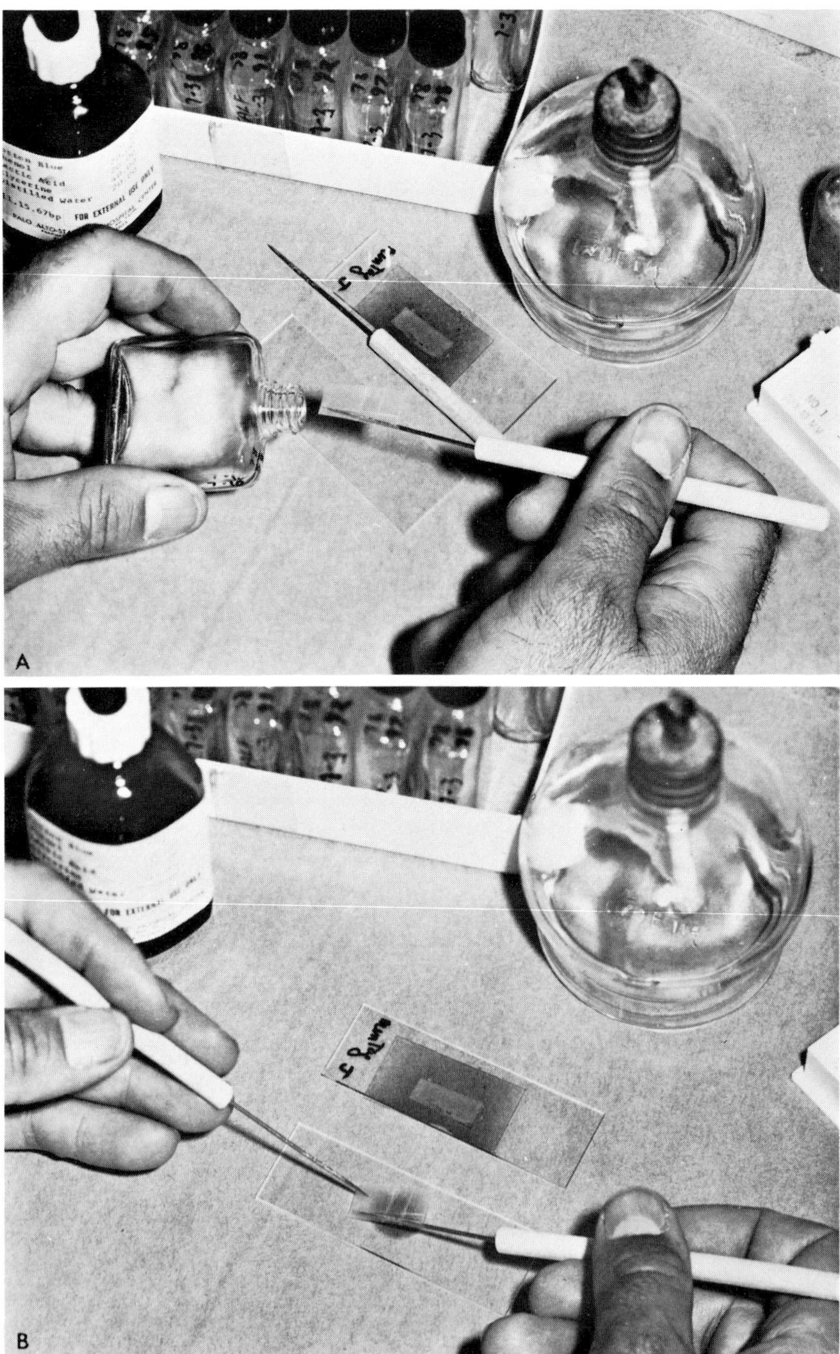


**Figure 10:4.** *A*, Inserting acetate tape "flag" into fungus culture bottle to pick up conidia. *B*, Tape is pressed down on a drop of lactophenol cotton blue stain. A coverslip is added and the preparation is ready for microscopic examination. Note completed slide preparation in the background.

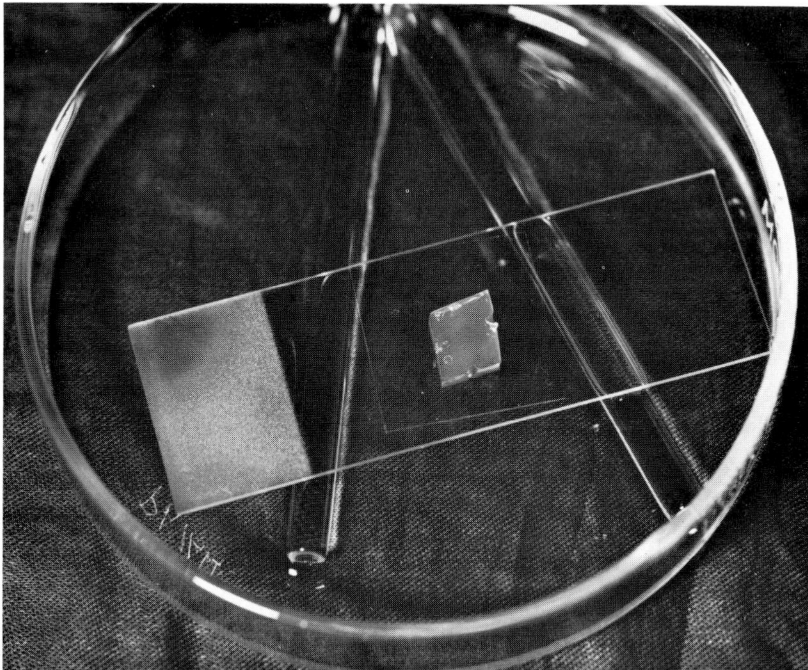

**Figure 10:5.** Moist chamber (Petri dish) for preparation of slide cultures. A small block of Sabouraud's agar is placed on a sterile slide and covered with a coverslip. Note indented edges of agar where inoculation took place.

In skin scales, the branched septate hyphae of one dermatophyte are very like those of another, and isolation and culture is necessary for certain identification. However, the arrangement of spores in or on the hair is of interest. In hair the downward growth of the fungus keeps pace with the growth of the hair, and never advances into the mitotically active area in the bulb (Fig. 10:1). The mycelium in the older portions of the hair may break up into a large number of spores. The way in which these arthrospores affect the hair is typical of certain fungi. This is less important in veterinary medicine, as most animal dermatophytes are of the ectothrix classification.

Ectothrix dermatophytes have arthrospores arranged on the outside of the hair shaft. Small spores (2 to 3 microns) not clearly visible by low power objective are arranged in masses or in a mosaic pattern. These hairs may fluoresce and are typical of *Microsporum canis*, *M. audouini* and *M. distortum*. Large spores (5 to 8 microns) in sparse chains outside the hair and visible with low power are usually not fluorescent. They are seen in *M. gypseum* and *M. vanbreuseghemi*. Intermediate spores (3 to 7 microns) in dense chains that do not cause fluorescence are seen with *Trichophyton mentagrophytes*, *T. verrucosum*, *T. rubrum*, *T. equinum* and *T. gallinae*.

Endothrix spores (5 to 8 microns) are found inside the hair shaft and cause the hair to break off or curl. They may be found in *T. rubrum*, which has been reported in dogs, but generally are typical of *T. tonsurans* and other infections more common in man.

## MYCOTIC DISEASES OF THE SKIN

Fungal diseases of the skin can be classified as deep and superficial mycoses. Most of the deep mycoses are infections of other systems with secondary cutaneous lesions. They include maduromycosis, histoplasmosis, blastomycosis and others and will only be mentioned here. The superficial mycoses produce diseases localized to the cornified parts of the skin, known as dermatomycoses.

### Dermatomycoses (Superficial Mycotic Infections)

The terminology used to classify dermatophytes is exceedingly complex because of the large number of synonyms. Dermatophytes can be categorized (Kaplan, in Marples) as zoophilic, those whose normal host is mammals other than man; anthropophilic, those whose normal host is man; and geophilic, those whose normal habitat is soil. Of the dermatophytes affecting animals almost all are of the genus Microsporum or Trichophyton. Three fungi cause 99 per cent of all clinical cases of ringworm in dogs and cats in the U.S.A. These are *M. canis*, *M. gypseum* and *T. mentagrophytes* (var. *granulare*). In cats, 98 per cent of cases are caused by *M. canis*, with 1 per cent due to *M. gypseum* and 1 per cent to *T. mentagrophytes*. In dogs, 70 per cent of cases are due to *M. canis*, 20 per cent to *M. gypseum*, and 10 per cent to *T. mentagrophytes*. Jackson (1968) reports a much higher incidence of *T. mentagrophytes* in the Florida area. Seven other dermatophytes are seen rarely in small animal practice and are shown in Table 10:1. This text will discuss identification details for the three major dermatophytes. For identification of other fungi the reader is referred to standard texts on mycology.

#### *MICROSPORUM CANIS*

This zoophilic fungus is by far the most common dermatophyte of dogs and cats. It also commonly produces disease in man, in whom it causes a more severe inflammatory reaction than anthropophilic species. *M. canis* is world-

TABLE 10:1. Dermatophytes in Small Animal Practice (Modified from Rebell et al.)

| *Dermatophyte* | *Dog* | *Cat* | *Monkey* | *Rabbit-Squirrel* |
|---|---|---|---|---|
| *M. canis* | usual | usual | frequent | occasional |
| *M. distortum* | reported | – | reported | – |
| *M. audouinii* | reported | – | reported | – |
| *M. gypseum* | frequent | occasional | reported | frequent |
| *M. vanbreuseghemi* | reported | – | – | reported |
| *K. ajelloi* | questionable | – | – | – |
| *T. mentagrophytes* | occasional | occasional | frequent | usual |
| *T. equinum* | reported | – | – | – |
| *T. verrucosum* | reported | – | – | – |
| *T. gallinae* | reported | – | – | – |
| *T. rubrum* | – | – | – | – |

There are reports of *T. schoenleini* infections in animals and birds in areas where this fungus is common.

wide in distribution. It is endemic in catteries, where all the young may be affected clinically. Adult cats may be asymptomatic carriers. Spores are small and present in masses on the hair shaft. The affected hairs frequently, but not always, fluoresce to a bright yellow-green because of a metabolite produced by the fungus.

**Colony Morphology.** The colony on Sabouraud's dextrose agar develops fairly rapidly, forming a white cottony or woolly, aerial mycelium. With age it becomes powdery with a central depressed area and sometimes shows radial folds (Fig. 25:1*A*). The pigment on the undersurface is yellowish orange, later changing to reddish brown. On potato dextrose agar the pigment is lemon yellow and is easily seen because of the sparse development of aerial hyphae. There are no special nutritional requirements, but unlike *M. audouini, M. canis* grows profusely on polished rice.

**Microscopic Morphology.** Macroconidia are usually produced in fair numbers and are characteristic (Fig. 10:6*A*). They are long, spindle-shaped and thick-walled with an asymmetric knob. The rough surface is particularly evident at the knob, and each macroconidium is composed of more than six compartments. Numerous clavate or elongated microconidia may be seen but are not diagnostic. Racquet hyphae and chlamydospores are present occasionally.

**Diagnostic Criteria.** The characteristic macroconidia and the yellow-orange pigment on the underside of the colony are definitive features.

### *MICROSPORUM GYPSEUM*

*Microsporum gypseum* is a soil-inhabiting fungus which occasionally infects man and animals. It is world-wide in distribution. Sporulation on the hair shaft is mainly ectothrix, but the spores are sparse and in chains. Fluorescence is rare but if present is very dull. In animals, thick, well-circumscribed, tightly adherent gray crusts are typical in clinical lesions. Chronic cases in the dog respond to treatment slowly.

**Colony Morphology.** The colony is rapid-growing with a surface texture like chamois because of the multitudes of macroconidia. The surface is rich cinnamon-buff in color centrally but terminates in a border of downy, white mycelium (Fig. 25:1*B*). The pigment on the undersurface is cream to tan in color. There are no special nutritional requirements.

**Microscopic Morphology.** Macroconidia are present in enormous numbers. They are large, thin-walled, ellipsoidal structures the shape of cucumber pickles (Fig. 10:6*B*). The surface is rough and up to six compartments may be present. Clavate microconidia may be seen but are not diagnostic.

**Diagnostic Criteria.** The characteristic macroconidia and colony morphology are definitive features.

### *TRICHOPHYTON MENTAGROPHYTES*

This dermatophyte has many variants. Its zoophilic form (var. *granulare*) is highly infectious and may transfer to man where it causes an inflammatory form of ringworm. It is more common in laboratory animals and horses than in dogs and cats. In the generalized form in the dog and cat it presents dry, scaly, diffuse lesions which are exceedingly resistant to treatment. It may also cause localized infections of canine nails (onychomycosis). Ectothrix chains of spores

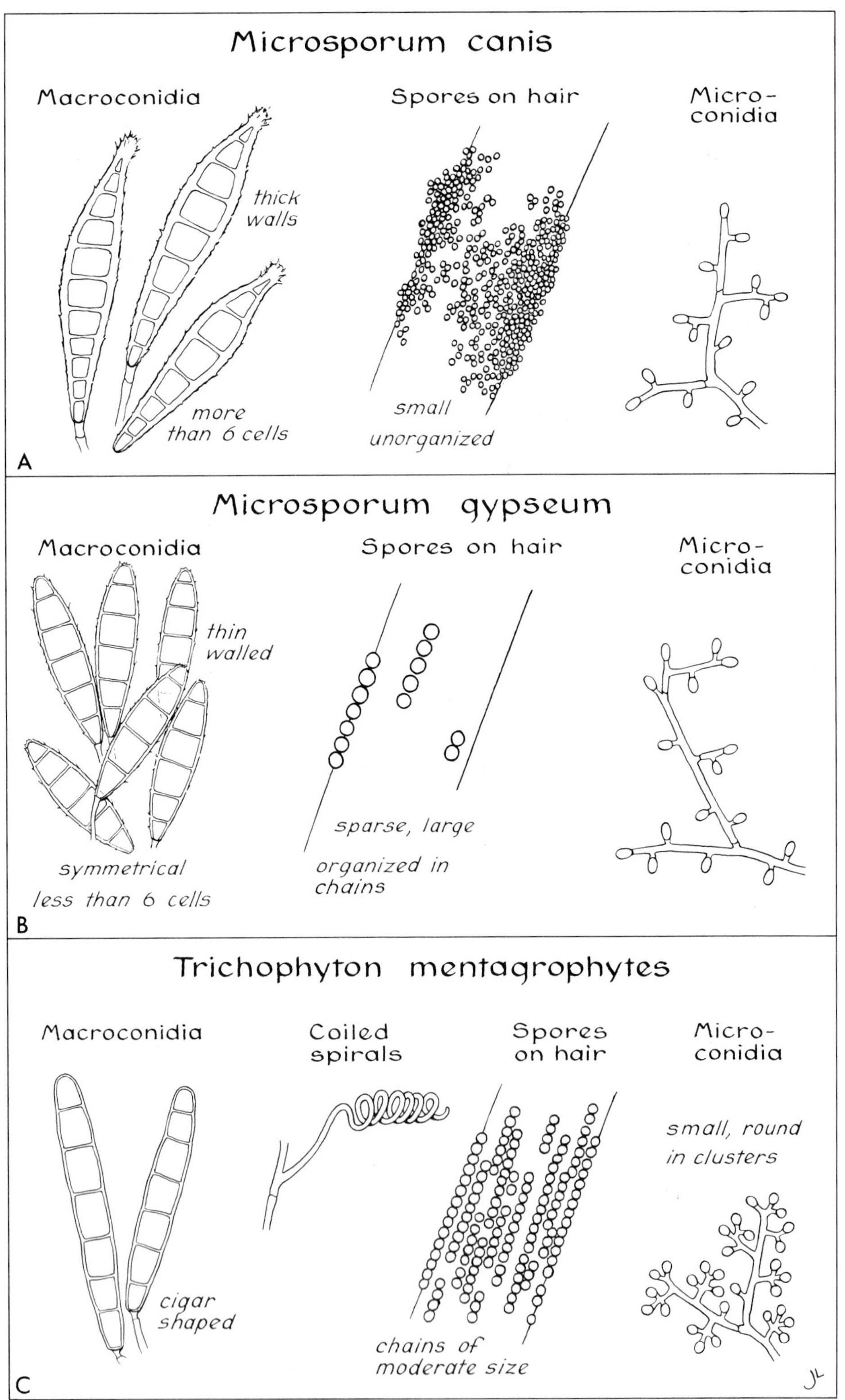


**Figure 10:6.** *A*, Characteristic microscopic morphology of *M. canis; B*, characteristic microscopic morphology of *M. gypseum; C*, characteristic microscopic morphology of *T. mentagrophytes.*

are found on the hair. There is no fluorescence. The distribution of *T. mentagrophytes* is world-wide.

**Colony Morphology.** The zoophilic form characteristically produces a flat colony with a white to cream powdery surface (Fig. 25:1*C*). The powder, which has the appearance of face powder sprinkled in concentric rings and rays, consists mainly of enormous clusters of microconidia. Some strains develop dark red pigment on the reverse side of the colony. No special nutritional requirements are known.

**Microscopic Morphology.** The zoophilic form of *T. mentagrophytes* has more abundant numbers of microscopic structures than anthropophilic or pleomorphic strains. Macroconidia are present in association with microconidia early in the life of the colony (Fig. 10:6*C*). Many strains also produce numerous coiled spirals, which are not unique to *T. mentagrophytes* but are often present more abundantly in this species.

The macroconidia are cigar- or club-shaped with thin, smooth walls. They have narrow attachments to the vegetative hyphae. Abundant small, round microconidia are often present in grape-like clusters.

**Diagnostic Criteria.** The colony morphology and typical small, round microconidia with coiled spirals are significant diagnostic features. Well-formed macroconidia are also typical.

### *TRANSMISSION OF DERMATOPHYTES*

When an animal is exposed to a dermatophyte, infection may or may not be established, and even if it is, disease in the form of skin lesions may not result. This situation has already been alluded to in *M. canis* infections in cats, but similar carrier states exist with many dermatophytes. It often appears that young animals (including man) are more susceptible to infection and are more likely to show clinical lesions than are adults. This difference may be caused by physiologic variations in the skin at different ages, or it may be from acquired immunity or hypersensitivity. There is some clinical and experimental evidence that infection may be enhanced or lesions intensified if the host is nutritionally (i.e., vitamin A-deficient) or otherwise debilitated. Once the disease is established it runs a course that may be uninfluenced by treatment and may resolve spontaneously. Following recovery a resistance to infection has been noted, and it is probable that acquired immunity plays a part in the epidemiology. There is no evidence of cross immunity between species of fungi.

Dermatomycosis has been transmitted by rubbing infected tissue into gently abraded skin, and it is assumed that natural infection is by contact. Contaminated brushes, combs and clippers may be important fomites.

### *THE SKIN'S RESPONSE TO DERMATOPHYTES*

In mild infections on glabrous skin the response is minor and easily missed. It causes mild hypertrophy of the horny layer. There is scant fungal growth and special stains may be needed to demonstrate fungi. As fungal growth becomes more prolific the entire epidermis may hypertrophy. These same hypertrophic changes occur in the hair follicles, but the root sheath is well cornified so the hairs become surrounded by wide collars of keratinized scales and hyphae. The bulge may produce a conical dilation of the opening of the hair follicle, a process which gives a false impression of papillomatous swelling. Mycotic infections invade hairs only in anagen, and grow down the follicle in keratin tissue to the "critical level" or fringe of Adamson where mitotic activity is evident (Fig. 10:1). (Dermatophytes do not survive in living cells). Mild congestion and edema of the dermal papilla may be seen, together with a mild lymphocytic infiltration. If the secondary bacterial infection occurs, microabscesses form in the superficial epidermis, together with suppurative folliculitis.

The gross appearance of dermatomycosis varies (Fig. 25:2). There are usually different degrees of scaling and encrustation of epithelial debris and loss of hair. The hair loss is not permanent unless the follicle is destroyed by secondary bacterial infection. Usually the hairs become brittle and break off near the skin surface, leaving a short stubby hair shaft which can be seen emerging through scales and crusts.

In the course of some "ringworm" infections, the organisms tend to die out in the center of the lesions and the skin then returns to normal, while those organisms at the periphery remain active. The reason for this phenomenon is unknown. A description of typical mycotic skin diseases is given on page 251.

## Candidiasis (Moniliasis)

*Candida albicans* is a simple, yeast-like fungus that reproduces by budding. It forms pseudomycelia and septate mycelia under proper conditions, but does not produce ascospores. Both yeast-like cells and mycelial elements occur in tissues, but colonies on solid media do not form aerial hyphae and therefore do not become fuzzy, but are soft creamy colonies like true yeasts. Although *C. albicans* can be grown on Sabouraud's dextrose agar at room temperature, ideally it should be incubated at 37° C. for 48 hours.

*Candida albicans* is generally considered to be a true saprophyte of the intestinal tract of warm-blooded animals. With lowered host resistance or after prolonged antibiotic therapy, it may produce serious local infections. On occasion it may extend from the digestive tract to the genitourinary tract or become systemic and involve the lungs, lymph nodes, liver or meninges.

Infection with the organism is rare in patients seen in small animal practice. It has a distinct predilection for mucous membrane, areas of mucocutaneous junctions or where moisture may persist and macerate the skin. On mucous membranes the lesions appear as thick, white, opaque plaques. On the skin these are less distinct and moist, red, eroded areas predominate: Clinical cases in dogs have been reported in the perineum, the external ear, the nail folds and the oral mucosa.

In man this infection may emerge after longtime therapy with broad-spectrum antibiotics. This condition has not been a problem in veterinary practice—perhaps because antibiotic therapy is usually of short duration. Nystatin is the drug of choice for topical treatment of *C. albicans* infections and amphotericin B has been suggested for systemic therapy. Chronic oral infections respond poorly to treatment and a guarded prognosis must be given. Candidiasis is an example of a fungus that usually causes mild superficial infection, but on occasion has produced deep, serious infections which may even be fatal. A description of canine candidiasis is given on page 345.

## Cutaneous Aspects of Deep Mycotic Infections

Whereas dermatophytes are parasites that exist in the dead, keratinized structure of the skin, geophilic dermatophytes and fungi that cause deep-seated mycoses are saprophytes of soil and vegetation, and they become parasitic by chance. Some of the diseases occur very rarely, and only in geographic localities where the fungus is endemic. In contrast to superficial fungus infections which are contagious, the deep-seated are not. They are poorly adapted parasites which reach a dead end in the living host. Superficial fungi tend to infect young animals but the deep-seated agents produce chronic disease in mature or aged animals. Allergic sensitization to some fungus infections can be demonstrated by making skin tests with extracts of the causative agent (i.e., Histoplasmin test).

Deep-seated fungus infections frequently produce tubercles, or tumor-like masses called infectious granulomas. They have necrotic centers in which spores, yeast-like cells, or hyphae may be demonstrated. These centers are outlined by thick, fibrous capsules which in turn are surrounded by epithelioid and multinucleated giant cells. Some deep mycoses infect only internal organs such as lungs, liver and spleen, but the entire group of diseases can be said to infect primarily tissues other than those of the superficial areas of the body. Several of the group, however, cause fistulas or otherwise involve the skin. These will be discussed briefly here, and the reader is referred to texts on mycology and infectious diseases for additional information.

### *MADUROMYCOSIS (MYCETOMA)*

Maduromycosis is a clinical entity characterized by nodular, mycotic granulomas of the skin and subcutis. It has a protracted course and responds poorly to therapy. A variety of fungi may cause the lesion. In the dog and cat *Curvularia geniculata*, and *Brachycladium spiciferum* have been identified.

The lesions appear as nodular or ulcerative granulomas or fistulas of the feet or lower extremities. The paws are swollen and painful, and produce a purulent exudate. The granules are usually pigmented brown or black from colors produced by the fungi, especially by the chlamydospores. Diagnosis can be made from histological sections or by culture of the organisms but no effective treatment is known.

### *SPOROTRICHOSIS*

This disease is caused by *Sporotrichum schenckii*, a fungus which is a soil saprophyte. It requires high humidity and a relatively warm climate for survival and is common along the coastal regions and river valleys of the southern United States. Systemic invasion occurs in dogs and cats. Most skin infections are introduced by wood splinters, briar scratches and other traumatic incidents. Firm spherical nodules form at the site and may spread along the lymph channels. They are painful and may ulcerate. The brown pus may contain cigar-shaped, yeast-like bodies but no mycelia. Cultures on Sabouraud's media are needed for positive diagnosis. The disease responds readily to systemic treatment with iodides for a period of at least one month.

### *NOCARDIOSIS*

This disease is caused by *Nocardia asteroides* and, besides systemic manifestations, may cause severe dermatologic lesions in dogs, most commonly on the legs. The lesions consist of nodules, ulcers, fistulas and abscesses. The edematous feet discharge a brownish red purulent exudate and there is cutaneous hypertrophy.

The organism is gram-positive, nonmotile and aerobic and is one of the pathogenic Actinomycetes. Usually a soil saprophyte, the organism can be grown on culture media as smooth, soft, orange colonies with long, thin mycelia (1 micron or less in diameter).

In cats, nocardiosis clinically produces pyothorax with a characteristic brown pus in the chest cavity. There is usually destruction of the lung tissue and a fatal outcome. Feline skin lesions, consisting of subcutaneous nodules, ulcers and cutaneous edema, may accompany the pleural affliction. Enlargement of the submandibular and cervical lymph nodes may be present with the disease in cats.

### *NORTH AMERICAN BLASTOMYCOSIS*

*Blastomyces dermatitidis* causes a chronic granulomatous, suppurative mycotic infection that may be generalized but is often confined to the skin and subcutaneous tissues or to the lungs. The disease is restricted largely to the Middle Atlantic and South Central states, and to the area of the Ohio and Mississippi valleys. It has been reported, though rarely, in dogs and cats (Menges, 1960; Easton, 1961). The organism is a spherical, thick-walled, budding yeast-like fungus in tissues or in cultures at 37° C. However, at room temperature it slowly develops typical mold-like filaments. In nature the organism is thought to be a self-sufficient soil saprophyte. The disease spreads by hematogenous routes, and a subcutaneous ulcerated nodule may be the first or the last sign to appear.

Treatment with amphotericin B may be effective but is long and painful, and the prognosis should be guarded to poor.

### *MISCELLANEOUS MYCOSES*

Many other internal mycotic infections are found in pet animals but they rarely affect the skin. These include: *Cryptococcus neoformans, Coccidioides immitis, Aspergillus fumigatus, Histoplasma capsulatum* and organisms belonging to the Phycomycetes.

## References

Bruner, D. W., and Gillespie, J. H.: *Hagan's Infectious Diseases of Domestic Animals.* Comstock Publishing Associates, Ithaca, N.Y., 1966.

Easton, K. L.: Canad. Vet. J. 2:350, 1961.

Henrici, A. T.: Characteristics of Fungus Diseases. Journal Bact. *39*:113, 1940.

Jackson, W. F.: Personal communication, 1968.

Jubb, K. V. F., and Kennedy, P. C.: *Pathology of Domestic Animals,* Academic Press, New York, 1963.

Kaplan, W.: Dermatophytosis. *In* Kirk, R. W.: Current Veterinary Therapy III, W. B. Saunders Co., Philadelphia, 1968.

Kligman, A. M.; Pathophysiology of Ringworm Infections in Animals with Skin Infections. J. Invest. Derm. *27*:171, 1956.

Marples, M. J.: The Ecology of the Human Skin. Charles C Thomas, Springfield, Illinois, 1965.

Menges, R. W.: Veterinary Medicine. 55:45, 1960.

*Rebell, G., Taplin, D., and Blank, H.: *Dermatophytes, Their Recognition and Identification.* Dermatology Foundation of Miami, Miami, Fla., 1964.

Stableforth, A. W., and Galloway, I. A.: Diseases Due to Bacteria. *In*: *Infectious Diseases of Animals.* Vol. I, Academic Press, New York, 1959.

Stewart, W. D., Danto, J. L., and Maddin, S.: *Synopsis of Dermatology.* C. V. Mosby Co., St. Louis, 1966.

*Wilson, J. W., and Plunkett, O. A.: *The Fungous Diseases of Man.* Univ. of Calif. Press, Berkeley, 1965.

*Suggested supplemental reading.

# ELEVEN

# *Cutaneous Parasitology*

Animal skin is exposed to attack by many kinds of animal parasites. Each species has a particular effect on the skin, which can be mild, such as the isolated fly or mosquito bite, or severe, such as generalized demodectic or sarcoptic mange. Although the skin's reaction to the infestation may be slight, a consideration of the common parasitisms must be included here because the dermatologist is the logical consultant in such cases.

When ectoparasites serve as vectors or intermediate hosts of bacterial, rickettsial or parasitic diseases they become more important. They may produce a severe local or systemic reaction by injecting poisonous venom into the skin (bee and wasp stings). The larvae of some parasites live in wounds or on macerated skin to produce a condition known as myiasis. The most serious dermatologic concern develops when the dermatosis produced by parasites living in or on the skin produces irritation and sensitization.

Some parasites live on the skin (chiggers and biting lice), subsisting on the debris and exudates which are produced on its surface. Others live on the skin but periodically penetrate its surface to draw nourishment from blood and tissue fluids (sucking lice and ticks). Still others live in or under the skin for at least part of their life cycle producing more severe cutaneous effects (demodectic and sarcoptic mites).

The skin's reaction to these insults varies from trivial to lethal but usually includes inflammation, edema and an attempt to localize the "foreign body," toxin or excretory products of the parasite. These secretions are often allergenic and cause itching and burning sensations.

Although many kinds of parasites affect animals, we will discuss only those in the following list, which includes the important skin parasites of dogs and cats in North America (Table 11-1).

## PROTOZOAN PARASITES

Leishmaniasis is caused by an oval flagellated, nonmotile protozoan, *Leishmania canis*, which is common in tropical countries. Dogs and rats are major reservoirs of importance for public health reasons. The sand fly is the chief vector. The parasite lives chiefly in endothelial cells of capillaries of the spleen,

TABLE 11:1. Common Skin Parasites

A. Protozoan parasites
    *Leishmania canis*
B. Helminth parasites
    1. *Rhabditis strongyloides*
    2. *Dirofilaria immitis*
    3. Schistosoma cercariae
C. Arthropod parasites
    1. Arachnida
        Acarina
            Argasid ticks (soft)
                *Otobius megnini,* (spinous ear tick)
            Ixodid ticks (hard)
                *Rhipicephalus sanguineus* (brown dog tick)
                *Dermacentor variabilis* (American dog tick)
                Ixodes sp.
                Amblyomma sp.
        *Dermanyssus gallinae* (poultry mite)
        *Eutrombicula alfreddugèsi* (chigger mites)
        *Cheyletiella yasguri*
        *Demodex canis*
        *Demodex felis*
        *Sarcoptes scabiei* (var. *canis*) (dog scabies)
        *Notoedres cati* (cat scabies)
        *Otodectes cynotis* (ear mites)
    2. Insecta
        Phthiraptera (lice)
            *Linognathus setosus* (sucking louse)
            *Trichodectes canis* (biting louse)
            *Felicola subrostratus* (biting louse of cats)
        Siphonaptera (fleas)
            *Ctenocephalides felis* (cat flea)
            *Ctenocephalides canis* (dog flea)
            *Echidnophaga gallinacea* (sticktight flea)
        Diptera (flies)
            *Cuterebra maculata* (skin bots)
            Calliphorids (blow flies)
            Sarcophagids (flesh flies)
            *Stomoxys calcitrans* (stable fly)
            Miscellaneous (Mosquitos, black flies and so on)
        Hymenoptera (bees, wasps, hornets)

liver, lymph nodes and bone marrow and produces a chronic malaria-like disease. If skin lesions develop, they are pruritic, indurated papules or nodules near the head and ears which may enlarge to 1 inch in size. Ulceration with the formation of brownish crusts is common, and healing with extensive scars takes place over a period of months.

The disease has been seen in several dogs imported into the United States from the Mediterranean region or Central and South America. Antimony compounds are suggested for therapy, but their effect may be inconsistent.

## HELMINTH PARASITES

### Rhabditic Dermatitis

Under filthy conditions, the free-living nematode *Rhabditis strongyloides* may invade the skin of dogs. The adults live in damp soil or decaying organic material such as straw bedding, and the life cycle is direct. The larvae (600 microns long) (Fig. 11:1) may be found in skin scrapings from affected animals or in their bedding. The lesions are usually confined to the abdomen, chest, extremities and areas which normally contacted the bedding. There is intense pruritus, and the lesions are hairless, with erythema, papules, pustules and, later, crusts and scales. The larvae, and also some parthenogenetic adult females, may be found in the hair follicles in histologic sections and there is subcutaneous inflammation with leukocytic and eosinophic infiltration of the corium (Baker, 1968). Diagnosis is easily accomplished by observation of the larvae in skin scrapings.

Treatment is simple and effective. Complete removal and destruction of bedding is mandatory. The beds, kennels or cages should be thoroughly washed and sprayed with 5 per cent DDT, 1 per cent chlordane or other insecticide. The patient should be given a shampoo to cleanse the skin and treated with 0.5 per cent chlordane or 1 per cent ronnel. The skin treatment should be applied three times, at intervals of ten to 14 days. In some cases the secondary pyoderma which is present will require careful treatment (see p. 323).

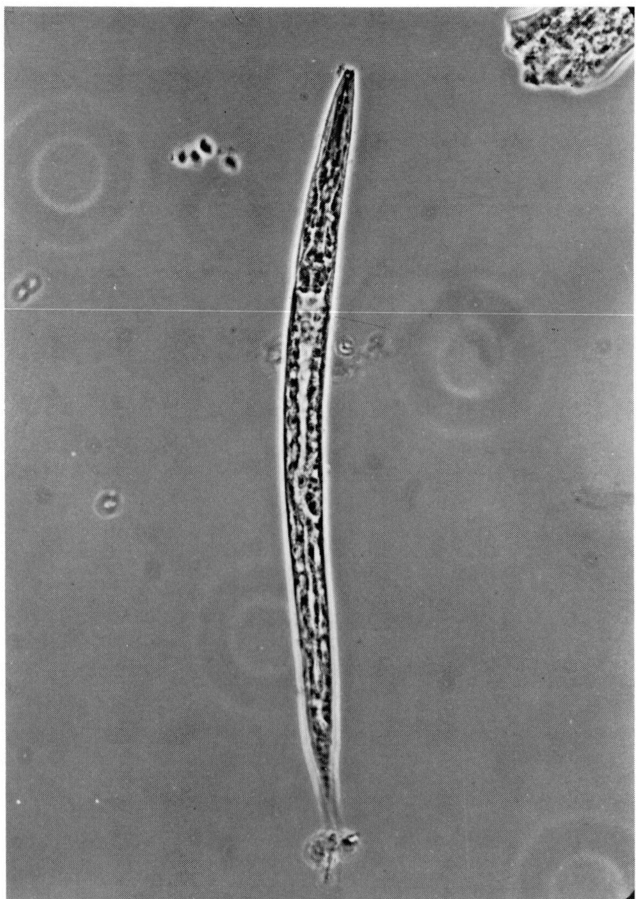

**Figure 11:1.** Larva of the free-living nematode, *Rhabditis strongyloides*. (Courtesy of Jay R. Georgi.)

### Ancylostomiasis

The larvae of *Ancylostoma braziliense* and *A. caninum* cause a characteristic serpiginous skin lesion in man called "creeping eruption." These larvae do not produce as severe skin lesions in the dog or cat since these are their specific hosts. Any skin invasion is incidental to completion of the normal life cycle with the larvae quickly abandoning the skin and proceeding to the digestive tract.

### Dirofilariasis

The larvae of *Dirofilaria immitis* are found in the blood and occasionally in the subcutaneous tissues. Dogs affected with these parasites have been observed to develop mild erythema and patchy alopecia of the front legs and chest. It has not yet been proved that the parasites cause these lesions.

### Schistosoma Dermatitis

Schistosoma cercariae of various ducks, shore birds, mice or muskrat hosts may penetrate the skin of man or of warm-blooded animals and produce a dermatitis. Since they are not in their natural host, they do not penetrate beyond the skin. In order for the cercariae to be present in the water a suitable snail host must be present. These are found in the North Central and Eastern states and on the East and West coasts of the United States. In order for animals to become severely affected it is necessary to have repeated heavy exposure, and the reaction tends to become a sensitization phenomenon.

The skin develops urticarial wheals, which are intensely pruritic. These subside to macules followed later by papules and pustules. The reaction is most severe two to three days after exposure and healing takes seven to ten days. The cercariae become walled off in the skin by an acute inflammatory reaction with infiltration of neutrophils, lymphocytes and eosinophils.

Palliative topical treatment of the lesions with antipruritic lotions may be helpful. Prevention of exposure by keeping animals away from contaminated ponds or treatment of these areas to kill snails may be effective.

## ARTHROPOD PARASITES

### Arachnids

Arachnids differ from insects in the absence of wings, the presence of four pairs of legs in adults and fusion of the head and thorax. With ticks and mites, the head, thorax and abdomen are fused so they have lost their external signs of segmentation. The mouthparts and their base, the capitulum, are attached to the anterior body by a movable hinge. This anterior segment is called the gnathosoma, the rest of the body, the idiosoma. There are separate sexes.

#### *PARASITIC TICKS*

Ticks differ from mites in their larger size, the hairless or short-haired leathery body, exposed armed hypostome and the presence of a pair of spiracles near the coxae of the fourth pair of legs. Most are not host specific. Ticks are divided into argasid or soft ticks and ixodid or hard ticks. The argasid are more primitive, less often parasitic, procedure fewer progeny and infect the premises occupied by their hosts. Ixodid ticks are more specialized, highly parasitic, produce more progeny and infest the open country frequented by their hosts.

**Argasid (Soft) Ticks.** These are more commonly parasites of birds, and are found frequently in warmer climates. In endemic regions, however, they may infest all types of wild and domestic animals. They have no dorsal plate, the sexes are similar, the capitulum is not visible dorsally and the spiracles lie in front of the third pair of unspurred coxae. Ticks of this class seldom travel far from their lairs and are often nocturnal feeders. Only one species will be discussed.

SPINOUS EAR TICK. This tick *(Otobius megnini)* is found in the external ear canal of dogs and cats, but its range is limited to the southern United States, especially the southwest. The larvae and nymphs infest the ear canal of the host, producing acute otitis externa, pain and occasional convulsions. Often the ear canals become packed with immature ticks, but in some cases only a few are found. The life cycle is described in Figure 11:2. Adults are fiddle-shaped with a constriction at the middle, but they are not spiny and do not feed since they are not parasites. The larvae, engorged on lymph from the ear canal, are yellow or pink. They are 1/8 inch long and spherical with three pairs of minute legs. The nymphs, which also inhabit the ear canal, are bluish gray with four pairs of yellow legs (Fig. 11:3). They are widest in the middle and the skin has numerous sharp spines.

Damage from spinous ear ticks results from the loss of blood and lymph. Also, severe irritation and secondary otitis cause vigorous head shaking and scratching. Neurologic signs, paralysis or convulsions have been reported in calves, sheep, donkeys and horses.

Treatment involves mechanical removal of ticks with forceps, spraying the coat with insecticidal materials such as DDT or malathion and treatment of the otitis externa with antibiotic, corticosteroid lotions such as Panolog.

Reinfestation is rarely a problem, but if it develops, destruction of the ticks' lair or nests is important. Spraying the sheds, grounds, wood piles and other "homesites" with 1 per cent ronnel, 0.25 per cent malathion or Kem dip may be effective. Repeated application in 30 days is necessary since complete eradication is difficult.

**Ixodid (Hard) Ticks.** Hard ticks possess a chitinous shield, the scutum, which covers the dorsal surface of the male and the anterior dorsal part of the female. The capitulum is visible dorsally at the anterior end and its base is important taxonomically. The sexes are dissimilar although both are blood suckers. It is beyond the scope of this text to identify ticks specifically, but because *Rhipicephalus sanguineus* (in comparison to Dermacentor) can reproduce easily in buildings and thus presents special control problems, a few key features for identifying genera will be given (Figs. 11:4 and 11:5).

Rhipicephalus is recognized by a vase-shaped base of the capitulum, elongated spiracles and in the male by triangular adanal plates. Coxae IV are no larger than the other three.

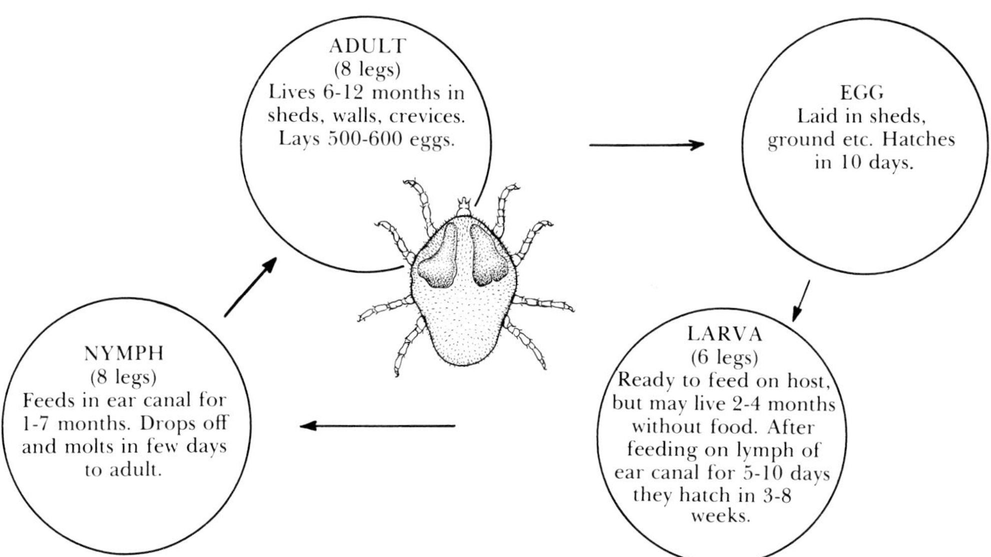
ADULT
(8 legs)
Lives 6-12 months in sheds, walls, crevices.
Lays 500-600 eggs.
EGG
Laid in sheds, ground etc. Hatches in 10 days.
LARVA
(6 legs)
Ready to feed on host, but may live 2-4 months without food. After feeding on lymph of ear canal for 5-10 days they hatch in 3-8 weeks.
NYMPH
(8 legs)
Feeds in ear canal for 1-7 months. Drops off and molts in few days to adult.

**Figure 11:2.** Life cycle of *Otobius megnini* (spinous ear tick) (five–12 months).

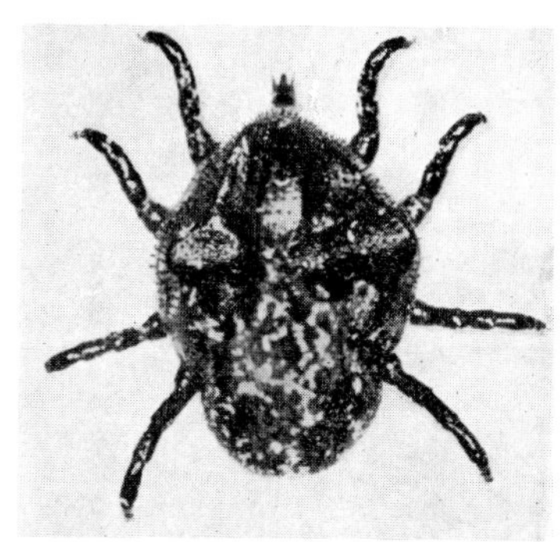

**Figure 11:3.** Nymph of *Otobius megnini,* the spinous ear tick. (From Monnig: *Veterinary Helminthology and Entomology.* Williams & Wilkins, Baltimore, 1962.)

IXODES
A
HÆMAPHYSALIS
h c
c.s.
p
4
3
2
1
b.c.
B
BOOPHILUS
C
AMBLYOMMA
D
RHIPICEPHALUS
E
DERMACENTOR
F

**Figure 11:4.** Capitula of various genera of hard ticks, ventral view, b.c., basis capituli; c, chelicera; c.s., sheath of chelicera; h, haustellum; p, pedipalps. (From Belding: *Textbook of Parasitology.* Appleton-Century-Crofts, N. Y., 1965.)

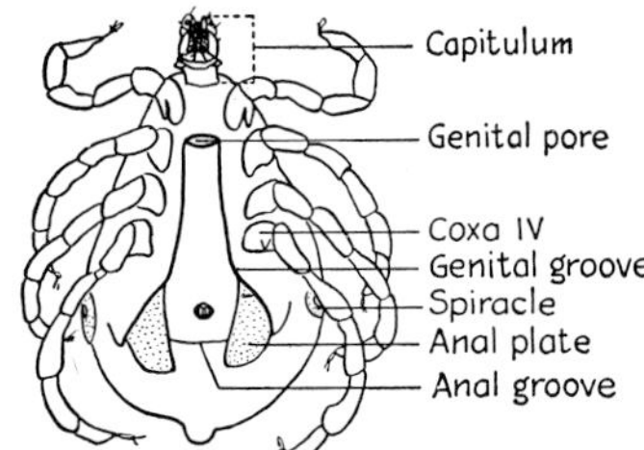


A RHIPICEPHALUS SANGUINEUS

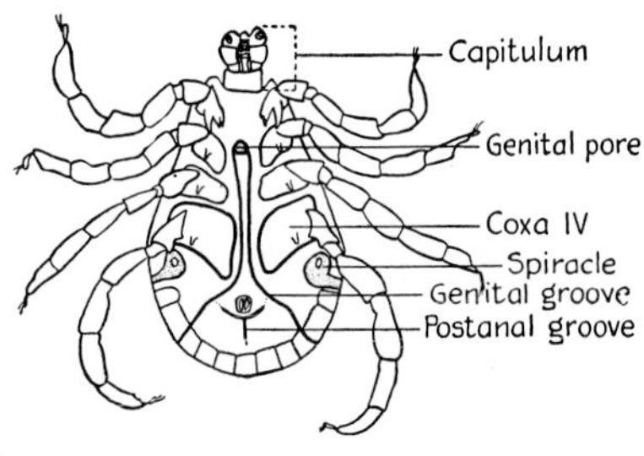


B DERMACENTOR ANDERSONI

**Figure 11:5.** Ventral view of various species of male ixodid ticks, showing genital and anal grooves, coxae and plates. Differential characteristics are indicated by heavy lines and dotted areas. (From Belding: *Textbook of Parasitology*, Appleton-Century-Crofts, N. Y., 1965.)

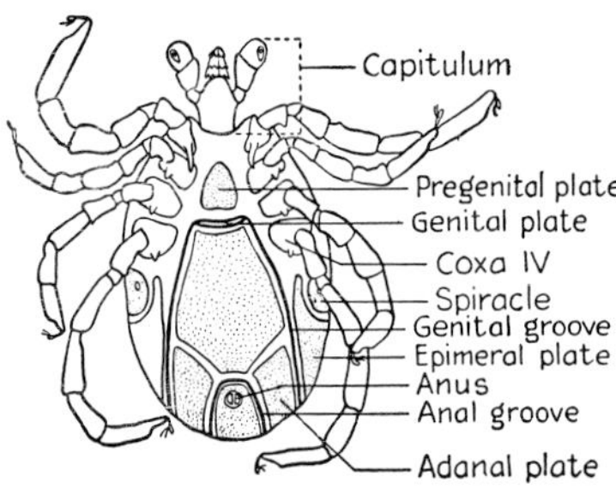


C IXODES RICINUS

Dermacentor ticks are characterized by the very large fourth coxae, the rectangular base of the capitulum and the ornate scutum.

The general life cycle of ixodid ticks is given in Figure 11:6, although each species may vary slightly in some details. Generally the life cycle requires three hosts, preferably animals of varied size for larva, nymph and adult, although some species pass through all stages on the same mammal. If the complicated life cycle is interrupted, the tick can survive for long periods or hibernate through the winter. Although the life cycle is usually completed in a single year it may be extended for two or three years.

While off the host these ticks infest ground covered with small bushes and shrubs. They resist cold but are susceptible to strong sunlight, desiccation and excessive rainfall. They do require a moist environment.

DAMAGE FROM TICKS. Ticks injure animals by the irritation of their bites,

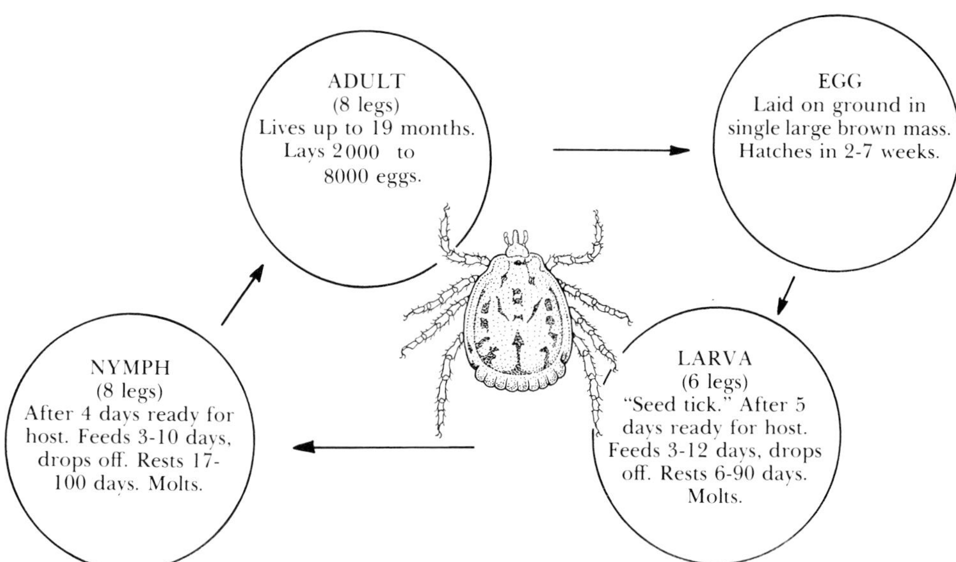


**Figure 11:6.** Life cycle of ixodid (hard) ticks (Two–24+ months).

by serving as vectors for bacterial, rickettsial, viral and protozoan diseases, and by producing tick paralysis through their poisonous secretions.

Tick paralysis has been produced by 12 ixodid species including *D. variabilis* and is seen in many hosts including dogs and cats. The paralysis is caused by a protein toxin produced by the salivary glands of the tick. It may be elaborated by ovarian function as it is associated with egg production. Individual ticks vary in their toxin-producing capacity, although those attached near the spine and neck seem to produce a more severe intoxication. The toxin affects the lower motor neurons of the spinal cord and cranial nerves and produces a progressive ascending flaccid paralysis.

TREATMENT AND CONTROL OF TICKS. In cases of tick paralysis, rapid recovery follows mechanical removal of the complete tick(s). When animals are infested by small numbers of ticks, picking them off is often simple and easy. An effective method is to soak the tick in alcohol or ether, grasp the head parts at the surface of the skin gently with a hemostat, and apply firm traction. Ticks are commonly found in the ears and between the toes. The collected ticks should be burned or soaked in alcohol until dead. Under no conditions should ticks be removed from animals by soaking them in gasoline or kerosene or by applying a lighted cigarette – the consequences to the host's skin are too severe.

With heavy or persisting infestations the dog may be treated topically with 4 per cent malathion powder, or 0.5 per cent solution. Ronnel (1 per cent) or Kem dip may be used effectively on the dog or the premises. Because of susceptibility to most topical insecticides, cats should be treated only with powders of methoxychlor (2 per cent) pyrethrin (1 per cent) or carbaryl (1 per cent).

Infestations of *Rhipicephalus sanguineus* in houses and kennels can often be controlled or eliminated by repeated spraying of woodwork, crawl spaces, pipe clearances and cracks with Kem dip or 2 per cent chlordane. In severe cases commercial exterminators should be employed.

Outdoor control measures can help limit ticks by controlling their hosts and by destroying or treating vegetation. The population of wild rodent hosts can be reduced by trapping or poisoning. Their habitat can be destroyed by cutting and burning brush and grass, by cultivating land and rotating pastures. In urban areas grass and shrubbed areas can be treated with 5 to 10 per cent toxaphene, chlordane or dieldrin dusts (or sprays) applied at the rate of 20 to 40 pounds per acre. This is applied in the spring and repeated once during midsummer.

COMMON SPECIES OF IXODID TICK AFFECTING DOGS AND CATS. *Rhipicephalus sanguineus.* The brown dog tick is widely distributed in North America and is the primary tick problem in many sections. This is because it can survive indoors because of its low moisture requirements, and can complete its life cycle with only one animal as host. Although its principal host is the dog, it is found on other canine and feline species, rabbits, horses and man. It requires three distinct hosts (but perhaps the same animal) in its life cycle. It can transmit babesiosis and anaplasmosis, *Rickettsia canis, Pasteurella tularensis* and can cause tick paralysis.

*Dermacentor variabilis.* The American dog tick also is widely distributed in North America but is especially common along the Atlantic coast in areas of shrub and beach grass. The adult tick's principal host is the dog but man, domestic animals and large fur-bearing mammals may be attacked. The immature tick's principal host is the field mouse, but other small rodents or larger mammals may be infested. It spreads Rocky Mountain spotted fever, St. Louis encephalitis, tularemia, anaplasmosis and causes tick paralysis.

*Other Ticks Which May Affect Dogs and Cats: Dermacentor andersoni* (Rocky Mountain wood tick), *Dermacentor occidentalis* (Pacific or West coast tick), *Ixodes scapularis* (black-legged tick), *Amblyomma maculatum* (Gulf Coast tick) and *Amblyomma americanum* (Lone star tick).

### PARASITIC MITES

Mites are members of the order Acarina. They are smaller than ticks and do not have a leathery covering; the hypostome may be unarmed and some mites have spiracles on the cephalothorax. Parasitic mites are chiefly ectoparasites of the skin, mucous membranes or feathers, but a few are endoparasites. They are world-wide in distribution, infest plants and animals, cause direct injury to animals and spread disease.

**Dermanyssus Gallinae (Poultry Mite).** This mite attacks poultry, wild and cage birds, and dogs as well as man. It is called the red mite but is only red when engorged with blood. At other times it is white, gray or black (Fig. 11:7). The engorged adult, which is the largest form, is only 1 mm. in size. It lives in nests and cracks in cages or houses and after a meal of blood lays up to seven eggs at a time. They hatch to six-legged nymphs which do not feed. After 48 hours these molt to eight-legged protonymphs which feed and 48 hours later molt to deutonymphs. These also feed and molt 48 hours later to adults. The whole cycle takes only seven days under ideal conditions but without feeding opportunities may last five months.

This mite affects dogs and cats only rarely and almost accidentally. They cause intense itching and erythema localized to the legs and back. Almost any insecticidal bath, dip or spray will eliminate the mites but treatment of the af-

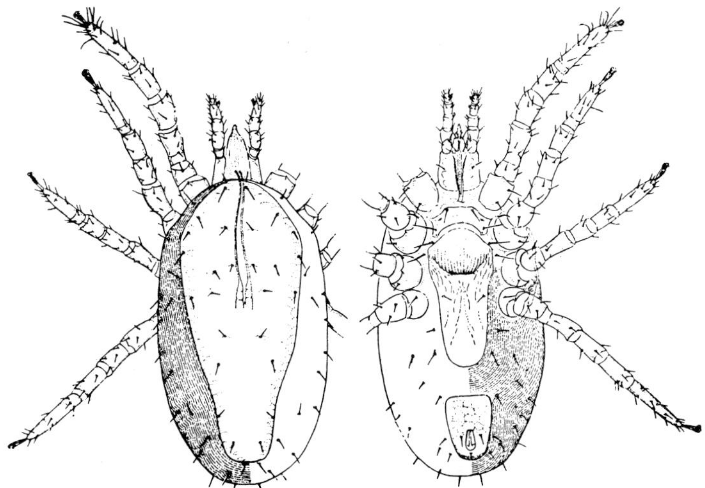

**Figure 11:7.** *Dermanyssus gallinoe* (Degeer). Left, dorsal view of female; right, ventral view of female. (From Monnig: *Veterinary Helminthology and Entomology.* Williams & Wilkins, Baltimore, 1962.)

fected premises which initiated the infection should be accomplished to prevent reinfestation.

**Eutrombicula Alfreddugèsi (North American Chigger).** The adult form is a scavenger living on decaying vegetable material. It is orange-red, about the size of the head of a pin and lives about ten months, producing probably one generation per year. The eggs are laid in moist ground, hatch to six-legged red larvae which are parasitic and feed on animals. They drop to the ground and become nymphs and finally adults (Fig. 11:8). The entire cycle is complete in 50 to 70 days but adult females may live over a year. The larvae crawl up the legs and attach themselves to the skin. The bite causes severe irritation and pruritus.

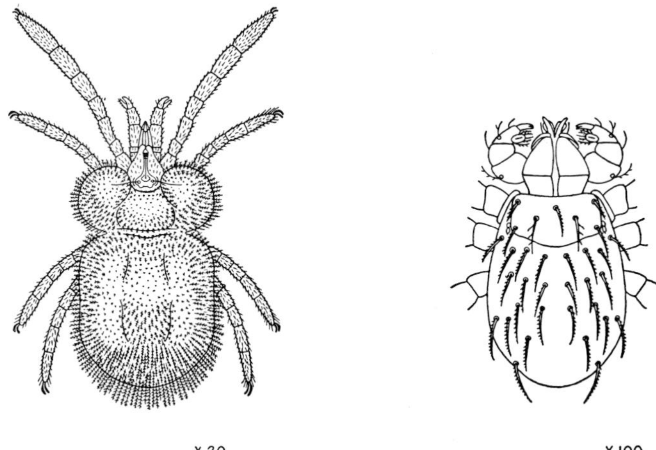


**Figure 11:8.** *A, E. alfreddugesi* (North American chigger) adult; *B, E. alfreddugesi* larva, dorsal view (legs omitted). (From Belding: *Textbook of Parasitology.* Appleton-Century-Crofts, N. Y., 1965.)

The affected skin remains soft, but the irritation produces scaling and alopecia. Mites have been found inside the external ear canal and pinna of cats and are easily distinguished from ear mites by their red color and tendency to adhere tightly to the skin.

**Cheyletiella Yasguri.** This large mite affects dogs, which are the important reservoir hosts (Ewing, 1968). Adults can be free living and thus infest kennel buildings for extended periods. The parasite is found commonly in puppies, especially on the rump and along the spine, the top of the head and the nose. It produces mild pruritus and, although the skin does not react acutely, yellow-gray scales of "dandruff" are abundant in the region. Careful inspection reveals the large mites (385 Microns) which have four pairs of legs bearing combs instead of claws (Fig. 11:9*A*). The most diagnostic feature is the accessory mouthparts or palpi which terminate in prominent hooks (Fig. 11:9*B*). It is easy and embarrassing to "miss" the diagnosis of the cause of the "dandruff" in these cases. Treatment of the puppies with almost any nontoxic insecticidal shampoo, dip, spray or powder is successful in controlling the infestation. It is desirable to remove the patients from their infested environment at least until it is thoroughly cleaned and sprayed with 5 per cent DDT or 2 per cent chlordane. It is difficult to completely eradicate these mites from the premises.

**Demodex Canis.** This is a parasite which is present in the hair follicles of almost all dogs and it is also found in some cats. Adults are elongated cylindrical mites with four pairs of short three-jointed legs, a short sucking capitulum and a long tapering abdomen. The female (40 × 300 microns) has a long vulva on the abdominal venter while the male (40 × 250 microns) has a penis protruding from the dorsal thorax. The adults burrow head downward into the hair follicles where dozens of mites may have congregated. The life cycle, which is spent entirely in the host, is incompletely understood. However, fusiform eggs hatch into small six-legged larvae, which molt into the eight-legged protonymphs. These in turn molt into deutonymphs which are larger, and finally into adults (Fig. 11:10*A*, *B*, *C*, *D* and *E*). Although the epizootiology of this parasitism is unknown, predisposing factors seem to be youth, short hair, and poor condition or debilitating diseases. Several clinical syndromes are recognized, and these are discussed on page 243.

**Sarcoptes Scabiei (var. canis) and Notoedres cati.** These two mites will be discussed together since they belong to the family Sarcoptidae and have many similarities. *Sarcoptes Scabiei*, var. *canis* adults are small (200 to 400 microns), oval, whitish mites with two pairs of short legs anteriorly which bear long unjointed stalks with suckers (Fig. 11:11). The stalks are of medium length in *Notoedres cati* (Fig. 11:12). Two posterior pairs of legs are rudimentary and do not extend beyond the border of the body. Except for the fourth pair of legs of the male Sarcoptes, each of which carries a suckered stalk, the posterior legs terminate in long bristles. The anus of sarcoptes is terminal whereas that of Notoedres is dorsal in location. The finely striated integument is ornamented dorsally with cones, spines, scales and bristles, which are of taxonomic importance.

Copulation occurs in the molting pocket on the surface of the skin. The fertilized female excavates a burrow at the rate of 2 to 3 mm. per day through the horny layer of the skin. She lays eggs behind her which hatch as larvae. These burrow out of the tunnel and travel along the skin. They form molting pockets in the surface and feed there. Nymphal forms also wander, but they may

*(Text continued on page 152.)*

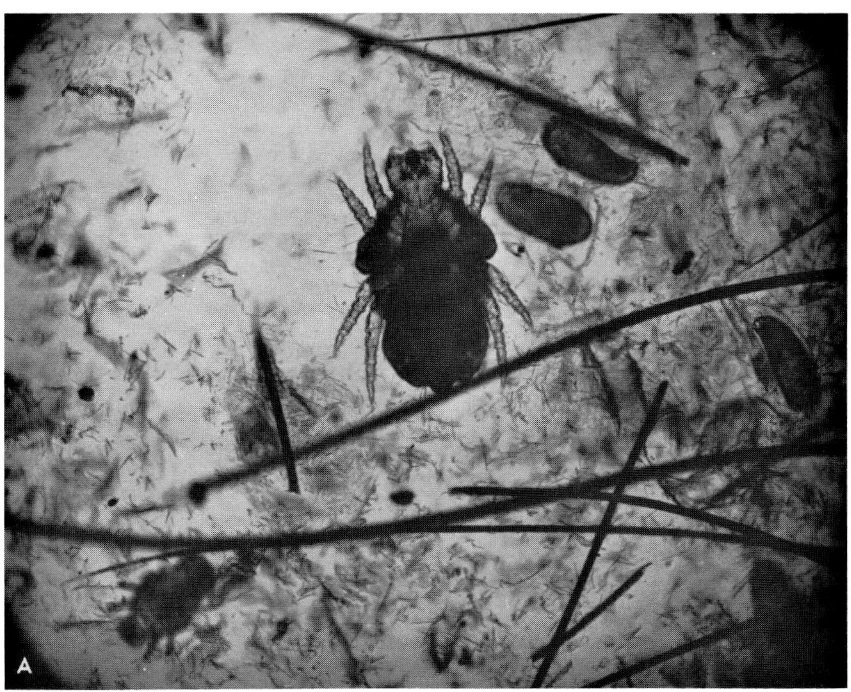


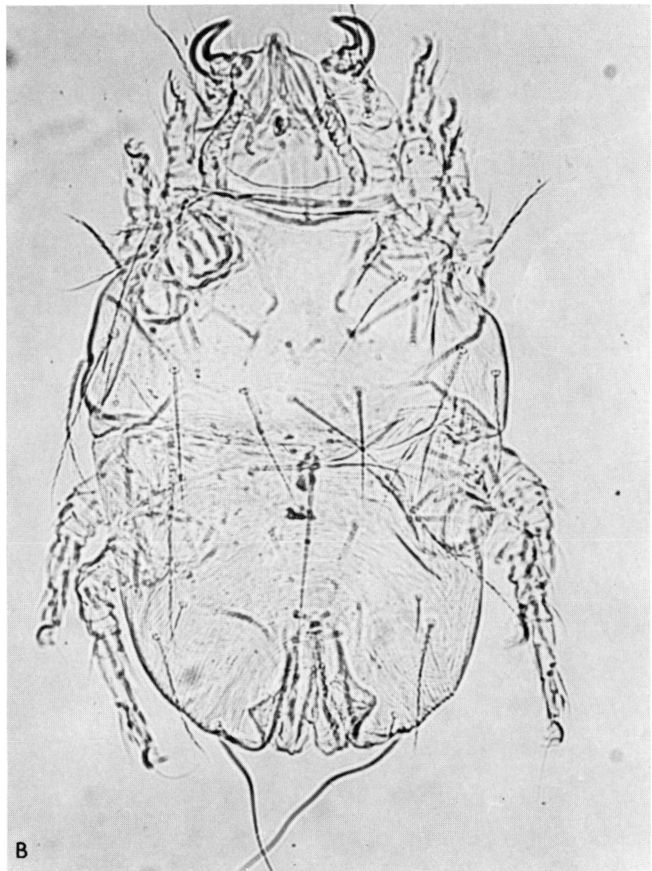


**Figure 11:9.** *A, Cheyletiella Yasguri* adult, larva and eggs from skin scraping. (Low power.) *B, Cheyletiella Yasguri* adult mite showing the diagnostic hooks of the accessory mouthparts.

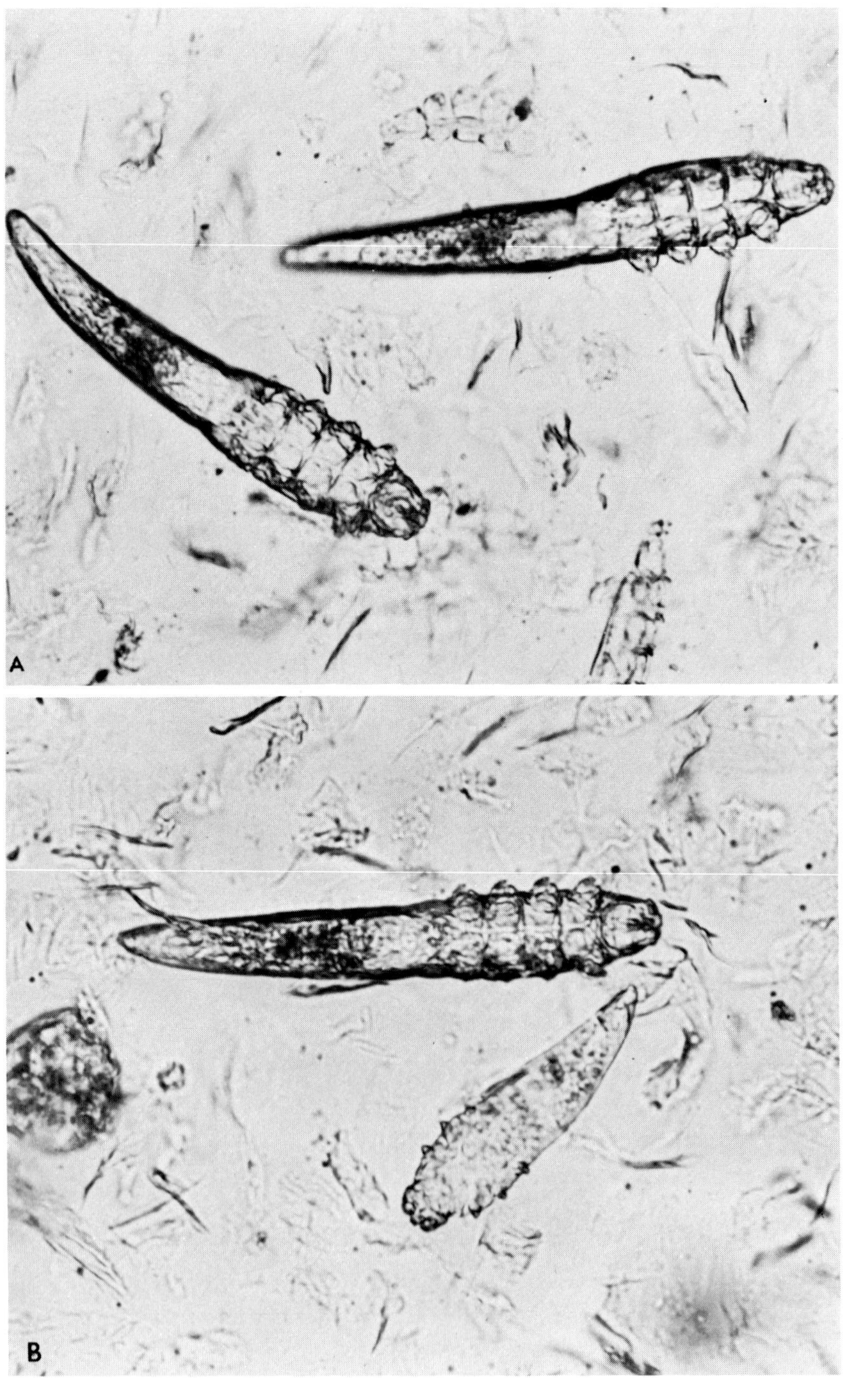


**Figure 11:10.** *Demodex canis* (× 500). *A*, Two adults (four pairs of legs); *B*, adult and larva (three pairs of stubby legs); *C*, nymph (four pairs of stubby legs); *D*, egg (arrow).

*(Illustration continues on opposite page.)*

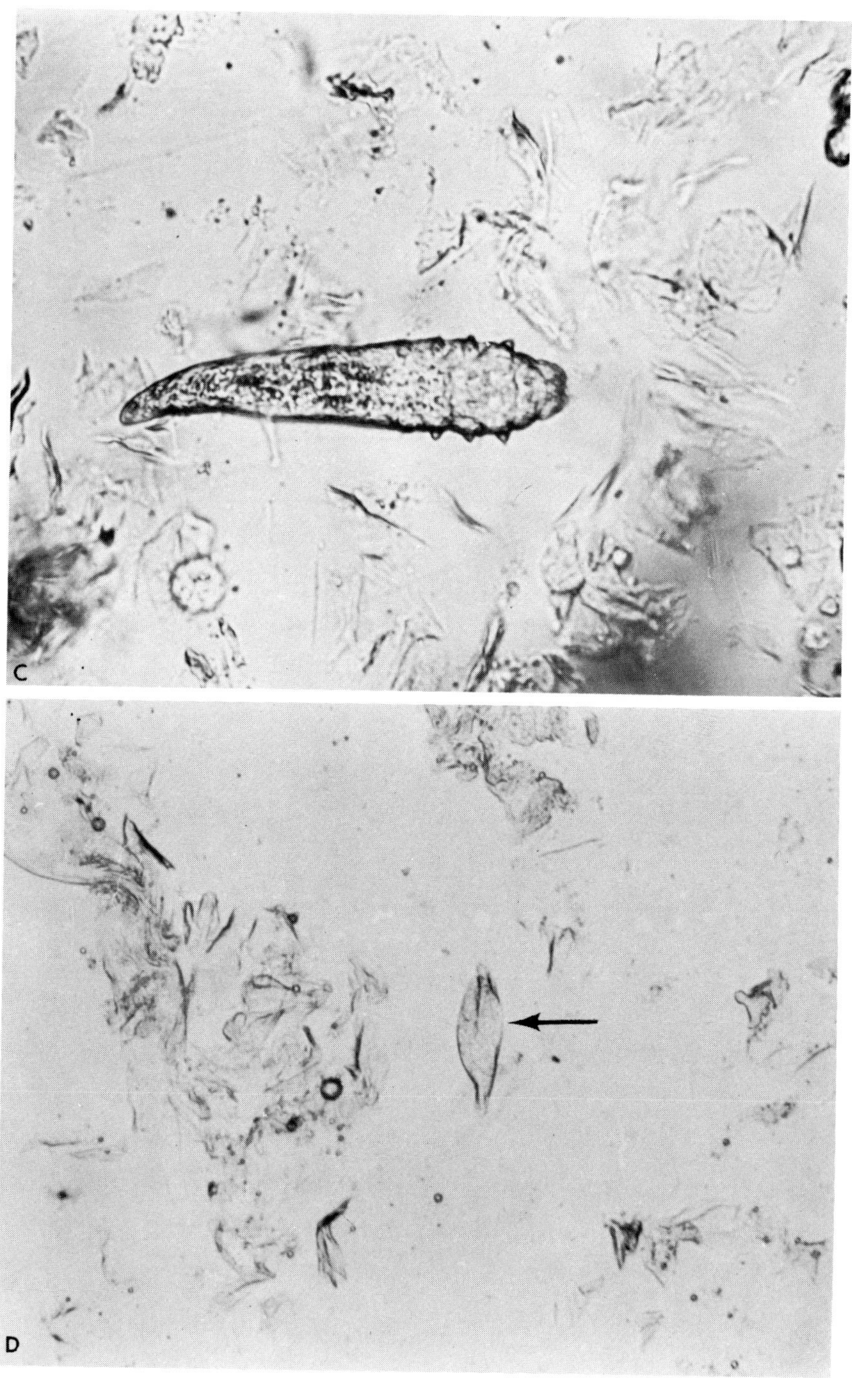


**Figure 11:10.** *Continued.*

*(Illustration continues on following page.)*

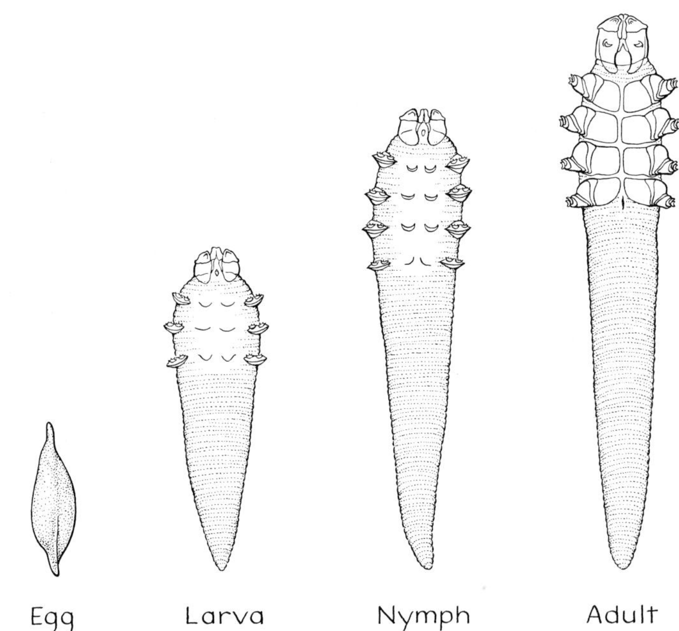


E

**Figure 11:10.** *E*, Adult and immature forms of *Demodex canis.*

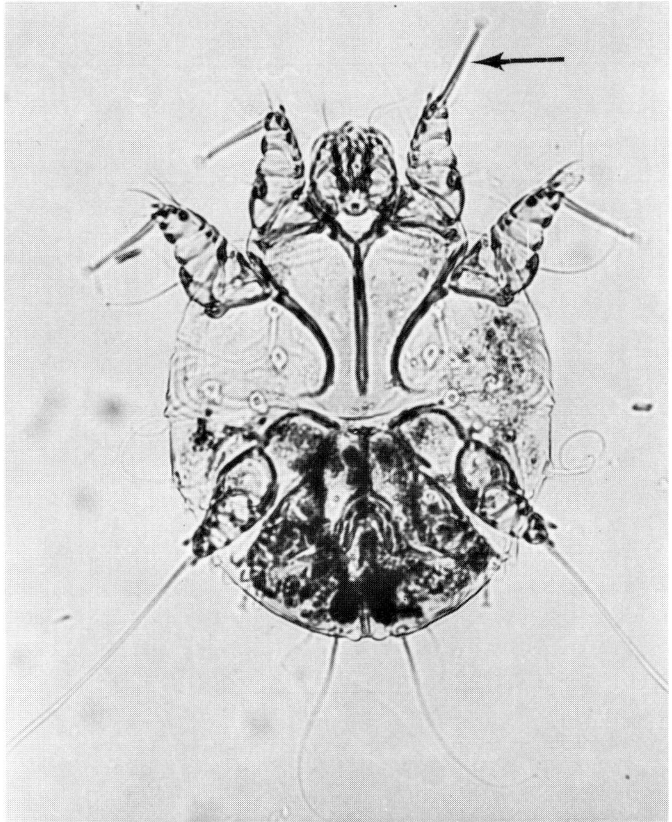

**Figure 11:11.** Adult *Sarcoptes scabiei* (var. *canis*). Note the long unjointed stalks and suckers.

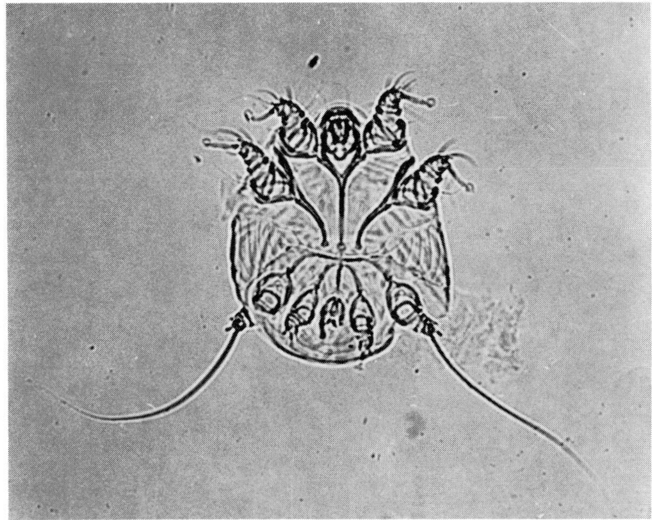

**Figure 11:12.** Adult *Notoedres cati.* Note the medium length stalks, the striated integument, and the lack of a terminally located anus. This mite is smaller than *Sarcoptes scabiei* (var. *canis*).

stay in the molting pocket until they reach maturity (Fig. 11:13). The mites prefer parts of the body that are not covered by much hair such as the ear flaps, elbows, face and extremities. However, as they spread, hair is lost and the entire body may become infested. The condition is highly contagious as it spreads by direct contact. Males, females, and hosts of all age groups are equally susceptible. The mites are sensitive to drying, however, and only live a few days off the host. *Sarcoptes canis* attacks primarily dogs, but can infest other hosts temporarily. It will affect man for a few hours, but only starts a pocket in the skin and soon withdraws and falls off the skin. In man a slightly pruritic pink papule remains for a few days as a result of this temporary parasitic infestation. *Notoedres cati* attacks cats, foxes and rabbits, and produces pruritic, crusted lesions of the face, ears, feet and perineum. Clinical aspects of scabies and notoedric mange are discussed on pages 329 and 315.

**Otodectes Cynotis (Ear Mites).** *Otodectes cynotis* is a psoraptid mite which does not burrow but lives on the surface of the skin. The mites do not pierce the skin for body fluids but feed on epidermal debris. They cause intense irritation and thick reddish brown crusts in the ears of dogs and cats. The ears become filled with a mixture of loose crusts and cerumen. Lesions may be restricted to the external ear canal, but mites are found on other areas of the body, so general treatment is necessary. It is highly contagious, and especially prevalent in the young. Many species of carnivores can be infested as the mites are not host-specific.

Adult mites are large, white and freely moving. The anus is terminal, they have four pairs of legs and all except the rudimentary fourth pair of the female extend beyond the body margin. All four legs of the male bear short, unjointed stalks (pedicles) with suckers. These are present on the first two pairs of legs of females.

The life cycle takes three weeks (Fig. 11:14). The egg is laid with a cement

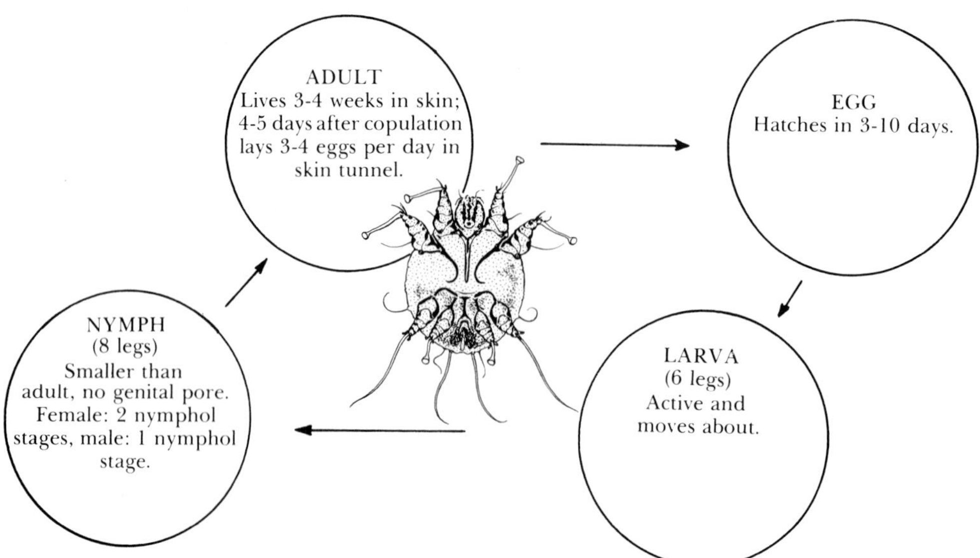


**Figure 11:13.** Life cycle of sarcoptid mites (17–21 days).

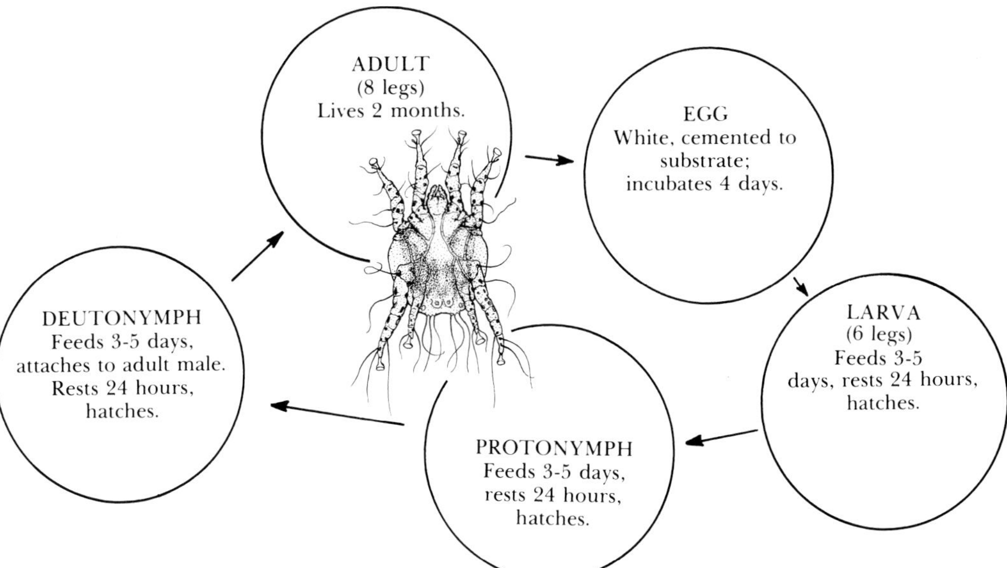


**Figure 11:14.** Life cycle of *Otodectes cynotis* (three weeks).

which sticks it to the substrate. After four days' incubation it hatches to the six-legged larva. This feeds actively for three to ten days, rests ten to 30 hours and hatches to the protonymph, which has eight legs although the last pair is very small. After a similar active and resting stage, this molts into the deutonymph. The deutonymph is usually approached by the adult male (Fig. 11:15) and the two become attached (end to end) by the pair of dorsal posterior suckers on the

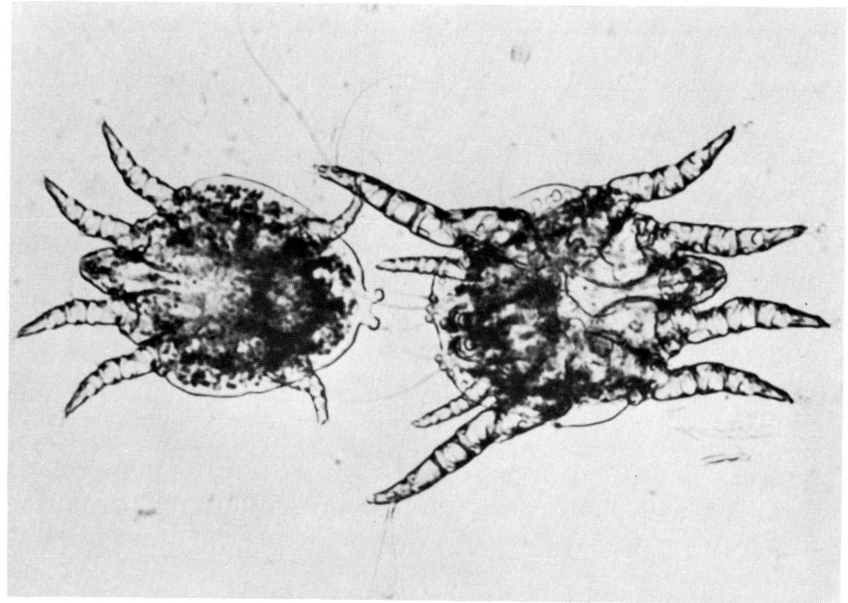

**Figure 11:15.** Larger male *Otodectes cynotis* mite approaching a deutonymph.

body of the nymph and those on the rear legs of the adult male. If a male adult is produced from the deutonymph the attachment has no physiological significance, but if a female emerges, copulation occurs at that moment and she will be egg-bearing. Females that are not attached to permit copulation at the moment of ecdysis do not lay eggs. Sexual dimorphism occurs only in the adult form. The first four legs of all stages bear unjointed, short stalks and suckers, but only the adult males have suckers on the rear legs.

## Insects

The numerous species of insects play important roles in the health of animals as vectors of disease and as irritants to the skin. Insects have a head bearing appendages and sensory organs such as antennae and simple or compound eyes. The structure of the masticatory mouthparts varies depending on the feeding habits. The thorax typically carries two pairs of wings and three pairs of legs. The abdomen is segmented and terminates in the male hypopygium or the female ovipositor. The body is encased in hard chitinous plates connected by flexible membranes. The life cycles of insects may be direct development, incomplete metamorphosis or complete metamorphosis. In the first type the newly hatched insect is a small replica of the adult. Incomplete metamorphosis occurs in primitive insects and the larvae differ from adults in size, proportion and lack of wings. Complete metamorphosis is found in more specialized species, the worm-like larvae differing from the adult in feeding habits. After several molts it pupates and emerges as an adult. The larvae and pupa possess characteristic hairs, bristles and appendages which are of taxonomic importance. The duration of adult pupal and larval stages varies with the species and the environment.

**Phthiraptera (Lice).** These are small degenerate, dorsoventrally flattened, wingless insects which do not undergo true metamorphosis. The eyes are reduced or absent and each leg bears one or two claws. There is one pair of spiracles on the mesothorax and usually six pairs on the abdomen. Lice are host-specific and spend their entire life on their host. They survive only a few days if separated. Lice are spread by direct contact or by contaminated brushes and combs. The operculated, white eggs (nits) are cemented to the hairs of the host. The nymph hatches from the egg, undergoes three ecdyses (molting) and becomes the adult (Fig. 11:16). The entire cycle takes 14 to 21 days.

Lice are divided into two suborders, anoplura or sucking lice and Mallophaga or biting lice.

ANOPLURA. These have mouthparts adapted for sucking the blood of the host. With heavy infestations they produce sufficient anemia to produce weakness, and some animals become distraught and ill-tempered because of the chronic irritation. The only species found commonly on dogs is *Linognathus setosus* (Figs. 11:17*A* and *B*, 11:18*C*).

MALLOPHAGA. These so-called biting lice feed on epithelial debris and hair but some species also have mouthparts adapted for drawing blood from their hosts. Since they are very active they may cause more irritation than sucking lice, and rubbing by the host may cause alopecia. *Trichodectes canis* (Fig. 11:18*A*) is the common biting louse of dogs. It may act as the intermediate host of the dog tapeworm, *D. caninum*. *Felicola subrostratus* infests cats (Fig. 11:19). *Heterodoxus spiniger* may be found on dogs in warm climates only (Fig. 11:18*B*).

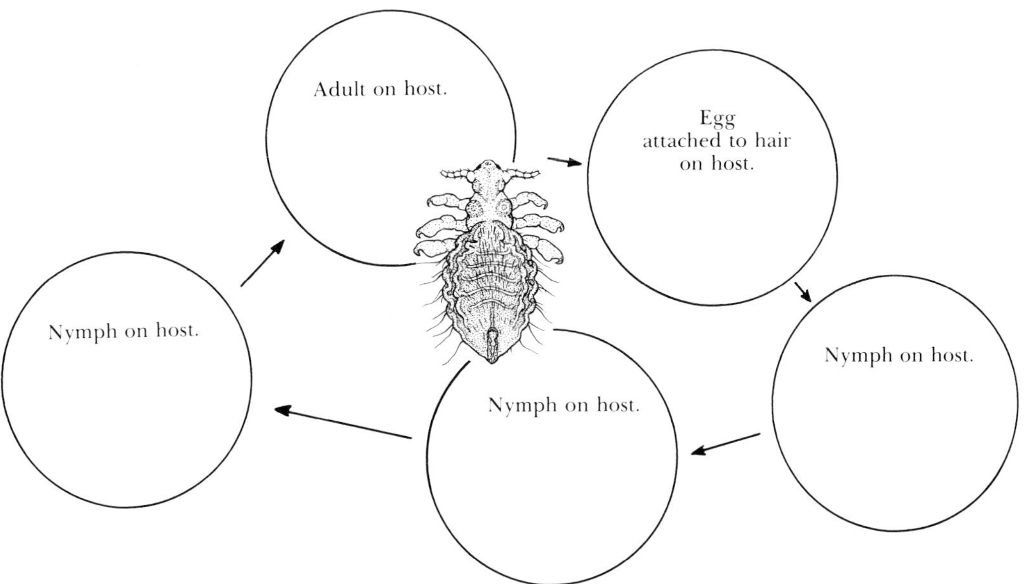


**Figure 11:16.** Life cycle of the louse (14–21 days).

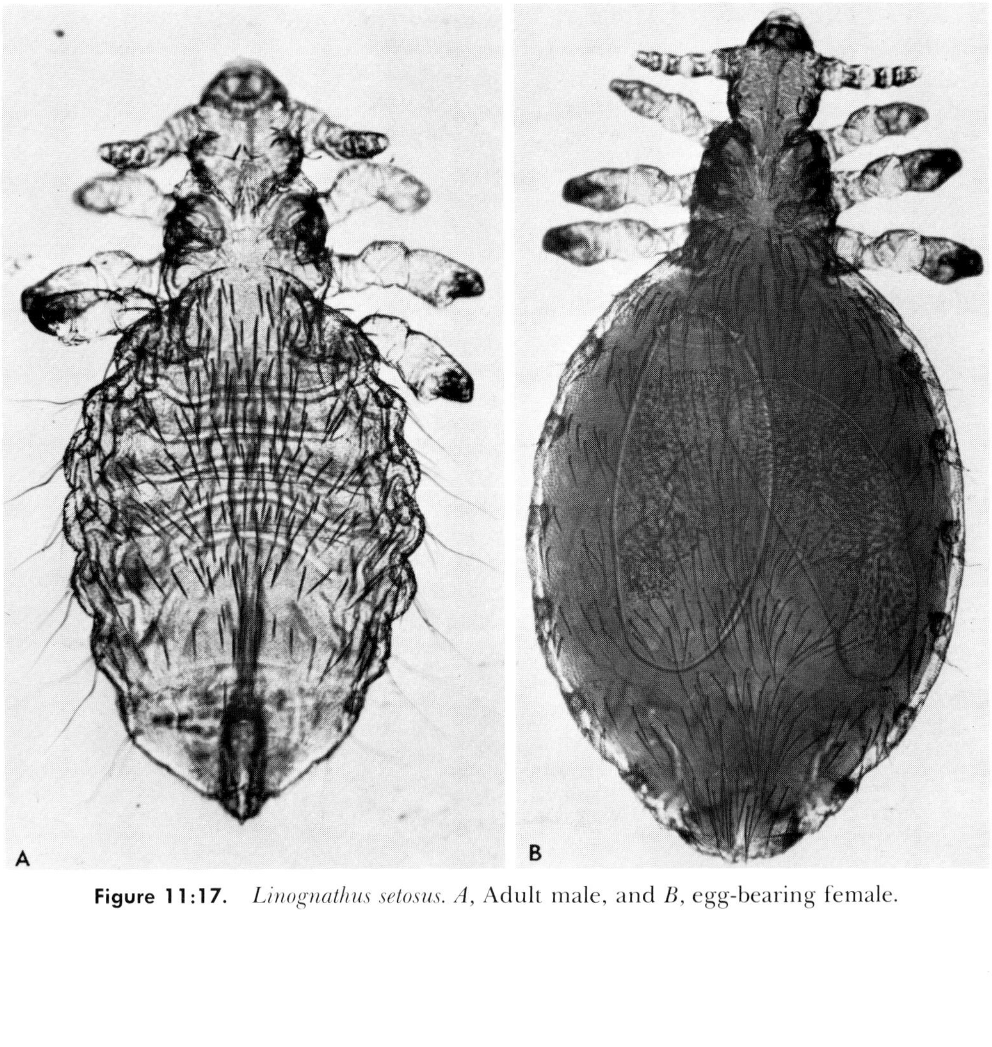

**Figure 11:17.** *Linognathus setosus. A,* Adult male, and *B,* egg-bearing female.

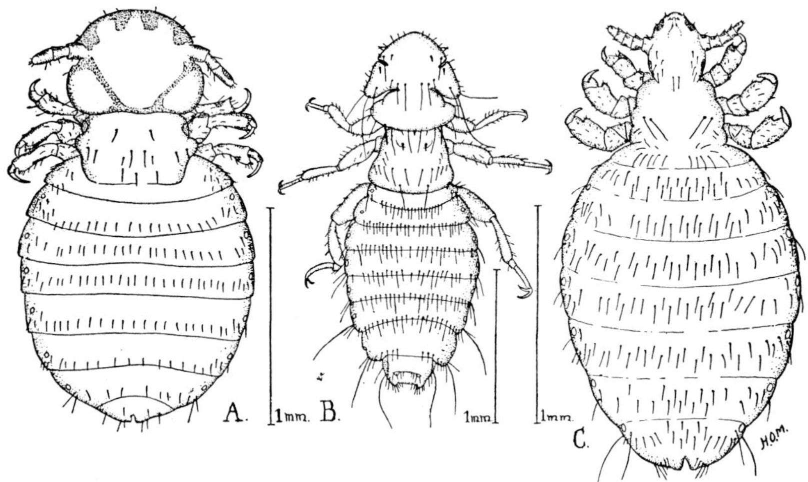


**Figure 11:18.** Dog lice. *A, Trichodectes canis; B, Heterodoxus spiniger; C, Linognathus setosus.* (From Monnig: *Veterinary Helminthology and Entomology.* Williams & Wilkins, Baltimore, 1962.)

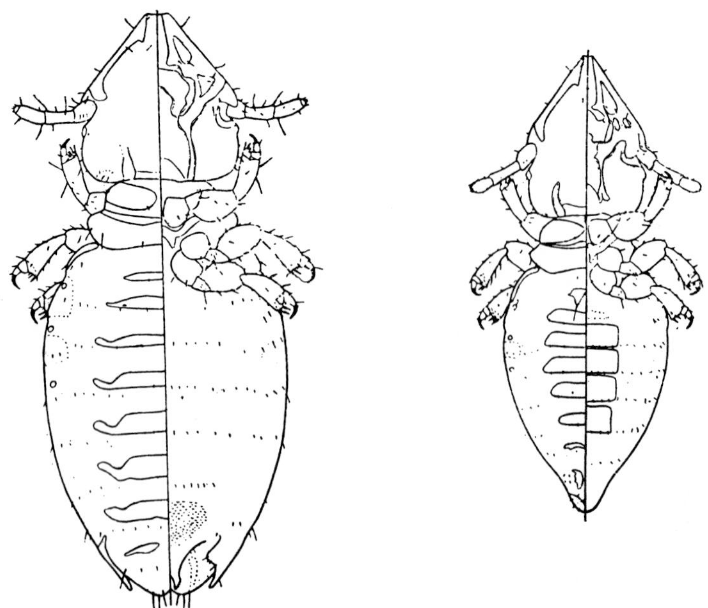

**Figure 11:19.** *Felicola (Trichodectes) subrostratus.* Female on the left, male on the right. (From Lapage: *Veterinary Parasitology,* 2nd ed. Charles C Thomas, Springfield, Ill., 1967.)

**Siphonaptera (Fleas).** Fleas are bloodsucking ectoparasites that feed sporadically on mammals and birds.

Fleas spend most of their life cycle off the host.

Fleas are small, brown, wingless insects with laterally compressed bodies (Fig. 11:20). Males are smaller than females, and the chitinous head bears antennae, eyes, combs and suctorial mouthparts (Fig. 11:21). The prothoracic and genal combs are useful taxonomically. Each segment of the three-sectioned thorax bears a pair of powerful legs terminating in two curved claws. This structure adapts fleas for powerful jumping which enables them to transfer from host to host.

Fleas develop by complete metamorphosis. The eggs, which are ovoid, white and glistening, are laid on the premises in cracks of buildings or on damp ground (Figs. 11:22 and 34:1*D*). Those which are laid on the host soon fall off. The female lays only three to 18 eggs at one time, but with frequent blood meals and frequent copulation she may lay several hundred over her life span of one year. Adult fleas separated from the host live only one to two months. Fleas do not live at altitudes higher than 5000 feet. They lay more eggs when the temperature reaches the range of 65° F. to 80° F., and when the humidity is high (70 per cent). After incubation of two to 12 days the egg hatches into the larva—an active white bristled worm with chewing mouthparts (Fig. 11:23). They ingest

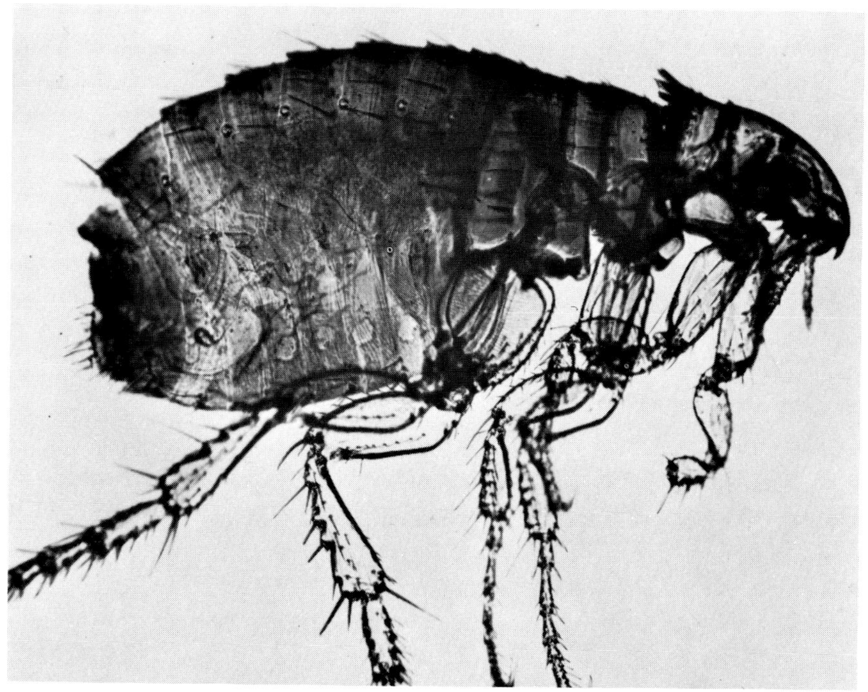

**Figure 11:20.** *Ctenocephalides felis*, adult.

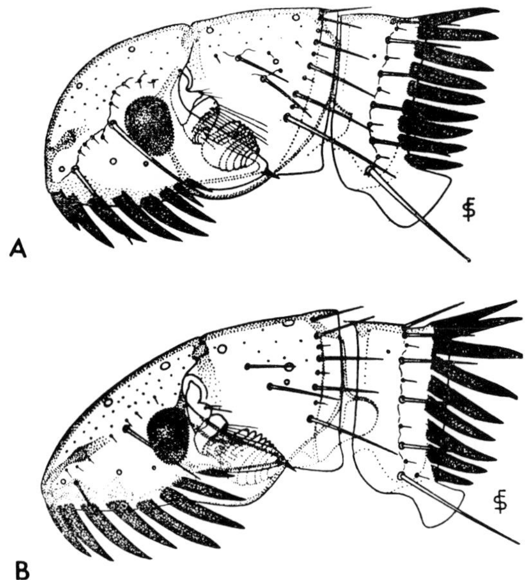


**Figure 11:21.** *A, Ctenocephalides canis.* Female. Head and pronotum, showing one of the antennae and the genal and pronotal combs. *B, Ctenocephalides felis felis.* Female. Head and pronotum, showing one of the antennae and the genal and pronotal combs. (From Lapage: *Veterinary Parasitology,* 2nd. ed. Charles C Thomas, Springfield, Ill., 1967.)

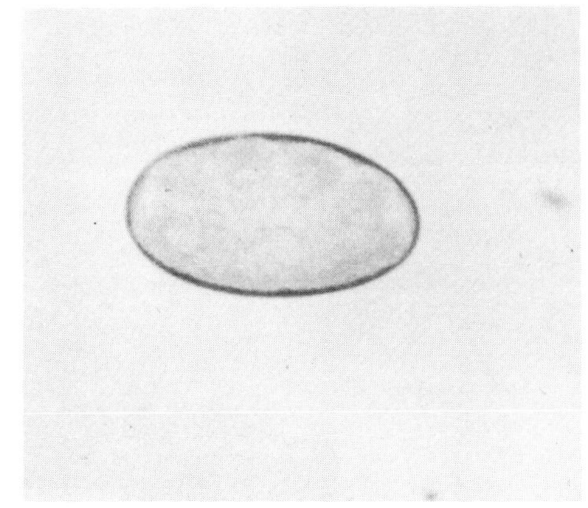

**Figure 11:22.** *Ctenocephalides felis*, egg.

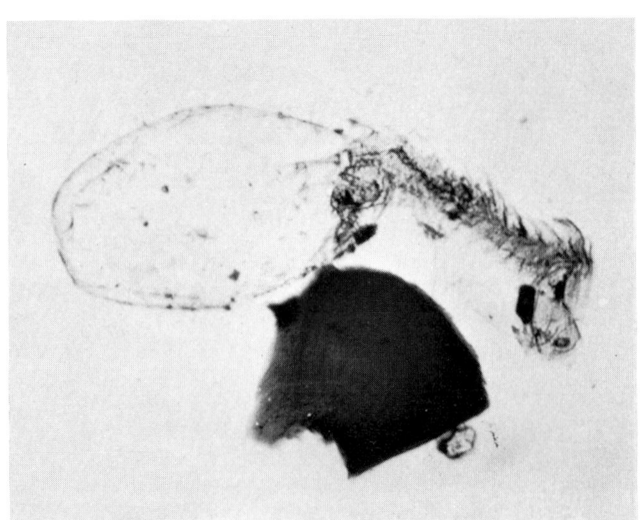

**Figure 11:23.** *Ctenocephalides felis*, larva emerging from egg. Dark mass is adult flea's fecal cast to be used as larval food.

fecal casts from adult fleas and thus may develop a reddish tinge. The posterior end has two hooked processes called anal struts which are used for locomotion. These distinguish a flea larva from that of a dipterous insect. Larvae grow and molt twice over a period of nine to 200 days. The third molt produces an opaque white larva which becomes quiescent and spins a loose whitish gray cocoon, inside which it pupates for seven days to one year. The adult flea breaks out of the cocoon and looks for a host on which to feed (Fig. 11:24).

ECHIDNOPHAGA GALLINACEA (Fig. 11:25). The sticktight poultry flea is found in warm climates. It also attacks dogs and cats. Adult fleas of the species are active at first but during copulation the female attaches herself to the skin of the host's face. She does not move rapidly but burrows into the skin and forms an ulcerated nodule in which she lays her eggs. The eggs hatch on the host but the larvae fall off and the life cycle of about one month is completed as described for other fleas.

Fleas produce severe skin irritation because of their frequent bites. The itching induces self-mutilation by the host. Flea saliva is highly antigenic in some individuals and produces an allergic dermatitis (see p. 287). Fleas may be mechanical vectors of many diseases and are important vectors of Pasteurella infections. The cat and dog fleas *(C. canis* and *C. felis)* also are intermediate host of the dog tapeworm *(Diplidium caninum)*. The sticktight flea produces special skin lesions of the face in addition to the effects mentioned above.

Without question, *C. felis* is the common flea of dogs and cats, with *C. canis* being found only occasionally. Sticktight fleas are rare. The human flea *Pulex irritans* and the rat flea, *Leptosylla segnis* may also attack dogs, cats and man. Some people are more susceptible to fleabites than others, and bites on man tend to be focused on the lower legs and trunk. The lesions are multiple red papules which are intensely pruritic.

FLEA CONTROL. Because fleas spend only short periods on their host the

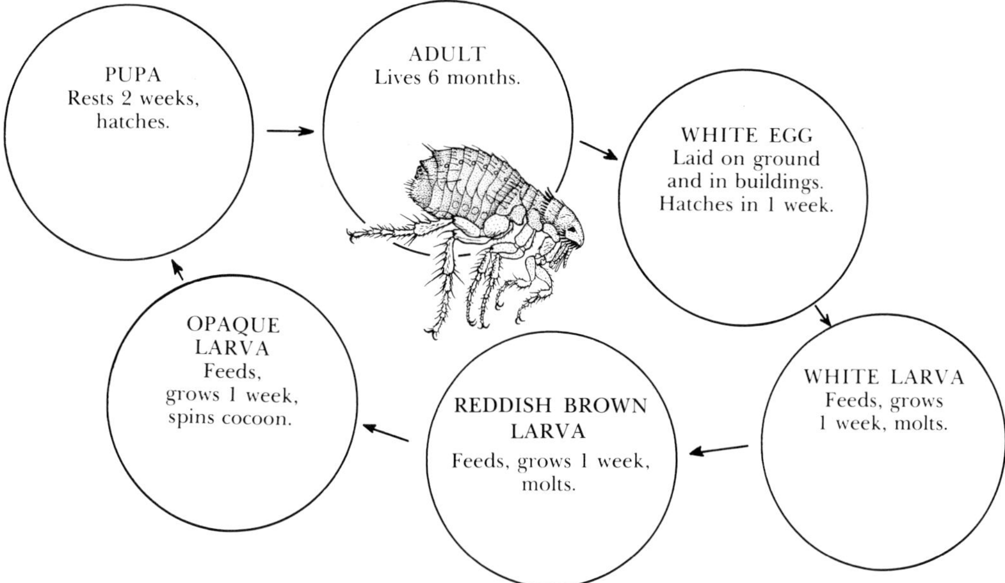


**Figure 11:24.** Life cycle of *Ctenocephalides felis* (three weeks to two years).

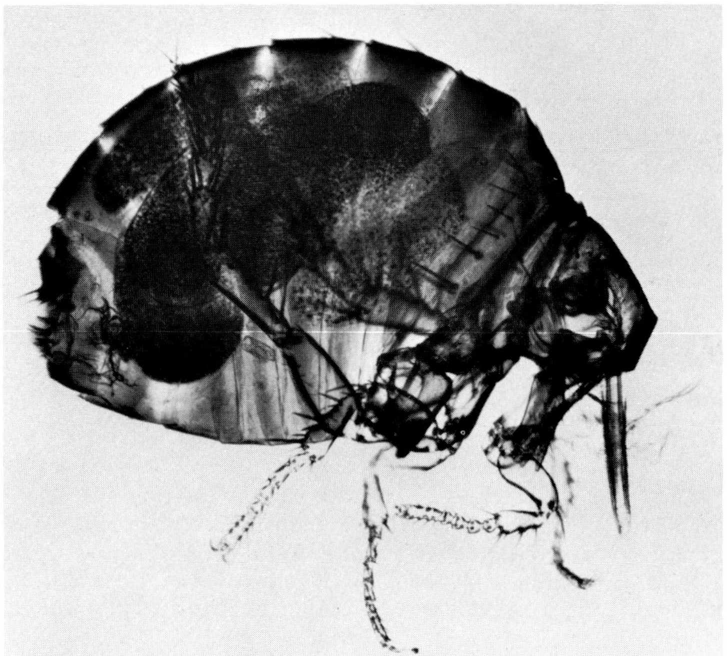

**Figure 11:25.** *Echidnophaga gallinacea* (sticktight flea), adult.

major effort for flea control must be directed to the premises where the eggs, larvae, pupae and some adults congregate. Damp, cool floors, especially those of dirt, sand or concrete, and cracks and crevices are favorite areas for flea development.

Because some stages of the life cycle may persist for months, treatments must be residual in effect or repeated periodically. Lindane .5 per cent spray or 1 per cent dust, chlordane 2 per cent or 0.25 per cent dichlorovinyl dimethyl phosphate (DDVP) sprays can be used effectively. Products used in the home should be tested for possible staining before application. Thorough vacuum cleaning with special attention to cracks, corners, rugs and upholstery is helpful if the contents of the cleaner are carefully burned afterward. In severe infestations one should secure a professional exterminator to treat the premises.

Elimination of fleas from animal hosts should coincide with treatment of the premises. Chlordane 0.5 per cent and malathion 0.25 per cent in sprays or powders can be used on dogs. Only 2 per cent methoxychlor, 1 per cent pyrethrin or 1 per cent carbaryl powders should be used on cats. Malathion 0.25 per cent spray may be safe for adult cats. Usually these treatments follow an initial bath with KFL shampoo, Seleen or Thionum with lindane. The powder or spray should be applied to the host every four days, and treatment of the premises should be repeated every two weeks. Flea collars containing DDVP may be helpful if the animal is not sensitive to the collar and develops a contact dermatitis (up to 10 per cent of cases).

**Diptera (flies).** Medically, flies form a most important order of arthropods, as they transmit or are intermediate hosts for many bacterial, viral, protozoan and helminth disease agents. However, their effects on skin are minor and are limited to bites (mosquitos, stable flies and deer flies) and to myiasis.

The reaction to insect bites varies, since some individuals are less attractive or less susceptible to certain flies. The local lesion is a sensitivity reaction that may become less severe with repeated exposures. The systemic reaction to injected antigen, however, often increases with repeated exposures (bees and fleas).

The primary lesion is a wheal or papule around a bleeding point. The reaction may be transient or persist for weeks. In the latter case a pseudoepitheliomatous hyperplasia develops, with scaling and alopecia. A dermal infiltrate of eosinophils, plasma cells and lymphocytes may be present.

CUTEREBRA MACULATA. The larval form of Cuterebra is a large (3/4 inch) "grub" which is found singly or in pairs in large subcutaneous pockets. The larva must have air so the cyst-like structures communicate to the surface by a fistula. The egg is laid in the soil, so the larva probably penetrates the host's skin directly. It parasitizes very young kittens, and puppies of breeds with a very dense hair coat, and many wild rodents. The seasonal incidence is July, August and September, but details of the life cycle are largely unknown.

Treatment involves incising or spreading the fistulous opening and extracting the "grub" by means of a mosquito forceps. Care should be taken to avoid crushing the larva as retained parts may produce allergic reactions. The infected wound should be treated but, even so, healing will be slow.

MYIASIS. The adult forms of many dipterous flies place eggs on the wet, warm skin of debilitated, weakened animals with draining wounds or urine-soaked coats. However, the attractive animals are not equally attractive at all stages to all flies. As the skin breaks down and liquefies it becomes attractive to other flies, and in some cases the initial larval infestation modifies the habitat to further attract a second or third species. Calliphorids (blow flies) and sarcophagids (flesh flies) are most common in small animal myiasis. True screw-worms, *Cochliomyia hominovorax*, have been eliminated from large areas of North America. They are obligate parasites of living tissue and never were common in dogs and cats. Specific identification is not important to the treatment of most myiasis cases. However, larvae can be kept until adult flies develop; or the posterior aspect of the larvae examined for posterior spiracles and stigmal plates which are taxonomically significant.

The larvae found in cutaneous myiasis are highly destructive and produce lesions over extensive areas with "punched out" round holes in the skin. These may coalesce to form broad defects with scalloped margins. The larvae may be found under the skin and in the tissues. Favorite locations are around the nose, eyes, mouth, anus and genitalia, or adjacent to neglected wounds. Myiasis is always a disease of neglect.

Treatment requires clipping hair away from the lesions and cleaning them with pHisoHex. The larvae must be meticulously removed from deep crevices and from under the skin. Nitrofurazone or other topical antibiotics should be applied to the wound and the rest of the animal's coat sprayed with 0.25 per cent malathion. Daily routine wound care is necessary and the patient should be housed in screened, fly-free quarters.

**Hymenoptera (Bees, Wasps, Hornets).** These venenating insects are not parasitic. They possess membranous wings and mouthparts for chewing, sucking or licking. The ovipositor of the female is adapted for stinging. She has paired venom glands which express a toxin during the sting. When bees and certain wasps sting, the tip of the abdomen and the whole poison apparatus breaks off and remains in the wound. The gland may continue to express poison, so the "stinger" should be removed from a bite as soon as possible. Other wasps and hornets may sting repeatedly as they remain intact. Local redness, edema and inflammation soon develop, and in some animals severe anaphylaxis. If cardiac and respiratory impairment result the patient may die.

The stinger should be removed if it can be located. In severe cases with urticaria, epinephrine should be given intramuscularly. With anaphylaxis, large doses of prednisolone and a rapid-acting antihistamine should be administered systemically. Hot compresses may relieve local pain. Subsequent bites or multiple bites make the reaction more severe.

## References

Baker, D. W.: Personal communication. 1968.

Belding, D. L.: *Textbook of Parasitology, 3rd edit.* Appleton-Century-Crofts, New York, 1965.

Brown, H. S., and Belding, D. L.: *Basic Clinical Parasitology, 2nd edit.* Appleton-Century-Crofts, New York, 1958.

Coles, E.: *Veterinary Clinical Pathology.* W. B. Saunders Co., Philadelphia, 1967.

Ewing, S. A.: Personal communication, 1968.

*Georgi, J. R.: *Parasitology for Veterinarians.* W. B. Saunders Co., Philadelphia, 1969.

Jubb, K. V. F., and Kennedy, P. C.: *Pathology of Domestic Animals.* Academic Press, New York, 1963.

*Lapage, G.: *Monnigs' Veterinary Helminthology and Entomology, 5th ed.* Williams & Wilkins Co., Baltimore, 1962.

*Lapage, G.: *Veterinary Parasitology,* Charles C Thomas, Springfield, Ill. 1956.

Nutting, W. B.: Studies on the Genus Demodex, Owen. Ph.D. thesis, Cornell University, 1950.

Sweatman, G. K.: Biology of *Otodectes cyanotis* the ear canker mite of Carnivora. Canadian J. Zool. *36*:849, 1958.

---

*Suggested supplemental reading.

# TWELVE

# *Dermatologic Allergy*

Skin diseases of allergic origin not only make up a large percentage of the dermatoses seen in small animal practice but are also among the most trying cases. The accompanying pruritus causes discomfort to the animal and annoyance to the owner. The veterinarian faces the problems of establishing the diagnosis, finding the offending allergen and providing relief from severe itching. A sound understanding of the basic principles of dermatologic allergy is therefore very helpful.

> Allergic skin diseases are among the most difficult to handle successfully.

Allergy is traditionally defined as a specific, acquired, and altered capacity to react to a foreign substance. This definition is more difficult to understand than the clinical manifestations. The "altered capacity to react" means that the body has produced a substance called an antibody, which reacts with a specific exogenous agent called an antigen to produce a reaction of tissue cells called an antigen-antibody reaction which is the basic mechanism of allergy.

Defining and understanding of the following terms is necessary: hypersensitivity, immunity, antigens, antibodies, immediate or delayed reaction, sensitization or hypersensitization, contact dermatitis and atopy. These terms are defined in the subsequent discussion of this chapter. In veterinary practice, such an understanding will prevent allergic dermatitis from degenerating into the "catchall" term that has been the fate of eczema.

## ALLERGY AND IMMUNITY

Allergy and immunity are closely related. The antigen-antibody reaction is a basic principle of both. In allergy the tissue reactivity is increased in such a way that the sensitization which is produced is harmful to the body. In immunity, however, the antigen-antibody reaction serves to protect the body from disease mechanisms. One might speculate, therefore, that allergic hypersensitivity is in reality an immune reaction that has been channeled to harm rather than help.

## ANTIGENS (ALLERGENS)

An antigen is any substance that stimulates antibody production when introduced into animal tissues. There are hundreds of environmental antigens, called allergens, which are capable of producing antibody formation. Some animals are more likely to develop allergy than others. When they are exposed to an antigen for the first time they develop antibodies to it. After a suitable induction period they will react to subsequent exposure to the same antigen. The interaction of antigen with antibody is an allergic reaction. Animals which are not sensitized in this manner, do not react to these antigens, and thus are not allergic.

Antigens in immediate reactions differ from those in delayed reactions. Immediate antigens are complex proteins of high molecular weight, produced by plasma cells which are circulating in the bloodstream. They can be transferred to other animals by serum injections. Delayed antigens are simple chemicals of low molecular weight that alone are not capable of producing allergy. They must combine with skin protein to form a complex which acts on lymphocytes to produce sensitized lymphocytes.

## ANTIBODIES

Antibodies are formed through exogenous stimulation by an antigen. Antibody formation occurs more easily in allergically predisposed animals. When such an animal is exposed to an antigen for the first time, it may develop antibodies to it. These antibodies will make it allergic to that antigen by a process called sensitization. The antibodies produced as a result of exposure to the antigen are highly specific for that antigen.

Antibodies found in immediate reactions are globulin fractions formed by plasma cells which circulate in the blood and can be transferred by serum injections. The antibody mechanism of delayed reactions is not understood. However, it is possible to transfer delayed hypersensitivity by transfusion of large numbers of viable lymphocytes.

## ANTIGEN-ANTIBODY REACTION

When an animal with antibodies for a specific antigen is exposed to that antigen, a reaction of tissue cells occurs and an allergic reaction results. (Fig. 12:1*A*) In a nonallergic animal antibodies do not form and no sensitization takes place (Fig. 12:1*B*).

### Immediate Reaction

The immediate type of allergic reaction develops in a few seconds or a few minutes from the time of exposure to an antigen. Seasonal pollinosis in dogs is an example of an immediate reaction in which there may be sneezing as well as pruritus. When the reaction involves the skin, there is usually erythema, whealing or urticaria. Anaphylactic shock, though rare in dogs, is a manifes-

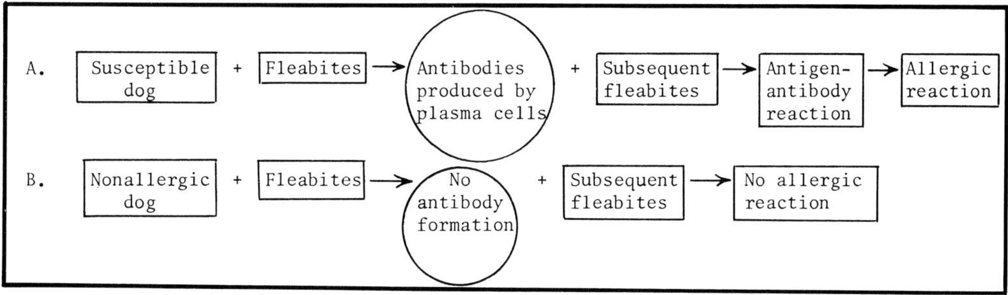


**Figure 12:1.** Susceptibility to allergy. In *A*, the dog acquired antibodies during the sensitization phase. This made it sensitive to flea saliva. When this dog was subsequently bitten by fleas and thereby exposed to a challenging dose of antigen, the antigen-antibody reaction was provoked. As a result of this sensitization, a later exposure caused allergic symptoms and lesions. Subsequent exposures compound the reaction and make it more severe. Further discussion of flea allergy dermatitis is found on page 287.

tation of an immediate reaction which can be fatal. It can occur in dogs hypersensitized to bee venom. In immediate reactions the sensitization occurs in "shock tissues," such as smooth muscle of blood vessels and bronchioles, mucus-secreting cells and mast cells. This is mediated by serotonin, histamine and other kinins. In the dog the shock organ is the liver, which reacts with severe vascular spasm (Fig. 12:2).

In the immediate reaction type of allergy, antigen-antibody complexes cause enzymatic degranulation of basophils and mast cells with the liberation of vasoactive amines. These amines cause increased permeability of capillaries through their action on the endothelial cells of blood vessels, and act on smooth muscle to produce spasm. Local tissue involvement causes inflammatory changes in blood vessel walls and finally breakdown of the antigen-antibody complexes. Histamine and serotonin, two of the amines involved, vary in their importance as etiologic agents in different species. Antihistamines protect against histamine effects, while the anti-serotonin compounds and cortisone block the serotonin effect. Acetylcholine, heparin, bradykinin and slow reacting substance are other agents which may play a role in immediate response allergic reactions.

### Delayed Reaction

In contrast to the immediate type, the delayed hypersensitivity results from the reaction of sensitized lymphocytes to the antigen without histamine release. For this reason antihistamines are without benefit in treatment of this type of allergic reaction (Fig. 12:3).

## ALLERGIC CONTACT DERMATITIS

Allergic contact dermatitis is always a delayed-reaction hypersensitivity. It results when the skin, which has previously been sensitized by an allergen (antigen), comes in contact with the same allergen again. The incubation period is the time from the initial sensitizing exposure to the allergen to the time of capa-

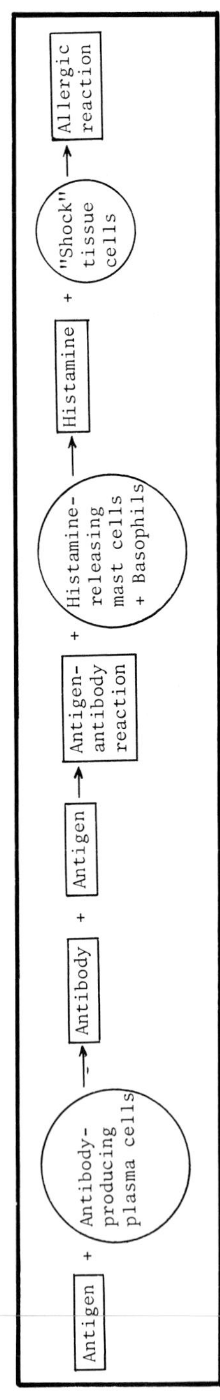


**Figure 12:2.** Immediate reaction.

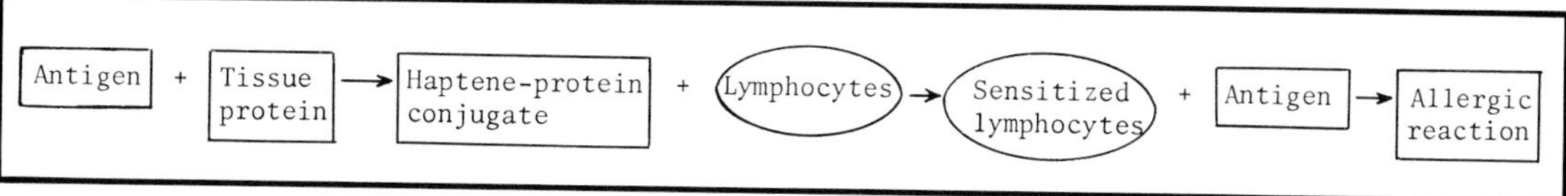


**Figure 12:3.** Delayed reaction. The delayed type of reaction occurs several hours to several days later. Allergic contact dermatitis is an example of the delayed type. The reaction of the skin consists of erythema, papule formation and pruritus.

bility of hypersensitivity reaction. This period varies from five to 21 days (Fisher, 1967). After this incubation period, the skin is ready to respond with allergic reactions to challenge by a contactant (allergen). The skin may remain sensitized from a few weeks in some animals to the entire life span in other individuals. Antibody formation has not been proved in allergic contact dermatitis. The hypersensitivity develops in the lymphoid cells where the antigens are concentrated. Large lymphocytes are produced that spread throughout the body and sensitize the skin to the antigen.

## Clinical Disease in Dogs

Susceptible dogs exposed to contact allergens experience a delayed type of hypersensitivity that results in allergic contact dermatitis. Although individuals of many breeds may become affected, it seems to be prevalent in wirehaired fox terriers, Scottish terriers, and French poodles. Contact dermatitis is one of the more troublesome canine skin diseases, and it frequently becomes a chronic problem. Intense pruritus causes complications of self-inflicted trauma. The difficult task of discovering and eliminating offending contactants depends on careful examination of the environment of the dog. A clinical description of a typical case is given on page 238. It should be noted that hyposensitizing injections are rarely effective as a means of controlling allergic contact dermatitis.

Intradermal allergy testing fails to diagnose contact allergens, and hyposensitizing injections are ineffective for controlling allergic contact dermatitis.

## Contact Allergens

Fisher (1967) lists numerous substances which are capable of causing allergic contact dermatitis in man. Animals do not contact as many allergens as man. Intradermal allergy testing is not indicated for diagnosis of contact allergens. Although patch testing is more reliable, too little testing has been done in dogs to really evaluate the problem.

Diagnoses have been circumstantial, and have depended on careful observation and elimination of suspected substances—one at a time. Sometimes initial exposure to likely allergens has produced characteristic lesions, giving some measure of proof. There have been reports of allergic contact dermatitis caused by leather harnesses, grasses, jasmine, lanolin, insect powders, collars and sprays, petrolatum, paint, fabrics, wool and fiber carpets, poison oak, rubber, and wood preservatives (Muller, 1967).

## ATOPIC DERMATITIS

Atopy is a hereditary allergic state characterized by pruritus, chewing at the feet, sneezing and lacrimation. Atopic dermatitis is an intensely pruritic, chronic skin disorder that occurs in animals with a predisposition to the condition. Characteristically, dogs scratch and rub their face, lick their feet, and show generalized pruritus. Criep (1967) reports that 10 per cent of the human population is atopic. Judging from the number of clinical cases of canine atopy, it is reasonable to assume that a large number of dogs are atopic too.

Atopy is an immediate type of hypersensitivity. Atopic dermatitis involves antibodies that have a special affinity for the skin and are called "skin sensitizing" antibodies. The principle characteristics of atopic dermatitis are:

1. It begins at a young age, usually by the time a dog is one year old.
2. The course is chronic.
3. Pruritus is always present.
4. Self-inflicted trauma results from the scratching.
5. Face rubbing and feet biting are common findings.
6. Seasonal recurrences are common (ragweed and other conditions).
7. There is a breed predilection for wire-haired fox terriers, Scottish terriers, Dalmatians and poodles.

Clinical manifestations and treatment of atopic dermatitis are described on page 234. Flea allergy dermatitis is described on page 287 and contact dermatitis on page 238.

More information has been collected recently about allergic dermatoses of animals. Previously, eczema became a "catchall" term for many pruritic skin disorders, especially atopic dermatitis.

At this point it may be possible to clarify the term eczema (Gr., "boiling over"), which has caused great confusion to veterinarians and dog owners. Before the word eczema was removed from the standard dermatologic nomenclature of the American Animal Hospital Association, the meaning fell somewhere between contact dermatitis, atopic dermatitis and allergic dermatitis. The morphology of atopic dermatitis is inflammatory in character but so is the morphology of allergic contact dermatitis. In retrospect, it becomes clear that the enigma that arose around eczema could hardly have been avoided, since atopy in dogs has only recently been recognized (Patterson et al., 1963; Schwartzman, 1965), and contact dermatitis is just now being defined in animals (Walton, 1965; Muller, 1967). Now, however, the terms eczema and eczematous dermatitis should be eliminated and such pruritic dermatoses should be more specifically placed into one of the following groups: atopic dermatitis, allergic contact dermatitis, or allergic dermatitis (fleas, pollen and similar causes).

## *References*

Allergy and Hypersensitivity, Basic Systems, Inc. Charles Pfizer & Co.

*Criep, Leo H.: *Dermatologic Allergy.* W. B. Saunders Co., Philadelphia, 1967.

Dermatology Committee Report, American Animal Hospital Association Committee Reports, Elkhart, Indiana, 1960.

*Fisher, A. A.: *Contact Dermatitis.* Lea & Febiger, Philadelphia, 1967.

Muller, G. H.: Contact Dermatitis, Arch. Derm. 96, Oct., 1967.

Patterson, R., Chang, W. W. Y., and Pruzansky, J. J.: The Northwestern University Colony of Atopic Dogs, J. Allergy. *34*: 455-459, 1963.

Schwartzman, R. M.: Atopy in the Dog, in: Rook, A. J., and Walton, G. S.: *Comparative Physiology and Pathology of the Skin.* F. A. Davis Co., Philadelphia, 1965.

Walton, G. S.: Contact Dermatitis in Domestic Animals, in: Rook, A. J., and Walton, G. S.: *Comparative Physiology and Pathology of the Skin.* F. A. Davis Co., Philadelphia, 1965.

---

*Suggested supplemental reading.

# THIRTEEN

# *Endocrine Imbalance*

Many hormones affect the skin and adnexa. Although this chapter is limited to endocrine influences on canine and feline skin, it must be remembered that hormones also have vital effects on the rest of the body. Small animal clinicians frequently see animals exhibiting skin changes caused by hormonal imbalance. Since partial or complete hair loss is common with these disorders, adequate treatment may improve their appearance dramatically. It is often difficult to determine the endocrine disorder responsible for such changes, for only a few laboratory tests for evaluation of endocrine function have thus far been standardized for dogs and cats. The effect of the major endocrine glands on the skin is further complicated by physiologic relations that exist between the pituitary and its dependent end-organs (Fig. 13:1). Hypothalamic signals, trophic homones, feedback systems and interactions between the individual endocrine glands present additional complexities.

Clinically, bilaterally symmetrical alopecia is usually the first noticeable sign of a hormonal dermatosis. Some endocrine abnormalities delay or stop anagen, and alopecia results when hairs in telogen are lost naturally by friction. In hypothyroid dogs, for instance, the telogen hairs can be easily epilated, but replacement does not occur unless the imbalance is corrected by renewed thyroid output or by supplemental thyroid administration.

Bilaterally symmetrical melanin pigment deposits accompany a few endocrine diseases. Axillary hyperpigmentation characterizes acanthosis nigricans (Fig. 20:1), just as gray pigmentation of the male genital area is highly suggestive of the male feminizing syndrome (Fig. 37:1).

Primary pruritus is not common in endocrine dermatosis; however, there may be itching caused by secondary bacterial infection, crusting or cutaneous calcinosis. At no time is such pruritus as severe or as prolonged as in cutaneous allergies.

Useful characteristics associated with endocrine disease are:

1. Bilaterally symmetrical alopecia;
2. Bilaterally symmetrical hyperpigmentation;
3. Lack of pruritus;
4. Chronic course.

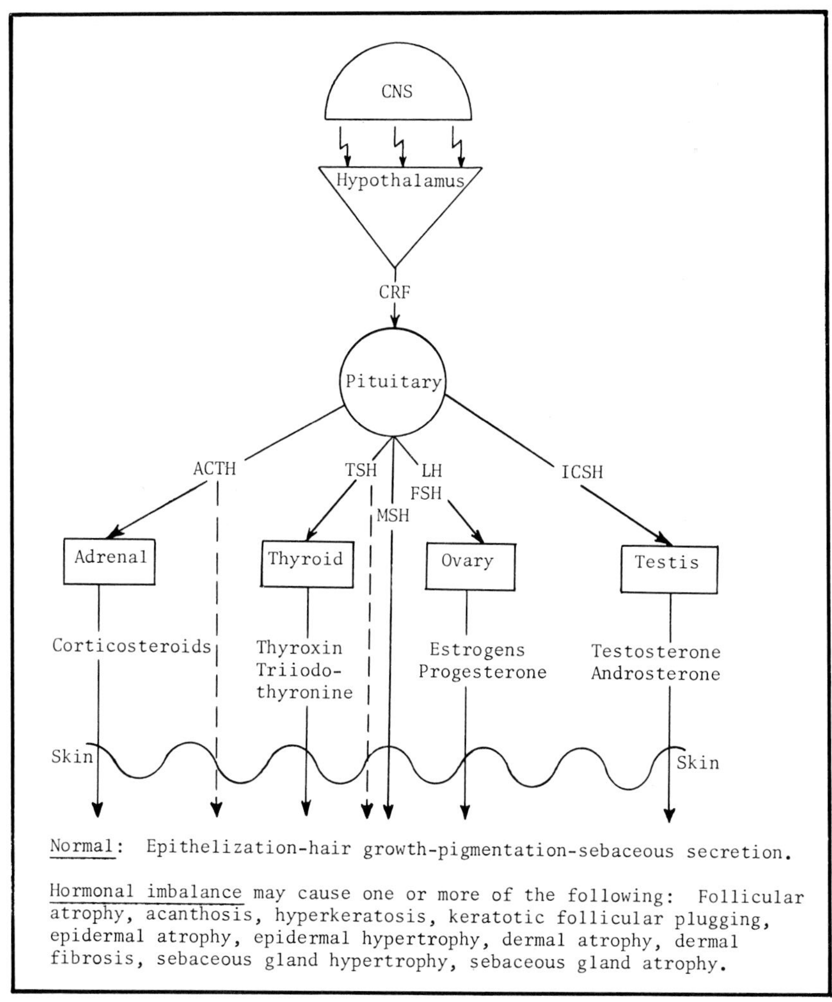


**Figure 13:1.** Endocrine influences on canine skin.

In addition to the four characteristic findings just listed, other secondary lesions may accompany hormonal dermatoses. Excess scaling and "greasiness" is a constant finding in acanthosis nigricans, the feminizing syndrome and certain ovarian imbalances. Ceruminous otitis externa may also accompany these conditions. A dry lusterless coat is found in such diseases as hypothyroidism and hyperadrenocorticism. Comedones form rapidly in conditions where increased androgenic or corticosteroid hormones may be present. Apocrine hyperhidrosis is a frequent finding in gonadal and pituitary imbalance. As endocrine dermatoses become chronic, it is common to see areas of epidermal hyperplasia (acanthosis) and plaques of lichenification.

The progress of an endocrine disease with cutaneous manifestation is usually chronic. As a rule, the disorder will develop slowly, gradually becoming more severe until it reaches a chronic stage. Endocrine diseases usually afflict the individual dog for the rest of its life, and hyperadrenocorticism may terminate fatally after running a course of many years.

The histopathologic skin changes produced by endocrine diseases may include follicular atrophy, acanthosis, hyperkeratosis, keratotic follicular plugging, epidermal atrophy, epidermal hypertrophy, dermal atrophy, dermal edema, dermal fibrosis, sebaceous gland atrophy, apocrine hidradenitis and calcinosis cutis. One or several of these changes may be present in a single disease.

Only those endocrine glands that have the greatest influence on the health and disease of the skin will be considered here. They are the pituitary gland, thyroid gland, adrenal gland, testes and ovary.

The parathyroids, thymus, islets of Langerhans of the pancreas and the pineal body will not be considered because we know little of the effects of their hormones upon the skin.

## THE PITUITARY GLAND (HYPOPHYSIS)

The anterior lobe of the pituitary gland has been called the "master gland," a term it deserves because it secretes trophic hormones which control many other endocrine glands. In the dog and cat it is an oval gland located at the base of the brain in the hypophyseal fossa. It is divided into the neurohypophysis and the adenohypophysis. The adenohypophysis consists of three parts: the pars tuberalis, the pars intermedia and the pars distalis. The pars distalis produces several trophic hormones which dramatically affect the skin either directly or through their effect on other endocrine glands (target glands).

The following hormones are produced by the pars distalis of the pituitary gland and influence the skin directly or indirectly:

ACTH – Adrenocorticotrophic hormone.
STH – Somatotrophic hormone.
FSH – Follicle stimulating hormone.
LH – Luteinizing hormone (female).
ICSH – Interstitial cell stimulating hormone (male).
MSH – Melanocyte stimulating hormone.
TSH – Thyroid stimulating hormone.

---

Two major skin diseases may be caused by pituitary imbalance: acanthosis nigricans (Possible TSH deficiency) and hyperadrenocorticism (so-called Cushing's disease)

---

In addition, pituitary hormones may indirectly affect the skin by their actions on target organs. Increased ACTH production causes increased cortisol production, which may cause slight hypertrophy of the skin and epilation in areas of wear. Conversely decreased ACTH is thought to cause alopecia and hyperpigmentation of the flanks and axillary areas. FSH causes a decrease in sebaceous gland activity and increased epidermal keratinization, perhaps via stimulation of estrogen production. Administration of sex hormones decreases gonadotrophic production of the adenohypophysis while castration or spaying increases its production. Genetically determined differences in the rate of secretion of growth hormones (STH) are presumably responsible for such unusual canine shapes as the achondroplastic breeds (dachshund) or the acromegalic breeds (St. Bernard). Certain skin diseases of endocrine origin, such as acanthosis nigricans, which predominate in dachshunds, might also be related to inherited differences in pituitary secretion.

A congenital hypopituitarism is sometimes, but very rarely, seen in German shepherds and puppies of other breeds. In these individuals the adenohypophysis presumably has failed to develop properly or has atrophied, and a dilated hypophyseal cavity or a cyst of Rathke's epithelium is found. Although affected pups appear to be normal at birth, they do not grow normally and are permanent dwarfs. They retain their fine "puppy hair," and later in life may develop a bilaterally symmetrical alopecia of the trunk and hind limbs. It is Belshaw's opinion that the clinical signs of some patients may be caused primarily by combined deficiencies of growth hormone (STH) and thyroid stimulating hormone (TSH), the latter resulting in secondary hypothyroidism. In other cases, gonadal and adrenocortical deficiencies may also be involved, but their relative importance in the clinical manifestations of the disorder has not been defined.

Pituitary tumors may result in dermatologic problems resulting from secondary hypothyroidism or hyperadrenocorticism, which they sometimes cause. Compression of the pars distalis by the tumor results in hypopituitarism, and hypothyroidism is usually its first clinically apparent effect. There is presumptive evidence that certain pituitary tumors (usually chromophobe tumors) may cause some cases of hyperadrenocorticism via excessive and uncontrolled secretion of ACTH. Pituitary tumors are usually the chromophobe cell type, or tumors of the pars intermedia; basophil and acidophil cell tumors are rare in the dog.

### The Feedback System

Pituitary function is controlled by chemical signals received through the blood stream and by neurologic signals from the hypothalamus. Through these two channels, the pituitary receives communications from its dependent end-organs, and a dynamic relationship exists which is called the feedback system. This complex interrelation is clearly shown by the ACTH-adrenocorticosteroid production ratio of the pituitary-adrenal axis. ACTH produced by the pituitary stimulates the production of cortisol by the adrenal cortex, and the presence of increased quantities of cortisol in the blood stream inhibits ACTH production. Cortisol, in addition, may have varying effects on TSH, FSH, LH, STH, and MSH production (Kupperman, 1963). As the target glands (testes, thyroid, adrenals) respond to the pituitary trophic hormones, they produce their own hormones which, in turn, inhibit the pituitary output of their respective trophic hormones. This is called "negative feedback control," and completes the cycle. Although the feedback control plays a major part in the normal control of target glands, both the thyroid and adrenal cortex (and possibly others) maintain a baseline level of function even in the absence of the pituitary.

## THE THYROID

The thyroid gland plays an important role in the health of the skin and in hair growth. There are two separate lobes in the dog, one on each side of the trachea in the region of the first to eighth tracheal rings. The main secretory unit of the thyroid is its follicle. It is round, lined with flat cuboid or columnar cells and has a lumen filled with fluid which contains thyroid hormone. The products of the thyroid cells are thyroxine and triiodothyronine. Hypothyroidism is one of the most common endocrine abnormalities in dogs, whereas hyperthyroidism is rare. Clinical signs of hypothyroidism are lethargy, and a tendency to obesity, even though food intake is low. The hair coat is thin, and the hairs are dry, lusterless and easily epilated. There is a tendency to bilateral alopecia. The skin is dry, rough and scaly, and occasionally hyperpigmented; the subcutaneous tissue may be doughy and indurated. A clinical description of hypothyroidism is given on page 296.

## Pituitary-Thyroid Interaction

Although the thyroid functions at very low levels after hypophysectomy, the presence of TSH is vital to normal synthesis and release of thyroxine.

The probable sequence of effects of TSH in the dog is (Rosenberg et al., 1965):

1. Stimulation of enzymatic hydrolysis of thyroglobulin resulting in a prompt increase in secretion of thyroxine and triiodothyronine, and in the release of inorganic iodide from the gland.
2. After a lag period, there is an increase in the rate of organification of iodide. As this increases, the intraglandular pool of $I^-$ decreases. This results in:
3. An increase in rate of uptake of $I^-$ from the blood.

## Thyroid Function Tests

When the clinical lesions resemble hypothyroidism, laboratory tests can be useful in confirming the diagnosis. The following tests may be helpful if performed and interpreted carefully. Choice of tests also will depend on the capabilities of laboratories readily available to the clinician.

### 1. RADIOACTIVE IODINE UPTAKE ($I^{131}$)

This test measures the thyroid uptake of radioactive iodine. The normal canine uptake is 10 to 30 per cent at 72 hours. A lower uptake indicates hypothyroidism, TSH deficiency or prior intake of large amounts of stable iodine ($I^{127}$).

### 2. PROTEIN-BOUND IODINE (PBI)

This test measures the iodine bound to plasma proteins which, under normal conditions, is chiefly iodine present in thyroid hormone bound to plasma proteins. It is essential to use a laboratory experienced in performing *canine* PBIs. Belshaw (1968) has obtained consistently good results with two laboratories.* Errors in the results of PBI can be caused by iodine contamination of glassware, or by prior administration of iodine-containing drugs and chemicals, such as anthelmintics or tincture of iodine. According to Belshaw, the PBI of normal dogs varies from 1.2 to 3.6 mcg./100 ml. with an average of 2.4 mcg./100

*Boston Medical Laboratory, Bay State Rd., Boston, Mass. 02115 and Leonard's Medical Laboratory, 4568 Mayfield Rd., Cleveland, Ohio 44121.

ml. (S. D. ±.6 mcg./100 ml.), as determined by these two laboratories. Hypothyroid dogs seldom have a PBI above 1.4 mcg.; however, the average PBI for hypothyroid dogs is 1.0 mcg./100 ml. (S. D. ±0.5 mcg./100 ml.). Bullock (1968) has found that TSH response may be a useful means of differentiating between hypothyroid and euthyroid dogs. Dogs with eventually proven hypothyroidism with an average increase of PBI of less than 0.5 mcg./100 ml., responded to a single dose of TSH whereas euthyroid dogs increased their PBI an average of 3.0 mcg./100 ml. (see TSH response test, following).

### 3. SERUM CHOLESTEROL

This test is not specific for thyroid function but serves a useful purpose because few diseases cause the high cholesterol levels found in many hypothyroid dogs. In about one-third of hypothyroid dogs, however, the serum cholesterol level is normal, so the test is not diagnostic. When it is elevated it tends to return to normal with thyroid replacement therapy. There my be occasional brief spurious elevations after the institution of adequate replacement therapy, but even so, the test may be useful in regulating the dosage of thyroid hormone.

Serum cholesterol levels may be moderately elevated in diabetes mellitus, nephrosis, hyperadrenocorticism, and in animals fed diets high in saturated fats. Normal fasting serum cholesterol levels in dogs range from 90 to 280 mg./100 ml. with 180 mg./100 ml. the average.

### 4. T-4 TEST

Preliminary testing and clinical evaluation indicate that the T-4 test may be a practical new test for measuring the thyroid function of dogs.

The T-4 test by competitive protein binding ($^{125}$T-4, TT-4, or Murphy Pattee test) measures the total serum thyroxine. In this test radioactive T-4 is displaced from thyroxine binding globulin by the addition of T-4 extracted from serum. (Kallfelz, 1969, and Murphy, 1965). Standardization is afforded by use of thyroxine standards and the results are recorded in terms of T-4 iodine. The several advantages of this assay include high sensitivity and accuracy when low T-4 levels are examined. Exogenous iodine compounds do not interfere with this test. Diphenylhydantoin (Dilantin), because of its strong selective binding to thyroxine binding globulin, can interfere and give spuriously high results.

Tentative findings from studies of dogs indicate that the normal T-4 is approximately 80 per cent of the PBI and ranges from 1.8 to 3.5 mcg. per 100 ml. (Kaneko, 1969).

### 5. TSH-RESPONSE TEST

Hypothyroidism in dogs is usually of primary origin, but it is occasionally caused by TSH deficiency (in hypopituitarism). Some aid in differentiation is provided by tests of the response to TSH administration.

Serum is collected for PBI determination followed immediately by an intramuscular injection of five to ten units of TSH (Thytropar, Armour). Twenty-four hours later, serum is again collected for PBI determination. According to Belshaw and Siegel (1968), the mean elevation in euthyroid dogs is 3.0 mcg./100 ml. above the pre-TSH value. Dogs with hypothyroidism secondary to hypopituitarism usually show a rise greater than 1.0 mcg. whereas those with primary thyroid atrophy or destruction have a response of 0.5 mcg. or less.

Response to TSH can also be measured using $I^{131}$ uptake. Control measurements are made 24, 48, and 72 hours after administration of the radioiodine tracer. TSH is then administered in doses of two to three units twice daily for two to three days followed by a single dose of five units with a second dose of radioiodine. Uptake measurements are again made at 24, 48, and 72 hours, with correction for residual radioactivity from the first tracer. Failure to significantly increase uptake following TSH indicates primary disease of the thyroid.

## THE ADRENAL GLAND

The adrenal glands of the dog and cat are small, oval structures located near the anteromedial surface of the kidney. Each gland consists of a cortex and a medulla, with each portion functionally distinct, and secreting separate hormones. The adrenals are two highly vascularized organs that secrete vital hormones. Their rich nerve supply is derived from the sympathetic system through the celiac plexus and the splanchnic nerves.

The cortex consists of three distinct zones, zona arcuata, zona fasciculata and zona reticularis. Various steroids are secreted by cells in each zone of the cortex, and several play important roles in maintaining the health of the skin and hair coat. Increase or decrease of these steroids can be responsible for producing varied cutaneous abnormalities. The corticosteroids exert a most dramatic effect on the skin. The glucocorticoids influence the skin in several ways, indirectly by regulation of blood glucose levels, protein metabolism and fat metabolism, and directly by reducing inflammation and decreasing hyperpigmentation.

The androgens, estrogens and progestogens produced by the adrenal cortex are sex steroids which theoretically could have important dermatologic effects.

### Increased Adrenocortical Production

Hyperadrenocorticism (Cushing's disease) is caused by an increased secretion of hormones by the adrenal cortex in the dog. The clinical aspects are discussed on page 292. The disease usually is caused by adrenocortical hyperplasia; less frequently by an adenoma or carcinoma of the adrenal cortex. Adrenocortical hyperplasia can theoretically occur as a primary disorder, but is probably almost always secondary to increased ACTH secretion, with or without pituitary tumor.

Adrenal hyperplasia is the most common cause in dogs. Although the patient may be presented because of hair loss, general signs are always present. They consist of polydipsia, polyuria, pendulous abdomen from muscle weakness, and lethargy.

## THE TESTES

The testes consist of an accumulation of seminiferous tubules enclosed by a fibrous membrane and a serous membrane. The tubules contain spermatogenic cells and Sertoli cells. Between lobules of tubules are interstitial cells which produce androgens.

Certain imbalances in the secretion of testicular hormones cause definite skin changes in dogs and cats. Since androgens are also produced by the adrenal glands, the testis alone cannot always be incriminated. One of the most unusual states is the feminization syndrome of male dogs. This produces a clinical picture resembling the Sertoli cell syndrome, but its exact cause is unknown. For a clinical description, see page 300.

Sertoli cell tumors of the testis (usually retained) produce feminization and skin changes consisting of alopecia, hyperpigmentation, and seborrhea. Removal of the tumor will reverse the cutaneous changes. The clinical aspects are described on page 383.

Since normal canine values for many androgenic, pituitary and adrenal hormones are not established, and since the test procedures are complex, the exact nature of some of the clinical syndromes are poorly understood.

## THE OVARY

The ovary consists of a medulla and a cortex. The medulla (zona vasculosa) contains muscles, nerves and lymphatics and does not produce hormones, whereas the cortex is the main source of female formones. Through pituitary gonadotrophic stimulation (FSH and LH) the ovary secretes estrogen and the corpus luteum secretes progesterone. Additional estrogenic hormones are secreted by the adrenal gland in both the male and female dog.

Imbalances of estrogens, both increased and decreased secretion, cause definite skin changes. Because specific tests and normal values have not been devised to assay female hormones of dogs and cats, this text will avoid the terms hypoestrogenism and hyperestrogenism and arbitrarily classify abnormalities as "ovarian dysfunctions." Bilaterally symmetrical alopecia and hyperpigmentation, lichenification, epidermal hyperplasia, epidermal atrophy, comedones and seborrheic changes are seen in various combinations. Many skin changes are accompanied by pseudocyesis, anestrus and vulvar enlargement. Many of these changes can be reversed by removal of the ovaries.

Cystic graafian follicles, cystic corpora lutea, and atrophic cysts may occur and influence both the genital organs and the skin.

Skin changes associated with ovarian imbalance vary greatly. In some cases there is atrophy of the hair follicles with resulting alopecia. In other cases there is hyperpigmentation, alopecia, hyperkeratosis, pseudocyesis and lichenification. In all cases the distribution patterns of the lesions are in the areas of the genitalia, mammary glands, and perineum. The flanks are frequently hyperpigmented and lichenified. Treatment depends on estimation of the cause. Ovariectomy is useful in many cases, and estrogen supplementation helps in others. As in any target organ dysfunction, the origin can theoretically be primary in the ovary or secondary through trophic stimulation by the pituitary gland. An irregular estral cycle plus some of the aforementioned cutaneous changes are important signs of ovarian imbalance. One should remember, however, that hypothyroidism also is a cause of reproductive disorders, lack of libido and other changes.

## MAJOR ENDOCRINE DERMATOSES

The following major endocrine dermatoses are distinct clinical entities and are described elsewhere in the text, as listed: hypothyroidism (p. 296), hyperadrenocorticism (p. 292), male feminizing syndrome (p. 300), ovarian imbalance (p. 318), acanthosis nigricans (p. 225) and feline endocrine alopecia (p. 277).

### *References*


Belshaw, B. E.: Personal communication, 1968.

*Brown, J. H. U., and Barker, S. B.: *Basic Endocrinology.* F. A. Davis Co., Philadelphia 1962.

Bullock, Leslie: Personal communication, 1968.

Kallfelz, F. A.: Comparison of the $^{125}$T-3 and $^{125}$T-4 tests in the Diagnosis of Thyroid Gland Function in the Dog. J.A.V.M.A., *154*:1, 1969.

Kaneko, J. J.: Personal communication, 1969.

Kupperman, H. S.: *Human Endocrinology.* F. A. Davis Co., Philadelphia 1963.

Miller, M. E., Christensen, G. C., and Evans, H. E.: *Anatomy of the Dog.* W. B. Saunders Co., Philadelphia, 1964.

Muller, G. H., et al., Endocrine Influences on Canine and Feline Skin. Dermatology Committee Reports, in 31st Annual Committee Reports of the American Animal Hospital Association. Elkhart, Indiana, 1964.

Murphy, B. P.: The Determination by Competitive Protein-Binding Analysis Employing an Anion-Exchange Resin and Radiothyroxine. J. Lab. Clin. Med., *66*:161, 1965.

Netter, F. H.: *Endocrine System and Selected Metabolic Diseases,* CIBA, 1965.

Schwartzman, R. M.: The Androgenic Dog. 13th Gaines Veterinary Symposium, Jan. 15, 1964.

Siegel, E. T.: Hyperadrenocorticalism and Hypoadrenocorticalis. *In* kirk, R. W. *Current Veterinary Therapy III.* W. B. Saunders Co., Philadelphia, 1968.

*Siegel, E. T., and Belshaw, B. E.: Laboratory Evaluation of Adrenocortical and Thyroid Function in the Dog. *In* Kirk, R. W. (Ed.): *Current Veterinary Therapy III.* W. B. Saunders Co., Philadelphia, 1968.

*Turner, C. D.: *General Endocrinology.* W. B. Saunders Co., Philadelphia, 1961.

*Rosenberg, I. N., Athans, J. C., and Isaacs, G. H.: Studies on Thyroid Iodine Metabolism. *In:* Pincus, G. (Ed.): *Recent Progress in Hormone Research.* Academic Press, New York, 1965, Vol. 21, pp. 33-72.

---

*Suggested supplemental reading.

# FOURTEEN

# *Skin Tumors*

## ETIOLOGY AND INCIDENCE

This chapter will include tumors of epithelial and connective tissue origin which affect the skin and subcutaneous tissues. Extensive data by Cotchin (Table 14:1) and Head (Tables 14:2 and 14:3) point up the importance of neoplasms of these regions. Cotchin reports that 37 per cent of canine tumors and 24 per cent of feline tumors involve the skin. There is no significant difference in incidence of skin tumors between sexes. Age does play a part, however. Histiocytomas, epulides and oral papillomas are seen commonly in dogs under two years of age whereas fibromas and generalized lymphosarcomas are encountered in young cats. The highest incidence of transmissible venereal tumor occurs during the years of greatest sexual activity. Otherwise skin tumors are more prevalent in dogs older than six years and in cats older than four years.

Skin tumors make up at least one-third of the tumors of dogs and about one-fourth of the tumors of cats.

TABLE 14:1. Systems of Origin of 4,187 Tumors of Dogs and 571 Tumors of Cats, Examined in the Period 1940-58 Inclusive*

| System of origin | Grand total | Dog % | Ranking order | Grand total | Cat % | Ranking order |
|---|---|---|---|---|---|---|
| Skin | 1,572 | 37.5 | 1 | 140 | 24.5 | 2 |
| Female genital† | 1,086 | 25.9 | 2 | 68 | 11.9 | 4 |
| Alimentary | 588 | 14.0 | 3 | 164 | 28.7 | 1 |
| Male genital | 299 | 7.1 | 4 | 0 | 0.0 | — |
| Skeletal | 164 | 3.9 | 5 | 47 | 8.2 | 5 |
| Lymphatic | 159 | 3.8 | 6 | 70 | 12.3 | 3 |
| Miscellaneous | 319 | 7.6 | — | 82 | 14.4 | — |
| | 4,187 | | | 571 | | |

*From Cotchin, E.: Some Tumours of Dogs and Cats of Comparative Veterinary and Human Interest. Vet. Rec., Vol. 71, No. 45, 1959.

†Including mammary gland.

TABLE 14:2. Skin Tumors: Age and Sex Distribution of Normal and Tumor-Bearing Dogs*

| Description | Sex | | | | Age in Years | | | | | | | | | | | | | | | | | | | | |
|---|---|---|---|---|---|---|---|---|---|---|---|---|---|---|---|---|---|---|---|---|---|---|---|---|---|
| | ♂ | ∅♂ | ♀ | ∅♀ | 0-1 | 1 | 2 | 3 | 4 | 5 | 6 | 7 | 8 | 9 | 10 | 11 | 12 | 13 | 14 | 15 | 16 | 17 | 18 | 19 | 20 |
| 'Normal' Population | 7693 | 3 | 4675 | 35 | 3901 | 1224 | 1113 | 963 | 734 | 645 | 579 | 533 | 585 | 495 | 494 | 381 | 359 | 173 | 110 | 62 | 28 | 17 | 6 | 3 | 1 |
| Papilloma: Oropharynx | 39 | | 12 | | 36 | 14 | 3 | | | | | | | 1 | | | | | | | | | | | |
| Skin | 54 | | 35 | | 16 | 7 | 6 | 8 | 3 | 6 | 4 | 5 | 8 | 7 | 1 | 1 | 4 | 6 | 3 | | 1 | | | | |
| Squamous-cell Carcinoma | 51 | | 37 | 1 | | 1 | | 6 | 5 | 7 | 4 | 8 | 10 | 12 | 8 | 6 | 4 | 4 | 2 | | 1 | | | | |
| Basal-cell Carcinoma: Superficial | 32 | | 18 | 1 | 1 | | 1 | | 5 | 5 | 6 | 6 | 6 | 6 | 4 | 4 | 3 | 4 | | | | | | | |
| Deep | 38 | | 19 | | | | 2 | 1 | 2 | 10 | 7 | 4 | 12 | 7 | 7 | 3 | 3 | 2 | | | | | | | |
| Glandular Tumour of Sweat Glands | 26 | | 15 | | | | | 3 | 2 | | 2 | 3 | 6 | 7 | 7 | 1 | 2 | 1 | 1 | 2 | | 1 | 1 | | |
| Sebaceous Papilloma | 123 | | 48 | | 1 | | 2 | 2 | 3 | 6 | 15 | 9 | 26 | 13 | 18 | 25 | 22 | 4 | 12 | 4 | 3 | 1 | 1 | | |
| Glandular Tumour of Sebaceous Glands | 25 | | 8 | 1 | | | 2 | | 1 | 1 | 2 | 3 | 5 | 3 | 1 | 3 | 7 | | 4 | | | | | | |
| Glandular Tumour of Perianal Glands | ·168 | | 12 | | | 1 | | 1 | 2 | 3 | 11 | 6 | 8 | 19 | 26 | 20 | 29 | 17 | 11 | 2 | 4 | 1 | | | |
| Glandular Tumour of Modified Sebaceous Glands | 36 | | | | | | | | | 1 | 4 | 1 | 3 | 5 | 3 | 1 | 5 | 3 | 1 | | 1 | | | | |
| Subcutaneous Tumours of Fibrous Tissue | 108 | | 60 | 1 | 1 | 1 | 1 | 1 | 5 | 6 | 11 | 12 | 22 | 26 | 24 | 25 | 16 | 5 | 7 | 2 | 5 | 1 | | | |
| Acquired Lipomatoid Mass | 36 | | 68 | | | | 1 | 3 | 3 | 7 | 5 | 6 | 10 | 10 | 13 | 7 | 13 | 4 | 11 | 3 | | | | | |
| Haemangioma | 30 | | 25 | | 1 | | | 1 | 2 | 4 | 5 | 4 | 3 | 10 | 7 | 5 | 4 | 2 | 4 | | | | | | |
| Generalized Lymphosarcoma | 67 | | 15 | | | 3 | 3 | 4 | 5 | 16 | 11 | 8 | 8 | 10 | 8 | 5 | 6 | 5 | 3 | | 1 | | | | |
| Mast-cell Tumour | 83 | | 62 | | | 3 | | 4 | 3 | 18 | 15 | 20 | 10 | 16 | 21 | 7 | 14 | 3 | 3 | | | | | | |
| Histiocytoma | 142 | | 64 | | 50 | 57 | 36 | 18 | 8 | 13 | 9 | 4 | 10 | 2 | 2 | 1 | 2 | 1 | | | | | | | |
| Melanotic Tumours | 127 | | 28 | | 2 | 1 | 1 | 1 | 4 | 7 | 15 | 8 | 16 | 12 | 15 | 14 | 8 | 8 | 7 | 2 | 2 | | | | |

*From Rook, A. J. and Walton, G. S.: *The Comparative Physiology and Pathology of the Skin.* F. A. Davis Co., 1965.

TABLE 14:3. Skin Tumors: Age and Sex Distribution of Normal and Tumor-Bearing Cats*

| Description | Sex | | | | Age in Years | | | | | | | | | | | | | | | | | | | | | |
|---|---|---|---|---|---|---|---|---|---|---|---|---|---|---|---|---|---|---|---|---|---|---|---|---|---|---|
| | ♂ | ⌀♂ | ♀ | ⌀♀ | 0-1 | 1 | 2 | 3 | 4 | 5 | 6 | 7 | 8 | 9 | 10 | 11 | 12 | 13 | 14 | 15 | 16 | 17 | 18 | 19 | 20 | 21 |
| 'Normal' population | 2436 | 1159 | 1508 | 390 | 2126 | 636 | 448 | 325 | 261 | 227 | 223 | 178 | 212 | 150 | 176 | 120 | 127 | 72 | 83 | 44 | 27 | 22 | 18 | 7 | 7 | 2 |
| Squamous-cell carcinoma | | 4 | | | | | 1 | | | | | | | 1 | 2 | | | | | | 1 | | | | | |
| Basal-cell carcinoma | 1 | 6 | 3 | | | | | 1 | 1 | 1 | 1 | | | | 2 | 1 | | 1 | 1 | 1 | 2 | | | | | |
| Ceruminous Adenocarcinoma | 4 | 3 | 1 | 1 | | | | 1 | 1 | | 1 | 2 | 1 | 1 | 1 | 1 | 1 | 2 | 1 | | | | | | | |
| Fibroma | 5 | 10 | 4 | | | 4 | 3 | 2 | 2 | 1 | 1 | 1 | | 1 | 1 | 1 | | 1 | | 1 | | | | | | |
| Generalized Lymphosarcoma | 7 | 9 | 1 | 2 | | 7 | 2 | 2 | 2 | 2 | 2 | 2 | | 2 | 2 | 1 | 3 | | | 1 | 1 | | | | | |
| Mast-cell tumors | 3 | 3 | 2 | | | | 1 | 2 | | 2 | | | 1 | 1 | | | | | | | | | | | | |

*From Rook, A. J. and Walton, G. S.: *The Comparative Physiology and Pathology of the Skin.* F. A. Davis Co., 1965.

One explanation for part of the age variability is the fact that young animals are susceptible to the virus-caused tumors, whereas older animals may have an acquired immunity. Viruses are known to cause lymphosarcoma in cats, oral papillomatosis and mastocytoma (mast cell leukemia) in dogs, and fibroma and myxomatosis in rabbits.

On the other hand the cause for the preponderance of tumors in mature or older animals is not known. Long latent periods may be needed, continual stimulation to carcinogens may be required, or it may take aging changes to induce tissue sensitivity.

Breed incidence is an interesting phenomenon for which no clear explanation is available. Boxers, cocker spaniels, Boston terriers, Scottish terriers and wire-haired fox terriers have a high incidence of skin tumors, whereas Pekingese and chows seldom have tumors. Giant breeds such as the Great Dane, St. Bernard, and Irish wolfhound have a high incidence of osteogenic sarcoma. It is conceivable that the latter is a result of trauma, as is possible in the higher incidence of mammary tumor in the posterior breast, but these are not established facts.

Congenital, non-neoplastic tumors such as the ocular dermoid, the dentigerous cyst and the dermoid sinus are not common. The dermoid cyst, which is prevalent in Rhodesian ridgeback dogs, is caused by a gene complex, so most individuals of this breed may carry some of the factors. The sinus is caused by incomplete dehiscence between the spinal cord and the skin after closure of the neural tube in embryologic development. On the surface it appears to be a minute opening with a tuft of hair protruding. A thin, hollow cord of skin at the midline connects the surface with the dura mater in the sacral region or the second or third cervical vertebra in the neck region. The sinus becomes filled with sebum, keratin debris and hair, and is often inflamed. Surgical dissection is the treatment of choice, but because of its deep attachments complete removal is not possible. Meningitis often complicates these cases.

It is probable that heredity is a factor in neoplastic disease but statistical proof is lacking. Parasites (*Spirocerca lupi*) appear to be a factor in sarcoma of the esophagus, but cases involving other parasites have not been documented. Topical application of tar, smegma and other carcinogens has been successful in producing tumors; and ionizing radiation and ultraviolet ray exposure from the sun cause keratoses and squamous cell carcinomas.

## GROWTH CHARACTERISTICS AND STRUCTURE

When the clinician is presented with an animal showing an abnormal skin growth he must decide what it is and what to do about it. In some cases no treatment is needed, but in others early recognition and proper therapy may be vital to a successful outcome. Any item of history or examination concerning the problem will be useful in making these decisions.

Most animals have predilections for neoplasms at particular locations. Thus basal cell carcinomas and apocrine adenomas have a high incidence on the face and head. Mastocytomas are most common on the hind quarters and the genitalia, while melanomas are found on the feet, face and mouth. Fibrosarcomas occur commonly in the mouth and mammary gland, and epidermal cysts are usual along the top of the back and neck.

TABLE 14:4. Distinguishing Between Benign and Malignant Neoplasms

| Criteria | Benign | Malignant |
|---|---|---|
| **Cellular Characteristics** | | |
| Cell size | uniform, normal | pleomorphic |
| Nuclear chromatin | normal | hyperchromic |
| Nucleoli | normal | large |
| Mitotic figures | few | numerous |
| **Tissue Characteristics** | | |
| Anaplasia | none (differentiated cells) | present (undifferentiated cells) |
| Stroma | usually abundant | may be scanty |
| Invasion of vessels | rare | frequent |
| Blood supply | adequate | may be "outgrown" by tumor or there may be marked vascularity |
| Necrosis and ulceration | unusual | common, often with hemorrhage |
| **Growth Characteristics** | | |
| Growth rate | slow | rapid |
| Growth limits | limited, often by capsule | unrestricted |
| Growth termination | may stop or regress | usually progressive |
| Growth mode | expansion, pedunculation | infiltration, destruction |
| Metastasis | never | common |
| **General Characteristics** | | |
| Recurrence after removal | rare | frequent |
| Constitutional effects | rare | common |

TABLE 14:5. Prognostic Classification of Skin Tumors

I. Method of Spread
- A. Metastatic
  - 1. Common
    - a. Early
      - Melanoma
      - Fibrosarcoma
    - b. Late
      - Squamous cell carcinoma
      - Apocrine and mammary adenocarcinoma
      - Mastocytoma
  - 2. Rare
    - Neurofibroma
    - Sebaceous adenocarcinoma
- B. Nonmetastatic
  - 1. Local recurrence possible
    - Basal cell carcinoma
    - Perianal adenoma or adenocarcinoma
    - Hemangioendothelioma, hemangiopericytoma
    - Transmissible venereal tumor
  - 2. Local recurrence rare
    - Papilloma
    - Lipoma
    - Fibroma
    - Hemangioma
    - Histiocytoma

II. Sensitivity to Ionizing Radiation
- A. Radiosensitive
  - Transmissible venereal tumor
  - Mastocytoma
  - Perianal gland adenoma or carcinoma
  - Basal cell carcinoma
  - Lymphosarcoma
- B. Nonradiosensitive
  - Melanoma
  - Fibrosarcoma
- C. Palliative response to radiation
  - Squamous cell carcinoma
  - Sebaceous, apocrine and mammary adenocarcinomas

The question of a tumor's malignancy, or potential malignancy, is difficult to answer in many cases, but Table 14:4 provides a common summation of criteria which may help in differentiation.

## TREATMENT

Although hormonal and ionizing radiation are useful treatments, they usually are adjunctive measures to the primary goal—surgical excision. Ross (1968) outlines the methods for handling specific skin tumors and emphasizes the importance of early surgery as ideal therapy. Section Six (p. 359) gives detailed information on the diagnosis and treatment of specific tumors. Table 14:5 shows a prognostic classification of skin tumors.

### *References*

Cotchin, E.: Some Tumors of Dogs and Cats of Comparative Veterinary and Human Interest. Vet. Rec. *71*:No. 45, Dec. 26, 1959, 1040-1054.

*Head, K. W.: Some Data Concerning the Distribution of Skin Tumors of Domestic Animals. In Rook, A. S., and Walton, G. S.: *Comparative Physiology and Pathology of the Skin.* F. A. Davis Co., Philadelphia, 1965.

Hopps, H. C: *Principles of Pathology.* Appleton-Century-Crofts, New York, 1959.

Lord, L. H., Cawley, A. J., and Gilray J.: Mid-Dorsal Dermoid Sinuses in Rhodesian Ridgeback Dogs—a Case Report. Jour. Amer. Vet. Med. Assn. 131: 1957, pg. 515.

*Moulton, J. E.: *Tumors in Domestic Animals.* Univ. of Calif. Press, Berkeley, 1961.

Mulligan, R. M.: *Neoplasms of the Dog;* Williams & Wilkins Co., Baltimore, 1949.

Ross, G. E.: Skin Tumors, In Kirk, R. W. (Ed.): *Current Veterinary Therapy III.* W. B. Saunders, Philadelphia, 1968.

*Suggested supplemental reading.

# DERMATOLOGIC THERAPY

*Section Four*

# FIFTEEN

# *Therapeutic Principles*

Successful treatment of skin diseases depends on accurate diagnosis and a thoughtful, integrated therapeutic program based on the individual requirements of the specific case. Over the years a complex array of nostrums has been devised by clinicians and touted by pharmaceutical houses until dermatologic pharmacy has attained the reputation of an occult art akin to witchcraft. A knowledge of basic principles and an understanding of phamacologic actions of a few key drugs permit the clinician to utilize skin medications effectively.

## TEN BASIC PRINCIPLES

1. **Make a correct diagnosis.**

A definitive diagnosis is vital to effective therapy. When it is necessary to await confirming laboratory results for a definite diagnosis, the case should be placed in a disease category and symptomatic therapy started.

2. **Avoid overtreatment.**

If in doubt undertreat the skin. Rest is important, while protection and mild medications give natural healing processes an opportunity to function. Skin should be handled gently, the hair clipped off, and crusts, scales, dirt and offending strong medications should be removed. Start treatment with bland, soothing preparations.

3. **Use simple medications.**

Complex formulations are seldom needed or desirable. Plain wet dressings or petrolatum give surprisingly good results in many instances.

4. **Select the best topical treatment for each dermatologic stage.**

For example, wet dressings are useful for acute inflammations or crusted lesions, and ointments are contraindicated for moist, weeping lesions.

5. **Do not change treatment too frequently.**

Allow medications to demonstrate their effectiveness before changing therapy. However, if no response is observed in seven to ten days, a reevaluation of the diagnosis and treatment is in order.

6. **Prevent self-inflicted trauma.**

Use emollients, antipruritics, sedatives, tranquilizers or mechanical protective devices, but avoid bandaging skin lesions unless absolutely necessary.

7. **Familiarize yourself with a few proved drugs and know their actions on the skin.**

A medicated shampoo, a soothing lotion, a drying powder, a washable cream and several ointments are sufficient for topical therapy of the common dermatoses. For complete understanding one must know the effect of the active ingredient *and* the vehicle.

8. **Learn the effect of dermatologic vehicles and select the correct one for each dermatosis.**

9. **Use fungicides for dermatomycoses only.**

Their keratolytic and irritating effect is usually undesirable in other skin and disorders.

10. **Remember systemic corticosteroid therapy gives only symptomatic relief.**

Prolonged use may cause serious consequences.

## OBJECTIVES OF THERAPY

Correct the specific cause if possible.

This may involve elimination of parasites, fungi or bacteria; correction of metabolic disorders; modification of hormonal imbalance; removal of neoplasms; management of allergy; supplementation for nutritional deficiencies; or protection from toxins or external irritants.

Treat the skin symptomatically.

TABLE 15:1. Objectives and Agents of Topical Skin Therapy

| *Objectives* | *Agent* |
|---|---|
| Relief of: Pruritus | Wet dressings, corticosteroids, systemic antihistamines |
| Dryness | Emollients |
| Pain | Systemic analgesics |
| Inflammation | Wet dressings, topical corticosteroids |
| Protection | Emollients |
| Alteration of blood flow | Wet dressings |
| Removal of: Bacteria | Antibacterials |
| Ectoparasites | Antiparasitics |
| Fungi | Antifungals |
| Crusts and scales<br>Exudates<br>Excess sebum | Clipping, wet dressings and detergents |
| Excess keratin | Keratolytics such as salicylic acid |

If a definite diagnosis cannot be made immediately, symptomatic treatment may be started. This implies external medication to relieve dryness, pain and pruritus and to remove exudates, crusts, scales and excess keratin. Protective films or emollients often are highly desirable.

The main objectives of topical therapy and the agents employed are listed in Table 15:1.

# SIXTEEN

# *Topical Treatment*

## CLEANING THE SKIN

The skin surface constantly accumulates debris. The skin surface film contains excretory products of skin glands, exfoliated flakes of the horny layer, and extraneous dirt on the normal skin, as well as excessive amounts of these, together with exudates, blood and crusts, in the normal skin. For health, the skin and coat should be groomed to minimize these accumulations (see Chapter 19). Proper skin and coat care is neglected, primary skin effects may result, or accumulations of debris may have adverse effects on the skin disease which is already present.

Most cases of skin disease which need topical medication require clipping, cleansing and application of therapeutic agents as logical steps to effective treatment. Clipping is most desirable to enable close scrutiny of the lesions. It also permits thorough cleansing and adequate and economical application of the desired medicament. In many cases complete removal of the coat may be necessary, but usually clipping the local area suffices. This should be done neatly to avoid disfigurement. If the hair over the involved area is clipped closely (against the grain with a No. 40 clipper), while a border around this is clipped less closely (with the grain), the regrowth of hair more quickly "blends" the area into the normal coat pattern. When the cosmetic effects of clipping may be severe they should always be discussed with the owner first to obtain approval. This is especially important when dealing with show animals or those with long coats such as Afghan hounds. All needless clipping should be avoided. After clipping, a vacuum cleaner can be used advantageously to remove all loose, dry hair and debris. The lesions are inspected carefully before deciding on further procedures.

Acute and subacute dermatoses, especially when vesiculation and oozing are present, are damaged by vigorous washing with soap and water. Topical cleansing should be avoided in these cases. In other instances wet dressings, warm oil baths and cosmetic cleansing creams can be used safely. For certain problems judicious use of alcohol or ether may be effective. Agents such as gasoline, paint remover and cleaning fluids should never be used on dog or cat skin. They are extremely irritating and highly toxic. Road tar on the feet or legs of dogs and cats can be treated satisfactorily by using scissors to cut off the large masses of tar and hair. The remaining tar is soaked in *vegetable* oil for 24 hours, which softens the mass. A simple shampoo then usually removes any residuum. Paint on the coat is best removed by clipping after the paint has hardened.

## HYDROTHERAPY

Plain tap water is one of the most effective agents in the treatment of skin diseases. It is often forgotten.

Water is a component of many lotions and may be applied also as wet dressings or in baths. Frequent periodic renewal of wet dressings (15 minutes on—several hours off) prolongs the effect; but if more continuous therapy or occlusive coverings are used, the skin temperature rises and an undesirable maceration occurs. If the wet dressing is left open this is less likely to happen. The water temperature may be cool or above body temperature and the effect thus can be modified as needed. Whirlpool baths, with or without detergents and antiseptics added, make gentle, effective cleaning possible. These treatments may be used to remove crusts and scales, to cleanse wounds and fistulas, to rehydrate skin (Fig. 16:1*C*) and to prophylactically manage patients prone to decubital problems, urine scalds and other ills. Ten to fifteen minutes of therapy once or twice daily is adequate. The patient should be toweled and placed in an air-stream drier to dry. Other topical medications can be applied later if needed.

With hydrotherapy it is the moisture which is specific, and various additives change effects only slightly. In general, water treatment removes crusts, bacteria and other debris and greatly reduces the possibility of secondary infection. It promotes epithelialization and allays the symptoms of pain, pruritus and burning.

## MEDICATIONS USED WITH WATER

Astringents, antiseptics or antibiotics added to water create effects in addition to the cooling and cleansing ones of compresses and baths.

*Aluminum acetate* (Burrows solution USP) is available commercially as Domeboro. It is drying, astringent and mildly antiseptic. The usual solution is 1:40 in cool water and soaks are repeated three times daily for 30 minutes.

*Magnesium sulfate* 1:65 solution (1 tablespoonful per quart of warm water) is a mildly hypertonic solution for wet dressings. Isotonic sodium chloride solution for wet dressings can be made by adding 1 teaspoonsful of table salt to 1 pint of water.

*Silver nitrate* 0.25 per cent solution may be applied to moist, weeping, denuded areas as an antiseptic, coagulant and stimulating agent. It should be used infrequently and sparingly.

*Antibiotic wet dressings* may be made from many antibiotics. Neomycin sulfate has excellent stability, is bactericidal and effective against many gram-positive and gram-negative bacteria. In man it has been known to cause sensiti-

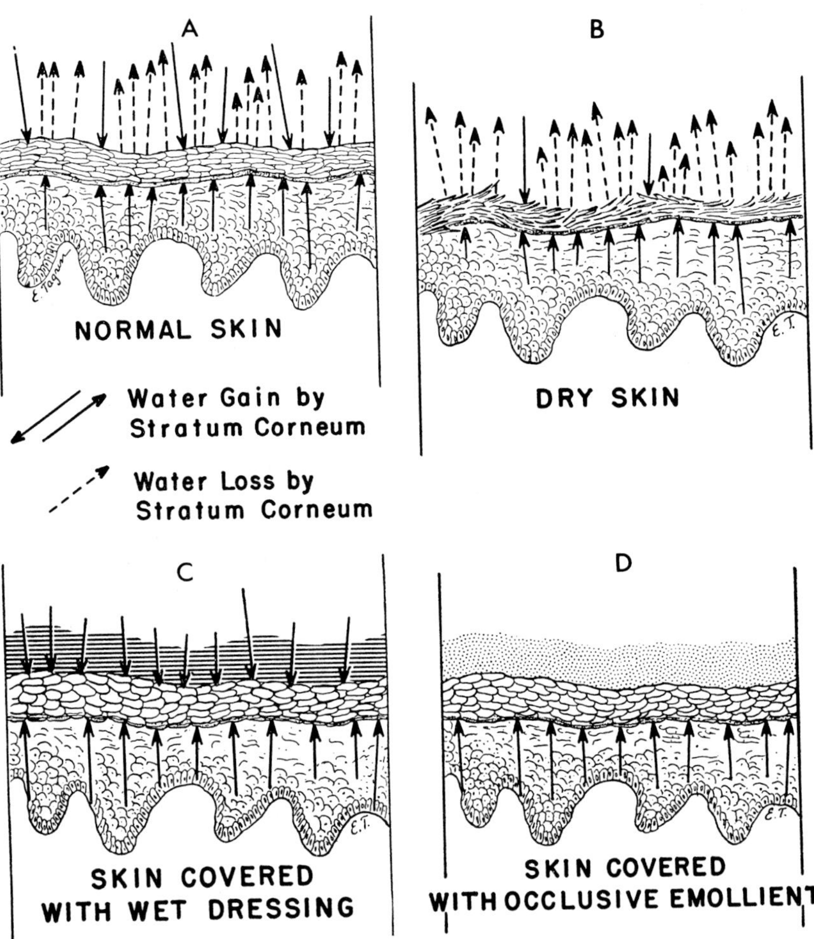


**Figure 16:1.** *A*, Water exchange through the stratum corneum of normal skin at equilibrium with the environment. Water is being received from the underlying tissues and from the environment. Also, water is being lost to the environment and there is a net transfer from the underlying tissues to the environment. *B*, Water exchange through the stratum corneum of skin which has been transferred from a high to a low environmental humidity. The water loss to the environment is temporarily increased and that received from the environment is decreased. The stratum corneum becomes dehydrated since the amount of water it can receive from the underlying tissues is limited. *C*, Water exchange through the stratum corneum when the skin is covered with a wet dressing. The stratum corneum hydrates since water is being received both from the underlying tissues and the external water. *D*, Water exchange through the stratum corneum when the skin is covered with an occlusive emollient. The stratum corneum hydrates since water is being received from the underlying tissues and water loss to the environment is prevented. (From Frazier and Blank: *A Formulary for External Therapy of the Skin.* Charles C Thomas, Springfield, Ill., 1954.)

zation, but this has not been reported in dogs and cats. Ordinarily 500 mg. is added to 25 ml. of saline for wet dressings and irrigating solutions.

*Bath oils* which are commonly used in human medicine (Nutraspa, Domol, Lubath) have limited use for animals. Products such as Alpha-Keri are available in aerosol spray, which can be applied to the dry coat and massaged to produce improved sheen. Solutions are also available to add to a small volume of water after a bath as a rinse. They contain dewaxed, oil-soluble fraction of lanolin, mineral oil and a nonionic emulsifier and produce a nice gloss after the coat dries. These products are available at pharmacies without prescription.

*Soaps and shampoos* are cleansing agents for the skin and hair. Soluble soaps are sodium (hard soap) or potassium (soft soap) salts of high molecular weight, monobasic aliphatic acids. In addition they usually contain preservatives, essential oils and coloring matter. The osmotic effect and detergent action of soaps may irritate the skin. Irritation is caused by the mechanical effect of the foam, emulsification of the skin oils and grease, and softening of the epidermis. The most blands soaps and shampoos are made from coconut or other vegetable oils. No matter how bland the soap, it should always be thoroughly rinsed from the skin. Coconut oil shampoo, hexachlorophene liquid soap USP (hexachlorophene 10 per cent in potassium soap) and pHisoHex NNR (Hexachlorophene 3 per cent in 18.4 per cent anhydrous detergent base) are examples of simple cleansing agents commonly used.

*Medicated soaps and shampoos* contain additional ingredients which supposedly enhance or add other actions to that of the shampoo. It is incongruous in some cases to add medications to a drug whose primary purpose is to remove substances from the skin. However, some medicaments may have enough opportunity for effect or for limited absorption during a prolonged shampoo and their addition may be justified (insecticides, salicylic acid, sulfur, tar, selenium, hexachlorophene).

*Soap substitutes* can be obtained in the form of detergents or of cleansing creams. Because these products do not foam vigorously they are not especially effective unless the hair has been removed. They cause little irritation to sensitive skin and are particularly effective in removing greasy films or glandular exudates such as sebum. pHisoderm, a hypollergenic emulsion containing entsufon, wool fat cholesterols, lactic acid and petrolatum, is an example of an aqueous detergent cleanser, while Nivea Creme or oil, emulsions of neutral aliphatic hydrocarbons in water with wool fat cholesterol, are examples of nonaqueous cleansing creams.

Although many types of solid debris can be removed from the skin by various soaps and detergents, removal of excess surface, keratinized epithelium is dependent on maceration of the scales. Here *alkaline* soaps or detergents are more effective. The removal of bacteria is effected by the electrical charge of the skin and the organisms. Since soap or markedly alkaline detergents make both skin and organisms more negative electrically, they are more efficient in removing bacteria than less alkaline detergents.

## LOTIONS AND LINIMENTS

Lotions and liniments are liquids for topical use in which medicinal agents are dissolved or suspended. Some are essentially "liquid powders," because when the liquid evaporates a thin powder film is left on the skin. Lotions tend to be more drying (because of their water or alcohol base) than liniments which have an oily base. These medications tend to be cooling, antipruritic and drying (depending on the base). They are vehicles for active agents such as sulfur and resorcinol. The liquid preparations can be applied repeatedly, but when they tend to "cake" or build up they should be removed gently by wet dressings. In general, lotions are indicated for acute oozing dermatoses and are contraindicated in dry, chronic conditions. Pellene and calamine are examples of lotions or liniments.

## POWDERS

Powders are pulverized organic or inorganic solids which are applied to the skin in a thin film. They may be added to liquids to form "shake lotions," or to ointments to form pastes. Some powders are inert (talc, starch, zinc oxide) and have a physical effect; others contain active ingredients which have a chemical or antibacterial effect (sulfur). Powders are used as drying agents, and to cool and lubricate intertriginous areas. The affected skin should be cleaned and dried before the powder is applied. Avoid powder build-up or caking, but if it occurs, wet compresses or soaks will remove the excess gently. On long-coated animals, a fine powder is an acceptable retention vehicle for insecticides and fungicides.

## CREAMS AND OINTMENTS

Creams, ointments, salves and pastes are mentioned here in order of increasing viscosity. All spread fairly easily and maintain contact between the drug and the skin. They act merely as vehicles in most cases, but may disrupt the horny layer so that penetration is enhanced, or interfere with water loss and glandular secretion. These effects may serve to hydrate the skin somewhat (Fig. 16:1*D*) but also may produce a folliculitis because of occlusion of pilosebaceous orifices.

Creams and ointments are mixtures of grease or oil and water which are emulsified with high speed blenders. Emulsifiers, such as Tween 80, and coloring agents and perfumes are often added to improve the physical characteristics of the product. Pastes are highly viscous ointments in which large amounts of powder are incorporated. While pastes may be tolerated on slightly exudative skin (the powder takes up water) in general, creams and ointments are contraindicated on oozing areas.

Creams and ointments function to lubricate and smooth roughened skin. They form a protective covering which reduces contact with the environment, and certain types may reduce water loss. They also serve to transport medicinal agents into follicular orifices and keep drugs in intimate contact with the horny layer. This type of medication should be applied with gentle massage several times daily to maintain a *thin* film on the skin. Thick films are wasteful, occlusive and messy to surroundings. Usually ointments disappear spontaneously, but thick films can be softened and removed by water or oil soaks and gentle massage.

Water washable ointment bases are those which can be readily removed with water (Carbowax 1500). Other bases are not freely water washable. It is important for the clinician to understand the uses and advantages of these types of bases because the total effect on the skin is caused by the vehicle as well as its "active" ingredient.

For soothing protection of inflamed skin, try simple white petroleum jelly.

The classification of vehicles by Frazier and Blank (1954) is given in Table 16:1.

*Hydrophobic oils* mix poorly with water. They contain few polar groups (-OH, -COOH and so on). These oils get in close contact with the skin and spread easily. Since they are hydrophobic, it is difficult for water to pass through a film of these oils and they are occlusive for the skin. They retain heat and water and more viscid forms (petrolatum) produce an uncomfortable sensation to the patient. The oily forms (mineral oil) are often incorporated into emulsion type vehicles.

*Hydrophilic oils* are miscible with water. They contain many polar groups, and those with the greatest number are most soluble in water. Although they are ointments in physical characteristics only, the polyethylene glycols are alcohols which are readily miscible with water. Polymers with a molecular weight greater than 1000 are solid at room temperature, but a slight rise to body temperature causes melting to form an oily film. Carbowax 1500 is such a product. It mixes with skin exudates well, is easily washed off with water and is less occlusive than other bases.

Emulsions are of two types: oil dispersed in water, and water dispersed in oil (Fig. 16:2). Although both are used as vehicles, the former type dilutes with water and loses water rapidly and therefore is cooling. The latter type dilutes with oil and loses its water slowly. In both cases once the water evaporates the action of the vehicle on the skin is no different from that of the oil and emulsifying agent alone. Thus the characteristics of the residual film are those of the

TABLE 16:1. Classification of Vehicles

| | |
|---|---|
| I. Anhydrous Vehicles | |
| A. Hydrophobic oils | |
| Oils of mineral origin | Petrolatum |
| Oils of animal origin | Lard |
| Oils of vegetable origin | Olive, castor oils |
| B. Hydrophilic oils | |
| Absorption bases | Hydrophilic petrolatum USP |
| (Mildly hydrophilic) | Aquaphor, Polysorb |
| Washable bases | Carbowax |
| II. Vehicles that Contain Water | |
| A. Water-in-oil emulsions | Hydrous wool fat |
| B. Oil-in-water emulsions | Hydrophilic ointment USP, cold cream, vanishing cream |
| III. Vehicles that Contain Powder | |
| A. Powder in hydrophobic oil | Zinc oxide ointment USP |
| B. Powder in hydrophilic oil | Starch in hydrophilic petrolatum |

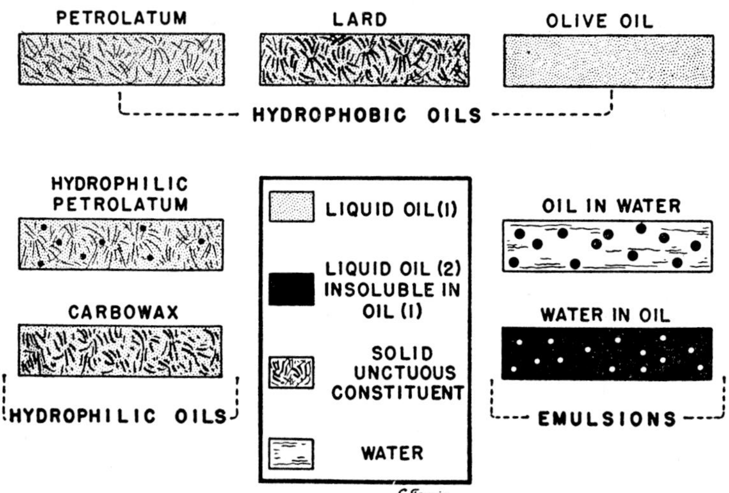


**Figure 16:2.** Physical structure of various types of ointment vehicles. (From Frazier and Blank: *A Formulary for External Therapy of the Skin.* Charles C Thomas, Springfield, Ill., 1954.)

oily phase of the vehicle. This can be illustrated by comparing cold cream and vanishing cream.

Cold cream is mostly oil with little water. The oils are of low melting point, so when the water evaporates a thick, greasy film is left on the skin. A vanishing cream, on the other hand, is mostly water with oils which have a high melting point. When the water evaporates a thin film of high melting point fat is left on the skin. This does not feel greasy.

## FACTORS WHICH INFLUENCE DRUG EFFECTS ON THE SKIN

Although the pharmaceutical characteristics of an ointment in the jar are important, the pharmacological action of the medication on the skin is paramount. When a drug is incorporated into a vehicle it may go into true solution and become molecularly dispersed, or it may be suspended in particles larger than molecules. These large particles are not in motion in the vehicle so those at the skin-ointment interface are the only ones available to the skin (Figs. 16:3 and 16:4). With a true solution (in oil or water) the molecules are in motion and theoretically all of the drug will be available to the skin. Other than affecting solubility, the vehicle itself has very little influence on quantitative variations of absorption through the skin, since no vehicle will "carry" through the skin a compound incapable of penetration.

Enhancement of penetration of the skin barrier by drugs may result from physical factors affecting the intact epidermal barrier, from cellular damage to it, or from its complete disruption. Thus skin which is pretreated with lipid solvents, with keratolytic agents or with Scotch tape "stripping" to remove the barrier zone will have increased absorption potentials. Moisture, too, is thought to enhance percutaneous absorption. Occlusive dressings cause retention of

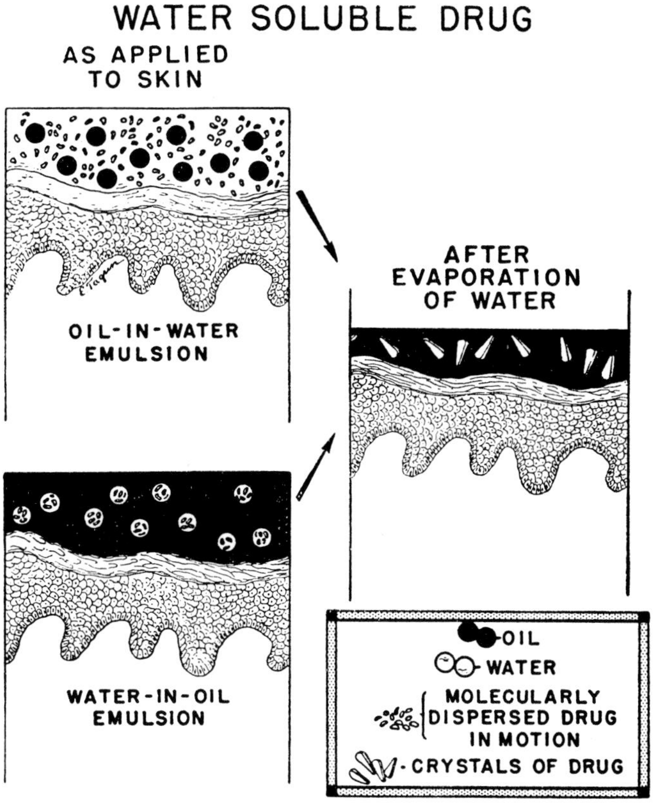

WATER SOLUBLE DRUG
AS APPLIED TO SKIN
OIL-IN-WATER EMULSION
WATER-IN-OIL EMULSION
AFTER EVAPORATION OF WATER
OIL
WATER
MOLECULARLY DISPERSED DRUG IN MOTION
CRYSTALS OF DRUG

**Figure 16:3.** The physical structure of oil-in-water and water-in-oil vehicles containing a water-soluble drug as they are applied to the skin and after the water has evaporated. (From Frazier and Blank: *A Formulary for External Therapy of the Skin.* Charles C Thomas, Springfield, Ill., 1954.)

OIL SOLUBLE DRUG
AS APPLIED TO SKIN
OIL-IN-WATER EMULSION
WATER-IN-OIL EMULSION
AFTER EVAPORATION OF WATER
OIL
WATER
MOLECULARLY DISPERSED DRUG IN MOTION

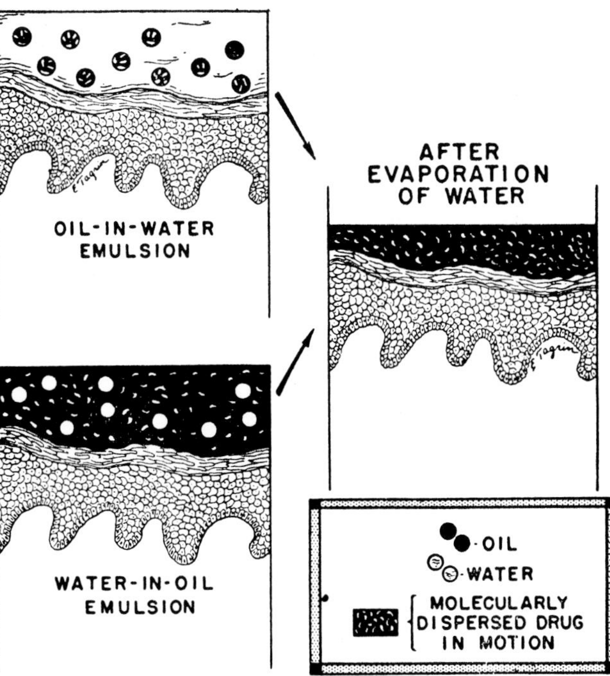

**Figure 16:4.** The physical structure of oil-in-water and water-in-oil vehicles containing an oil-soluble drug as they are applied to the skin and after the water has evaporated. (From Frazier and Blank: *A Formulary for External Therapy of the Skin.* Charles C Thomas, Springfield, Ill., 1954.)

moisture and softening or maceration of the horny layer with increased absorption resulting.

Variation in concentration of ingredients causes variation in absorption. Although increased concentration sometimes causes increased absorption, certain compounds (caustic) in high concentrations produce crusts on the skin surface which hinder penetration. (See also Chapter Two, Physiology of the Skin, p. 37.)

## EMOLLIENTS, KERATOLYTICS AND DRY SKIN

Emollients (cold cream or Nivea Creme) are agents which soften or soothe the skin, and keratolytics are agents which promote separation or peeling of the horny layer of the epidermis. Both types of drugs are useful in hydration and softening the skin.

"Dryness of the skin" is recognized when any one of the following are present: roughness of the surface, inflexibility of the horny layer or fissuring with possible inflammation.

Normal skin is not a waterproof covering but is constantly losing water to the environment by transpiration (Fig. 16:1*A*). This loss is dependent on body temperature, on environmental temperature and on relative humidity (Fig. 16:1*B*). The barrier layer of the epidermis is the major deterrent to water loss, although the normal lipid film on the surface plays a minor role too. This film is derived from sebum and from degenerated epidermal cells. Dry keratin is highly insoluble and can be soaked in oil for months without any effect. If it is immersed in water for a short period, however, it quickly softens.

The hydration of keratin is a basic principle of softening skin.

If all cells at the surface of the skin desquamated completely and evenly the surface of the skin would remain smooth. They are lost in flakes and patches, however, so the skin surface is rough. This is accentuated when excessive use of soap and defatting agents removes lipids and causes the alternation of excess hydration and drying. This allows clumps of cells to be loosened prematurely and fissures to form accentuating the skin roughness. Sebum on the skin or externally applied lipid films have a tendency to make the surface feel smoother. The flexibility of keratin is related directly to its moisture content. Since the barrier in the epidermis limits water which the horny layer can receive from below, its moisture content is dependent on the environment. Water content of the horny layer can be increased by occlusive dressings to prevent loss (Fig. 16:1*D*), by adding water with baths or wet dressings (Fig. 16:1*C*) or by using hydroscopic medications to attract water (glycerine). For maximum softening, the skin should be hydrated in wet dressings, dried and covered with an occlusive hydrophobic oil (petrolatum). Nonocclusive emollients are relatively ineffective in retaining moisture.

Keratolytic agents do not dissolve keratin, but soften excessively keratinized tissue so it can be removed mechanically. Excessive hydration causes maceration and such tissue is removed easily. Salicylic acid is a keratolytic agent which is present in many ointments. Ointment under an occlusive dressing causes water to accumulate in the horny layer. Some of the moisture leaches salicylic acid out of the ointment and the resulting reduction of the skin pH allows the keratin to absorb more water than at its normal pH. Thus the cornified epidermis is macerated and can be removed.

## ANTIPRURITICS

Antipruritic agents attempt to provide temporary relief of itching, but no really satisfactory medication exists. Corticosteroids, systemically and topically offer much help, but they are not without risk. Antihistamines systemically are useful in urticaria, but topically they are useless. Topical anesthetics may be partially effective but they may be toxic or have sensitizing potentials (phenol 0.5 per cent, tetracaine, lidocaine 0.5 per cent).

Cool wet dressings are often helpful and in general any volatile agent provides a cooling sensation which may be palliative. This is the basis for menthol (1 per cent) thymol (1 per cent) and alcohol (70 per cent) in antipruritic medications. In addition, menthol has a specific action on local sensory nerve endings.

## ANTIBACTERIAL AGENTS

*Alcohol* (ethyl or isopropyl) is effective for rapid killing of organisms on the skin. They are used on unbroken skin only in concentrations of 50 to 100 per cent. For germicidal effect the skin should be kept wet with alcohol for at least two minutes.

*Quaternary ammonium compounds* are bactericidal for gram-positive organisms but are not effective against spores, many gram-negative organisms, and some staphylococci. They are inactivated by proteins, phospholipids and soaps.

*Hexachlorophene*, when incorporated in soap and used repeatedly for washing the skin, reduces the gram-positive flora of skin. Three days' use is necessary before effects are evident.

*Antibiotic medications* are used topically for many types of skin infections. Wet dressings are not popular on account of the difficulty of maintaining the effect; therefore most medications are incorporated in ointment bases. Specific agents should be used which have been indicated by antibiotic sensitivity tests. Penicillin, streptomycin and the sulfanilamides have a high index of sensitization and should therefore be avoided. Neomycin (5 mg./gm.), bacitracin (500 units/gm.), polymyxin B (5000 units/gm.), and tyrothricin (0.5 mg./gm.) are antibiotics commonly used topically. Neomycin, however, has a high sensitizing index in man so use care in handling it. Nitrofurazone (0.2 per cent) is an antibacterial agent which is effective in liquid or dressing form.

## ANTIFUNGAL AGENTS

Systemic antifungal agents are usually the treatment of choice since local therapy of dermatomycoses in dogs and cats is not highly effective. Because of the heavy hair coat and the organisms' habitat deep in the hair follicle, contact with topical agents is incomplete. Clipping the hair and use of liquid, low viscosity vehicles is helpful in obtaining more penetration. Some cases have thick keratin scales, and keratolytic agents may promote good contact. Powder vehicles are of little value, and creams are useful only on glabrous areas. Iodine solutions are fungicidal, but some forms are highly irritating if used repeatedly. Vioform cream, however, is a nonirritating form of iodine. Sodium hypochlorite solution (0.5 per cent), diluted 1:20 may be used safely on all animals, and commercial lime-sulfur solutions diluted to 2.5 per cent are also effective. Salts of undecylenic and caprylic acids may be useful. Tolnaftate, which is effective on the glabrous skin of man, is much less effective on the hairy skin of dogs and cats. Nystatin suspension and amphotericin B suspension appear to be useful for Monilia infections.

## ANTIPARASITIC AGENTS

A host of products are available for use on dogs and cats. The active ingredients are incorporated into dips, shampoos, sprays, powders and lotions. Many of them would be highly toxic if applied in a vehicle which promoted absorption, or in a form which enabled the animal to ingest quantities by licking the medication. Cats are especially prone to licking habits and are particularly susceptible to toxic reactions with chlorinated hydrocarbons and organic phosphate products.

With the emphasis on new, more effective drugs we sometimes forget that sulfur and its derivatives are excellent parasiticides. The commercial lime sulfur solution mentioned on page 454 is safe for dogs and cats and is a cheap, effective treatment for several mite infestations, as well as being fungicidal, bactericidal and antipruritic. Sulfur dressings and 10 per cent sulfur ointment USP are other forms of sulfur medications. Citrine ointment (mercury nitrate) and Goodwinol ointment (rotenone) are safe to use near the eyes and can be prescribed for sarcoptic and demodectic mange.

Of the chlorinated hydrocarbons, 5 per cent DDT powders, 0.25 per cent chlordane dips and 2 per cent methoxychlor powder are useful for fleas and lice. However, only the methoxychlor is safe to apply to cats. A mixture of benzyl benzoate and lindane (Mulzyl) may be used topically on dogs (not cats) for sarcoptic or demodectic mange.

Chemicals which are cholinesterase inhibitors are of two kinds, the carbamate compounds and the organophosphates. Carbaryl (1-naphthyl methyl carbamate) is safe for dogs and cats in proper dose and is known under the trade name of Seven. In 3 to 5 per cent concentrations it is used in Diryl, SOK, and Kemic dusts and in numerous sprays at 0.5 per cent concentrations.

The organophosphorus compounds are exceedingly toxic. Although malathion may be safe to use on feline adults, none of this group should be applied to kittens, and many of the group are toxic to all cats. Dioxathion, Delnav, p-dioxane-2-3-diyl ethyl phosphorodithioate; dichlorvos, DDVP, Vapona, 2-2-dichlorovinyl dimethyl phosphate; ronnel, Ectoral, 0,0-dimethyl-0-(2,4,5-trichlorophenyl) phosphorothioate are closely related compounds which are used alone or in combination for fleas, lice and ticks for dogs. Dichlorvos is volatile and has a quick kill while ronnel, malathion and dioxathion give long residual action. These products make excellent agents for treatment of infested premises where residual effect is important.

Two of the organophosphates, ronnel and trichlorfon, have been given to dogs orally as parasiticides, but their expense and somewhat uncertain action have diminished their general popularity.

## TOPICAL ANTI-INFLAMMATORY AGENTS

Wet dressings, previously discussed, are among the simplest and safest agents to reduce inflammation. In recent years topical corticosteroid preparations have been used effectively and safely to reduce inflammation. There is little evidence to suggest that they have caused dissemination of cutaneous infections, but if they are used in the presence of known infections, specific antibacterial, or antifungal agents should be added to the preparation.

In high concentration, in abraded skin or under occlusive dressings, there may be absorption of small amounts of these steroids but they have not produced untoward effects. The most commonly used topical corticosteroids are methylprednisolone Medrol (0.25 to 1 per cent), hydrocortisone (0.25 to 1 per cent), prednisolone (0.5 per cent), dexamethasone (Decadron 0.25 per cent), triamcinolone acetonide (Kenalog 0.1 to 0.25 per cent) and fluocinolone acetonide (Synalar 0.025 per cent).

## MISCELLANEOUS TOPICAL PREPARATIONS

Several active ingredients are used in topical medications without any real understanding of their mechanism of action. Although their indications are empirical, practical experience has shown them to be effective anti-inflammatory agents. These compounds have variable effects with different strengths, and some are characteristically milder than others. They are listed here starting with mild drugs and progressing to stronger ones.

*Salicylic acid* (0.1 to 2 per cent) is said to be keratoplastic or to exert a favorable influence on the new formation of the keratinous layer, and it is indicated in oozing acute dermatoses. In 5 to 20 per cent concentrations, however, salicylic acid acts as a keratolytic, which may be beneficial in thick, scabby keratotic dermatoses.

*Resorcinol* (0.1 to 2 per cent) in compresses and lotions is astringent and somewhat anti-inflammatory. In high concentrations, it, too, is keratolytic and even caustic.

*Sulfur* is similar to resorcinol in its general effects. Strakosch (1943) has shown that the action of sulfur on the skin is mainly twofold, keratoplastic and keratolytic. He obtained the best keratolytic action when sulfur was incorporated in petrolatum. (This is in sharp contrast to the findings with salicylic acid, which produces its effect faster when employed in an emulsion base.) Sulfur's keratolytic effect results from its superficial effect on the horny layer and the formation of hydrogen sulfide. The keratoplastic effect is caused by the deeper action of the sulfur on the basal layer of the epidermis. This effect also was produced by giving sulfur orally or by injection, but the best keratoplastic changes occurred when sulfur in an emulsion base was applied topically. Ten per cent precipitated sulfur in lotions or ointments may intensify epidermal peeling, and is useful for seborrheic and intertriginous dermatoses. Weaker concentrations in other vehicles may be used effectively for bacterial, fungus and parasitic infections.

*Ichthammol* (ichthyol) is a black tar material obtained from bituminous shale. It may be combined with zinc oxide powder to form a thick ointment. Preparations containing ichthammol are mildly astringent but concentrations of 2 to 20 per cent rarely irritate. They are useful for folliculitis and superficial infections such as carbuncles.

Other weaker drugs are used for the treatment of minor inflammations, as astringents, or for stimulation of ulcers and granulation tissue. These include tannic acid (2 to 5 per cent), scarlet red (2 per cent), bismuth subnitrate and subgallate (10 per cent) and benzoin (10 per cent).

## CHEMICAL CAUTERY

Stronger medications may destroy surface tissue and thus may be useful to destroy granulation tissue or to cauterize fissures or ulcers and hasten healing.

*Phenol* (90 per cent) is useful and can be neutralized with alcohol. *Silver nitrate* sticks ($AgNo_3$ 75 per cent and $KNO_3$ 25 per cent) do not penetrate deeply but form a thick superficial crust. *Trichloracetic acid* (75 per cent), a powerful coagulant which does not form thick crusts, is preferred by many dermatologists.

*Tar preparations* are derived from coal or wood distillation. They have important actions in dermatoses of the so-called "chronic eczema" type, but in addition to their antieczematous action they constrict blood vessels, paralyze nerve endings and have antibacterial effects. In concentrated form they may be quite irritating. With repeated use many are carcinogenic, but this would not be a practical problem with normal application. Protracted use also may cause chronic folliculitis and keratosis, and high concentrations used over large areas may cause systemic poisoning. Birch tar, juniper tar and coal tar are crude products listed in order of increasing irritability. Coal tar solution (5-10-20 per cent) produces a milder, more readily managed effect.

Popular veterinary ointments which incorporate some of the principles just listed include Pragmatar (Norden) (Cetyl alcohol, coal tar, sulfur and salicylic acid in an emulsion base), sulfur ointment (USP), ichthammol ointment (USP), zinc oxide and Thuja.

## PHYSICAL THERAPY

Heat and cold are rarely used as treatment modalities in small animal dermatology.

Light treatment is usually of minor importance, too, but ultraviolet has been advocated to produce mild erythema which is said to be beneficial for acne, seborrhea, alopecia and so on. Regulation of dosage is difficult and this treatment, too, should be relegated to antiquity. Sunlight is about the only practical way to apply this therapy.

X-ray therapy does have important benefits to contribute to treatment of skin tumors and acral lick dermatitis. Not all cells are equally sensitive to radiation, so these rays act selectively. Cells which divide rapidly, such as carcinoma cells, the basal cells of the hair papilla and the vascular endothelium, are damaged more easily than those of the balance of the skin. X-ray beams that are "filtered" through aluminum or copper sheets to remove soft rays penetrate deeply into the tissues because of their short wave lengths. Radiation delivered at about 80 kv. with little or no filtration (½ mm. Al) has longer wave lengths and its energy is dissipated very superficially.

Before considering x-ray therapy for a patient, the clinician must be certain:

1. The treatment has good potential for benefit and little potential for harm.
2. No other safer form of therapy will suffice.
3. Proper, safe equipment and facilities are available so:
   a. exact dose can be administered.
   b. The patient can be anesthetized or restrained for therapy without exposure to personnel.
   c. Proper shielding of unaffected parts is provided.
4. Adequate records will be kept for future references.

If these points can be accomplished X-ray therapy may be considered.

In superficial skin diseases such as acute pyoderma, certain dermatoses, rodent ulcer in cats, acral lick dermatitis, acne and externa otitis; or in slightly deeper inflammations such as cellulitis, elbow pyoderma or subcutaneous abscesses, soft to medium rays are helpful. The usual dosage is 300 to 500 R, (HVL 1 mm. A1) repeated within three days (total 600 to 1000 R). In deeper, more chronic inflammations the individual dosage may be 300 R but with filtration up to 0.5 mm. copper, and repeated at three- to four-day intervals for a total dose of 1000 to 1500 R.

In deeper conditions, primarily to deliver tumoricidal doses of radiation, a much larger total dosage is needed. Malignant lesions may require 2000 to 4000 R for effect, but the various types have specific sensitivities. With these higher doses, shielding of unaffected tissue is vitally important, and treatment of the lesion from different angles is desirable to spare tissues that can not be shielded.

*Perianal gland tumors* are highly sensitive to radiation. Castration causes marked regression too. Benign lesions (adenoma) receive 1000 to 2000 R; malignant lesions (adenocarcinoma) should receive 2000 to 4000 R.

*Transmissible venereal tumors* also are exquisitely radiosensitive, so this method is an excellent treatment. Dosage of 1000 to 2000 R produces complete remission.

*Mastocytoma* is usually radiosensitive but multiple sites and rapid extension complicate the treatment problems. Usual dose is 2000 to 4000 R.

*Squamous cell carcinoma* may be sensitive, but some tumors are highly resistant. If surgical excision is not possible, 3000 to 4000 R may be beneficial.

*Malignant melanoma* should be removed surgically by wide excision. Since it metastasizes very early, secondary palliative radiation may be temporarily useful. Dosage is 3000 to 4000 R.

*Fibrosarcoma* should be treated surgically if possible, but palliative radiation therapy, 3000 to 4000 R, may be used adjunctively.

*Neurofibrosarcomas* are highly resistant to radiation therapy.

## References


Arundell, F., and Farber, E. M.: *Cutaneous Medicine: Diagnosis and Management.* Handbook, Dept. of Dermatology, Stanford University School of Medicine, 1966.

Blank, I. H.: The Mechanisms of the Action of Emollients and Keratolytics on the Skin. *In* Sternberg, T. H. and Newcomer, V. D. (eds.): *The Evaluation of Therapeutic Agents and Cosmetics.* McGraw-Hill, N. Y., 1964.

*Frazier, E. N., and Blank, I. H.: *A Formulary for External Therapy of the Skin.* Charles C Thomas, Springfield, Ill., 1954.

Lewis, G. M., and Wheeler, C. E.: *Practical Dermatology, 3rd Edit.* W. B. Saunders Co., Philadelphia, 1967.

Merck Veterinary Manual, 3rd Edit., Merck & Co. Rahway, N. J., 1967.

Pascher, F.: *Dermatologic Formulary, 2nd Edit.* Hoeber Medical Div., Harper & Row, New York, 1957.

*Pillsbury, D. M., Shelley, W. B., and Kligman, A. M.: *Dermatology.* W. B. Saunders Co., Philadelphia, 1956.

Radeleff, R. D.: *Veterinary Toxicology.* Lea & Febiger, Philadelphia, 1964.

Robinson, H. M., and Robinson, R. C. V.: *Clinical Dermatology.* Williams & Wilkins Co., Baltimore, 1959.

Siemens, H. W.: *General Diagnosis and Therapy of Skin Diseases.* Univ. of Chicago Press, Chicago, Ill., 1958.

Strakosch, E. A.: Studies on Ointments. Archives of Dermatology and Syphilology *47:* 216-225, Feb., 1943.

*Welsh, A. L.: *The Dermatologist's Handbook.* Charles C Thomas, Springfield, Ill., 1957.


---

*Suggested supplemental reading.

# SEVENTEEN

# *Systemic Treatment*

## MEDICATIONS

*Antibiotics* are effective in the treatment of pyoderma, cellulitis, infected wounds and superficial mycoses. The specific drug is selected on the basis of sensitivity tests. The dose is determined on a basis of the patient's weight and route of administration. The following antibiotics are used commonly in dermatology.

Penicillin, alone or in combination with streptomycin, is indicated for cellulitis, wound infections and as the initial treatment of pyodermas. Oral forms are inexpensive but procaine penicillin is invariably given by daily intramuscular injections. Beware of urticarial reactions which occur in a few animals.

Synthetic penicillins often are more effective than penicillin against penicillinase-producing organisms (Staphylococcus). Oxacillin sodium, nafcillin sodium and cloxacillin are drugs in this category. Ampicillin, another synthetic, is not effective against penicillinase producers. It covers the usual gram-positive organisms, and a number of gram-negative bacteria including Proteus, Escherichia, Salmonella and Shigella.

The tetracyclines are bacteriostatic, but effective against a broad spectrum of organisms. There is little difference in the action of the various tetracyclines. They are usually given orally as their intramuscular administration often causes pain and local necrosis. Severe yellow discoloration of puppy teeth results from prolonged use of tetracycline during pregnancy or early life.

Chloramphenicol is also a bacteriostatic broad-spectrum antibiotic. Its indications in man are tempered by its notoriety for producing blood dyscrasias. Since these problems have not been prevalent following its use in small animals, it is prescribed more freely. Oral or intramuscular administration can be employed for infections due to Staphylococcus and to Salmonella, *E. coli* and other gram-negative bacilli.

*Sulfonamides* are bacteriostatic agents which characteristically affect only bacteria in the process of multiplication. Although there are many sulfonamides which are absorbed following oral use, the total effect of dosage with any one is the same. The major differences are in absorption and excretion times. These drugs should not be used topically. Their main dermatologic indication is for early use in acute infections caused by gram-positive bacteria. Generally, they should not be given for more than ten days. Most sulfonamides are available in

0.5 gm. tablets; and sulfadimethoxine, sulfasoxazole and triple sulfas (combinations of three sulfonamides) are veterinary favorites.

*Antifungal agents* for systemic use are highly selective.

Griseofulvin is a fungistatic antibiotic obtained by fermentation from several species of Penicillia. Absorption following oral dosage is enhanced if a microcrystalline form is used, and if it is given with food of high fat content. This also helps to alleviate the gastrointestinal distress which may be a side effect. Active griseofulvin is deposited in the horny layer of the skin and in the hair and nails *as they are formed.* It does not penetrate dead keratinous structures which are already formed.

Griseofulvin is active against all known species of Microsporum, Trichophyton and Epidermophyton. It is not effective against *Candida albicans* or deep mycotic agents.

Prolonged therapy is necessary for cure, so it should not be prescribed haphazardly. For proved dermatophytic diseases maintain the full dose for eight weeks, and for chronic cases continue oral therapy until cultures are negative. Do not use it for nonfungal dermatoses. For onychomycosis, maintenance doses of up to eight months are sometimes necessary.

Amphotericin B is a nephrotoxic drug which must be given by injection. It is the primary hope for blastomycosis, coccidioidomycosis, histoplasmosis and cryptococcosis.

*Central nervous depressants* employed may be of three types: sedatives, tranquilizers and analgesics.

Sedatives such as phenobarbital and pentobarbital may be used orally in mild doses for sedative effects, or in higher dosage as hypnotics. Their popularity has decreased, however, with the advent of tranquilizers.

Tranquilizers on the market are numerous. Pick one or two and understand their actions thoroughly. They are effectively used to control patients and to prevent self-mutilation. The ideal state of tranquilization causes the patient to sleep, yet he can be aroused to eat and to walk around. Chlorpromazine, promazine, perphenazine can be given orally or by injection. Propiomazine is effective by injection; however, a few drops on the tongue are absorbed from the oral mucosa. It is not absorbed from the gastrointestinal tract. Trimeprazine is a phenothiazine derivative which may have antipruritic properties too.

*Hormonal medications* are an enigma. Dosage levels are critical, and maintenance of continual, uniform levels as replacement therapy may be crucial to a proper response. Only a few preparations are prescribed effectively for specific skin effects.

Thyroid hormones can be used successfully for replacement therapy, although several weeks may be needed to obtain the initial response. Desiccated thyroid extract, L-triiodothyronine and sodium levothyroxine are oral replacement hormones, while thyroid stimulating hormone must be given by injection. The injections do not lend themselves to long term management of hypothyroidism, but may be useful in the initial management of acanthosis nigricans. The proper use of oral preparations is an inexpensive, practical solution to hypothyroidism in the dog and cat. The shelf life of desiccated thyroid is limited; therefore, it is important to purchase it in small quantities and from a reliable pharmaceutical manufacturer.

Sex hormones are useful in rare cases. Testosterone is indicated after castration for Sertoli cell tumors, and for the male feminizing syndrome. It also is used successfully in conjunction with thyroid extract for treating the hormonal alopecia of male cats. Androgenic hormones increase sebum production and the formation of comedones, so the use of these hormones is contraindicated in seborrhea.

Estrogens or diethylstilbestrol have unpredictable effects on the skin. They tend to reduce sebum production and may merit a trial in seborrhea. Although the cause of the ovarian imbalance syndrome is unknown, a cautious trial with estrogenic replacement hormone may be justified if hypoestrogenism is suspected.

Testosterone in oil USP, repositol testosterone, testosterone cyclopentylpropionate (TCP) for injection and fluoxymesterone (Halotestin) for oral use are androgenic preparations. Popular estrogenic substances include diethylstilbestrol in oil USP, estradiol cyclopentylpropionate (ECP), repositol stilbestrol, in injectable forms and diethylstilbestrol and Premarin in oral forms.

Adrenocortical hormones have potent effects on the skin and are commonly prescribed in dermatologic therapy. The most obvious effect is a marked reduction of itching, probably produced by decrease of inflammation or through inhibition of antigen-antibody reactions. This symptomatic treatment removes one of the major complaints of the patient (and its owner). The drug can be used effectively, but is all too often abused by over-use. Iatrogenic endocrine imbalances have occurred.

The anti-inflammatory effect on the skin is most important in dermatology. Topical or systemic medication causes a reduction of erythema, and inflammatory cells and rapid resolution of many dermatoses. In the presence of infection these steroids should be combined with appropriate antibacterial agents. With hypoadrenocorticalism the increased pigmentation (rare in dogs) may be reduced by proper replacement therapy.

There are many adrenocortical hormones available for systemic use. Most are effective in appropriate oral injectable formulations. Hydrocortisone, prednisone, prednisolone, methylprednisolone (Medrol), dexamethasone (Azium), triamcinolone acetonide (Vetalog) and fluocinolone acetonide (Synalar) are popular preparations.

## NUTRITION

*Nutritional factors* which influence the skin are exceedingly complex. It is obvious, however, that for proper skin health and function, the diet must be complete in all essential nutritional factors. When deficiencies are produced experimentally they often result in cutaneous disorders; but these are seldom characteristic enough to allow specific diagnosis. Furthermore, the interaction of nutrients is such that a deficiency of one item may upset delicate balances, and the skin manifestation may be the result of the imbalance rather than the initial deficiency. For these reasons it is felt that a complex diet of well-balanced, wholesome and fresh ingredients is the proper approach to providing adequate nutrition for skin health. It is necessary in some cases to modify the diet or to use nutritional supplements to improve skin health, but the cliche "Add more fat to the diet" is an overworked suggestion which seldom is helpful.

Nutritional factors influencing the skin are complex. There is no simple supplementation program which cures a skin disease.

General overeating leads to obesity which may cause intertriginous dermatitis and bacterial infections, or by increasing the fat layer make heat dissipation more difficult.

General malnutrition, on the other hand, causes the skin to become dry, inelastic and scaly. It may become more susceptible to infection and show hemorrhagic tendencies and pigment disturbances. Undernourishment can develop through interference with intake, absorption or utilization; through increased requirements or excretion; or through inhibition by antisubstances.

Specific nutritional factors are most difficult to evaluate; a great number of nutrients have been determined to have an influence on skin health. These include amino acids and protein, vitamins and minerals.

## Amino Acids and Protein

Protein deficiency edema is an extreme condition. Some species however, have shown skin lesions from diets deficient in methionine, cystine, tryptophane, and phenylalanine-tyrosine.

The polyunsaturated fatty acids (linoleic and arachidonic) are essential for most species, but arachidonic acid can be manufactured in animal tissues from linoleic acid. Only a severe deficiency of these nutrients produced dry hair, dry, scaly skin and susceptibility to infections (Hansen and Wiese, 1943).

Safer et al. (1965) have reported that excessively high carbohydrate levels produce dermatoses with pruritus.

## Vitamins

The members of the B-complex group seem to be important, as skin lesions have been reported from feeding diets deficient in thiamine, riboflavin, nicotinic acid, pyridoxine, panthothenic acid, biotin, inositol, para-aminobenzoic acid and folic acid.

Vitamin A is essential to integrity of epithelial tissues. A deficiency may cause follicular hyperkeratosis whereas excesses of five to ten times the amount needed for growth are reported to produce more lustrous coats (Bradfield and Smith, 1962).

Vitamin E is a natural antioxidant which helps inhibit the oxidation of fats and other nutrients such as vitamins A, D and pyridoxine.

## Minerals and Other Supplements

Robertson reported that diets high in calcium and low in zinc produced emaciation, poor growth, and skin lesions on the abdomen and extremities consisting of three to six small areas of alopecia, crusting and superficial desquamation. The entire coat was dull and rough. The lesions were reversed by lowering the level of calcium or increasing the level of zinc.

Although many nutritional supplements are available commercially which are touted as products to improve skin health and hair sheen, few of them really work except in cases of severe nutritional needs. In these cases steps to provide a fresh, well-balanced diet are usually more effective therapy.

One type of supplementation has somewhat more merit, and often does produce improvement in skin and coat. It contains a combination of polyunsaturated fatty acids, vitamins A, E and pyridoxine, and zinc. Although this synergistic combination may produce its effects with two to three weeks' supplementation, the basic diet of affected animals should be modified so that improvement is maintained without the need of prolonged supplementation.

## References

Bradfield, D., and Smith, M. C.: Nutrient Requirements of Dogs *in* Nutrient Requirements of Domestic Animals No. 8. National Academy of Science, National Research Council, 1962.

Hansen, A. E., and Wiese, H. F.: Studies with Dogs Maintained on Diets in Fat. Proc. Soc. Biol. Med. *52*:205, 1943.

Hawkins, W. W.: Antivitamin B6 in Diet of Dogs. Science *121*:880, 1955.

Krehl, W.: Borden's Review of Nutritional Research. *18*:1-5, 1957.

Monson, W. J.: Nutritional Considerations in Skin and Coat Maintenance. Vet. Med. Jan.: 54-56, 1965.

Robertson, B. T., and Burns, M. J.: Zinc Metabolism and Zinc Deficiency Syndrome in the Dog. Am. J. Vet. Res. *24*: 997-1002, 1963.

*Rothman, S.: *Physiology and Biochemistry of the Skin*, University of Chicago Press, 1954.

Safer, E. D., Jones, H. L., and Zimmerman, C.: Management of Dermatologic Conditions in Animals—A Review. Vet. Med. Oct.: 1028-1033, 1965.

*Suggested supplemental reading.

# EIGHTEEN

# *Skin Surgery*

The dermatologist who employs surgical treatment for diseases of man usually performs minor techniques on skin which is relatively hairless, therefore the cosmetic effects are crucial. Most procedures appear complex because avoidance of scarring is a primary consideration. In veterinary dermatology one should of course avoid disfigurement, but because of the dense pelage, small scars are relatively unimportant.

With any surgical procedure it is necessary to clip the hair closely, wash the surface of the skin carefully with soap and water, defat with ether swabs several times and apply an alcohol-base skin antiseptic. Tincture of Zephiran is a satisfactory solution to use and the skin should be kept wet with Zephiran for at least two minutes.

*Skin biopsy* procedures have been discussed on page 102.

*Excision* of small tumors and other lesions is a minor procedure which often can be done on an outpatient basis, but usually is better performed if the animal is held in the hospital for several hours. This enables one to use tranquilization, sedation or general anesthesia as needed to promote control and relaxation of the patient. Patients requiring extensive surgery with plastic repair procedures and grafts need to go to the operating room with complete aseptic routine. Even minor cases, however, must be handled with proper preparation, sterile instruments and other measures to accomplish a scrupulously *clean* operation.

Sedation with Demerol (5 mg./lb. i.m.), propiopromazine (0.2 mg./lb. i.v.), or Numorphan (0.1 mg./lb.) plus chlorpromazine (0.5 mg./lb. i.v.) should be used, together with local anesthesia. This can be subcutaneous infiltration of 0.5 per cent Xylocaine for deeper lesions or surface refrigerants such as ethyl chloride or Freon (Frigiderm) sprays for superficial ones. With the Numorphan-chlorpromazine combination alone analgesia usually is adequate for minor surgery.

The lesions should be outlined by elliptical scalpel incisions extended through the skin and the specimen dissected free of underlying tissue with scissors. Subcuticular catgut sutures, or fine nylon or stainless steel sutures, in the skin will produce good approximation with minimal scarring. Sutures approximating small incisions can be removed in seven days.

*Skin grafts*, flaps and procedures to reduce lines of tension influencing suture lines will not be considered here. These naturally fall into the realm of plastic surgery and readers are referred to the works of Spreull for complete information.

*Electrosurgery* requires specialized equipment which is designed to destroy superficial tissue in a manner which allows reepithelialization without formation of scar tissue. Most techniques are simple, have almost no danger of infection and no danger of dehiscence. Several forms of electrosurgery are used.

*Fulguration* is a monoterminal technique using Oudin current (high voltage, low amperage). A single active electrode is held a distance from the lesion and superficial destruction is caused by a spark arcing into the tissue. Destruction is by dehydration.

*Electrodesiccation* is similar to fulguration except that the electrode is inserted into the tissue before the current is applied. Special surgical diathermy units may be used for bipolar electrocoagulation or for cutting currents. These are expensive, complex electrical units that are eminently effective. They must be periodically inspected to assure safety and freedom from interference with radio or television communications.

With any electrosurgical unit it is necessary to avoid usage in the vicinity of explosive or inflammatory agents, and to avoid overheating surrounding tissues. When alcohol or ether is used to prepare the skin, the area should be thoroughly dried before introducing the current. When electrocoagulation is used to stop hemorrhage of nail beds, it is easy to overheat the area and cause subsequent deformity or lack of growth of the nails. Many units need to be grounded to the patient. This must never be overlooked, and good contact between the patient and the ground plate can be assured if saline or alcohol is used to wet the hair contacting the plate.

*Electrolysis* is used for permanent destruction of the hair follicle and is used in dogs only to destroy extra eyelashes (districhiasis). A continuous battery current (0.5 to 2.0 milliamperes) is utilized with the patient the positive pole and the needle the negative pole. The needle is inserted into or very close to the hair follicle and the current applied. It is a relatively painless procedure, but complete restraint is necessary because of the delicate manipulation it entails.

*Tattoo* marks are applied to dogs' ears and inner rear flanks to serve as a means of identification, or to unpigmented regions such as the eyelids or the dorsal nasal area to prevent sunlight exposure. General short-acting anesthesia is needed to control the patient. The tattoo ink must be inserted into the superficial layers of the dermis for lasting effects. If profuse hemorrhage occurs at tattooing much of the ink will be washed out. If the ink particles are deposited too superficially they will be shed with the epidermis, and if placed too deep they will be removed by the circulation. Several applications at one to three month intervals may be needed to build up a heavy layer of ink to properly shield unpigmented areas of skin (nose). In some severe cases of nasal solar dermatitis an annual "touch-up" tattoo is needed.

The Nicholsen tattooing needles, with or without the vibrator, can be used to push the ink particles into the skin or a clamp type tattoo punch can be used to apply numerals. Ink is applied to the skin before needling, and ink is gently rubbed into the area afterward.

A clinical case involving tattoo for nasal solar dermatitis is illustrated on page 306.

*Refrigeration* is used rarely in veterinary dermatology. Liquid nitrogen, if available, might be useful for removing warts. Ethyl chloride or Freon are helpful local anesthetics, and also are used to toughen tissue for "crisp" removal of biopsy specimens. The principle of superficial freezing is used in human dermatology to toughen the epidermis for dermabrasion procedures.

## Reference

Spreull, J. S. A.: Principles of transplanting skin in the dog. A.A.H.A. Scientific presentations, 34th Annual Meeting, 1967, American Animal Hospital Association, Elkhart, Ind. pp. 235-243.

# NINETEEN

# *Care of the Skin and Hair Coat*

Although it is true that the skin is a reflection of general health, many vigorous, normal pets have unkempt hair coats—mainly because of neglect. The veterinarian is vitally concerned with the health of his patient's skin, but he should leave the styling, grooming and cosmetic aspects of its hair coat to others. We do not visit a physician for a haircut; neither should we take our dog to the veterinarian for a trim. (However, some veterinarians do employ others to operate separate grooming facilities.) Styles change and variations in clipping can enhance or mask aspects of conformation which compliment the animal's appearance. These nuances are the province of owners, breeders, handlers and commercial grooming establishments. Much of the following discussion is presented here as background for students, or for transmittal to clients.

## GROOMING PROCEDURES IN VETERINARY PRACTICE

In everyday practice, clinicians are often faced with the need to clip, shave or otherwise alter a patient's coat for medical reasons. The cosmetic effects may be drastic and if not carefully explained may provoke intense client resentment. Shaving prior to surgical procedures is of course understandably important, but needlessly clipping the hair over a vein for a simple intravenous injection may produce a hairy defect which will be unsightly for several months. Hair removed from Afghans may take as long as 18 months to replace.

Remember the cosmetic effects of clipping hair and try to avoid drastic disfigurement.

Even necessary clipping can be made less obvious if the area is blended into the normal coat by beveling the edges of the lesion. Then as hair regrows the line of demarcation is not so abrupt and not obtrusive.

Proper use of the groomer's tools to remove hair mats and snarls will often obviate extensive clipping. Most clients sincerely appreciate initial attempts to remove crusts, debris and mats by grooming procedures rather than by hasty clipping. However, when harsh methods are indicated they must be used.

## Routine Grooming Care

Dog and cat breeds have many different coat types, so generalization of grooming details is difficult. A few important principles can be emphasized – the most critical being frequency of care. When a schedule of grooming is found to suffice for keeping the pet "looking sharp" it should be adhered to religiously. It is better to spend a few minutes regularly than many hours sporadically. Part of the impetus to do the job depends on motivation, so making it easy is important. If proper facilities, effective tools and a cooperative patient are combined, the task of grooming can be fun. A solid, convenient table with a nonskid surface, or a grooming stand with a chair is necessary. It should be located in a quiet area free of distractions. The proper grooming tools should be clean and in good repair. Comb, brush, nail clipper and file, towels, cotton and swab sticks are the vital implements needed for most breeds. Shampoo, ear cleaning solution, hair lotion and flea spray are necessary too. Specialized tools, to be described later, are essential for grooming and conditioning some coats.

The animal and his training can make a world of difference in the ease of grooming. Regular habits of good behavior during grooming, established early in life, result in complete cooperation. Most properly trained pets thoroughly enjoy their grooming care.

Prospective pet owners should contemplate grooming problems before purchasing a pet. If time and expense are likely to be problems one should not choose a pet from a long-haired, wiry or woolly-coated breed, but instead select a short-coated, easy-to-groom animal. An owner should perform simple daily or weekly grooming chores himself, but he should periodically take advantage of professional grooming service. The grooming needs of five typical coat types will be discussed later.

## Grooming Tools

Various grooming implements are needed (Fig. 19:1), the number and type depending on the breed and coat type.

*Electric clippers* especially designed for small animals are best. They should have changeable heads and a selection of different-sized blades. Clippers should be held gently on the skin surface and moved slowly. The moving parts should be clean, sharp and well lubricated. If the blades become hot, are forced, or are pointed down at the skin, severe irritation and "burns" may result. The delicate skin of the genital, eye and ear regions is most susceptible. Clipping against the "lay" of the hair produces a shorter cut with any blade than cutting with the hair. Clipping blades are numbered – the larger the number the closer the cut is made to the skin and the more hair is removed. The No. 40 blade produces a shaven appearance when used against the hair. Only a slight stubble is left when it is used with the hair. No. 15 also cuts closely. No. 10 blades leave enough hair to show the natural color of the coat. These two (Nos. 15 and 10) have general

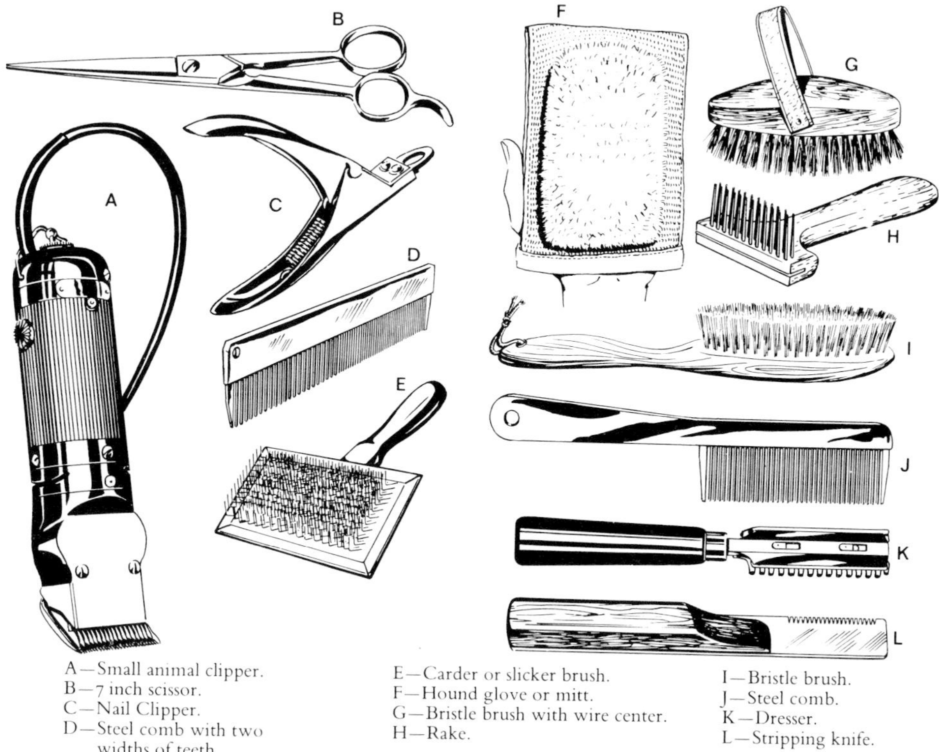


**Figure 19:1.** Grooming implements. (From Miller: *Know How to Groom Your Dog.* By Permission of Pet Library Ltd., a subsidiary of Sternco Industries, Inc., New York City)

purpose uses, especially around the face, feet and ears of many breeds. No. 7 blade leaves hair about 1/4 inch long and No. 5 leaves about 1/2 inch. These latter blades (Nos. 5 and 7) are used for "machine clipping" wiry-coated breeds.

Dogs should be carefully introduced to the clipper the first time. The owner can be helpful in this step by training at home. By holding an electric razor near the dog and rubbing it over his coat several times daily he will soon become accustomed to its vibration and noise. Gentle firmness and frequent short "breaks" for relaxation are necessary during the clipping sessions.

*Shears* are often used in conjunction with a comb. A barber scissors about 7 inches long with blunt tips is used to trim long hair and whiskers around the eyes, ears, face and feet. It is often needed to remove mats and tags. A thinning shears has one solid blade and one serrated blade so that large bulky coats can be thinned without obvious signs. It is well to insert the shears deeply under the surface of the coat to avoid destroying the external color of coats where the undercoat and the outer coat are different colors.

*Combs* should have rounded teeth to avoid scratching the skin. Combs should always be inserted their full depth into the coat to perform efficiently. Different tooth-spacing is needed for each coat type. Metal, plastic and bone combs are available. The material is not as important as the comb's design.

The *rake* is an instrument which is especially useful in hacking through the heavy mats in a badly tangled coat. The rake has a single row of long metal teeth set at right angles to the handle. It can inflict serious wounds, especially inside the hock and thigh, and should be used with the utmost care.

A *carder* is a square "board" with a short handle. It has bent, fine-wire teeth set close together. The teeth are placed near the skin and the carder twisted outward from the skin. This serves to loosen the coat, and to remove dead hair and some of the hair mats.

*Brushes* may be used the same way on long coats, and if the hair is meant to stand away from the skin the hair should be brushed (with short strokes) against its natural growth. Smooth-coated dogs should be brushed with the "lay" of the hair. Some groomers feel that nylon or synthetic bristles accumulate static electricity and cause hair breakage. They prefer natural pig bristles or soft wire brushes. Brushes for longer coats have wider-spaced, longer bristles which are firmly set into the rubber base handle.

*Hound gloves* have a palm consisting of boar hair, wire or fiber bristles. They are used on short-haired dogs to remove the dead undercoat and to give polish to the outer coat.

*Stripping combs* are also referred to as "dressers." They may be a type with a razor blade encased in serrated teeth, or merely a serrated metal blade attached to a wooden handle. These instruments are used to help "pull out" dull, dead hair. Hair is grasped between the thumb and the comb and removed with a twisting motion. Chalk is sometimes used on the coat to make the hair easier to grip firmly. If the hair is grasped between the thumb and forefinger and extracted, the process is called "plucking." The purpose of stripping and plucking, as applied to terrier type breeds whose coats are "blown" (loose or ripe), is to remove the dead hair and retain the live. When these animals are "clipped" with a No. 5 or No. 7 blade, both live and dead hairs are shortened. Although the machine clip is fast it is obviously much less desirable.

*Hand rubbing and toweling* are used to rub out dead hairs, to stimulate skin circulation and to give a gloss or glow to the hair.

## Special Grooming Needs Prior to Bathing

Prior to bathing the nails should be clipped or filed to keep them short. Only the Chihuahua breed can be tolerated (in shows) with moderately long nails. All other breeds should have the nails kept short to keep the feet compact and tight. With frequent filing the quick will recede and the nail can be maintained properly.

Teeth should be scaled periodically with a hook-shaped tartar scraper. Occasional scrubbing with cotton dipped in sodium bicarbonate helps keep them white. Periodic ultrasonic cleaning under deep sedation is recommended. The intervals between these procedures varies from three months to 18 months with the individual's tartar-building capacity.

The anal sacs should be palpated and expressed if necessary prior to bathing so any soilage can be removed during the bath. Placing cotton over the anus and pressing forward and together to express the sacs is reasonably effective. A more complete expression of sac contents can be performed by inserting a gloved finger into the rectum to express each sac separately.

The ears, too, should be cared for during bathing. Excess hair should be plucked from the external ear canal if cerumen accumulates and irritation is present. The process of plucking may cause irritation in normal ears. A cotton swab dampened with alcohol will usually serve admirably to remove waxy exudates. Pledgets of cotton should be placed firmly in each ear canal to block the entrance of soap and water. After the bath the cotton is removed and the ears carefully examined, and cleaned and dried thoroughly if necessary.

## Bathing

In addition to the foregoing, the dog's eyes should be protected from soap during bathing by applying a small amount of boric acid or cod-liver-oil ointment into the conjunctival sac. If the dog is unkempt and severely matted the tags and mats should be cut out *before* they are wet.

All long-coated dogs should be combed out completely before bathing.

The dog is placed in a raised tub and wet completely with warm water. A shower spray hose is almost essential for easy bathing. Use a bland, liquid coconut-oil shampoo for most dogs. Powdered detergents especially designed for dogs are very effective and rinse off easily without leaving a dull film. However, they should be dissolved completely before application and only used in small amounts. The shampoo is applied to the neck and topline of the dog. More water is added and a vigorous lather is worked up. Rub the lather into short-haired dogs, but squeeze it into long coats as rubbing may mat the long hair excessively. The dog's face should be washed carefully and rinsed carefully. Then the entire coat is rinsed thoroughly. A second lathering and rinse may be needed to wash the dog until the water runs off clear. The hair should squeak. Special vinegar, lemon or bleaching rinses are not recommended except for special problems. However, a small amount of Alpha-Keri or similar oil can be added to a pan of water for the last rinse and will add gloss to the coat.

Squeeze the coat to eliminate water, wrap the dog in a towel and lift him from the tub to a table. Short-coated dogs can be toweled almost dry and then pinned into a large towel to help "set" the coat smoothly. Pin towel under abdomen and at neck. Dogs with long coats should be placed in a stream of warm air and the coat combed, brushed and fluffed as needed to accomplish the desired effect. All animals should be protected from chilling during a bath and for several hours after, until thoroughly dry.

All breeds should be bathed before major trimming or stripping sessions as this loosens dead hair. The frequency of a grooming routine depends on the breed and the individual's needs. It is necessary to keep animals clean, but baths tend to soften those coats which should be hard and wiry and may remove natural oils so the coat becomes dull. Products such as Alpha-Keri, Mr. Groom, or St. Aubrey Coatasheen or Coat Dressing often work wonders in restoring luster and keeping hair manageable.

#### DRY BATHS

To avoid the drying influence of water baths, dry cleaner products can be used which are reasonably effective, especially in long coats. Talc, boric acid powder, or superior special products such as St. Aubrey powder can be dusted into the coat and then thoroughly brushed out. With a careful job the coat is left clean and lustrous. However, shampoo and water baths are still the most effective way to really clean the coat.

### Grooming Needs of Individual Coat Types

For grooming purposes dogs' coats can be divided into five types: the long coats, the silky coat, the nonshedding curly coat, the smooth coat, and the wiry coat. Special grooming greatly enhances the appearance of each dog, but he must have a good natural coat and good conformation for the best effect. The ability to grow a good coat depends largely on inherited factors. Medications, lotions and special nutrients, either internal or external, have only limited effects on the coat of a healthy dog.

#### THE LONG COAT WITH UNDERCOAT

Typical breeds include Newfoundlands, German shepherds, collies, Old English sheepdogs, Siberian huskies and Samoyeds.

Necessary implements include natural bristle brush, Hinds 3060 wire brush, regular and fine Resco combs.

Bathe twice yearly—in spring and fall. Save the coat during the winter. Comb and brush the coat forward over the top and sides, backward over the flanks. Use a fine comb, with the hair, under the chin and tail and behind the ears. Dry cleaning with powder brushed through the hair is effective.

#### THE SILKY COAT

Typical breeds include spaniels, Afghans, Maltese and Yorkshire terriers, setters, Lhasa apso and Pekingese.

Necessary implements include Hinds or St. Aubrey wire brushes, medium and fine steel comb, natural bristle brush, Oster clipper with blades Nos. 7, 10 and 15, Duplex stripping knife and barber scissors.

While all long coats require frequent regular brushing, silky coats in addition require fairly frequent bathing to prevent mats and skin irritation. To brush out these coats lift the hair with the hand and comb or brush down until it is free of snarls to the skin. Spaniels grow two or three coats per year and should be stripped or clipped about every three months.

#### THE NONSHEDDING CURLY OR WOOLLY COAT

Typical breeds include poodles, Bedlington terrier and Kerry blue terriers.

Necessary implements include Oster clipper with Nos. 7A, 10 and 15 blades, natural bristle brush, fine, medium and coarse steel combs (Twinco or Resco), and scissors.

The three breeds listed above must be clipped every six weeks for best appearance. The puppies should be exposed to grooming from eight weeks of age so they will accept the clippers. The first clip should be between eight and 12 weeks of age, when just the face, feet and tail are shaved. Use only the scissors under the tail as the skin is very tender there and easily irritated.

White, silver and apricot poodles seem to have especially sensitive skin. A soothing lotion such as Mercaptocaine or Nivea Creame should be applied to areas of possible abrasion.

Since dead and loose hairs from these coats are mostly secondary hairs which become enmeshed in the coat, neglect causes a felt matting. All dead hair must be completely combed out before bathing.

Routine care of this group includes daily combing and wire brushing or carding.

#### *THE SMOOTH COAT*

Typical breeds include the hounds, the retrievers, dachshunds, Dalmatians, beagles, whippets, Doberman pinschers, smooth terriers and boxers.

Necessary implements include only a hound glove or a rubber hound brush and scissors.

Dogs of this group should be bathed only when necessary for cleanliness. The scissors are used to trim off the tactile hairs on the face or to shape the fringes of hair on the tail, ears and brisket. The coat can be rubbed to shiny sleekness using the hound glove, the hands or towels. This also removes dead hairs.

#### *THE WIRY COAT*

Typical breeds include the wire-haired fox terrier, Welsh terrier, Airedale terrier, Lakeland terrier, schnauzer and Sealyham terrier.

Necessary implements include Oster clipper blades Nos. 7, 10, and 15, a Duplex stripping knife, a Hinds slicker brush, fine and medium steel combs, a hound glove and barber scissors.

Pups of these breeds should be started on a grooming routine at four months of age by trimming the head, ears and tail. As adults they require machine clipping every six to eight weeks or hand stripping every 12 weeks.

A special problem is presented by attempting to pull a coat that isn't loose. The skin will become sore by such treatment. Scissoring around the eyes, ears and tail should be done carefully to avoid lacerating those areas. Blunt-pointed scissors are useful to prevent eye lacerations.

The fingers can best be used to pluck excess hair from the vicinity of the eyes.

### Special Grooming Problems

*Mats* can usually be teased apart and combed out if they are small. Very small ones behind the ears and under the legs can be cut off. Larger mats can be slit with a special knife and then teased with one or two teeth of a comb. Some badly neglected long-coated cats or dogs may have an almost complete covering of felt matting. These mats do not form close to skin. The only solution to some of these unfortunate cases is general anesthesia and complete, close clipping. Extreme care is necessary to avoid cutting or irritating the skin. Sometimes the teeth of a comb can be slipped between the mat and the skin so the mat can be safely scissored.

*Tar* or *paint* imbedded in the coat may be difficult to remove. Small deposits should be allowed to harden and then cut off. Tar masses can be soaked in vegetable oil for 24 hours (bandaged if needed) to soften and then washed out with soap and water. *Never* use paint removers or organic solvents such as kerosene, turpentine, or gasoline to remove tar or paint! Ether may be used carefully for small areas.

*Odors* about a coat usually originate from places such as the mouth, ears, feet or perineum. These should be checked and washed carefully. A rinse with a dilute chlorophyl solution or dilute sodium hypochlorite (in a white animal only) may help remove traces of odors. Highly scented dressings and sprays are objectionable to many people and do not reliably mask odors. The odor of skunks can be greatly ameliorated with a soap and water bath, and a rinse in *dilute* ammonia water. (The tomato juice soak is effective but messy.) Once the dog dries the odor will be gone, but when wet, the hair may have a faint skunk scent for several weeks.

## Comments on Grooming Cats

The grooming implements used for dogs generally serve adequately for cats too. However, grooming details have special application which are outlined here. From the grooming standpoint, cats have three types of coats—the short hair, single coat; the short hair, double coat; and the long hair.

*The short hair, single coat* is typified by the Siamese, Burmese, Havana brown, rex, korat and the domestic shorthair. These cats can be bathed in shampoo and water, quickly dried to avoid chilling, and brushed and combed against the hair to remove dead hair. Final brushing is with the hair. A fine metal comb and natural boar bristle brush are the only implements needed.

*The short hair, double coat* is typified by the Abyssinian, Manx, Russian blue and the American shorthair. The double coat is composed of two sets of hair. The long guard hair gives the coat its color, and the dense, short undercoat provides warmth. Both sets of hair are essential in these breeds. The basic coat care of this group is similar to that used for single coats except that caution must be employed as over-grooming can destroy the coat.

*The long hair* is typified by Persians and Himalayans. Several sizes of metal combs and a boar bristle brush are necessary for grooming these breeds. The kittens should be started with grooming at four weeks of age.

Older kittens and adults can be bathed with mild shampoo and water. Place them on a slanted window screen in a tub. (They feel secure on the wire and stay put, yet water passes through easily.) Rinse well and dry quickly with a towel and a warm air blower. It is important to comb and brush the hair against the grain as it is being air-dried. This fluffs the coat and gives it body. Do not bathe frequently and not within two weeks preceding a show.

Mats tend to form behind the ears, and under the chin, front and rear legs and tail. The skin under the mat becomes irritated. Mats can be prevented by daily combing and brushing.

Some breeders dry clean the coats, with powder or talc sprinkled into the coat and carefully brushed out with an up and away from the body motion. If powder is left in the hair it resembles unsightly dandruff and is highly objectionable.

Never clip the ruff or tail of a long-haired cat. The eyes and nasal area should be cleaned to remove exudates which may accumulate.

### *SPECIAL FELINE GROOMING PROBLEMS*

A cat's nails should be clipped only if necessary. They soon grow out again and are honed sharply.

Cat's ears are much less prone to infection than dogs, but they should always be checked and cleaned if needed.

The large supracaudal organ on the dorsal surface of the tail is a mass of hyperactive sebaceous glands which may cause trouble if neglected. Breeders call the problem "stud tail," although it occurs in both sexes. A waxy, unsightly accumulation builds up in the area if proper hygiene is neglected. The exudate can be removed by applying powder to soak it up, by applying a thin oil to soften it, or by sponging the area with alcohol or detergents as solvents. Following this preparation, the oil usually can be brushed or washed off satisfactorily. Periodic cleansing should prevent any future problem.

## *References*

Bandy, A. D.: Personal communication. 1968.
Mahoney, J.: Personal communication. 1968.
*Miller, D.: *Know How to Groom Your Dog.* The Pet Library Ltd., New York, N.Y.
*Saunders, B.: *How to Trim, Groom and Show Your Dog.* Howell Book House Inc., New York, 1967.
Spath, S.: Personal communication. 1968.

*Suggested supplemental reading.

# CANINE AND FELINE DERMATOSES

*Section Five*

# TWENTY

# *Acanthosis Nigricans*

Acanthosis nigricans is a chronic disorder occurring mostly in dachshunds. It is characterized by hyperpigmentation, alopecia, rugose thickening and lichenification of the axillary skin. In advanced cases, the condition involves the legs, flanks and chest (Fig. 20:1*C*).

## SIGNIFICANT FACTS

1. The cause of acanthosis nigricans has not yet been definitely established; however, an endocrine "imbalance" is suspected. There is a popular theory that decreased production of thyroid stimulating hormone (TSH) by the pituitary gland is a major etiologic factor.

2. The disease occurs mostly in dachshunds, but is also seen in other breeds.

3. In obese individuals the lesions are more severe; however, friction of the axillary area alone is not the cause because most other short-legged, obese dogs do not have acanthosis nigricans.

4. Prognosis for complete recovery must always be guarded. Most cases respond favorably to intense and systematic treatment, but recurrences are frequent.

## LESIONS AND COURSE

1. The juvenile stage is easily overlooked. As early as six months of age, affected dogs have a small brown patch in both axillae. There is no discomfort, and the skin is normal except for these hyperpigmented spots (Fig. 20:1*A*).

2. As the disease advances, a bilaterally symmetrical patch in the axillae becomes grayish black, thickened, lichenified, and develops a greasy surface film that has a seborrheic, rancid odor (Fig. 20:1*B*).

3. Although there is no pruritus or discomfort in the earlier stages, secondary infection causes erythema and mild pain.

4. The disease progresses to an advanced stage afflicting the legs, chest, flanks and neck. Deep folds appear on the anterior and medial surfaces of the legs. The axillae and forelegs are involved first, then the hindlegs, and eventually the unsightly "tarsal flaps" appear. The entire ventral body surface is

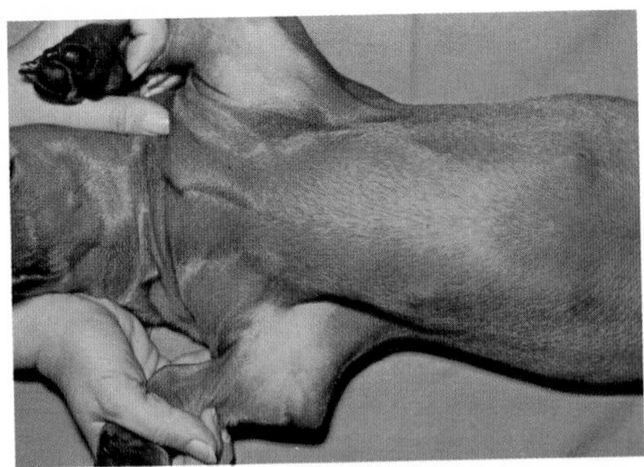

**Figure 20:1.** Acanthosis nigricans.

*A.* Juvenile stage. Note the small hyperpigmented patches in the axillae of this six-month-old dachshund.

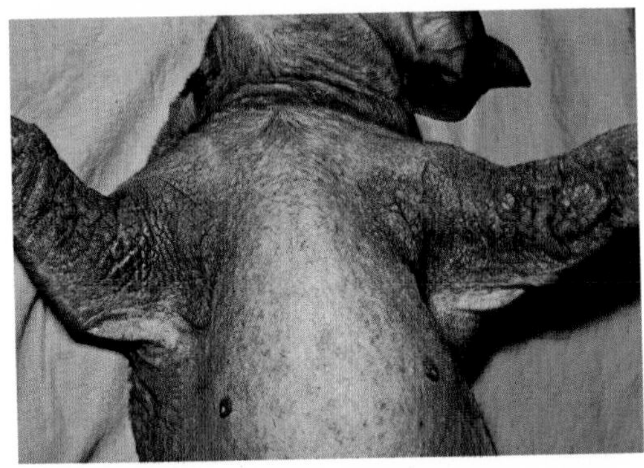

*B.* Severe hyperpigmentation and lichenification in a five-year-old dachshund.

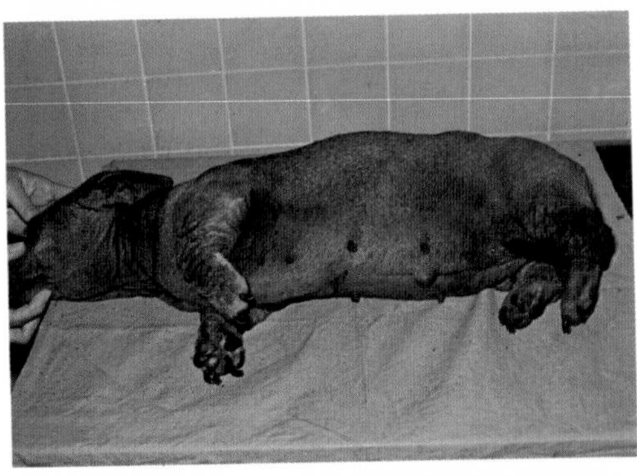

*C.* Chronic, advanced stage in a 13-year-old dachshund.

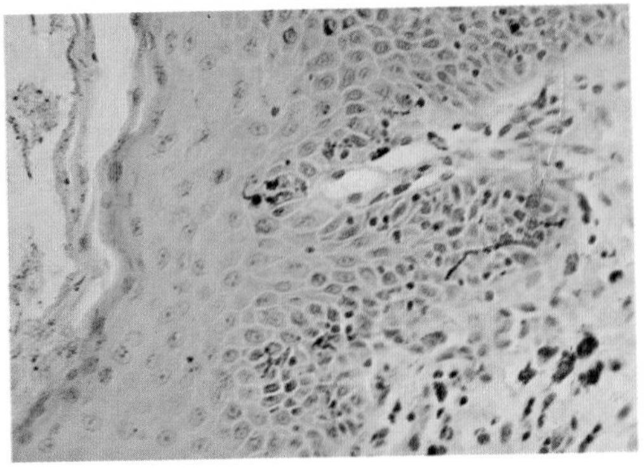

*D.* Epidermis showing an acanthotic, elongated rete ridge and parakeratotic horny layer. Note the increased melanin pigment in the basal layer and upper dermis. (High power.)

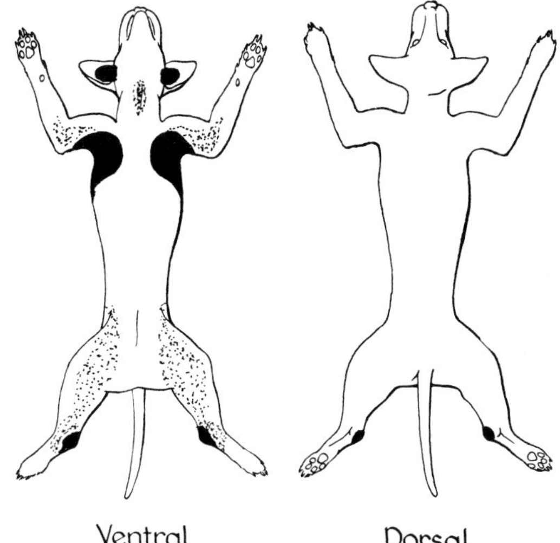


**Figure 20:2.** Acanthosis nigricans distribution pattern.

affected in extremely advanced cases. The dorsal surface, fortunately, remains relatively normal except for seborrheic scales (Fig. 20:1*C*).

5. In the advanced stage, seborrhea is present as a complicating factor.

## HISTOPATHOLOGY

As the name implies, there is marked acanthosis and increased deposit of melanin pigment in the upper dermis and the basal layer of the epidermis. The epidermal surface is wavy, covered with a parakeratotic horny layer, and some of the epidermal crevices are filled with keratin. Prominent rete ridges can be seen. There is atrophy of the apopilosebaceous units, with the remaining hair follicles devoid of hairs and filled with keratin and sebum (Fig. 20:1*D*).

## DIFFERENTIAL DIAGNOSIS

Lesions of acanthosis nigricans always start in the axillae.

1. The feminizing syndrome of male dogs shows ventral hyperpigmentation and lichenification, but lesions begin on the lower abdominal area and the flanks. Sertoli cell tumors produce similar lesions.

2. Some ovarian "imbalances" also affect the perigenital area and lower abdomen, causing hyperpigmentation and lichenification.

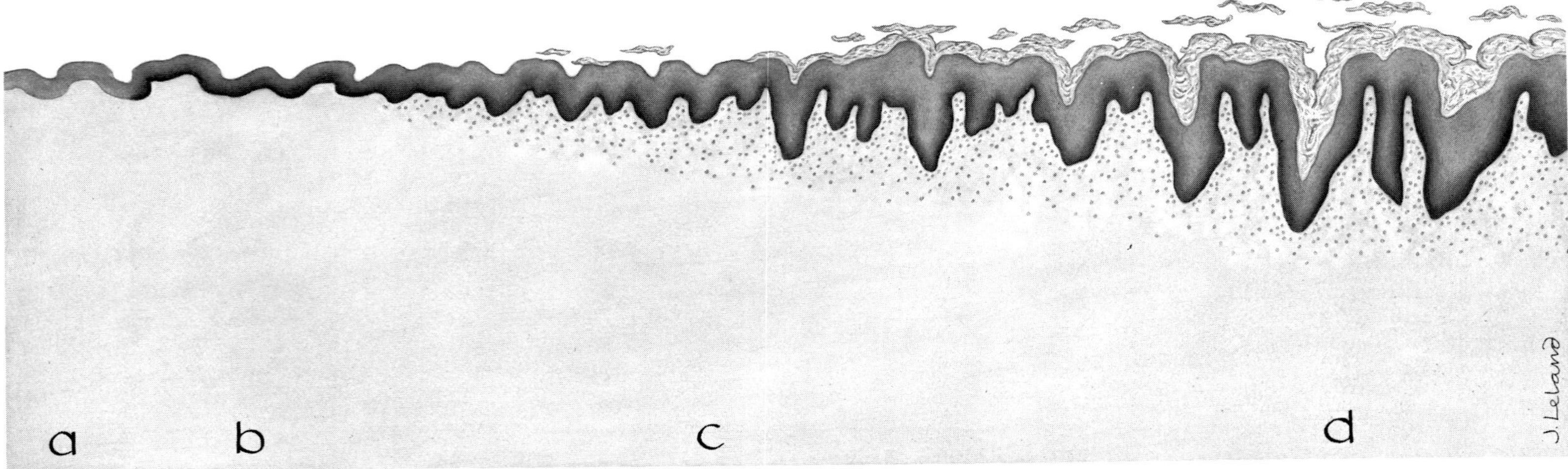


**Figure 20:3.** Acanthosis nigricans dermogram. *a.* Normal skin. *b.* In the early stage, hyperpigmented patches appear in the axillae. *c.* Elongated rete pegs, acanthosis, hyperpigmentation, hyperkeratosis and mild dermal infiltration account for the thickened, gray, lichenified skin of more advanced cases. Scales and a greasy film form on the surface. *d.* In the chronic stage, the skin in many ventral areas of the body becomes thickened and the changes shown in *c* are even more pronounced.

3. In advanced cases of gonadal imbalances ventral hyperpigmentation, hyperkeratosis and lichenification are common. An accurate case history is necessary to establish the order of appearance of the lesions.

## CLINICAL MANAGEMENT

### A. Systemic Treatment

1. Thyroid inhibitory drugs decrease hormone production of the thyroid gland, thereby stimulating the anterior pituitary gland to produce more thyroid stimulating hormone (TSH). There is a reciprocal relationship between the thyroxine circulating in the blood and the production of TSH by the pituitary gland. Administration of an antithyroid agent (propylthiouracil USP or methimazole USP) aids in providing a beneficial dermatropic effect in acanthosis nigricans through increased TSH production by the pituitary gland.

Propylthiouracil USP—Dosage is 5 mg./lb. of body weight daily. One 100 mg. tablet daily can be used for the average dachshund until lesions have been reversed. Thereafter, a small daily maintenance dose may be needed if lesions return.

Preliminary experience has failed to show undesirable side effects from prolonged maintenance therapy. Lifelong maintenance therapy has not been studied sufficiently at this time to recommend it without reservations.

2. Corticosteroids are useful because of their anti-inflammatory effects.

3. Appropriate broad-spectrum antibiotics should be given systemically only if there is secondary bacterial infection.

### B. Local Treatment

1. The first objective is to cleanse the affected skin and remove excess sebum, epidermal debris and bacteria. An antiseborrheic shampoo containing selenium sulfide is especially useful.

2. Topical corticosteroid ointments containing antibiotics, such as Panolog, are useful.

3. For lichenified, seborrheic skin, Pragmatar ointment is helpful. It should be applied once every other day for four to eight days.

### *Suggested Reading*

Börnfors, S.: Acanthosis Nigricans in Dogs. Acta Endocr. (Kbh), Supplement *37*:1-63, 1958.

Muller, G. H.: Acanthosis nigricans. *In* Kirk, R. W. (ed.): *Current Veterinary Therapy III*, W. B. Saunders Co., Philadelphia, 1968, p. 285.

# TWENTY-ONE

## *Acral Lick Dermatitis*
### *(Lick Granuloma, Acral Pruritic Nodule)*

Acral lick dermatitis produces a thickened, firm, oval plaque on the anterior surface of the lower foreleg or hindleg caused by the dog's persistent licking.

### SIGNIFICANT FACTS

1. This lesion occurs primarily in large breeds (Doberman pinschers, Great Danes, Labrador retrievers and others).
2. Boredom may be a major cause. Many of these large dogs are alone all day. When this factor is not present, other causes such as foreign bodies, or carpal or tarsal joint pain, have to be considered.
3. The lesion usually occurs in dogs over five years of age.
4. Secondary bacterial infection seldom occurs on the surface of the lesion, since licking keeps it clean. Purulence develops only in fistulas below the surface or under the crusts on the skin.

### LESIONS AND COURSE

1. At first, constant licking causes alopecia.
2. Next, the epidermis erodes and with sensory nerve exposure a lick-itch-lick cycle develops.
3. Finally ulceration develops and licking keeps the ulcer from healing.
4. Epitheliomatous hyperplasia accounts for the nodular plaque that is characteristic of the disease. Formerly, this stage was mistakenly called a granuloma or tumor. It is not neoplastic.
5. In almost all cases the lesion is single and unilateral (Fig. 21:1*A*).
6. The most common site is the anterior carpal or metacarpal area (Fig. 21:1*B*). Next in frequency are the anterior radial, metatarsal, tarsal, or tibial regions.
7. Chronic lesions become hard, thickened nodules with an ulcerated surface and a hyperpigmented halo (Fig. 21:1*C*).

**Figure 21:1.** Acral lick dermatitis.

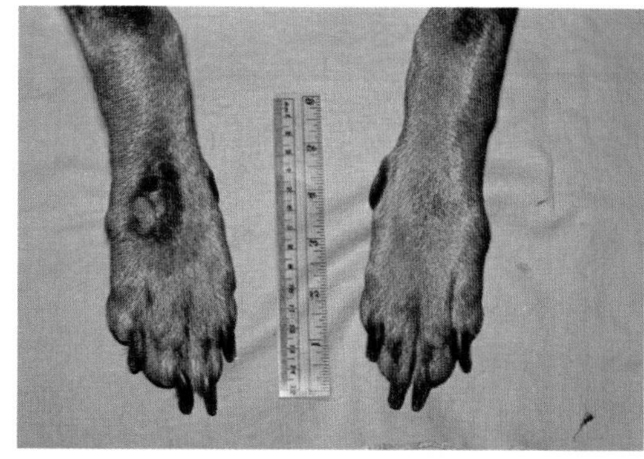

*A*. Unilateral appearance on anterior metacarpal region.

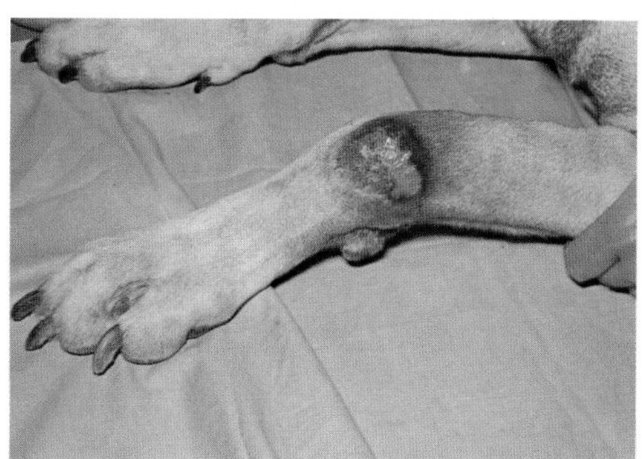

*B*. The carpal area is commonly affected.

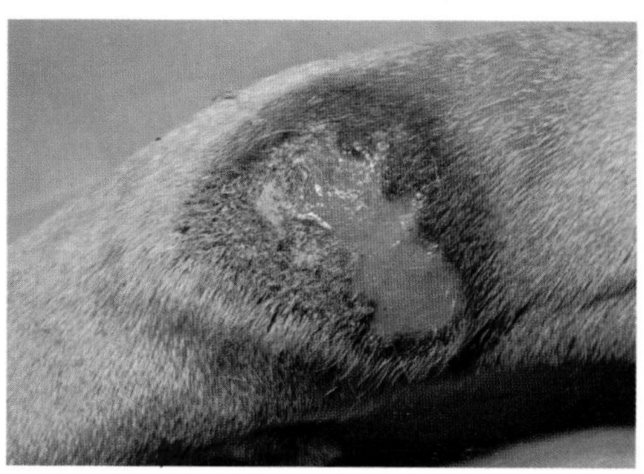

*C*. Close-up of *B* shows the thickened nodule with the characteristic ulcerated epidermis surrounded by a hyperpigmented halo.

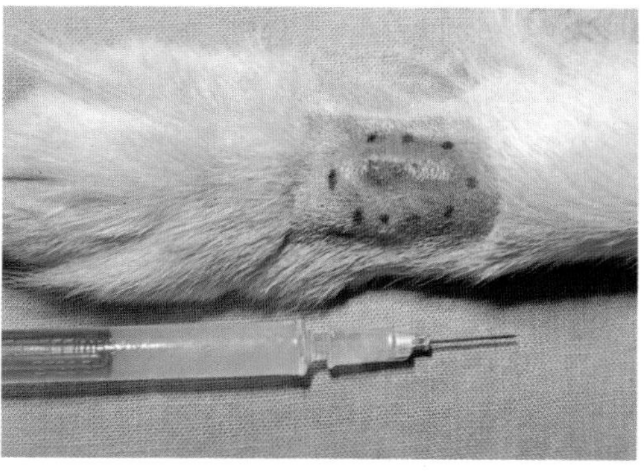

*D*. Blue dots mark the needle entrance of area to be infiltrated with intralesional corticosteroid.

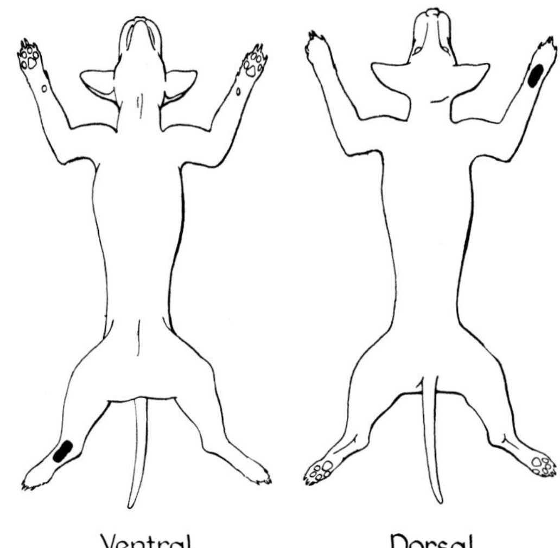


**Figure 21:2.** Acral lick dermatitis distribution pattern.

## DIAGNOSTIC AIDS

Biopsy of chronic lesions will show a consistently characteristic histopathologic appearance.

## HISTOPATHOLOGY

The most striking feature of an acral lick dermatitis is the inflammatory, plasma cell infiltration surrounding the apocrine sweat glands.

The epidermis is acanthotic and hyperkeratotic. In the follicles the hairs have been replaced with keratin plugs. A nonspecific inflammatory infiltrate is present in the upper dermis along with vascular dilatation. The epidermis is missing in the ulcerated areas and the exposed dermis shows fibroblastic hypertrophy.

## DIFFERENTIAL DIAGNOSIS

1. Dermatomycosis. The oval or circular configuration of the nodule resembles a ringworm lesion, but can easily be differentiated with a fungus culture.

2. Neoplasms. Certain tumors, especially histiocytomas and mastocytomas, may be mistaken for an acral lick dermatitis if they occur on the anterior surface of the leg. Biopsy will make the diagnosis.

## CLINICAL MANAGEMENT

1. Vigorous and radical therapy is usually required to resolve the lesion. However, for early lesions more conservative measures can be tried first.

2. The simplest method is topical corticosteroid therapy. An ointment such as Panolog is applied four times a day with gentle massage. Unfortunately the dog often will lick the drug off quickly.

3. If diversion can be provided for the dog (more exercise, human companionship or a canine playmate) he may break the lick-cycle habit.

4. Intralesional corticosteroids (such as triamcinolone acetonide, 2 mg./cc.) once a week for three to four weeks are useful in early lesions (Fig. 21:1*D*), or in lesions that are too large for surgical removal.

5. X-ray therapy alone or in conjunction with surgical removal often will break the lick cycle.

Schedule of Radiation Dosages

| *Area (sq. cm.)* | *Total Dose* | *Half-Value Layer* | *Treatments* |
|---|---|---|---|
| 1 | 750 R | 1.0 mm. Al | 1 |
| 1 to 5 | 750 R | 1.0 mm. Al | Total of two treatments at four to seven day intervals |
| 5 to 15 | 750 to 1000 R | 1.0 mm. Al | Total of three treatments at four to seven day intervals |

6. Elizabethan collars or other methods of physical restraint are effective only while in place. The dog usually licks the lesion again as soon as the device is removed.

7. Tranquilizers and sedatives can be used as an ancillary therapy, but they are not curative.

Surgical excision immediately after the initial diagnosis saves disappointment from failure of conservative therapy.

8. Surgical excision of the entire lesion is the treatment of choice. It is easily and quickly accomplished if the lesion is small enough to allow surgical repair without undue skin tension. Always close the incision with mattress sutures and use bandages or protective devices to prevent removal of the sutures or trauma by the dog before healing is complete (at least ten days).

9. If the lesion is too large for surgical removal the following measures can be taken.

a. Intralesional injections of triamcinolone acetonide.
b. X-ray therapy.
c. Topical corticosteroids (Panolog) four times a day for several months.
d. As a last resort, the lesion can be excised and replaced with a full thickness skin graft.

## *Suggested Reading*

Roberts, I. M.: Acral Pruritic Granuloma. *In* Kirk, R. W. (Ed.): Current Veterinary Therapy III. W. B. Saunders Co., Philadelphia, 1968, pp. 289-290.

Schwartzman, R. M., and Orkin, M.: *A Comparative Study of Skin Diseases of Dog and Man.* Charles C Thomas Co., Springfield, Ill., 1962, pp. 198-204 (Acral pruritic nodule).

# TWENTY-TWO

# *Atopic Dermatitis*

Atopic dermatitis is a hereditary, immunologic disorder accompanied by sneezing, lacrimation and pruritus or paw licking.

## SIGNIFICANT FACTS

1. An atopic dog is one who, by hereditary predisposition, is more likely than other dogs to develop immediate-type hypersensitizations to common allergens.
2. The disease starts between one and three years of age.
3. The atopic dog's skin is easily inflamed by hypersensitivity to one or more allergens, such as ragweed, other pollens, wool, housedust, flea saliva, molds and trees.
4. The majority of atopic dogs have allergic rhinitis (Fig. 22:1*A*) and sneeze frequently. Conjunctivitis is also common.
5. There is a breed predilection for wire-haired terriers, Dalmatians, West Highland white terriers, beagles and poodles.
6. White dogs' hair turns a characteristic rust color in areas that are licked. (This is an important diagnostic clue and is a result of the continued moisture in the area.)
7. A seasonal recurrence of pruritic episodes occurs frequently.

## LESIONS AND COURSE

Pruritus is the main complaint.

1. Pruritus causes severe biting and scratching by the dog (Fig. 22:1*C*).
2. There is generalized erythema with certain areas being affected more than others, depending on the allergens involved.
3. The affected areas are dry, erythematous and excoriated (Fig. 22:1*D*).
4. White scales form and reddish brown crusts result from the self-inflicted trauma.

**Figure 22:1.** Atopic dermatitis.

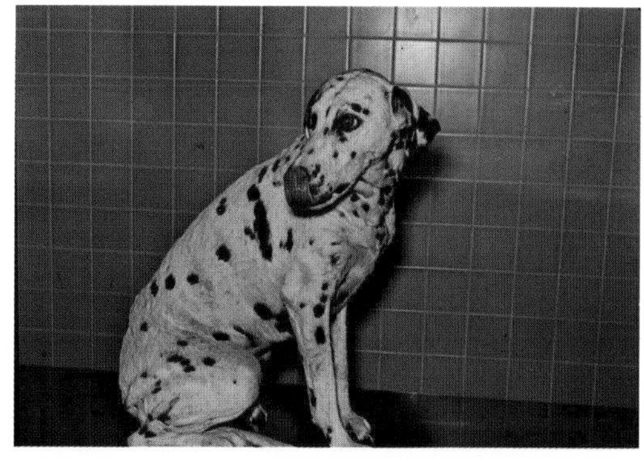

*A.* Affected Dalmatian with rhinitis and discolored hair of the flanks and feet caused by continual licking.

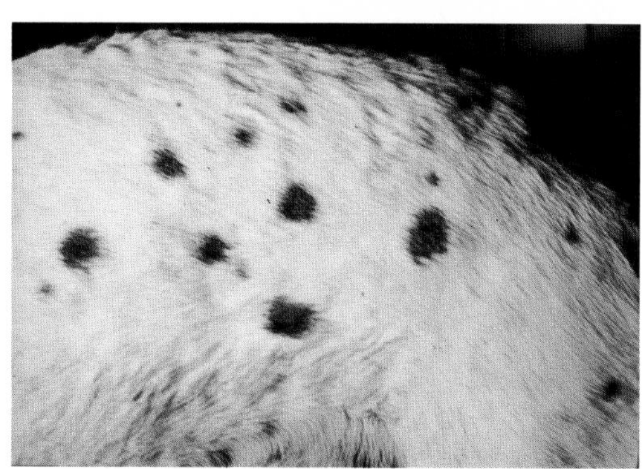

*B.* Close-up of lumbodorsal region of dog in *A* showing rough hair coat caused by erythema, papules and wheals (the latter is uncommon in atopic dogs).

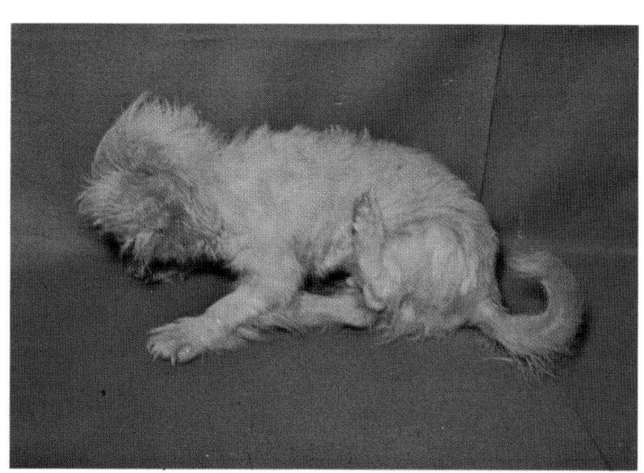

*C.* White dog showing general eyrthema and intense itching.

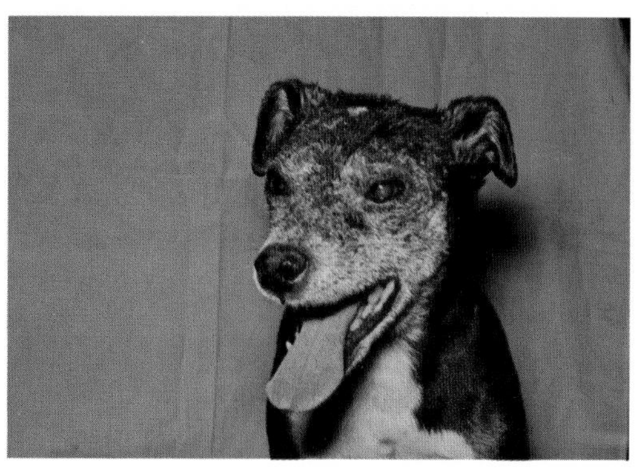

*D.* Face of terrier with atopic dermatitis whose skin has dry crusts, erythema and excoriations from scratching.

5. The course may be seasonal at first, but as the dog adds new allergens to his existing ones over the years, the disease becomes a continuous affliction.

6. Hyperhidrosis (apocrine sweating) is common in atopic dogs.

## DIAGNOSTIC AIDS

1. Intradermal allergy testing is widely used in atopy of man and may also be of value in animals. An allergy testing kit (EVSCO) is now available.

2. A careful case history is essential. With luck, an offending substance can sometimes be discovered in the dog's environment through careful "detective work."

## HISTOPATHOLOGY

Through the course of the disease there is great variation in the histopathology. There is always capillary dilatation. In the epidermis, spongiosis is common, but the main dermal reaction is an inflammatory infiltrate. In chronic disease, the epidermis becomes parakeratotic and acanthotic. Diagnosis of atopy cannot be made through histopathology alone.

## DIFFERENTIAL DIAGNOSIS

1. Allergic contact dermatitis is localized to areas in contact with the offending allergen.

2. Primary irritant contact dermatitis is very localized and usually transitory.

3. Seborrheic dermatitis consists of scaly, greasy patches without severe pruritus.

## CLINICAL MANAGEMENT

1. Systemic corticosteroids give consistently good relief from pruritus. The type of drug and dosage must be selected to suit the needs of the individual patient. It is not unreasonable to maintain the atopic dog on therapeutic corticosteroid levels for two to four weeks during pruritic episodes. However, the temptation to keep the dog continuously on corticosteroids must be resisted.

2. Antihistamines are of little value when compared to the effects of corticosteroids.

3. Hyposensitization, preceded by allergy testing, has been used. An evaluation of this method will be possible only after it has been used in clinical practice for several years. Its success will depend on the clinicians' ability to diagnose atopy, the efficacy of the testing kits and the hyposensitizing injectables, and the excellence of the clinical technique.

## *Suggested Reading*

Patterson, R., Chang, W. W. Y., and Pruzanski, J. J.: The Northwestern University Colony of Atopic Dogs. J. Allergy *34*:455-459, 1963.

Schwartzman, R. M.: Atopy in the Dog. *In* Rook, A. J. and Walton, G. S.: *Comparative Physiology and Pathology of the Skin.* F. A. Davis Co., Philadelphia, 1965, pp. 557-559.

# TWENTY-THREE

## *Contact Dermatitis*

Contact dermatitis is an inflammatory skin reaction caused by direct contact with an offending substance.

### SIGNIFICANT FACTS

1. The disease is divided into two types: primary irritant contact dermatitis and allergic contact dermatitis.

2. Primary irritant contact dermatitis causes cutaneous inflammation in all dogs and cats exposed without requiring an allergic response. A number of primary irritants such as soaps, detergents, insecticidal sprays, strong acids and alkalis are potential causative agents.

2. In allergic contact dermatitis susceptible dogs exposed to contact allergens experience a delayed type of hypersensitivity. The contact allergen is nonirritating to dogs that have not previously formed antibodies to it.

### LESIONS AND COURSE

1. Irritating and allergic substances come in contact with and may produce dermatitis in those areas where the hair coat is thin or missing. The abdomen, chest, axillae (Fig. 23:1*C*), flanks (Fig. 23:1*B*), interdigital spaces, legs, perianal area and eyelids are the most susceptible areas.

2. Only when the offending agent is liquid are hairy regions involved.

3. Patches of erythema and papules represent primary lesions (Fig. 23:1*C*). Vesicles are rarely present in dogs and cats. As the disease progresses crusts and excoriations occur.

4. Intense pruritus promotes severe self-trauma in the form of scratching and biting. Acute moist dermatitis and eventual ulceration frequently obliterate primary lesions.

5. Single episodes are common in primary irritant contact dermatitis, as in scrotal involvement from soap that is not rinsed off (Fig. 23:1*D*).

6. Seasonal recurrence results from exposure to pollens and flowers.

**Figure 23:1.** Contact dermatitis.

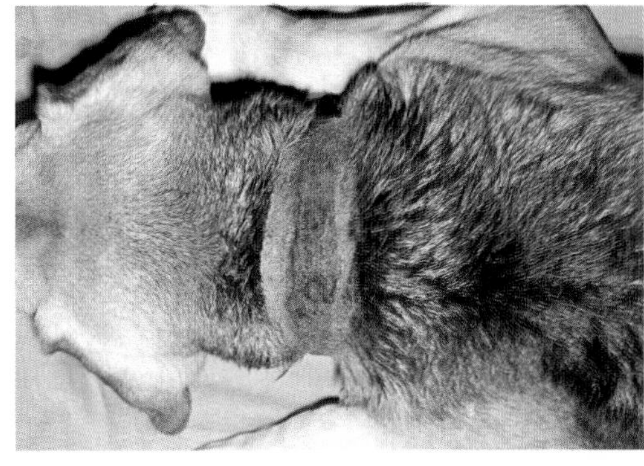

*A. Flea Collar Dermatitis.*

A contact dermatitis caused by a flea collar containing an organic phosphate insecticide (2,2-dichlorovinyl dimethyl phosphate and related compounds).

Severe cases, such as the one illustrated, require up to three months to heal even after removal of the offending collar. During the healing process there is excessive scaling and hyperpigmentation.

Severe systemic toxicity can be very serious and even fatal in some cases.

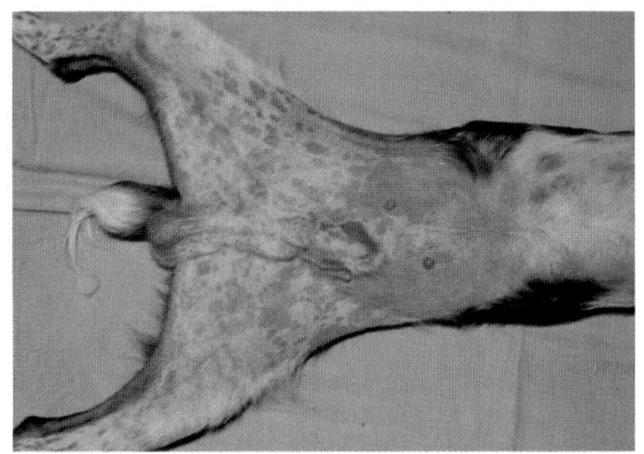

*B.* Allergic contact dermatitis affecting the glaborus skin, with papules and patches of erythema.

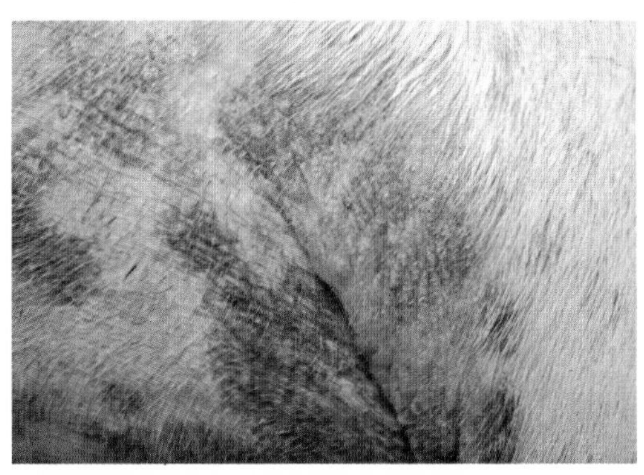

*C.* Axilla of affected dog shows erythema and papules—the primary lesions.

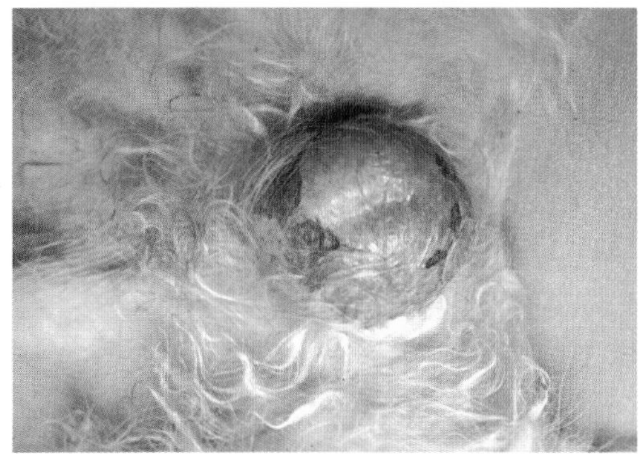

*D.* Irritant contact dermatitis affecting the scrotum—an area of delicate skin which commonly reacts to noxious substances.

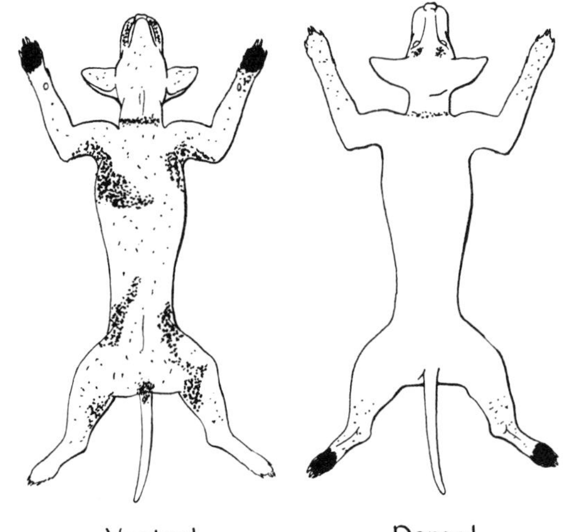


**Figure 23:2.** Allergic contact dermatitis distribution pattern.

## DIAGNOSTIC AIDS

1. Patch testing.
2. Obtaining an accurate history.

## HISTOPATHOLOGY

In general, contact dermatitis presents an acute dermatitic reaction with a marked increase of inflammatory cells in the upper dermis.

## DIFFERENTIAL DIAGNOSIS

1. Atopic dermatitis includes many features of contact dermatitis but is differentiated by its prolonged course, lifelong affliction, paw licking, lacrimation, sneezing and generalized pruritus.

2. Dermatomycosis has more circumscribed, circular lesions and fewer diffuse patches. Pruritus is minimal. Culture or microscopic examination will reveal fungal elements.

3. Seborrheic dermatitis is usually chronic with more scaling and very little pruritus.

4. Solar dermatitis characteristically affects hairless exposed anatomic areas such as the nose and ears in actinically predisposed individuals.

## CLINICAL MANAGEMENT

Find the offending substance and remove it.

1. The difficult task of discovering and eliminating offending substances depends on careful examination of the environment of the dog. Soap, flea collars, poison oak, grasses, pollens, insect powders, petrolatum, paint, wool, carpets, rubber, and wood preservatives are examples of contact allergens.
2. If the location of the initial inflammation can be correlated with an agent that came in contact with that area, the cause can sometimes be found.
3. When the contactant cannot be found, relief depends on systemic and topical therapy.
4. Corticosteroids can be administered systemically for one to several weeks. They often must be repeated during recurrences.
5. Topical treatment consists of wet dressings, baths, emollients (Nivea Creme or lotion) and corticosteroid ointments and lotions.

### *Suggested Reading*

Muller, G. H.: Contact Dermatitis in Animals. Arch. Derm. *96*: 423-426, 1967.

# TWENTY-FOUR

## *Demodectic Mange*

### *(Demodicidosis, Demodicosis, Demodectic Acariasis, Follicular Mange, Red Mange)*

Demodectic mange is an inflammatory skin disease of young dogs, characterized by the presence of larger than normal numbers of demodectic mites. (See also pages 146, 148, 149, and 150.)

### SIGNIFICANT FACTS

1. The mite, *Demodex canis* (Leydig, 1859), is part of the normal fauna of canine skin and is present in very small numbers in most healthy dogs. The skin of dogs with demodectic mange, however, is ecologically favorable to the reproduction and growth of demodectic mites. They seize this opportunity to colonize the hair follicles, and populate the skin by the thousands. The resulting alopecia and erythema is known as demodectic mange.

2. Two general types of demodectic mange are recognized: localized and generalized. The course and prognosis of the two types are vastly different.

3. Demodectic mange occurs almost exclusively in young dogs (three months to one year). When the disease is seen in older animals, they have been afflicted with it since their youth. Rarely, the disease has been seen to start spontaneously in dogs as old as ten years.

4. There is a predilection for short-haired breeds, especially dachshunds, beagles, boxers, English bull dogs, Boston terriers, basset hounds and Chihuahuas.

5. Puppies acquire mites from their mother during the nursing periods. Mites have been obtained from the skin of two-day-old puppies, but prenatal transmission has not been proved.

6. A hereditary predisposition is suggested by certain breeders' ability to predict which litters will develop the disease. Beagle kennels are especially plagued by such tendencies. The elimination of known disease carriers from the breeding colony is helpful in decreasing the incidence of affected litters.

## LESIONS AND COURSE

### A. Localized Demodectic Mange (Squamous)

1. A patch of skin develops mild erythema and partial alopecia. There is no pruritus and the area may be covered with fine silvery scales.

2. One to five patches can be present.

3. The most common site is the face, especially the periocular area and the commissures of the mouth (Fig. 24:1*A*). Next in order of occurrence are the forelegs. More rarely one or more patches are seen on the trunk (Fig. 24:3).

4. Most cases occur at three to six months of age.

5. Many cases heal spontaneously without treatment, while other early cases progress into the generalized form.

6. When the disease is controlled, hair will begin to regrow within 30 days. After this, recurrences are rare because the skin apparently has become an unfavorable habitat for the mites' rapid reproduction.

### B. Generalized Demodectic Mange

1. Although the localized type is a mild clinical disease, generalized demodectic mange is one of the most severe canine skin diseases. It can terminate fatally.

2. The disease begins as a localized case but, instead of improving, it gets worse. Numerous lesions appear on the head, legs and trunk (Fig. 24:1*C*). Each patch gets larger and some coalesce to form plaques (Fig. 24:4).

3. Generalized squamous demodectic mange is likely to become secondarily infected with bacteria (usually *Staphylococcus aureus*) and develop a complicating pyoderma. Acute pyogenic reactions occur and after many months develop into chronic cases with crusted, pyogenic, hemorrhagic lesions on much of the body (Fig. 24:1*C* and *D*). The abdomen is least affected. Pustules commonly form around the head and throat and this accounts for the synonym, "pustular demodectic mange" (Fig. 24:1*F*).

4. Hypersensitivity to either the mites or the bacteria apparently develops in the generalized type. Erythema, edema and pruritus are often present on the paws; in fact, interdigital pyoderma is a common complication.

5. Because of the obstinate nature of the disease at this stage, some owners request euthanasia for their dog.

## DIAGNOSTIC AIDS

1. Skin scrapings will reveal mites. Deep scrapings are not needed—a much better method is to place a drop of mineral oil on the lesion, firmly squeeze a fold of skin, and gently transfer material expressed from the hair follicles to a microscope slide. The larger the ratio of immature forms (ova, larvae and nymphs) to adults, the more guarded the prognosis should be (Fig. 24:2). Finding unusually numerous active adults is an unfavorable sign too. It is necessary to standardize the skin scraping procedure to obtain uniform results with this method.

2. Biopsy also will reveal mites in the hair follicles (Fig. 24:1*H*).

3. Culture and antibiotic sensitivity testing is valuable in pustular demodectic mange to properly guide antibiotic therapy.

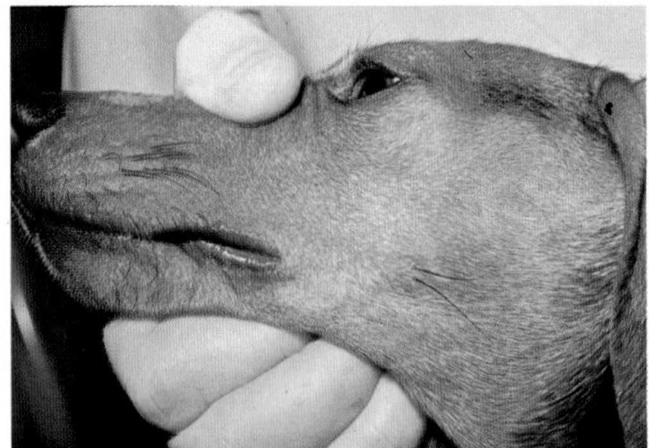

**Figure 24:1.** Demodectic mange.

*A.* Localized demodectic mange. A single alopecic patch at the commissure of the lips.

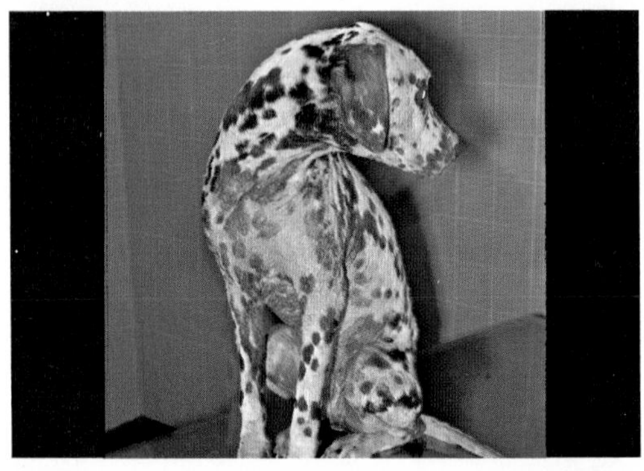

*B.* Generalized, squamous demodectic mange. Reddish discoloration is the reason for the former name, "red mange."

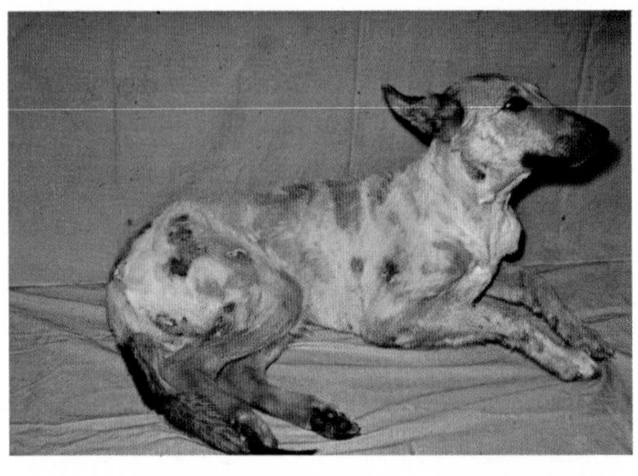

*C.* Generalized pyogenic demodectic mange. Distribution of lesions in a rapidly advancing case.

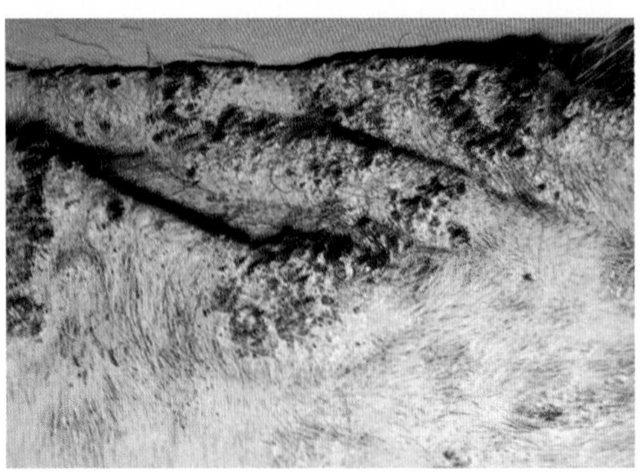

*D.* Close-up of skin from a very advanced case. *Staphylococcus aureus* and *Demodex canis* simultaneously inhabit this area.

**Figure 24:1.** Demodectic mange (continued)

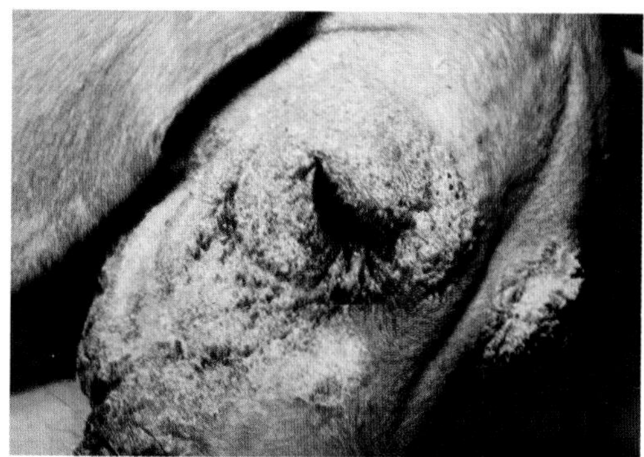

*E.* The face of a dachshund with chronic, pyogenic, demodectic mange.

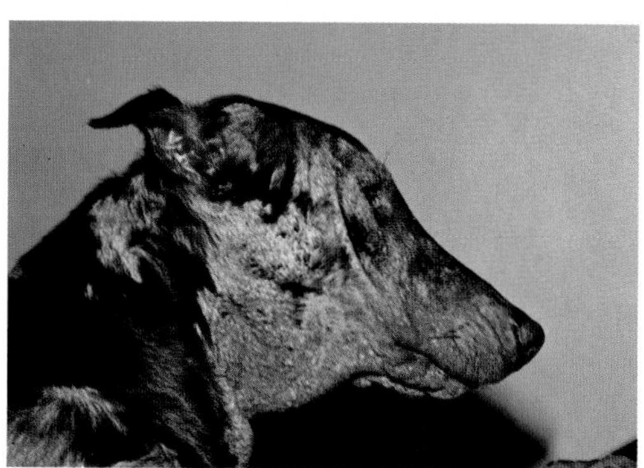

*F.* A nine-month-old Doberman pinscher whose once beautiful face is disfigured by the effects of the disease. The loose fold of skin at the throat containing numerous pustules is characteristic.

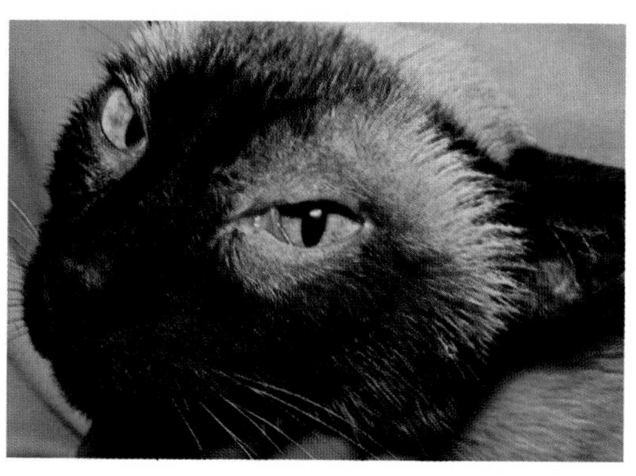

*G.* Demodectic mange in a cat. Only the eyelids and periocular area are affected. Infections with *Demodex cati* are usually mild.

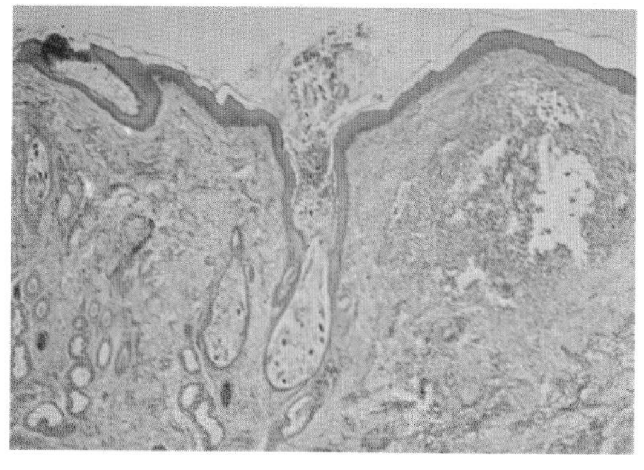

*H.* Section through a demodectic pustule, showing two parasitized hair follicles in the center. Note that the follicular orifice is closed with a plug of keratin and dead mites. On the right is an intradermal abscess. (Low power.)

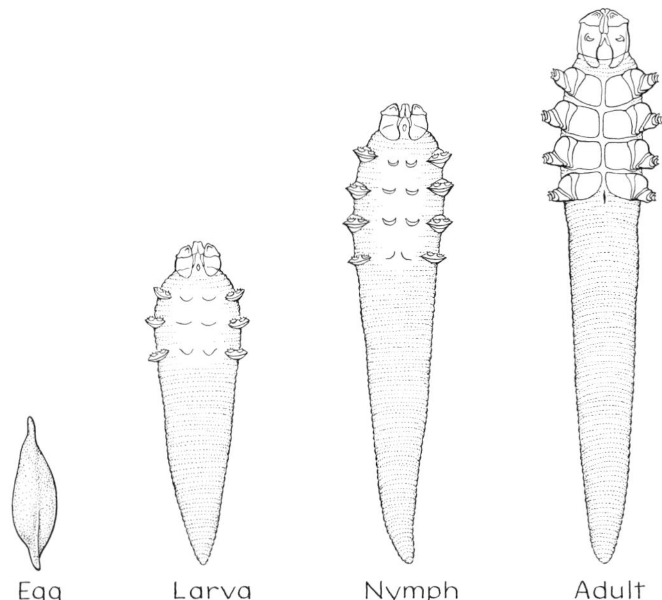


**Figure 24:2.** Adult and immature forms of *Demodex canis*.

## HISTOPATHOLOGY (FIG. 24:1*H*)

The most striking features are dilated hair follicles, devoid of hair but filled with mites and keratin. In localized demodectic mange the perifollicular inflammatory infiltrate is minimal, but in the generalized form it is more pronounced. A plug, consisting of keratin, debris and dead mites, closes each follicular orifice. The epidermis is acanthotic with mild hyperkeratosis. In generalized, pustular demodectic mange, intradermal abscesses are common. Hair follicles rupture and become abscessing sinuses. In the generalized type histologic lesions resemble those of pyoderma but in addition have mite-filled hair follicles.

## DIFFERENTIAL DIAGNOSIS

Since skin scrapings easily reveal mites in demodectic mange, it is seldom confused with other diseases. However, it is important to remember that a few mites (usually without eggs or immature forms) can be found in much normal skin, or in skin scrapings from other diseases. This is especially true of scrapings made on dogs' faces.

1. Generalized pyoderma may resemble demodectic mange.

2. Dermatomycosis resembles patches of localized, squamous demodectic mange. Differentiation is made by skin scrapings, KOH preparations, mycotic culture and the Wood's light.

3. Superficial abrasions in young dogs sometimes resemble the erythematous patches of localized demodectic mange. Conversely, demodectic mange may be mistaken for abrasions.

4. Acne on the face of young dogs sometimes resembles pustular demodectic mange, and certain demodectic pustules on the abdomen and inside surface of the thighs resemble canine acne lesions. Differentiation can be made by skin scrapings or by biopsy.

5. Allergic contact dermatitis exhibits erythematous papules that occasionally resemble pustular demodectic mange.

## CLINICAL MANAGEMENT

The treatment of demodectic mange should be individualized in each case. A different therapeutic regimen is required for the localized and for the generalized types. The generalized, pustular type is particularly difficult as it exhibits a multitude of lesional combinations, each of which may respond favorably to one therapy although it may be damaged by another.

Many drugs have received credit for demodectic mange cures that, in reality, were spontaneous recoveries.

### A. Localized Demodectic Mange

1. Apply an acaricidal preparation (such as Goodwinol ointment, benzyl benzoate, or Canex) once daily to the affected areas. Also available are lotions and emulsions containing various acaricidal combinations of lindane, rotenone, benzyl benzoate and benzene hexachloride (Mulzyl, Benzyl-Hex, Milvonique, Furaspor).

2. The daily rubbing required to apply topical medications frequently causes more hairs to fall out of parasitized follicles. Hence, the owner should be warned that the lesion may at first appear more hairless and larger in size after a few days of treatment. Improvement can be expected in two to three weeks as hair growth returns.

3. The majority of localized demodectic mange cases recover in three to eight weeks and recurrence is rare.

### B. Generalized Demodectic Mange

All cases of generalized demodectic mange begin as localized types. Although there is a generalized squamous form and a generalized pyogenic form, they are really stages of one disease. Most generalized squamous cases will become infected with *Staphylococcus aureus*, thereby turning into the pyogenic type.

1. Avoid overtreatment! The skin is highly inflamed and very sensitive. Strong medications and vigorous rubbing and scrubbing will add further insults to the diseased skin and could be a major contributing factor toward producing a hopeless case.

2. Gently clip all hair on the affected areas and remove matted crusts. Submerged baths (15 to 30 minutes) and wet dressings will help loosen crusts

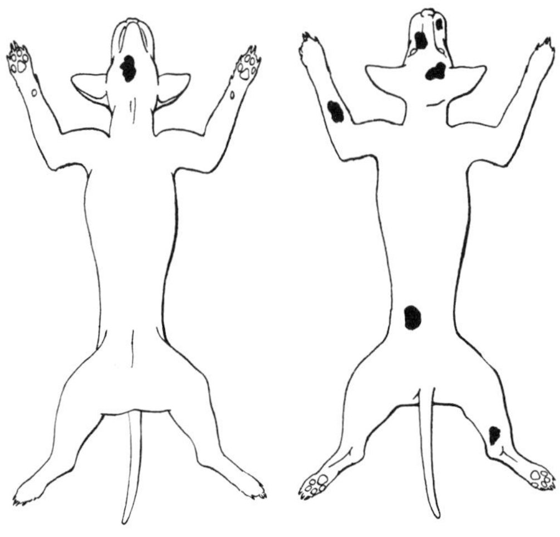


**Figure 24:3.** Localized demodectic mange distribution pattern.

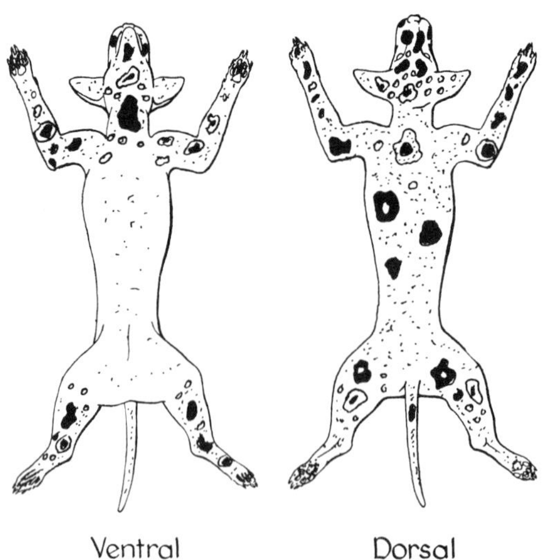


**Figure 24:4.** Generalized demodectic mange distribution pattern.

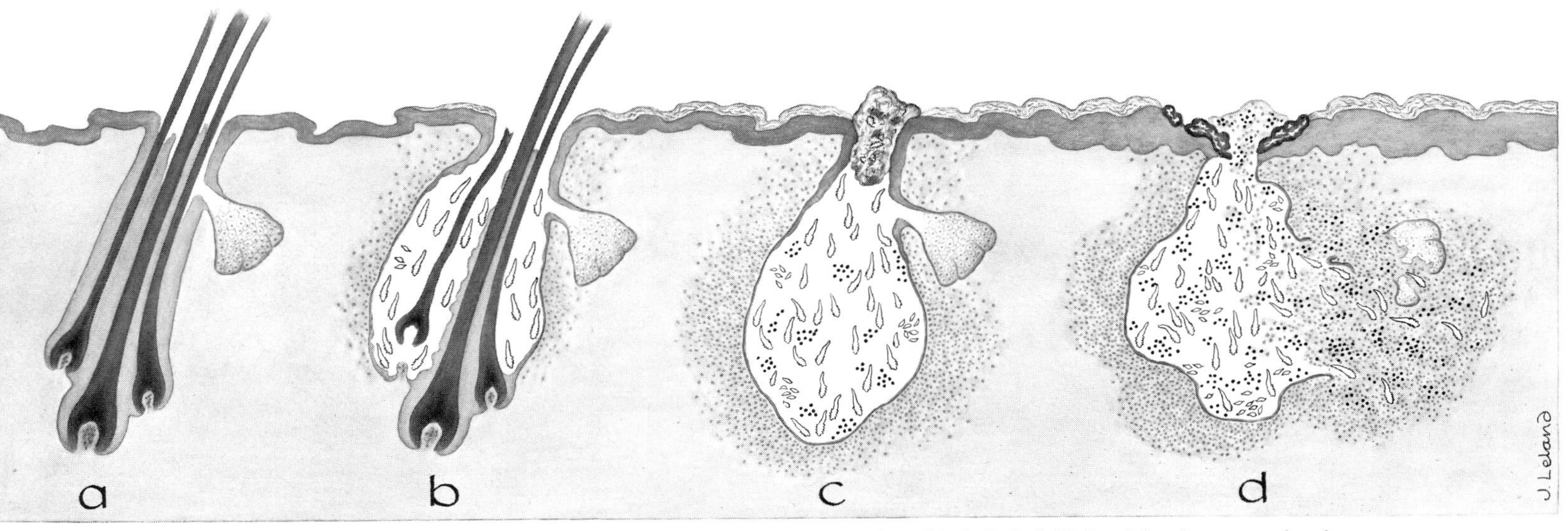


**Figure 24:5.** Demodectic mange dermogram. *a.* Normal multiple hair follicle with sebaceous gland. *b.* Localized demodectic mange. One hair follicle is shown with a small colony of *Demodex canis.* A few eggs are seen and one accessory hair is degenerating and partly broken. A very mild perifollicular infiltrate develops as the follicle dilates. *c.* Pustule formation in *generalized pyogenic demodectic mange.* The hairs are gone, and a comedo, consisting of keratin, sebum, debris and dead mites, plugs the follicular orifice. The ballooning hair follicle accommodates the expanding mite colony, which is packed with numerous adult mites, immature forms and eggs. The clusters of black dots represent *staphylococci* that have invaded the hair follicle. *d.* The ballooned hair follicle ruptures and transforms into a pustule, and later an intradermal abscess. (Figure 24:1*D* shows many gross lesions in this stage.) The sebaceous gland disintegrates. At this stage there is exudation through the follicular orifice. Some abscesses break through the epidermis separately. The epidermis is acanthotic, hyperkeratotic and crusted. Thousands of similar lesions produce the clinical appearance of generalized pustular demodectic mange.

and dissolve dried exudates. This can be followed by a gentle shampoo with pHisoHex or Seleen.

3. Dip or rinse the entire body once a week with an acaricidal preparation, such as ronnel or D.D.V.P. (Vapona). At least four weekly applications are needed.

4. In affected areas free of pyoderma, a topical benzyl benzoate preparation can be used daily. However, on pyogenic lesions the application of ointments and lotion is contraindicated because it can spread the infection to previously uninvolved hair follicles.

5. Follow-up treatment with a medicated shampoo containing selenium sulfide or a similar ingredient once a week is useful.

6. Antibiotic treatment for the accompanying deep pyoderma is most important. A bacterial culture on blood agar will reveal *Staphylococcus aureus* in most cases and an antibiotic sensitivity test will influence the correct selection of antibiotics. Chloramphenicol, Prostaphlin, Unipen, Oleandomycin and Lincocin are antibiotics often useful for treating the Staphylococcus infection secondary to demodectic mange.

7. Systemic acaricidal therapy has been advocated for many years. Since before the turn of the century scientists have searched for an oral or injectable drug that will kill demodectic mites. Although many preparations have achieved a period of popularity, none have maintained their rating and most have been relegated to history when their ineffectiveness became evident. Examples of such drugs include trypan blue intravenously, arsenical injections, griseofulvin and various organic phosphates. No doubt, the spontaneous recovery of some cases of demodectic mange has been attributed to some systemic medication. But any experienced clinician can recall hopeless cases, at the point of euthanasia, that have been on so-called systemic acaricides for weeks or months without improvement. Disophenol injections have been suggested recently, but results so far are not encouraging. It is the authors' sincere hope that a really effective acaricidal drug will become available which can reach the mites in the skin.

8. Corticosteroids are useful in reducing inflammation and pruritus in generalized demodectic mange when the feet are erythematous and edematous. However, in this disease, corticosteroids can be dangerous as well as useful. Along with their comforting effect, they reduce the body's defense against bacterial infection, and severe pyodermas may become uncontrollable. The clinician must use his best judgment in deciding whether or not to use corticosteroids.

9. Estrogenic hormones decrease sebum production and therefore decrease available food for the mites (who are thought to live on sebum and keratin). Either estrogen or stilbestrol can be used. The androgens, which increase sebum production, are always contraindicated. Thyroid does not seem to have any effect on the mites or the disease.

10. Time is always on the clinician's side because demodectic mange tends to be a disease of young dogs and they may improve spontaneously after sexual maturity. If sensible therapy, without overtreatment, can be used until the dog is mature there may be hope for apparently hopeless cases.

*Feline demodectic mange* is caused by *Demodex cati*. It is a rare disease which usually affects the eyelids and periocular area (Fig. 24:1*G*). It is the localized type of demodectic mange and is usually self-limiting. A mild ointment containing rotenone (Goodwinol) speeds recovery and has a soothing action on the erythematous, alopecic patches. Although generalized cases have been reported in older literature, the authors have seen only the localized form.

# TWENTY-FIVE

## *Dermatomycosis*

### *(Ringworm, Superficial Fungal Infection, Dermatophytosis)*

Dermatomycosis is an infection of the skin by a dermatophyte (fungus).

### SIGNIFICANT FACTS

1. Three fungi cause 99 per cent of all canine and feline dermatomycoses: *Microsporum canis*, *Microsporum gypseum* and *Trichophyton mentagrophytes*. In cats 98 per cent of all cases are caused by *M. canis*. In dogs 70 per cent are caused by *M. canis*, 20 per cent by *M. gypseum*, and 10 per cent by *T. mentagrophytes*. (Other dermatophytes are listed on page 128.)
2. Dermatophytes are transmitted to dogs and cats from other animals, from man or from the soil.
3. Some dermatophytes prefer animals as their host and are called zoophilic. These often cause less inflammatory reactions than geophilic fungi (which normally inhabit the soil) or anthropophilic fungi (which prefer man).
4. Dermatophytes live only on the nonviable keratin of the skin, hair and claws. They do not invade the living layers of the skin.
5. Fungal infections invade hairs only in the anagen stage of the hair growth cycle.
6. Young animals are more commonly affected than older ones.

### LESIONS AND COURSE

1. The classical "ringworm" lesion is a rapidly growing circular patch of alopecia varying from 1 to 4 cm. in diameter (Fig. 25:2*A*).
2. Variations are common, however. Lesions can be oval, irregular or diffuse in shape (Fig. 25:2*B* and *D*). Sometimes large portions of the body are affected, especially in chronic *M. gypseum* and *T. mentagrophytes* infections (Fig. 25:2*D*, *E* and *G*).
3. Although some lesions are barely discernible scaly patches, others are raised erythematous plaques. Under crusts, fungal infections often develop sec-

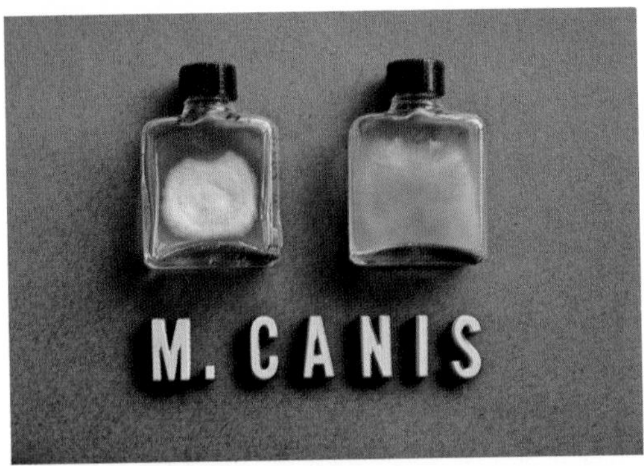


**Figure 25:1.** Dermatophyte colony morphology.

*A. Microsporum canis* grows as a whitish, coarsely fluffy spreading colony which develops a deep yellow pigment on the underside. This pigment appears during the first week of growth, but becomes dark and dull with aging.

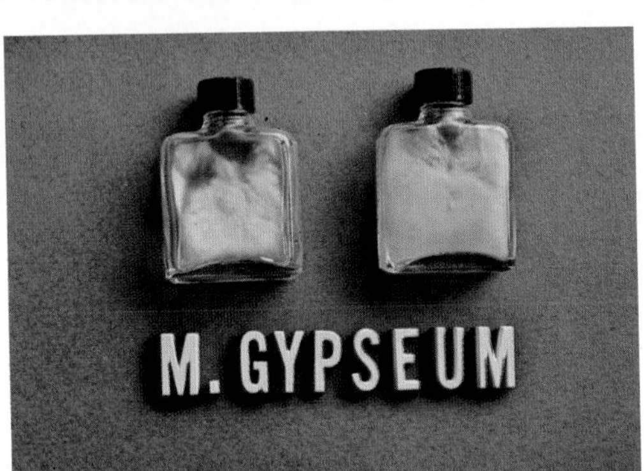


*B. Microsporum gypseum* characteristically has rapidly spreading colonies whose surface is a rich cinnamon-buff color with the texture of chamois. The underside is a light buff color.

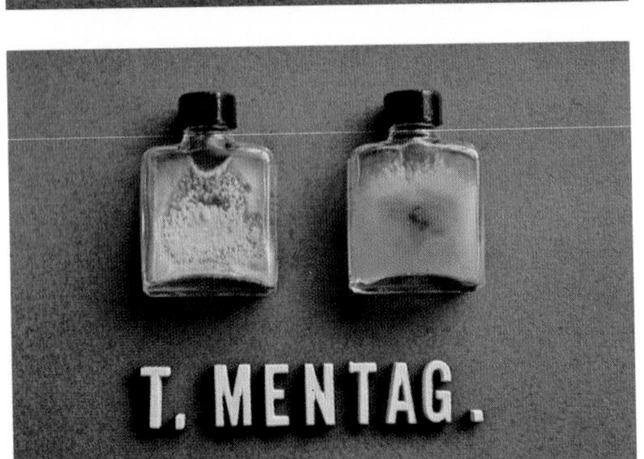


*C. Trichophyton mentagrophytes* has two colony types. The zoophilic form (illustrated) produces a flat colony with a yellowish buff or cream-colored, powdery surface. The powder appears to be sprinkled in concentric rings or rays. The underside may be tan or dark brown. The anthropophilic form consists of a dense, downy white colony.

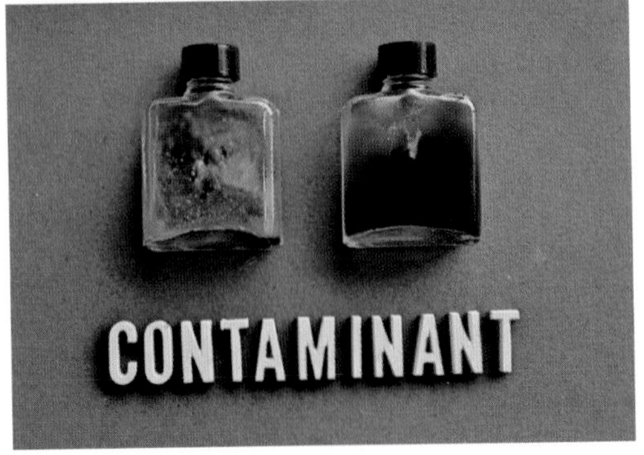


*D.* Contaminants or saprophytes can usually be recognized by their dark or black colonies.

ondary bacterial infections. When the crust is removed, the circular area of skin is usually honeycombed with small oozing holes (Fig. 25:2*C*).

4. Hair growth in affected follicles continues and there is no permanent hair loss unless the follicle is destroyed by secondary bacterial infection.

5. The course varies from self-limiting, acute infections that last two to four weeks, to chronic dermatomycoses that establish themselves on the skin for many months or even years.

## DIAGNOSTIC AIDS

The following tests are described in detail in the chapter on laboratory procedures:

1. Wood's light examination for fluorescence causes only certain strains of *M. canis* to produce a positive yellow-green color. Other dermatophytes of dogs and cats do not fluoresce and about 40 per cent of *M. canis* infections are negative to ultraviolet waves (see p. 98).
2. Potassium hydroxide preparation (see p. 95).
3. Mycotic culture is the most accurate method (see p. 96).
4. Skin biopsy and staining with PAS stain (p. 102).
5. Impression smears are especially useful for the yeast *Candida albicans* (p. 100).

## HISTOPATHOLOGY

The epidermis responds to the fungal invasion with acanthosis, parakeratosis and hyperkeratosis. Epidermal ridges become prominent and irregular. An inflammatory infiltrate appears in the upper dermis accompanied by advancing dermatophyte invasion within the keratinized structures. Mycotic elements (spores and mycelia) are present in the nonviable hair and keratinized layers of the epidermis and hair follicle only.

## DIFFERENTIAL DIAGNOSIS

1. Seborrheic lesions frequently mimic the circular lesions of ringworm. Differentiation is made by the course of the lesions and by evaluating the entire skin of the body rather than the individual lesions.
2. Demodectic mange, especially its localized form, also develops circular lesions. A skin scraping quickly differentiates the conditions.
3. Abrasions of circular shape may resemble ringworm lesions.
4. Contact dermatitis of the paws is frequently mistakenly called a "fungus infection."

## CLINICAL MANAGEMENT

1. Griseofulvin is the drug of choice. The dose of the microcrystalline form (Fulvicin u/f) is 10 mg./lb. of body weight daily. This can be administered

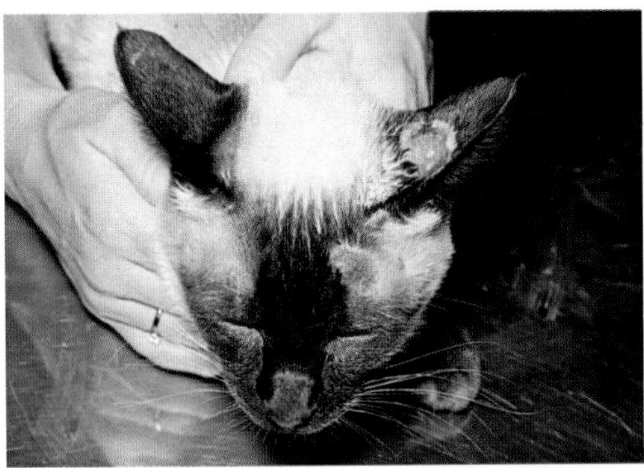

**Figure 25-2.** Dermatomycosis.

*A*. Classic "ringworm" lesions in a cat caused by *Microsporum canis.*

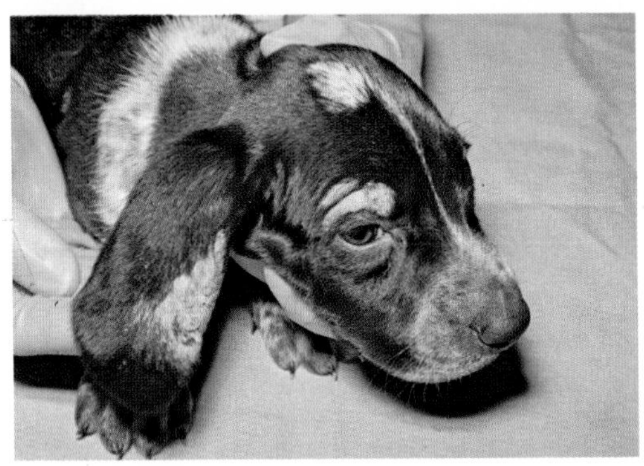

*B*. *Microsporum canis* infection in a pointer puppy whose litter mates were also affected. Note the relative lack of inflammation caused by a zoophilic dermatophyte in a dog.

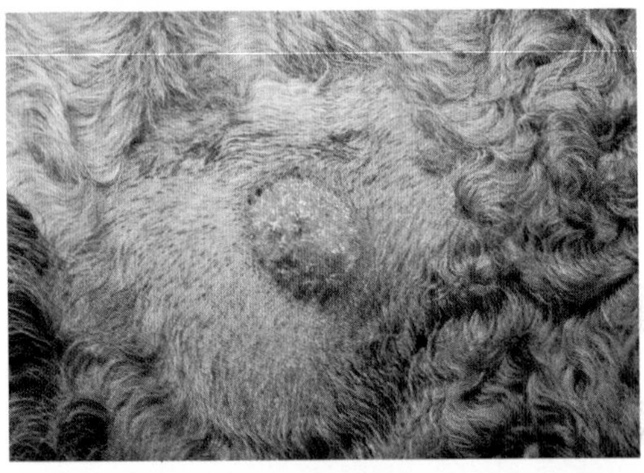

*C*. *Microsporum canis* infection in a French poodle. The circular, red, slightly elevated plaque became apparent when the crust was removed and the surrounding area was clipped.

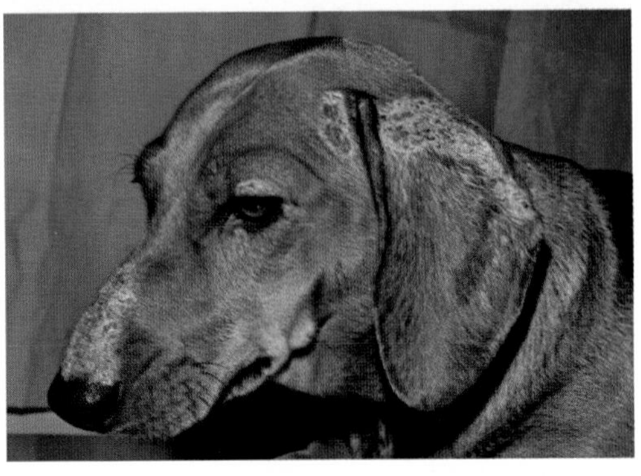

*D*. *Microsporum gypseum* caused a chronic fungal infection in this dachshund, who apparently contracted the geophilic dermatophyte by rooting in the ground with his nose. Eight months of griseofulvin therapy were required to control this stubborn infection.

**Figure 25:2.** Dermatomycosis (continued)

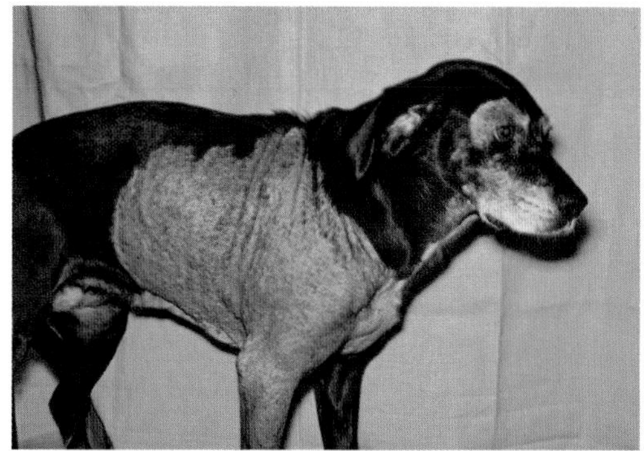

*E. Trichophyton mentagrophytes* (var. *granulare*) caused this extensive, almost generalized dermatomycosis of two years' duration. Hair loss resulted from the disease – area was not clipped.

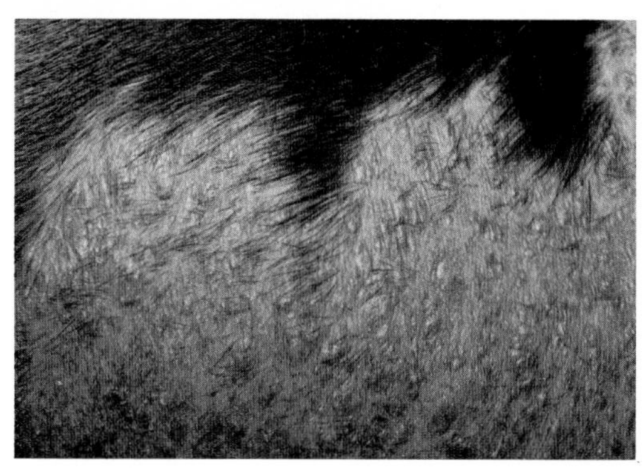

*F.* Close-up of skin from *E* showing the papular, erythematous alopecia. A few pustules and vesicles can be seen in the area.

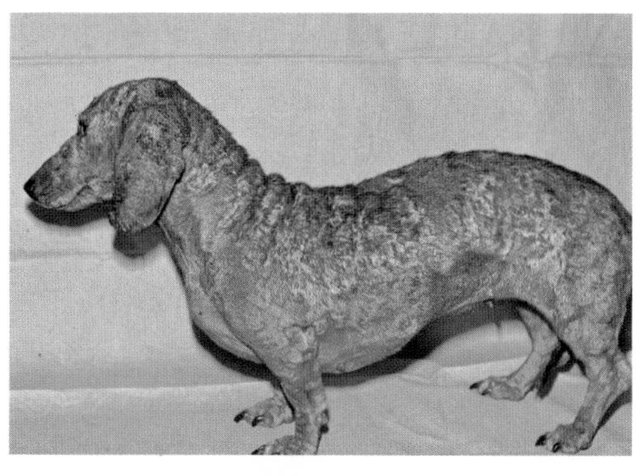

*G.* Generalized *Trichophyton mentagrophytes* infection complicated by secondary bacterial infection. Note the self-inflicted trauma at the ear margins caused by shaking the head.

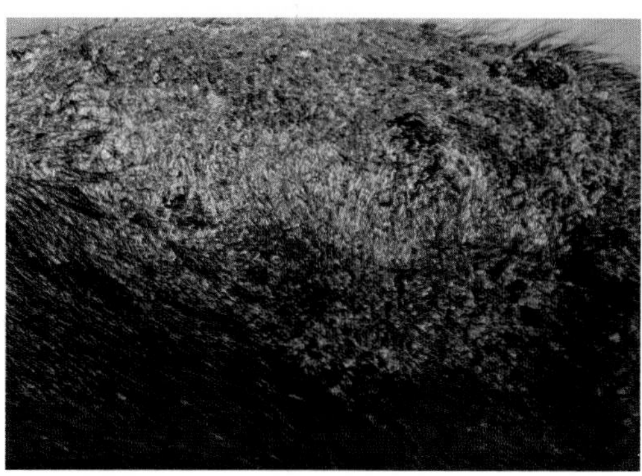

*H.* Close-up of skin from the back of a dog with a *Trichophyton mentagrophytes* infection that covered 90 per cent of its body for 18 months. Note the extensive scaling and crusting. Affected toenails of this dog are shown in Fig. 38-1, B.

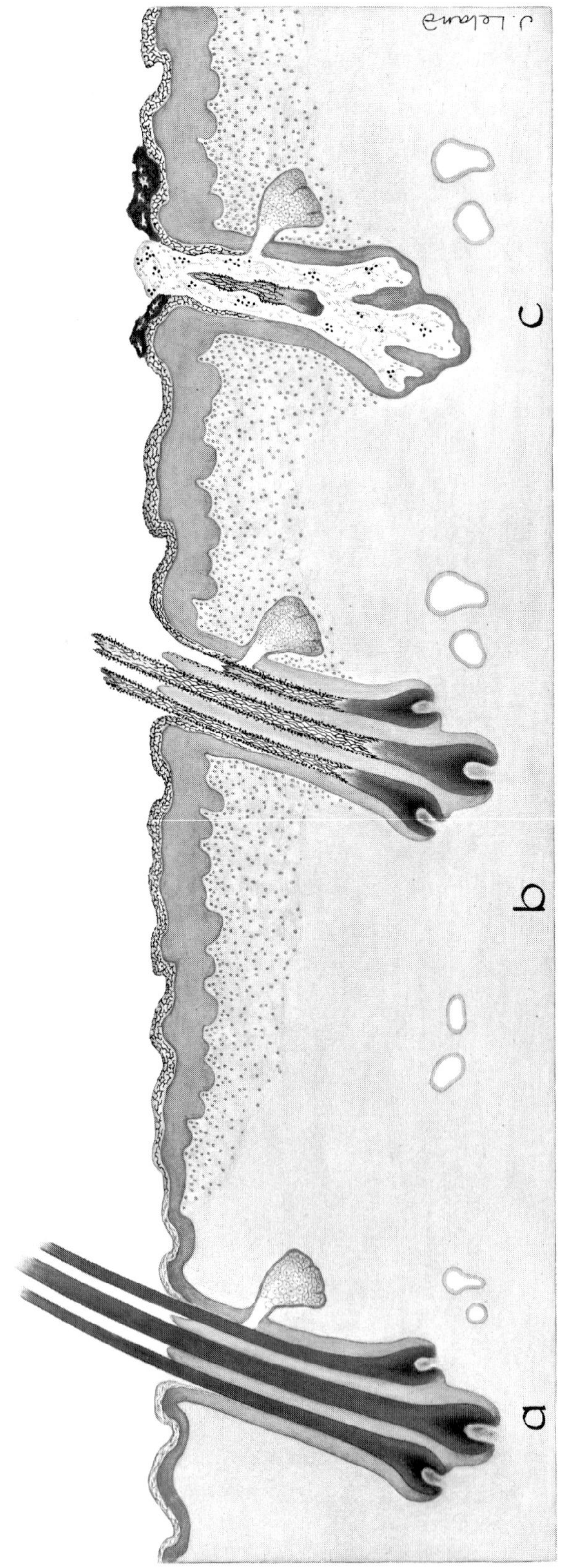


**Figure 25:3.** Dermatomycosis dermogram. *a.* Normal hair follicle. *b.* There is invasion of the hair follicle by a dermatophyte. Mycelia and spores can be seen affecting only the keratinized portions of the skin and appendages. There are acanthosis and inflammatory infiltration. The third hair is broken off, but hair roots are intact. Fungi are growing downward on the hair, stopping at Adamson's fringe—a zone just above the area of keratin synthesis. No fungi can be seen in the living cells of the dermis or epidermis. *c.* Secondary bacterial infection has caused partial destruction of the hair follicle. Hairs have been lost, a follicular plug has formed and crusts appear on the epidermal surface. The general histologic picture is that of a subacute to chronic dermatitis.

daily or in several massive doses. The massive dose consists of totaling the calculated daily dose for ten days and giving it at one time. It must be repeated every ten days until laboratory methods or clinical examinations show the skin is free of mycotic infection.

| *Body weight* | *Daily dose* | *Massive dose Repeat four times at 10 day intervals* |
|---|---|---|
| 5 lb. | 50 mg. | 500 mg. |
| 10 lb. | 100 mg. | 1000 mg. |
| 25 lb. | 250 mg. | 2500 mg. |
| 50 lb. | 500 mg. | 5000 mg. |

2. The affected area should be shaved to avoid reinfestation from infected hairs. Gentle cleansing with pHisoHex or Weladol is useful to prevent secondary bacterial infection.

3. Dipping or rinsing with captan is a useful adjunct to griseofulvin treatment. A dip prepared from a 1:200 dilution of 45 per cent technical captan is safe for dogs and cats. One or two dips a week can be given until clinical improvement appears.

4. Numerous topical fungicidal and fungistatic ointments are in common use. Most of these are keratolytic agents (salicylic acid, undecylenic acid) which remove the keratin "soil" the fungus needs to grow in. Other preparations (Whitfield's ointment) cause inflammation which interferes with the dermatophytes' normal activity. Recently an ointment containing tolnaftate (Tinactin) has been very useful in human dermatomycoses and is of value on the glabrous skin of dogs.

5. Avoid treatment with irritating preparations as they may encourage secondary pyoderma.

6. Prophylaxis: Griseofulvin can be used prophylactically on exposed animals. One massive, single dose (see item 1) is highly effective. Infected animals should be isolated from contact with people or pets. It is necessary to sterilize or destroy bedding, leashes and other contaminated equipment.

## *Suggested Reading*

Kaplan, W.: Dermatophytosis. In Kirk, R. W. (Ed.): *Current Veterinary Therapy III.* W. B. Saunders Co., Philadelphia, 1968, pp. 279-283.

Rebell, G., Taplin, D., and Blank, H.: *Dermatophytes.* Dermatology Foundation of Miami, 1964.

# TWENTY-SIX

# *Ear Dermatoses*

## *Fly Dermatitis*

Adult male and female stable flies (*Stomoxys calcitrans*) are peculiarly adapted for attacking the skin of the host and sucking blood. The rasping teeth and blades of the labella tear open the skin, and the labella and whole proboscis are plunged into the wound to suck blood. This entire action is highly irritating to the host and conducive to spreading disease.

The flies usually attack the face or ears of dogs. The multiple bites are commonly found on the tips of the ears (Fig. 26:1*A*) or at the folded edge of the skin in dogs whose ears are tipped over (such as shelties, collies and others). Erythema and hemorrhagic crusts from oozing serum and blood are typical lesions. Afflicted dogs are always housed outdoors, and often confined where they can not escape the fly attacks.

Ordinary fly repellents (6-12), fly or flea spray, or pastes made of flea powder (Diryl) and applied to the affected skin help prevent repeated bites. The patient should be housed inside during the day if possible until the lesions heal. Topical medications such as Panolog ointment may be beneficial.

The source of the flies should be investigated, and straw piles, manure pits and other likely areas can be sprayed with DDT every three weeks to help decrease the fly population.

## *Otitis Externa*

Otitis externa is an acute or chronic inflammation of the external ear canal.

### SIGNIFICANT FACTS

1. Approximately 80 per cent of cases involve long-eared dogs, and especially spaniels, poodles, Kerry blue terriers and breeds with abundant hair

growth in the ear canal. Of the erect-eared breeds, the German shepherd is especially prone to ear infections.

2. Water dogs may develop *Candida albicans* or Pityrosporum infections if the ear canals are not dried out, but the primary bacterial invaders in most otitis cases are Staphylococcus and Streptococcus species. Secondary infections follow caused by Proteus, Pseudomonas or Corynebacterium.

Poor air circulation in the ear canal favors infection.

## LESIONS AND COURSE

1. Types of otitis are classified as erythematous, ulcerative, purulent, ceruminous and hyperplastic, but many of these are stages of a single infection.

2. Early inflammations are characterized by erythema and swelling of the skin. This becomes ulcerated and secondary infection produces a purulent exudate (Fig. 26:1*B*). With seborrhea and certain hormonal imbalances an increase of sebum collects in the canal and ceruminous otitis results. Chronic infection often results in hyperplastic or cauliflower growths on the skin surface, but in advanced cases the cartilaginous tissue may become ossified.

3. Foreign bodies, water, tumors and parasites all have a marked effect in prolonging otitis infections and they are often the inciting cause.

## DIAGNOSTIC AIDS

The cause of the inflammation must be searched for diligently. Careful inspection of the canal for awns, fox tails and mites is essential. If ulcerative or purulent otitis is present antibacterial cultures and sensitivity tests are most helpful. Removal of accumulated hair and irrigation of the ear canal with water will often reveal foreign objects not previously visible.

## HISTOPATHOLOGY

In otitis there is epidermal hyperplasia, acanthosis, formation of rete ridges, hyperkeratinization of hair follicles, hyperemia and epithelial ulceration. The dermis is fibroplastic, the sebaceous glands are smaller and displaced by dilated ducts of the prominent ceruminous glands. These are often filled with a colloidal, eosinophilic material.

## DIFFERENTIAL DIAGNOSIS

This is rarely in doubt, the only question being the etiology.

## CLINICAL MANAGEMENT

Treatment depends on the cause, but these principles generally apply:

### 1. Acute Otitis

a. Look carefully for awns or other foreign bodies, parasites, or a history of water, soap or medications being applied.

b. In the erythematous stage, x-ray therapy is useful, but bland medications such as Panolog, or Fulvidex are practical, effective medications which should be *gently* applied every day.

c. Do not probe, swab or otherwise traumatize this delicate lining.

### 2. Chronic Otitis

a. General anesthesia, followed by clipping of hair around the ear and careful, thorough irrigation of the ear canal with dilute pHisoHex solution, is essential. (This should be preceded by a culture for bacteriologic examination if it is indicated.)

b. The canal is completely dried by aspiration with a tube connected to a siphon or vacuum pump. Gentle blotting may be indicated too.

c. The canal is inspected thoroughly with a magnifying otoscope.

d. Any ulcers should be cauterized with 5 per cent silver nitrate on a swab.

e. Antibiotics should be used topically (and systemically if indicated) according to sensitivity results. Neomycin, polymyxin, chloramphenicol and gentamicin are often effective. Nystatin is indicated only for candidiasis, and griseofulvin is not indicated topically.

f. Treatment is applied daily or three times weekly for two to three weeks.

### 3. Refractory Cases

a. Always check for an eroded tympanum with possible otitis media.

b. Surgical drainage of the external canal by one of the aural resection techniques or external ear canal ablation may be necessary. These techniques are successful in a high percentage of chronic infections. They should be utilized when chronic cases have relapsed three or four times, and before hyperplastic otitis develops.

c. Ceruminous otitis is usually a local manifestation of a generalized skin disease (see Seborrhea p. 333). Thoroughly cleansing the canal weekly with Fosteen or defatting agents may be helpful, or aural resection may provide air and sebum drainage and help ameliorate the problem. However, unless the general skin problem is controlled, efforts on the ear are only palliative. Ceruminolytic agents (Sebumsol, Debrisol, Cerumite and others) are useful if instilled into the affected ears at regular intervals.

d. Hyperplastic otitis is best treated by "scalping off" the cauliflower growths parallel to the cartilage and controlling hemorrhage by simple cautery or pressure bandages. Since this condition is usually caused by chronic purulent otitis, measures should be directed to eliminating the infection and to opening or obliterating the ear canal.

### *Suggested Reading*

Fraser, G.: Otitis Externa. *In: Progress in Canine Practice,* Part Three, Modern Veterinary Reference Series, American Veterinary Publications, Santa Barbara, California.

Kirk, R. W.: Otitis Externa in the Dog. Veterinary Scope, 1957, Vol. II, No. 3.

# *Otodectic Mange (Ear Mites)*

Otodectic mange is caused by infestation with *Otodectes cynotis* mites.

## SIGNIFICANT FACTS

Although most of the mites are found in or near the ears, they may occasionally inhabit other areas of the body, especially the tail.

1. The mites are large, white in color and easily observed with a magnifying otoscope. They may also be demonstrated by placing some of the ear exudate on a dark surface. The mites can be seen as white specks walking away.
2. Although the entire life cycle (egg, larva, nymph, adult) is spent on the host and may be completed in one month, this mite is not highly host-specific. It infests dogs, cats and foxes. (See life cycle of ear mites p. 152.)
3. It is highly contagious between animals in close contact, and entire litters of kittens and puppies are frequently affected.

## LESIONS AND COURSE

1. In early cases there are few signs except a dry, dark, waxy exudate in the ear canals (Fig. 26:1*C*).
2. Pruritus is intense and constant head-shaking and ear-scratching are observed. The posterior surface of the ears may be severely excoriated by scratching.
3. The external ear canal is usually secondarily infected by bacteria so that purulent otitis results.
4. Hematoma of the ear flap may be a sequela to the vigorous head-shaking of long-eared dogs.

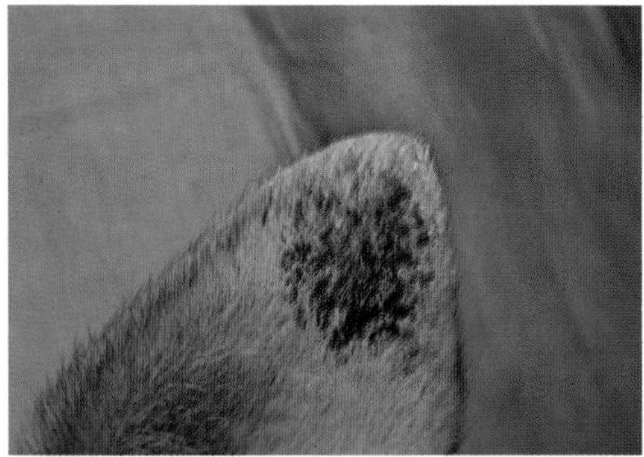

**Figure 26:1.** Ear dermatoses.

*A.* Fly dermatitis on a German shepherd's pinna. Hemorrhagic crusts form oozing serum and blood results from the rasping mouthparts of stable flies.

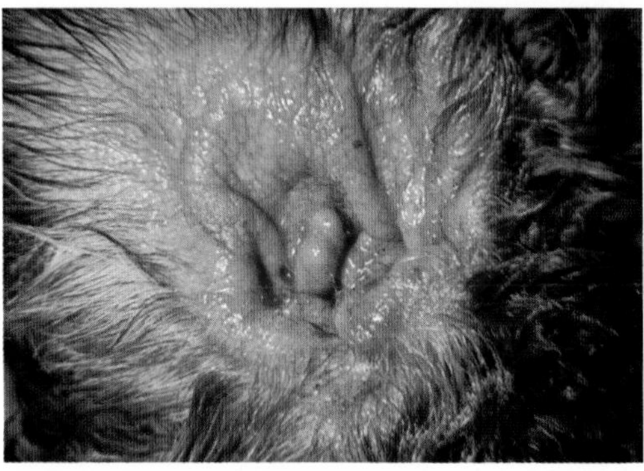

*B.* Otitis externa in a dog. There are edema, erythema and purulent exudation.

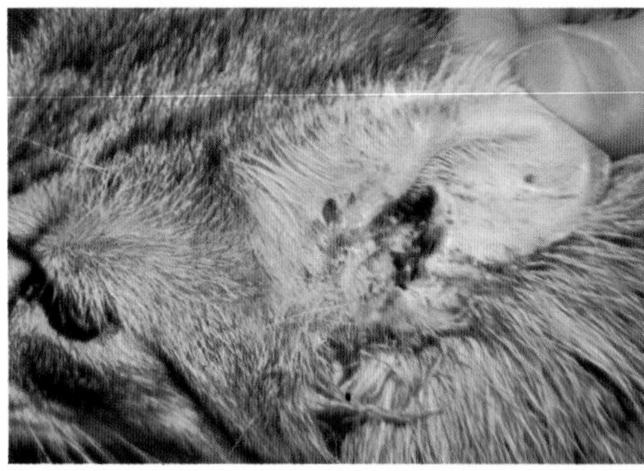

*C.* Dark brown, waxy exudate and crusts in the ear of a cat with ear mites *(Otodectes cynotis).*

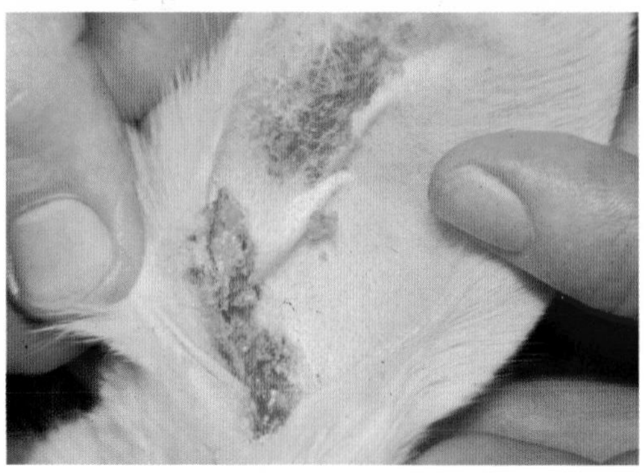

*D.* Firmly adherent crusts characteristically form in rabbit's ears infested with ear mites *(Chorioptes cuniculi).* (Figures B, C, and D courtesy of R. L. Collinson.)

## DIAGNOSTIC AIDS

1. Direct observation of the mites by magnifying otoscope or examination of the ear exudate is necessary for diagnosis.

2. Cerumen and crusted material from the ear can be mixed with mineral oil and examined microscopically.

## HISTOPATHOLOGY

In chronic cases the histologic changes observed are those described under otitis externa.

## DIFFERENTIAL DIAGNOSIS

Uncomplicated otitis externa, pediculosis, notoedric mange and moniliasis of the ear canal are some of the conditions to be differentiated. As the mites are easy to find in all cases, a positive examination will substantiate the diagnosis. However, mites may be present secondarily, too.

## CLINICAL MANAGEMENT

1. One part Canex in three parts mineral oil is a safe effective treatment for puppies or kittens. Polyderm can be used sparingly in the ear canal of mature individuals. Either preparation is applied after thorough cleansing of the canal with Fosteen or pHisoHex and water.

2. The entire coat should be dusted or sprayed with an insecticide such as Diryl, SOK, or a malathion aerosol preparation.

3. Both the preceding steps should be performed once or twice weekly for three weeks. All susceptible animals on the premises should be treated. The environment need not be treated.

4. When otitis externa is present the ears should be treated as described on page 260.

5. A number of ear mite medications are available commercially (Cerumite, Mitox) which combine acaricidal preparations with antibiotics and sometimes corticosteroids. They are more expensive than the simpler medications described previously, but are often useful for complicated cases.

# TWENTY-SEVEN

# *Eosinophilic Ulcer*

*(Rodent Ulcer)*

Eosinophilic ulcer is a chronic localized inflammation which may affect the lips, oral mucosa or skin of cats.

## SIGNIFICANT FACTS

1. This condition presents three different clinical syndromes, although their histologic appearance is similar. One affects the upper lip, another the hard and soft palates, and the third involves the skin of the abdomen, legs and feet.

2. The actual cause is unknown, but it seems to be associated with chronic irritation, especially licking.

3. The lesions may be spread by constant licking, too, as cats with affected lips have developed lesions on the flanks, or legs, and kittens nursing from queens with lesions of the abdomen have developed lip and nasal lesions.

## LESIONS AND COURSE

1. Lesions and course of each of the three syndromes vary.
   a. The lesion of the upper lip usually develops opposite a point of contact with a canine tooth. It starts as an area of erythema with a raised border. The surface of the lesion is often smooth and pale pink or red in color (Fig. 27:1*A*). In more advanced cases the surface is ulcerated (Fig. 27:1*B*). The lesion may progress to a squamous cell carcinoma of the lip and nose (Fig. 27:1*C*), but it is not clear if this is an actual change in morphology or if the early carcinoma merely resembles the eosinophilic ulcer.
   b. The lesion within the mouth is usually multiple, and consists of light, off-colored, well-circumscribed plaques with a rough, nodular surface.
   c. The skin lesions commonly are found on the abdomen, thighs and feet. They are hairless, moist red areas that are well circumscribed, and covered by a glistening film of exudate.
2. In many cases regional lymph nodes are enlarged.

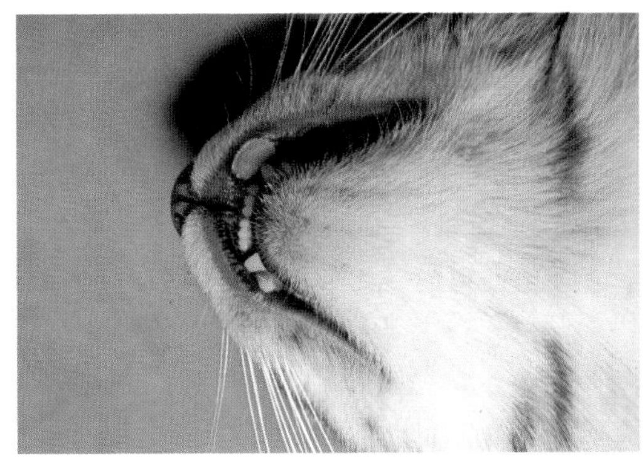

**Figure 27:1.** Eosinophilic ulcer.

*A.* Unilateral ulcerated lesion on the upper lip opposite the lower canine tooth.

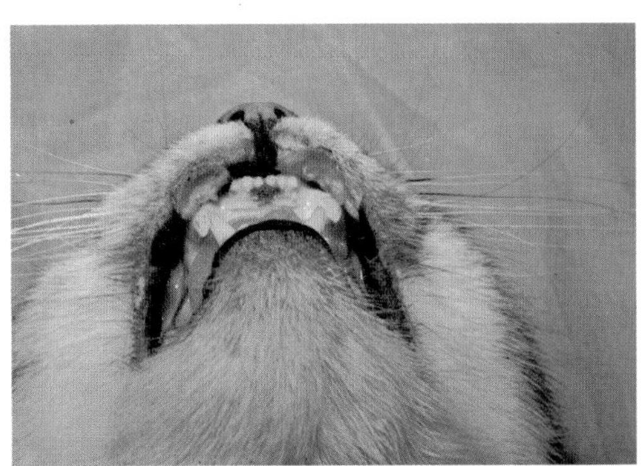

*B.* Bilateral ulcers that are chronic and necrotic.

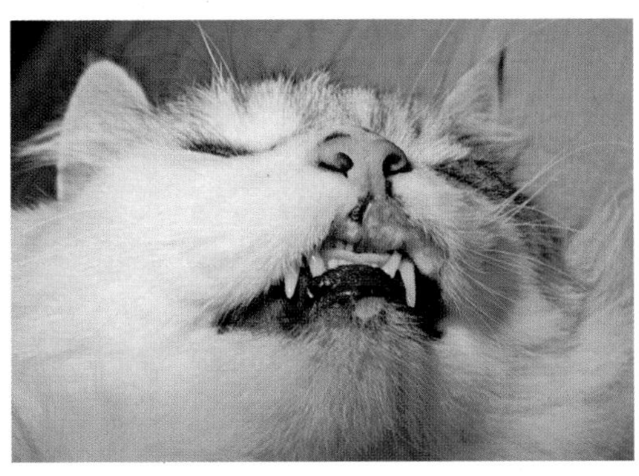

*C.* Ulcer that has developed into a squamous cell carcinoma.

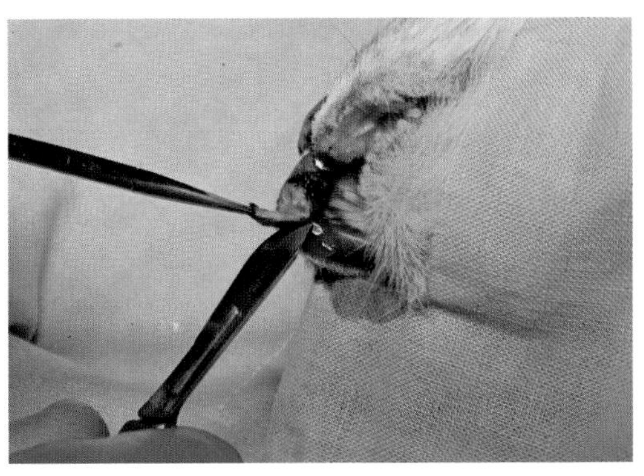

*D.* Surgical excision of the lesions shown in *B* is made with an incision directed horizontal to the surface but just below the lesion.

3. All lesions are chronic and sometimes have been present for more than a year before they are presented for treatment.

4. The circulating eosinophils are increased to 16 to 20 per cent in some patients.

## DIAGNOSTIC AIDS

Although the clinical appearance of eosinophilic ulcer is often diagnostic, positive diagnosis depends on histologic examination.

## HISTOPATHOLOGY

The lesions may show pseudoepitheliomatous hyperplasia which falsely suggests squamous cell carcinoma. The typical histologic lesion is a dense infiltration of eosinophils and histiocytes around the capillaries.

## DIFFERENTIAL DIAGNOSIS

1. The eosinophilic ulcer must be distinguished from fibrosarcoma, and squamous cell carcinoma. This usually requires histologic diagnosis.

2. Granulating wounds of the lip also may present a similar appearance, but they heal readily.

## CLINICAL MANAGEMENT

1. Careful surgical excision of the lip lesion often produces gratifying results. The superficial tissue is removed with special care to excise the marginal areas. With large lesions one must be careful not to produce deformities of the lips.

Skin lesions can be excised easily in most cases.

The palate lesions do not lend themselves to surgical treatment.

2. Large lesions and those of the mouth and pharynx often respond well to x-ray therapy repeated three times at seven day intervals (150 to 300 R dose, HVL 0.3 mm. Cu). Concurrent systemic corticosteroid therapy is often used.

3. Intralesional injections of triamcinolone acetonide repeated weekly for four or five treatments may also be beneficial, especially on the lip and cutaneous lesions.

4. Preventing the trauma of licking by using restraint collars for skin lesions or by filing down the opposing canine teeth may reduce irritation and enhance healing.

### *Suggested Reading*

Conroy, J. D.: *Diseases of the Skin in Feline Medicine.* American Veterinary Publications, Santa Barbara, 1964.

# TWENTY-EIGHT

## *Epidermoid Cyst*

### *(Epidermal, Keratinous or Sebaceous Cyst)*

Epidermoid cysts are firm nodules in the dermis or hypodermis that are lined with stratified squamous epithelium without secretory appendages.

## SIGNIFICANT FACTS

1. They are formed by a degenerative change in a hair follicle, by cystic changes in the ducts or cells of sebaceous glands, or by trauma which displaces epidermal fragments into the hypodermis.

2. Epidermoid cysts are especially common in Kerry blue terriers (Fig. 28:1*C*), boxers, English springer spaniels, cocker spaniels and fox terriers, and less common in cats.

3. There is no age or sex predilection.

## LESIONS AND COURSE

1. The cyst is round and encapsulated but fluctuates on pressure. It may be attached to the skin (dermis) and move with it, or located under the skin and move independently.

2. Approximately 60 per cent of cysts are solitary nodules, but the rest are multiple (Fig. 28:1*A*). They are located on the legs, chest, neck and back. Their size ranges from 1/4 inch to 2 inches in diameter.

3. When incised, a grayish white cheesy material exudes which resembles toothpaste (Fig. 28:1*B*).

4. The course is benign as the cysts enlarge very slowly. They may become irritated or ulcerated by external trauma from collars or by scratching.

## DIAGNOSTIC AIDS

1. The clinical appearance is highly suggestive, especially if the contents are typical. However, microscopic examination of the cyst wall is needed for positive diagnosis.

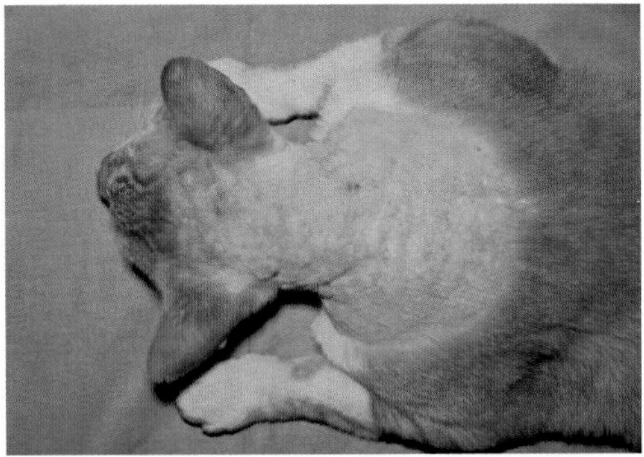

**Figure 28:1.** Epidermoid cyst.

*A.* Multiple epidermoid cysts on the neck of a cat. Area has been clipped.

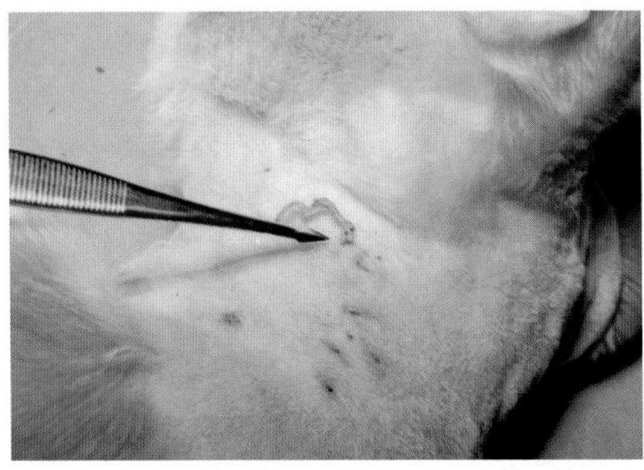

*B.* When incised the cyst matrix can be expressed as a grayish white cheesy material resembling toothpaste.

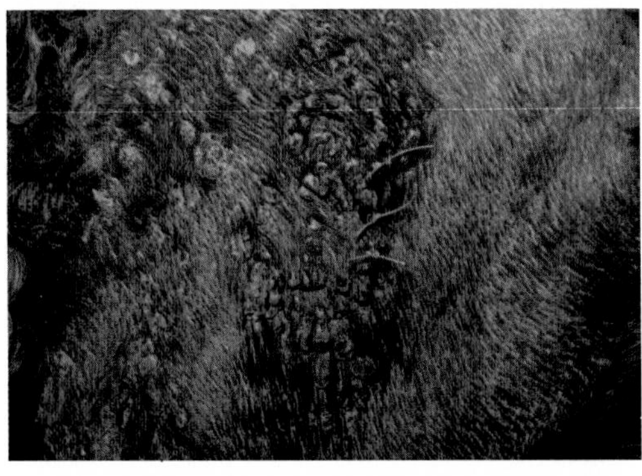

*C.* Multiple epidermoid cysts from the skin of the thorax of a Kerry blue terrier. Sutures mark site of biopsy.

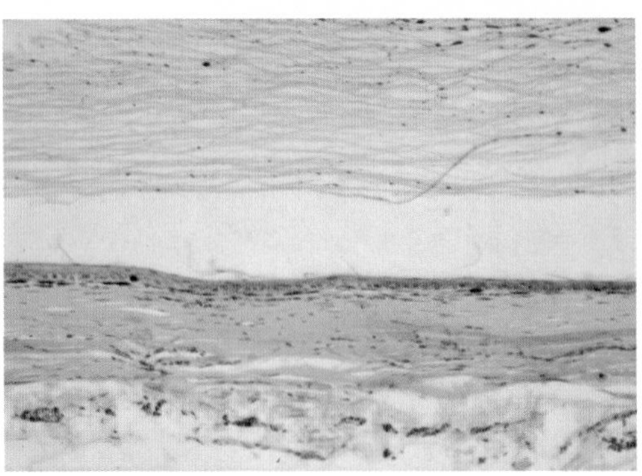

*D.* Histologic section of wall of epidermoid cyst showing central keratin (above) surrounded by stratified squamous epithelium. (High power.)

## HISTOPATHOLOGY (FIG. 28:1*D*)

1. The cyst is lined by stratified squamous epithelium, which encloses concentrically arranged rings of keratin. If the cyst is ruptured and some of the keratin and cholesterol debris escapes into surrounding tissues, it is highly irritating and initiates a severe granulomatous reaction, with foreign body giant cells and foamy macrophages accumulating.

## DIFFERENTIAL DIAGNOSIS

1. Dermoid cysts are probably developmental defects, as they are lined by epidermis with appendages.
2. Pilonidal sinuses or dermoid sinuses are developmental defects on the dorsal midline of Rhodesian ridgeback dogs.
3. Lipomas may simulate sebaceous cysts closely, and although the texture on palpation may be different, surgical excision may be necessary for differentiation.
4. Early forms of mastocytoma, basal cell tumor, squamous cell carcinoma and calcifying epithelioma are firm and do not fluctuate on palpation.

## CLINICAL MANAGEMENT

Epidermoid cysts should be completely excised.

1. Complete surgical excision is simple and curative. Various methods of cautery, curettage and other destructive measures have been employed but are not recommended. With multiple cysts where excision is impractical, surgical incision of the cyst wall and expression of the contents give only temporary improvement, but it is sometimes a necessary expedient.

### *Suggested Reading*

Conroy, J. D.: Epidermal Cysts. *In Kirk, R. W. (Ed.): Current Veterinary Therapy III.* W. B. Saunders Co., Philadelphia, 1968.

Moulton, J. E.: *Tumors in Domestic Animals.* University of California Press, Berkeley, 1961.

# TWENTY-NINE

## *Eyelid Diseases*

The eyelids are complex folds of skin susceptible to many structural and functional disorders which can, in turn, affect the eyeball (globe) itself.

### ANATOMY

Canine and feline eyelids consist of an upper eyelid, a lower eyelid, a third eyelid (membrana nictitans), a row of cilia in the upper lid only, the orbicularis oculi muscles, nerves, blood vessels, lymphatics and the following glands:

1. Meibomian glands (tarsal glands) are modified, large sebaceous gland units that produce a viscous, oily secretion.
2. Glands of Zeis are sebaceous glands associated with cilia.
3. Glands of Moll are modified apocrine sweat glands associated with cilia.
4. Glands of the third eyelid (nictitans glands, harderian glands) are masses of lymphoid tissue located on the inner surface of the membrana nictitans.
5. In addition there are accessory lacrimal glands in the eyelids which discharge tears into the conjunctival sac and contribute to the precorneal film. The largest of these in the dog is the superficial gland of the membrana nictitans, also known (erroneously) as the gland of Harder.

### DISEASES

1. Entropion (inversion or turning in) and ectropion (eversion or turning out) of the lid margins are best corrected by surgery. Chronic conjunctivitis or other disease of the eye that may result in distortion of the lid should also receive attention.
2. *Hordeolum* (sty). A hordeolum is an acute, painful pyogenic infection of a sebaceous gland of the eyelid. Two types are recognized:
   a. The external hordeolum (Zeissian sty) involves the glands of Zeis and the cilia on the outer eyelid.
   b. The internal hordeolum (meibomian sty) involves the meibomian gland on the inner surface of the eyelid. The internal type is the most common hordeolum in dogs. Treatment consists of incising the abscess

**Figure 29:1.** Eyelid diseases.

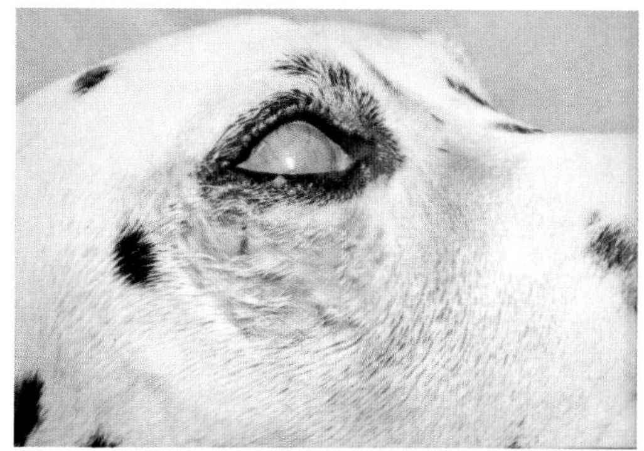

*A.* Mycotic blepharitis *(M. canis)* affecting the lower lid. The keratitis is secondary.

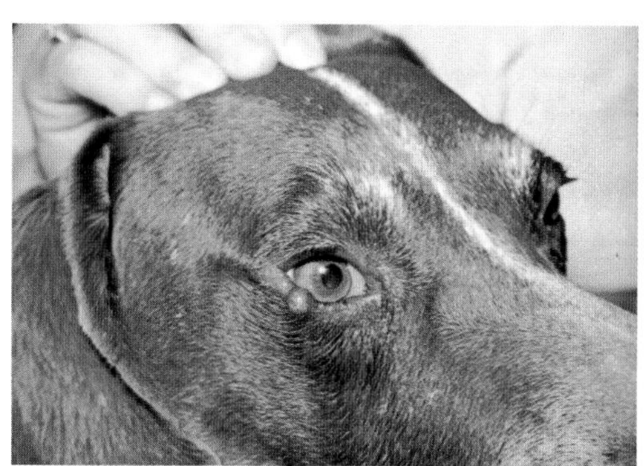

*B.* Chalazion, chronic inflammation of a meibomian gland – external appearance.

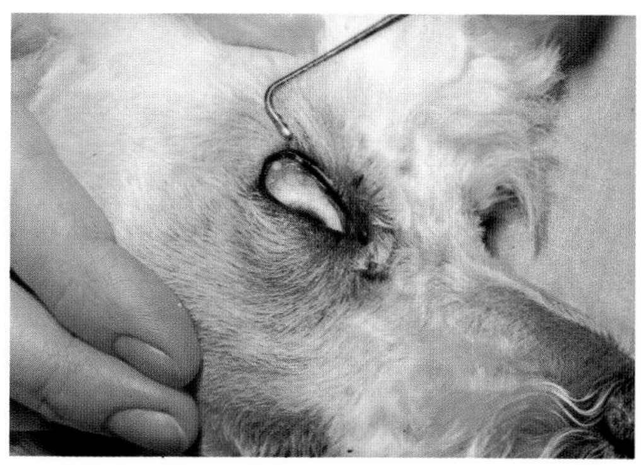

*C.* Chalazion, internal view of the early stage. A cystic meibomian gland has a similar appearance.

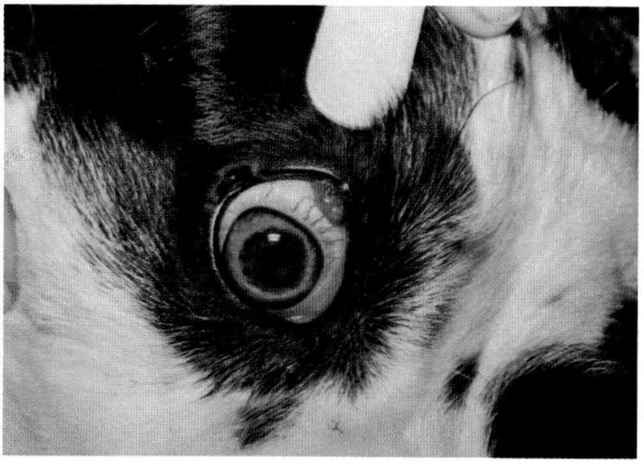

*D.* Sebaceous adenoma, upper eyelid.

and applying an antibiotic ointment. Appropriate systemic antibiotics are useful when the hordeolum is caused by staphylococci.

3. *Chalazion* is a chronic inflammation of a meibomian gland (Fig. 29:1*B* and *C*). It appears externally on the lid's skin surface as a painless nodule and internally on the palpebral conjunctiva as a yellow, smaller nodule. The irritation from the inner swelling causes conjunctivitis. Treatment consists of incision and curettage of accumulated sebaceous material. Large chalazia should be excised completely to prevent recurrence.

4. *Blepharitis* is an erythematous, crusted inflammation of eyelid *margins*, often accompanied by a mucous discharge. Many generalized skin diseases will extend to the lids, producing an inflammation that can be named after its cause.

a. *Seborrheic blepharitis* is characterized by greasy scales and flakes on the lids. Corticosteroid ointments are valuable symptomatic treatment (see p. 207).

b. *Mycotic blepharitis* occurs when a dermatomycosis extends to the lids and cilia (Fig. 29:1*A*). It is usually caused by *M. canis, M. gypseum,* or *T. Mentagrophytes.* Systemic griseofulvin is the treatment of choice (see p. 206).

c. *Demodectic blepharitis* is very common in young dogs. An alopecic, frequently erythematous patch on the upper or lower lid will usually yield demodectic mites when skin scrapings are made. As long as the condition remains localized and free of staphylococcus infection it is not serious. For treatment, a mild rotenone (Goodwinol) ointment, applied once a day, is sufficient. The cornea should be protected with ophthalmic ointment when irritating medication is used on the eyelids.

d. *Distemper blepharitis* accompanies most cases of canine distemper. It is closely related to the conjunctivitis that is common in distemper, and there is a copious mucous eye discharge. The eyes should be cleansed frequently and an antibiotic ointment (such as chloramphenicol ointment) used three times a day. A similar blepharitis accompanies some other acute infectious diseases of dogs and cats.

5. *Trichiasis* is an abnormal position or direction of the cilia resulting in epiphora, mucous eye discharge, and sometimes corneal vascularization and even corneal ulceration. Treatment consists of meticulous electro-epilation of the involved cilia.

6. *Distichiasis* is a condition in which aberrant cilia are found on the lid. They may emerge from the openings of the meibomian glands or the lower-lid margin.

7. *Nictitans gland hypertrophy* is seen as a bright red nodule protruding into the medial canthus from under the third eyelid. It is most common in Boston terriers and cocker spaniels. Although the condition may be unilateral, the opposite eye frequently becomes involved later. Surgical removal of the protruding nictitans gland is a simple operation that gives excellent results. It is most important to avoid damage to the third eyelid itself during this surgery.

## Suggested Reading

Magrane, W. C.: *Canine Ophthalmology.* Lea & Febiger, Philadelphia, 1965, pp. 49-71.

Roberts, S. R.: *Ocular Disorders in Canine Medicine.* American Veterinary Publications, Santa Barbara, California, 1968, pp. 765-772.

# THIRTY

# *Feline Acne*

Feline acne is an eruption on the chin of the cat that is characterized by comedones, pustules and folliculitis.

## SIGNIFICANT FACTS

1. Feline acne is restricted to the area of the chin and the margins of the lips.

2. Cats clean their bodies meticulously by direct licking. However, they use their saliva-moistened front paws to cleanse the face. Some cats have difficulty washing the chin in that manner, so surface lipids and dirt accumulate. This predisposes to comedo formation (Fig. 30:1*C*).

3. Only certain cats develop feline acne. Affected cats are those which may routinely fail to clean the chin sufficiently and have a seborrhea-like skin condition in which comedones form easily.

## LESIONS AND COURSE

1. The lesions consist of comedones, papules, pustules and small cysts. Edema of the entire chin is sometimes seen and in severe cases multiple folliculitis progresses to pyoderma.

2. The course can be acute or chronic. Acute episodes are likely to be presented for treatment, but chronic cases may be overlooked until they become severe. Although acne may respond to treatment, recurrences should be expected.

3. An explanation for the periodic occurrence of feline acne may be associated with the cat's shedding cycle. Acne starts when hairs are in the telogen phase, and the comedo forms because the telogen hair is unable to push out the keratin plug and keep the follicle open (Montgomery, 1962).

## DIAGNOSTIC AIDS

Inspection of the cat's chin provides visual evidence which is diagnostic. In case of doubt, a skin biopsy shows characteristic acne-like lesions which confirm the diagnosis.

**Figure 30-1.** Feline acne.

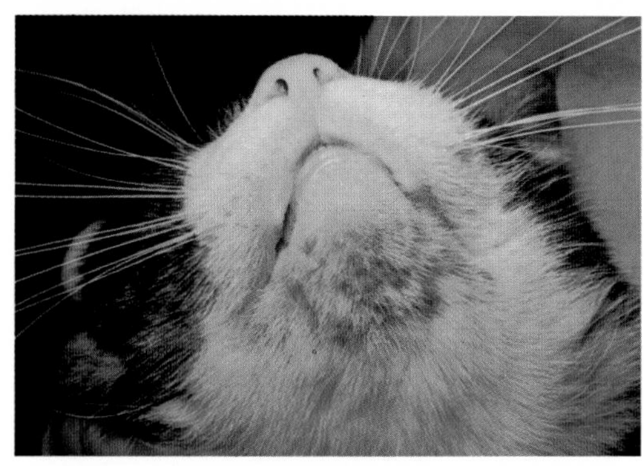

*A.* Early case with erythematous folliculitis.

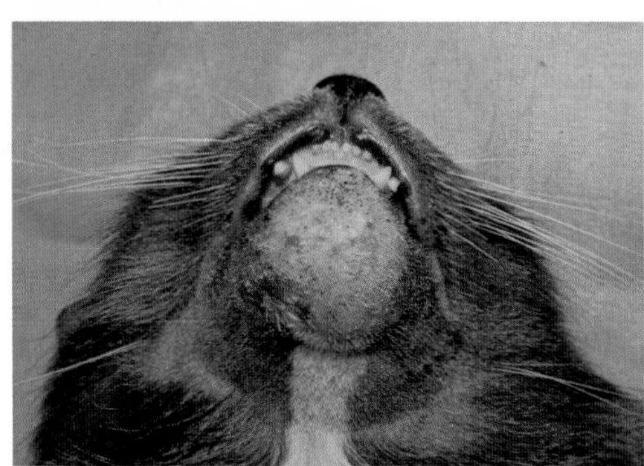

*B.* Advanced case with edema of the chin, alopecia and pustule formation. Hair has been removed from periphery of lesion for better visualization.

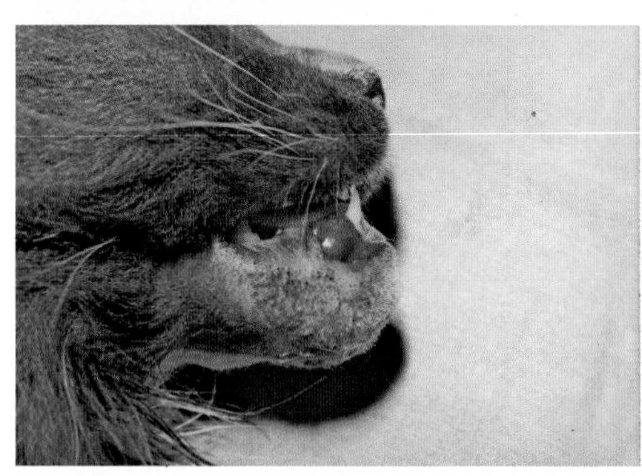

*C.* Side view of *B* clearly shows grayish-black comedones and edema of the entire chin.

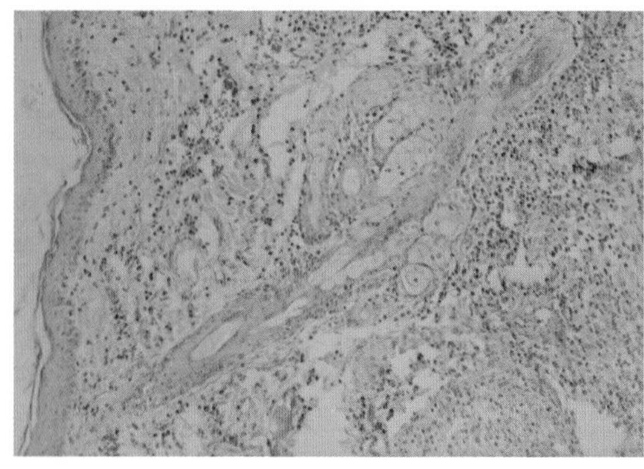

*D.* Biopsy from cat in *B* and *C* showing the acne-like folliculitis. Note the perifollicular inflammatory infiltrate. Surface of skin is at left. (Low power.)

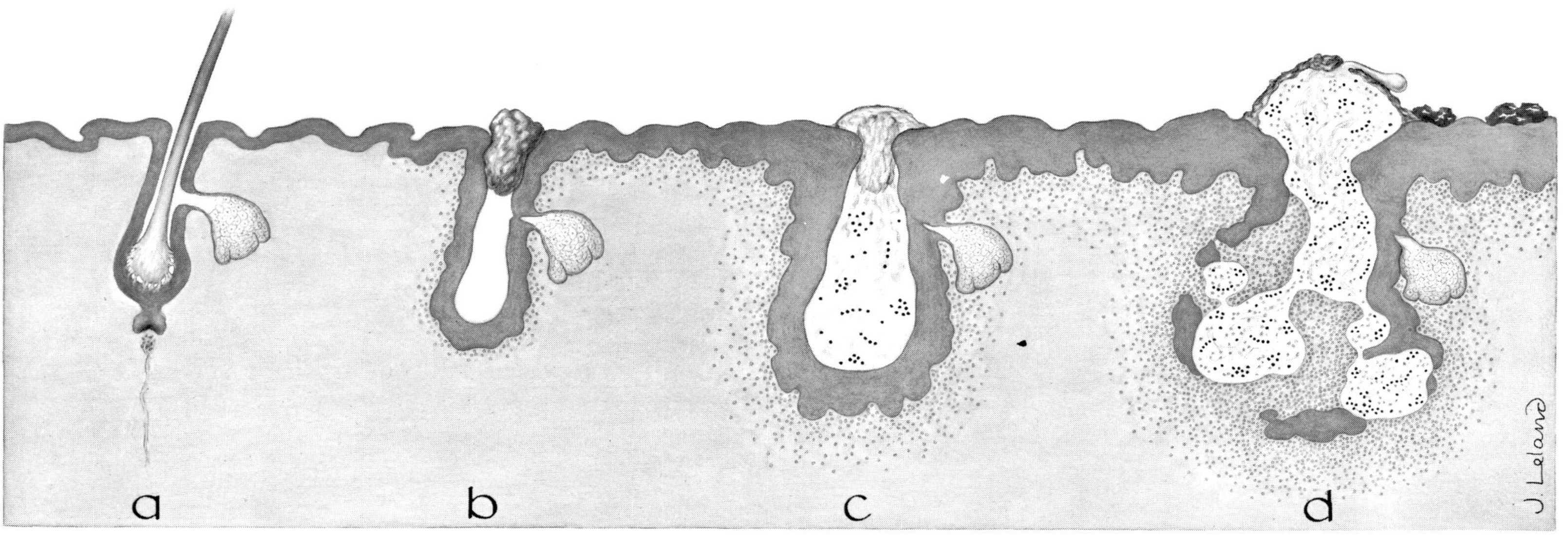


**Figure 30:2.** Feline acne dermogram. *a.* Hair follicle in telogen. *b.* The hair has been shed and a comedo plugs the follicular orifice. The epidermis is slightly acanthotic, and a mild perifollicular infiltrate forms. *c.* As bacteria (black dots) invade the follicle, acanthosis and inflammation increase. The follicle dilates, and a pustule begins to form. At the same time, the comedo disintegrates. *d.* Pustule formation is complete. The thin crust at the former follicular opening is breaking away as the first drop of pus oozes out. The former follicle is now a small intradermal abscess surrounded by a dense inflammatory infiltrate. This represents the severe form of feline acne on the chin.

## HISTOPATHOLOGY (FIG. 30:1*D*)

Following the formation of a keratin plug at the follicular orifice, there is a mild perifollicular infiltrate of neutrophils. The epidermis becomes acanthotic and the hair follicles begin to disintegrate. A subepidermal abscess results. In some cases the plugged follicles form cysts filled with keratin and sebum.

## DIFFERENTIAL DIAGNOSIS

Since cats (especially uncastrated males) frequently develop fight wounds, feline acne lesions can be mistaken for traumatic abscesses. Dermatomycoses, which are common on the head, also need to be differentiated from acne.

## CLINICAL MANAGEMENT

1. The acute stage responds to antibiotic therapy. Tetracycline, 100 mg. b.i.d. for one to two weeks, is effective. Penicillin is the second choice drug.

2. Topically, an antibiotic cream containing neomycin, polymyxin and bacitracin is useful. Neomycin-corticosteroid lotions or creams can also be used effectively.

3. Cleansing the affected area is essential to remove sebum and bacteria. This can be accomplished by daily gentle washing with a soap or soap substitute containing an antibacterial agent. Rubbing alcohol can also be used for this purpose. Certain acne cleansers available commercially for acne vulgaris of man are useful for the removal of feline comedones.

---

For prophylaxis, the owner should clean the cat's chin daily with alcohol or soap and water.

---

### *Suggested Reading*

Montgomery, G. L.: In: *Histopathology of the Skin*. Williams & Wilkins, Baltimore, 1962, p. 480.

Pillsbury, D. M., Shelley, W. B. and Kligman, A. M.: *Cutaneous Medicine*. W. B. Saunders Co., Philadelphia, 1961, pp. 273-281.

# THIRTY-ONE

# *Feline Endocrine Alopecia*

Feline endocrine alopecia produces a pattern of bilaterally symmetrical hair loss affecting the hindquarters of cats. It can be corrected by hormone therapy.

## SIGNIFICANT FACTS

1. It is a comparatively rare skin disease that should be easily recognized by clinicians.
2. Although the cause of this alopecia has not been proved, hair will regrow if both thyroid and sex hormones are administered empirically. Research is needed to determine whether both thyroid and sex hormones are actually deficient.
3. The disease seems to be most common in altered male cats, but is also seen in spayed females. It is rarely seen in unaltered males and unspayed females.
4. The cats appear to be normal except for the partial alopecia.

## LESIONS AND COURSE

1. The areas of noticeable alopecia are located from the sternum posteriorly, with sparing of hair on the lower legs and the dorsal midline (Fig. 31:1*C*).
2. In the affected areas, the hairs are fewer and shorter than normal.
3. The hair does not usually regrow without treatment.
4. The skin of the affected areas is not pruritic, scaly or inflamed, but the few remaining hairs are dry, brittle and stubby.
5. The condition occurs most commonly in mature cats.
6. The onset of hair loss is rapid, but once it reaches a certain stage it does not progress to total alopecia.

## DIFFERENTIAL DIAGNOSIS

1. Dermatomycosis is not bilaterally symmetrical.
2. Feline flea allergy dermatitis is intensely pruritic and characterized by

**Figure 31:1.** Feline endocrine alopecia.

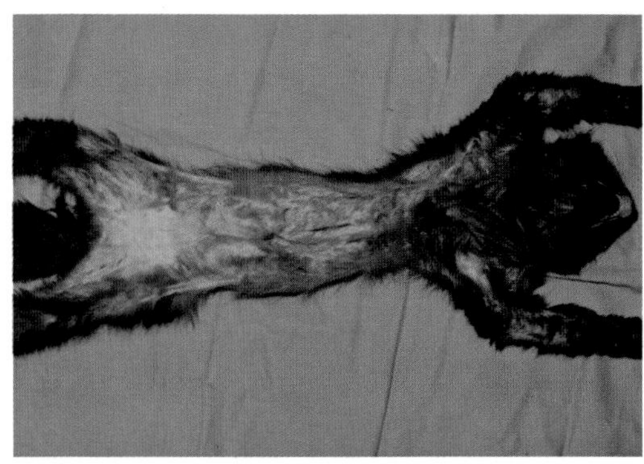

*A.* Ventral view showing characteristic bilateral alopecia without skin reaction or lesions.

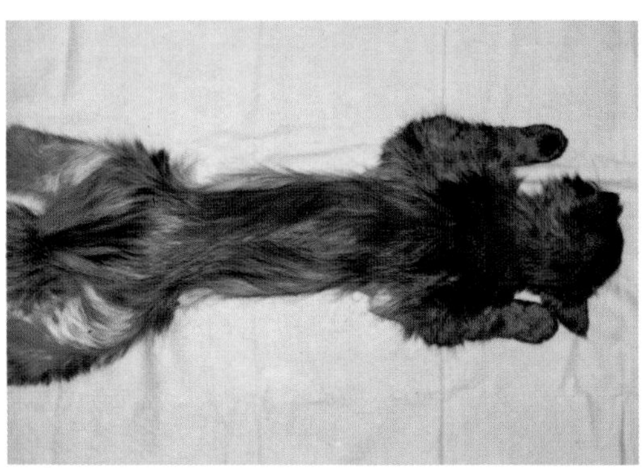

*B.* Bilateral alopecia showing normal hair along the dorsal midline.

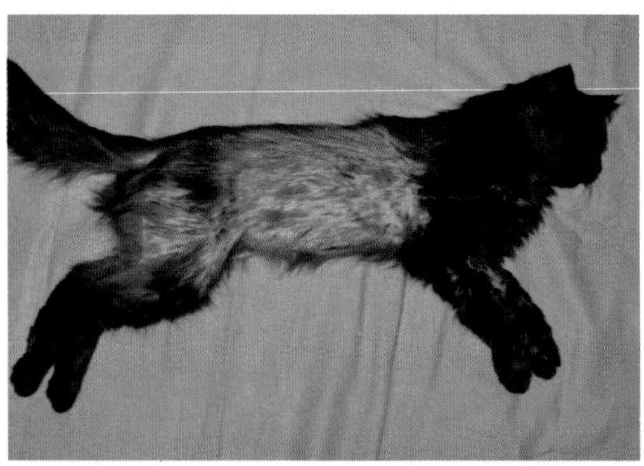

*C.* Characteristic alopecia from the sternum posteriorly, sparing hair on the lower legs.

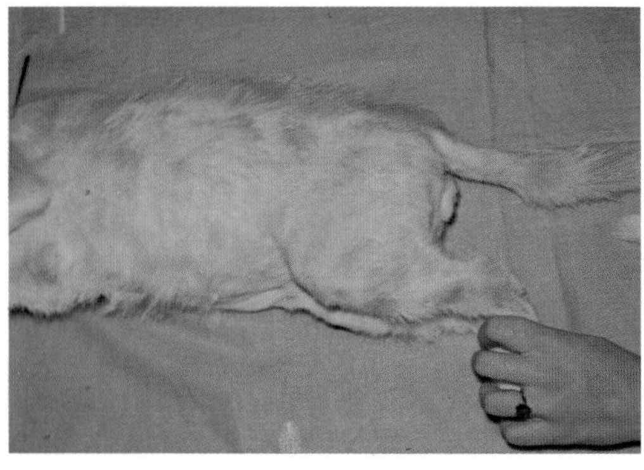

*D.* Similar case to *C.*

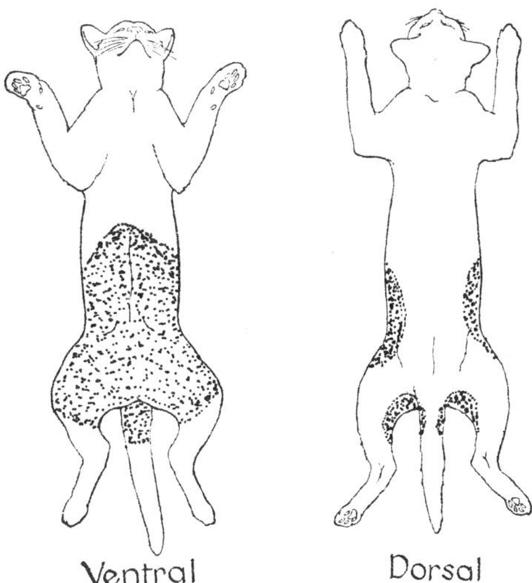


**Figure 31:2.** Feline endocrine alopecia distribution pattern.

miliary crusts and erythema in addition to some alopecia on the posterior dorsal portion of the body.

## CLINICAL MANAGEMENT

1. Oral thyroid supplementation is given to all cats (desiccated thyroid USP 2 gr./day orally for three to six months). Use fresh thyroid tablets. *Or*: Synthroid 0.1 to 0.3 mg. daily for three to six months.

2. Altered male cats should receive 2 mg. of testosterone per day orally (Halotestin). Testosterone may cause "spraying of urine." If so, the medication should be discontinued temporarily. Spayed females should receive 0.1 mg. of stilbestrol per day orally. Discontinue temporarily if cat goes into estrus, and *do not administer for more than 30 days*. Some females respond better to testosterone therapy.

3. Continue both medications simultaneously (caution with stilbestrol!) until hair has regrown. Some cats will then be cured, but others will lose their hair again after medication is discontinued.

4. For cases with recurrent hair loss, maintenance medication is necessary. The dosage required varies with individuals, but should be kept at the lowest levels consistent with good results.

# THIRTY-TWO

# *Feline Flea Allergy Dermatitis*

## *(Miliary Dermatitis, Feline Eczema)*

Feline flea allergy dermatitis is a specific skin disease of cats caused by hypersensitivity to fleabites and characterized by pruritus, erythema and the formation of miliary crusts.

### SIGNIFICANT FACTS

1. The disease affects only cats that are bitten by fleas, and its seasonal occurrence coincides with increases in flea infestations in the summer.
2. In warm climates homes remain infested with fleas all year but susceptible cats have a milder form of the disease in the winter.
3. Numerous causes and names have been associated with this disease. It is the authors' observation that most cases of feline eczema, miliary dermatitis or fish eater's eczema are in reality feline flea allergy. There is no substantial evidence to support beliefs that testosterone deficiency, biotin deficiency, food allergies or fat deficiency are etiologic factors.
4. Male and female cats are equally affected whether they have been neutered or not.
5. There is a marked increase in histamine and mast cells in the skin of cats with feline flea allergy dermatitis.

### LESIONS AND COURSE

Crusted lesions are concentrated on the lower back and spinal region.

1. The primary lesion is an erythematous papule covered by a small reddish brown crust (Fig. 32:1*C*).

**Figure 32:1.** Feline flea allergy dermatitis.

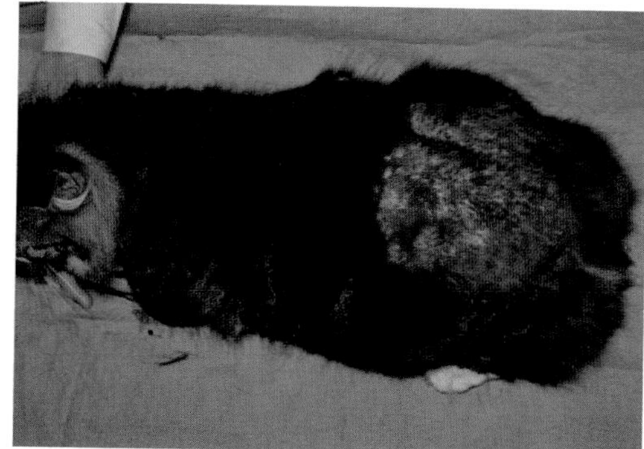

*A.* Numerous miliary lesions clustered on the back of this cat. Area has been clipped in Figures *A*, *B*, *C* and *D* to expose lesions.

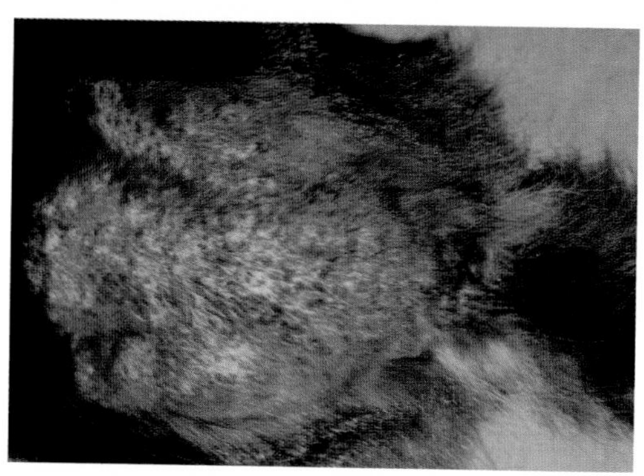

*B.* Closer view of the lower back of *A*.

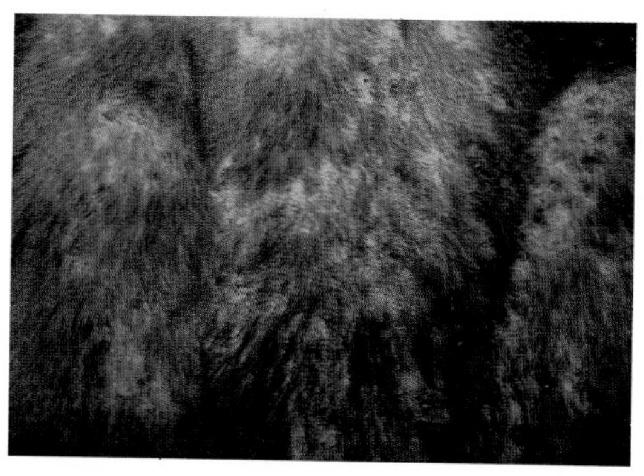

*C.* The individual miliary lesions are shallow excoriations covered with a small brown crust. Some crusts have been removed to show the lesion's base.

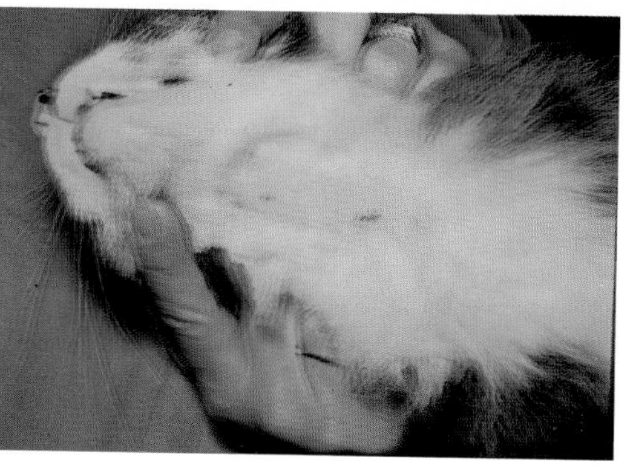

*D.* Other common sites of the miliary lesions are the neck and throat.

2. Numerous such miliary lesions are located on the back. The lower back and spinal regions are most severely affected (Fig. 32:1*A*) and the neck is the next most commonly affected area (Fig. 32:1*D*). In severely affected animals the entire body may be covered with lesions, with only the head and extremities being spared.

3. The back, neck and throat are the favorite feeding grounds of the flea and therefore the most common sites of lesions.

4. The constant and severe pruritus causes cats to bite, lick and scratch themselves.

5. Self-inflicted trauma results in excoriated patches.

## DIAGNOSTIC AIDS

1. Palpation of the small, crusted lesions, the typical distribution pattern, the case history and the presence of fleas are usually sufficient to make a positive diagnosis.

## HISTOPATHOLOGY

The parakeratotic, acanthotic epidermis is covered with a dried fibrinous exudate, which contains erythrocytes and neutrophils. In some areas of the epidermis there is spongiosis. In the upper dermis there is an infiltration of neutrophils, mast cells and macrophages. Vascular dilatation is present too.

## DIFFERENTIAL DIAGNOSIS

1. Lick or eosinophilic granulomas of neurodermatitis have a different distribution pattern and lack generalized pruritus.

2. Multiple, small, crusted puncture wounds on the neck and back may resemble miliary lesions but are not accompanied by pruritus.

## CLINICAL MANAGEMENT

1. Flea eradication is carried out in a manner similar to that described under canine flea allergy dermatitis (p. 159).

2. A good flea powder (Diryl, SOK) should be applied twice a week, or flea collars designed for cats should be prescribed.

3. Corticosteroids given systemically counteract the pruritus and allow the miliary lesions to heal completely. Prednisolone, 2.5 mg. orally twice a day for two to four weeks, is usually effective.

4. All other cats and dogs in the same household (though they may not be allergic to fleabites) must also be deflead simultaneously or they will act as flea reservoirs.

5. Recurrences are the rule if affected cats are again bitten by fleas.

### *Suggested Reading*

See the discussion of flea allergy dermatitis of dogs in Chapter 34 (p. 287). Most of its text and the dermogram apply to the feline form of the disease. Also, see the discussion of fleas (Ectoparasites) in Chapter 11 (p. 136).

# THIRTY-THREE

# *Feline Solar Dermatitis*

## *(Carcinoma of the White Ears of Cats)*

Feline solar dermatitis is a chronic dermatitis of the white ears of cats, which is caused by repeated sun exposure. It can develop into a squamous cell carcinoma.

## SIGNIFICANT FACTS

1. The disease occurs in white cats or in colored cats with white ears. Blue-eyed white cats are most susceptible.

2. Actinic damage to the ear tip occurs from repeated sunburn and exposure to solar ultraviolet waves of the 3000 Angström unit band. This erythema-producing band of sunlight is not filtered by thin clouds.

3. The disease occurs mostly in warm, sunny climates such as California, Florida and Hawaii.

## LESIONS AND COURSE

1. The earliest sign is erythema of the margin of the ear's pinna (Fig. 33:1*A*). The hair is lost in this area, making it even more accessible to solar radiation. There is almost no discomfort to the cat at this stage.

2. In susceptible cats the first lesions can occur as early as three months of age. Lesions become progressively worse each summer.

3. The advancing lesions consist of severe erythema of the pinna, peeling of the skin and formation of marginal crusts. At this stage cats show pain and will further damage their ears by scratching.

4. The margins of the lower eyelids often are affected, especially in white, blue-eyed cats.

5. A squamous cell carcinoma develops in many cases on the ears and in rare cases there has been metastasis to the regional lymph nodes. Carcinomatous change may occur, usually after six years of age but sometimes as early as three years.

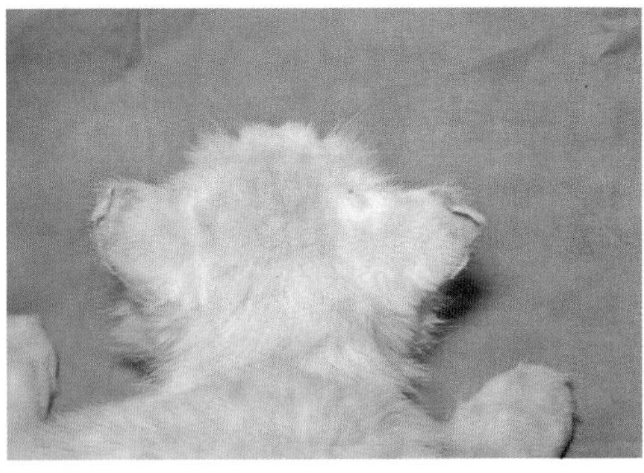

**Figure 33:1.** Feline solar dermatitis.

*A.* Sunburned erythematous margins of the pinnas precede the more serious stage of the disease. Note the characteristic curling of the tips.

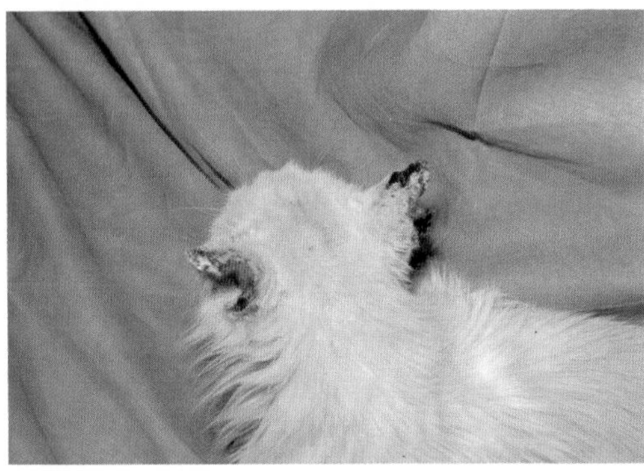

*B.* This 14-year-old cat had the disease for several years until a squamous cell carcinoma developed on both ears.

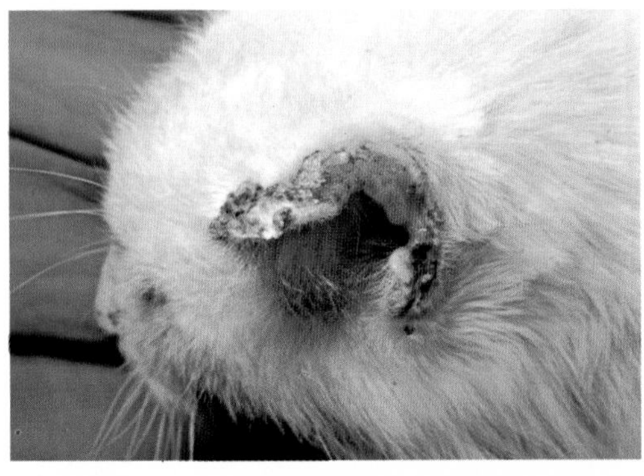

*C.* Close-up of cat in *B* showing the carcinomatous margin of the pinna.

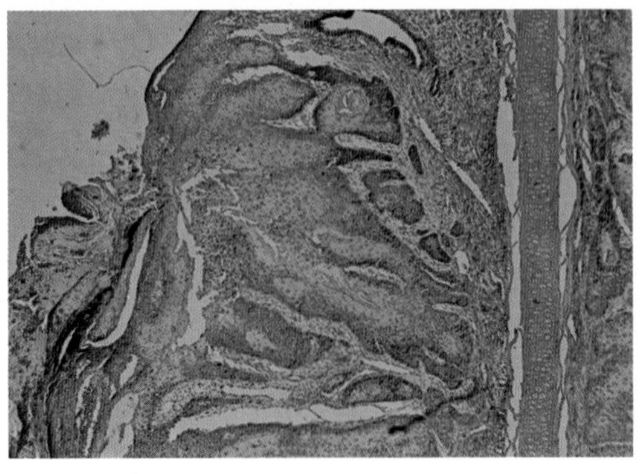

*D.* Biopsy of ear in *C.* Squamous cell carcinoma extends to the cartilage. Note the crust covering the tumor mass. (Low power.) (Epidermal surface is at left.)

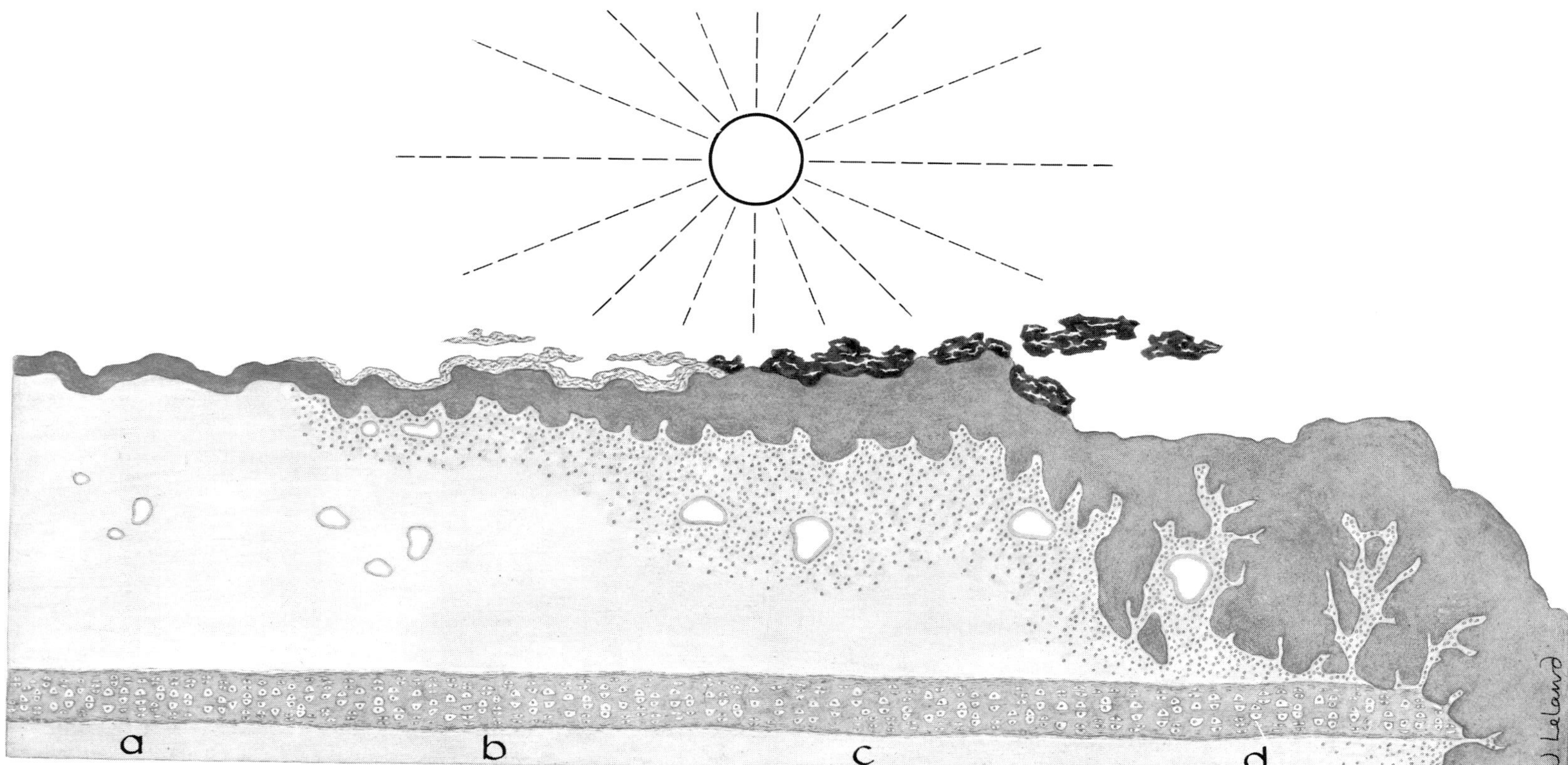


**Figure 33:2.** Feline solar dermatitis dermogram. *a.* Normal skin and cartilage of the ear's pinna. *b.* Sunburned skin showing mild acanthosis, scaling and vascular dilatation. *c.* With increasing solar radiation, the skin responds with more acanthosis, inflammation, hyperemia and crusting. *d.* Squamous cell carcinoma formation results from continued actinic effects on susceptible skin. Masses of neoplastic epidermal cells invade the dermis to the level of the cartilage. Skin and cartilage are eventually replaced by the squamous cell carcinoma.

6. The squamous cell carcinoma appears as an ulcerating, hemorrhagic and locally invasive lesion. It is partially crusted and in advanced cases destroys the pinna in a "rodent-ulcer" manner (Fig. 33:1*B* and *C*).

## DIAGNOSTIC AIDS

Biopsy of the lesion is valuable to determine whether the disease is in the erythematous phase or whether it has developed into a squamous cell carcinoma.

## HISTOPATHOLOGY (FIG. 33:1*D*)

In the early stages there is spongiosis of the epidermis, and edema, hyperemia and nonspecific inflammatory infiltration of the upper dermis. With squamous cell carcinoma formation, the epidermal surface is ulcerated and the dermis is invaded by nests of polyhedral epithelial tumor cells. In a disorganized manner these cells resemble the stratum spinosum. Their nuclei vary moderately in size and mitotic figures are frequent. The masses of tumor tissue extend to the level of the cartilage in advanced cases (see Figure 33:1*D*, p. 284).

## DIFFERENTIAL DIAGNOSIS

1. Severe ear mite infestation will sometimes cause an erythema similar to that of early solar dermatitis; however, mite eradication allows the lesion to heal.

2. Fight wounds on the ear, especially those with crusting and granulation, resemble solar dermatitis. They heal nicely, however, with antibiotic therapy.

## CLINICAL MANAGEMENT

1. Keep affected cats out of the sunshine from 10 a.m. to 4 p.m. when the ultraviolet rays are most damaging.

2. Protect ears during the summer with mild sun creams and lotions.

3. Once a carcinoma has developed, surgical excision of the affected portion of the pinna is necessary. Radical amputation of the pinna is necessary for advanced cases, but the cosmetic result is surprisingly satisfactory after the hair has regrown. In amputations it is important to achieve good skin to skin apposition over the cartilage so that hair can cover the margin.

---

Early amputation of the pinna saves further trouble, is usually curative and gives surprisingly good cosmetic results.

---

# THIRTY-FOUR

# *Flea Allergy Dermatitis*

*(Canine)*

Flea allergy dermatitis is a specific skin disease of dogs caused by hypersensitivity to fleabites and characterized by pruritus, self-inflicted trauma and acute moist dermatitis.

## SIGNIFICANT FACTS

1. This is one of the most common canine skin diseases in parts of the country where fleas are numerous. It is almost unknown in areas that are free of fleas, such as high altitude regions.

2. A hypersensitivity reaction occurs when a dog who has become sensitized to flea saliva (allergen) is challenged by new fleabites.

3. The sensitization reaction produced in flea allergy dermatitis depends on a hapten (incomplete antigen) from the flea's saliva combining with the skin's adjuvant (from collagen) to form a complete antigen (Feingold et al., 1968).

4. Both immediate and delayed reactions occur in flea allergy dermatitis. The probing of the flea, even without taking a blood meal, causes an immediate reaction. Delayed reactions occur later and are the important factors. Frequently there is an urticarial response to fleabites when many previous fleabites flare up after five days. This is not a true urticaria but only a delayed reaction to former bites (Feingold et al., 1968).

5. There is no sex or breed predilection. Affected dogs are usually over six months of age.

## LESIONS AND COURSE

Pruritus is the main symptom, and lesions are concentrated on the lower back.

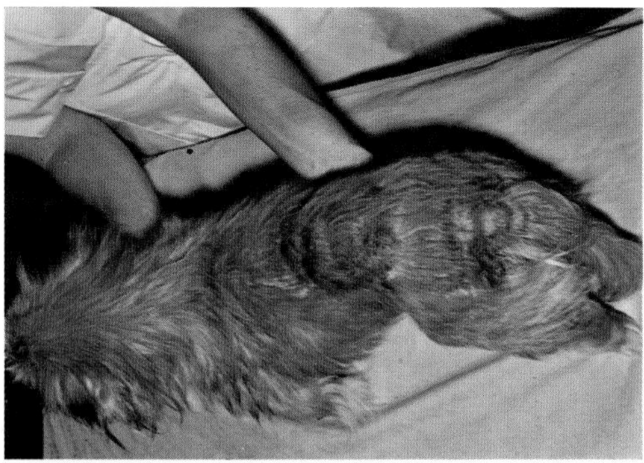

**Figure 34:1.** Flea allergy dermatitis (canine).

*A.* Chronic flea allergy dermatitis in a Pekingese, showing alopecia, hyperpigmentation and cutaneous hypertrophy on the lower back and tail base.

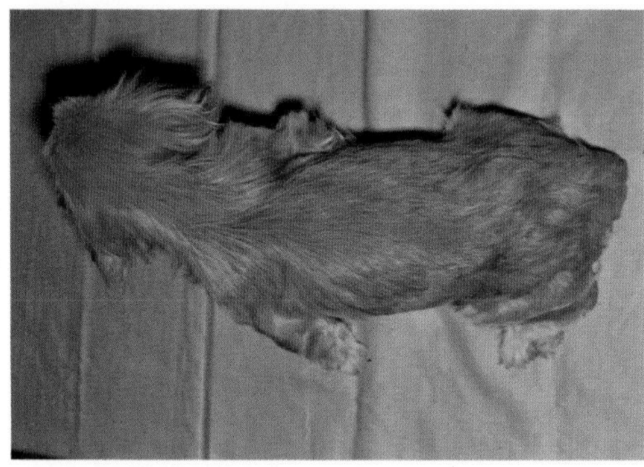

*B.* Same dog as in *A* showing that hair has regrown completely after eight months of treatment consisting mostly of flea eradication.

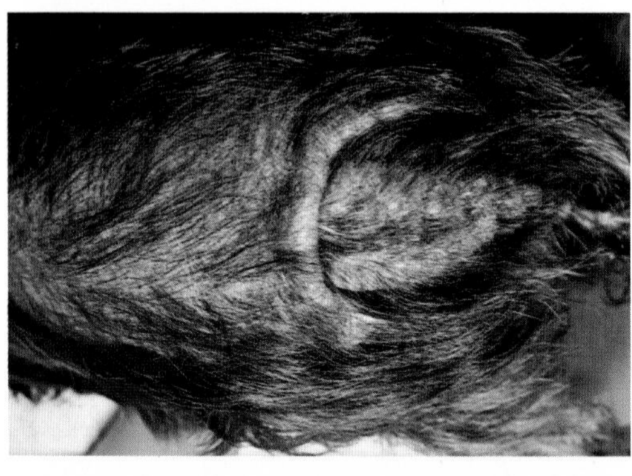

*C.* After many seasons of affliction, area of the lower back and tail becomes hairless, thickened, gray and folded.

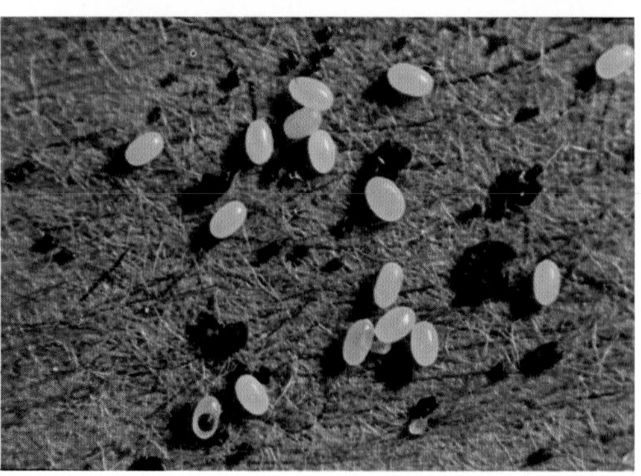

*D.* Macrophotograph of white flea eggs and dark brown flea fecal crusts on a piece of blue paper. Newly hatched flea larvae find the available fecal crusts a handy source of food.

1. Early lesions consist of wheals and erythema at the site of fleabites; however, they are often hidden by the hair coat.

2. Most lesions are the result of self-inflicted trauma in the fleas' favorite feeding grounds: the base of the tail, the dorsal lumbosacral area, the medial surfaces of the hindlegs, and the ventral pelvic area.

3. Lesions consist of erythema, papules, pustules and crusts.

4. Patches of acute moist dermatitis appear as self-inflicted excoriations become infected. The most frequently affected and most typical area is the lower back and the base of the tail (Fig. 34:1*A*).

5. After a dog has had flea allergy dermatitis for many years, the skin of the affected regions becomes hairless, thickened, gray and folded (Fig. 34:1*C*). Pruritus then is not as intense as in the earlier stages.

## DIAGNOSTIC AIDS

1. The distribution pattern (Fig. 34:2), clinical appearance and the history are the most important diagnostic aids.

2. Intradermal allergy testing can be tried; however, results are not conclusive.

## HISTOPATHOLOGY

Flea allergy dermatitis has the histologic appearance of chronic dermatitis. The epidermis shows acanthosis, parakeratosis, hyperkeratosis and irregular epidermal pegging. An inflammatory infiltrate is seen in the upper dermis. There is pilosebaceous degeneration and some follicles are plugged with

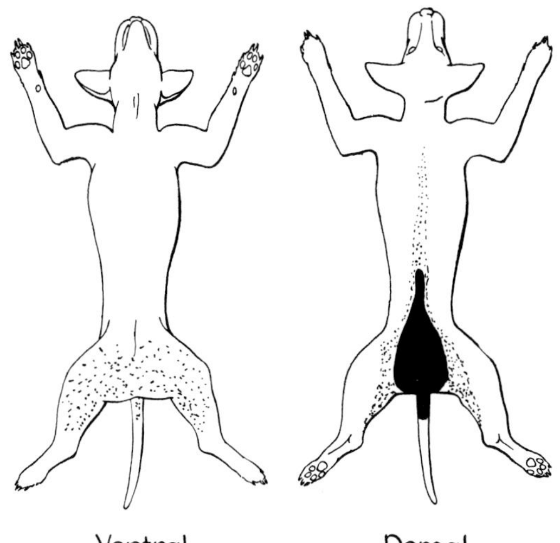


**Figure 34:2.** Flea allergy dermatitis (canine) distribution pattern.

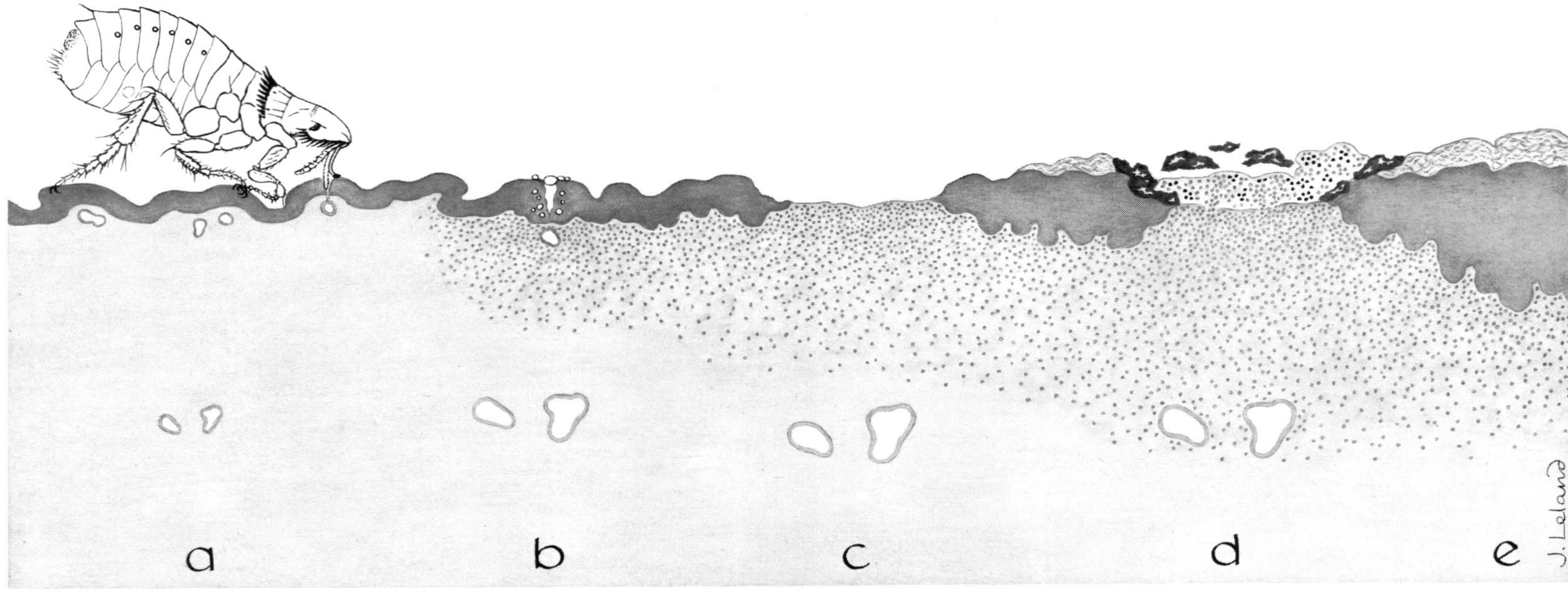


**Figure 34:3.** Flea allergy dermatitis dermogram. *a.* A flea feeds on normal skin by penetrating the epidermis with its sharply toothed laciniae. Without entering the puncture wound, blood is sucked up along a tube formed by the labrum-epipharynx and the laciniae. Saliva enters the wound during this blood sucking process. *b.* A saliva-filled puncture wound remains in the skin, and in animals hypersensitized to flea saliva an antibody-antigen reaction takes place (immediate type). *c.* Excoriation with dermal inflammatory infiltration results from self-inflicted trauma. *d.* Acute moist dermatitis develops on an excoriated lesion. There is superficial bacterial infection with massive dermal inflammation, exudation and crust formation. *e.* Chronic flea allergy dermatitis causes thickening of the skin with acanthosis, hyperkeratosis and lichenification. The thickened epidermis presents a formidable obstacle to future penetrations of the skin by the flea's mouthparts.

keratin and cellular debris. In the immediate reaction eosinophils are found. In the delayed reaction there is an infiltrate in the dermis containing many lymphocytes. In older lesions plasma cells are found.

## DIFFERENTIAL DIAGNOSIS

1. Atopic dermatitis is characterized by licking of the paws, lacrimation, sneezing or axillary scratching. None of these signs are characteristic of flea allergy.

2. Allergic contact dermatitis is found on the ventral body areas where the hair coat is sparse.

3. Primary irritant dermatitis often causes pruritus and acute moist dermatitis, but in a single, local acute episode which quickly subsides when contact with the irritation is discontinued.

## CLINICAL MANAGEMENT

1. Flea control is essential. Flea powders, flea sprays, flea dips and flea collars should be used on the animal. A flea eradication program for the property is necessary. (For details see Chapter 11, page 159.) The dog's owner can be given the pamphlet, Controlling Fleas, U.S. Dept. of Agriculture, Home and Garden Bulletin No. 121 (5¢ at U.S. Government Printing Office, Washington, D.C. 20402).

2. Corticosteroids in reasonably small doses provide relief from pruritus. Oral administration of 2.5 mg. of prednisolone twice daily for two weeks gives effective relief. Some other corticosteroids that can be given orally or by injection are dexamethasone, flumethasone, methyl prednisolone, triamcinolone and triamcinolone acetonide. Steroid therapy, although it controls pruritus, should not be prolonged; the dog's interests are better served by flea control.

3. Flea antigen has given only fair results because presently available antigens contain whole flea extracts. When antigens made from flea saliva (or its synthesized equivalent) become available commercially, hyposensitization should be much more effective.

4. Topical treatment. In most cases, systemic corticosteroid therapy and flea control measures are sufficient to permit recovery from the disease. Topical skin applications are useful in cases in which the skin is excoriated, infected or chronically thickened. Topical ointments containing corticosteroid-neomycin combinations (Panolog) are useful. In chronic cases with excess scaling, antiseborrheic shampoos (such as Seleen) help to cleanse the skin surfaces and open plugged hair follicles.

### *Suggested Reading*

Feingold, B. F., Benjamini, E., and Michaeli, D.: The Allergic Responses to Insect Bites. Ann. Rev. of Entomology *13*, 1968.

Kissileff, Alfred: The Dog Flea as a Causative Agent in Summer Eczema in dogs. J. Am. Vet. Med. Assn. *93*:21, 1938.

Muller, George H.: Flea Allergy Dermatitis. Small Animal Clinician *1* (6): 185-191, 1961.

Muller, George H.: Flea Allergy Dermatitis. *In* Kirk, R. W. (Ed.): *Current Veterinary Therapy III*, W. B. Saunders Co., Philadelphia, 1968.

# THIRTY-FIVE

# *Hyperadrenocorticism*

## *(Cushing's Disease)*

Chronic adrenocortical hyperfunction is characterized by dry, bilaterally symmetrical alopecia, thin skin, and such systemic manifestations as polydipsia, polyuria, a pendulous abdomen and muscular weakness.

### SIGNIFICANT FACTS

The clinical manifestations are the result of increased secretion of glucocorticoids (cortisol) by the adrenal glands.

The cause of hyperadrenocorticism can be adrenal, pituitary or iatrogenic.

1. The adrenal cause is either bilateral adrenal hyperplasia or a unilateral functional neoplasm of the adrenal gland.
2. Hyperadrenocorticism can be secondary to pituitary imbalance—either pituitary hyperplasia or a chromophobe pituitary adenoma.
3. Iatrogenic hyperadrenocorticism results from prolonged administration of large amounts of adrenocorticosteroids (Belshaw, Bloom, 1968).

### LESIONS AND COURSE

1. Early cases have a diffuse alopecia. The remaining hairs are dull, dry and easily epilated.
2. The bilaterally symmetrical alopecia affects the lateral surface of the trunk, the back, and the chest and abdomen. The head and extremities are covered with normal length hair except in extremely advanced cases. The alopecia is more dramatic in long-haired dogs.



3. Circular macules and patches that form on the trunk are characterized

**Figure 35:1.** Hyperadrenocorticism.

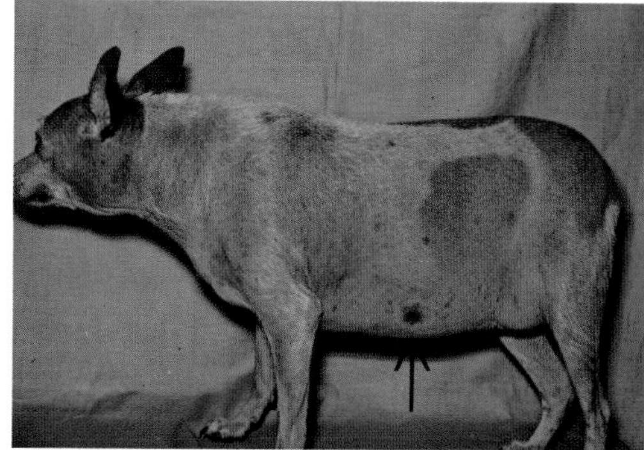

*A.* The patient is often lethargic, with a pendulous abdomen and muscle weakness. A circular macule with a hyperpigmented center surrounded by a rim of peeling keratin is characteristic (*arrow*).

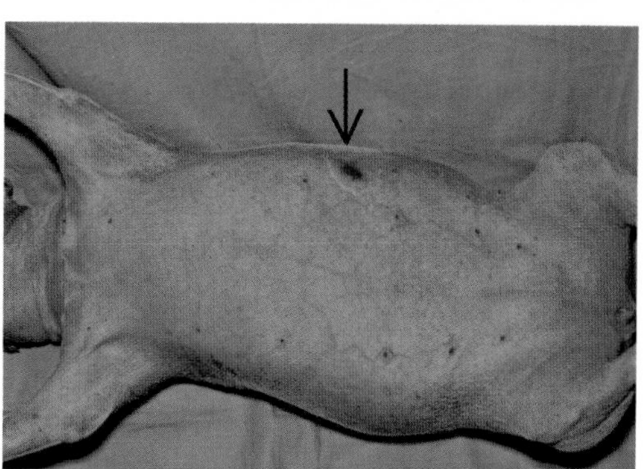

*B.* The distended abdomen has prominent blue veins, shows alopecia, and has skin that is cool to the touch. (Ventral view of patient in *A.*)

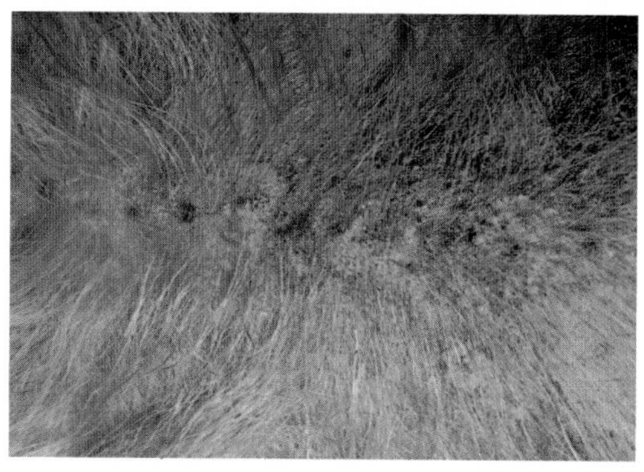

*C.* A row of dark blue firm nodules (calcinosis cutis) can be seen in the middle of the illustration.

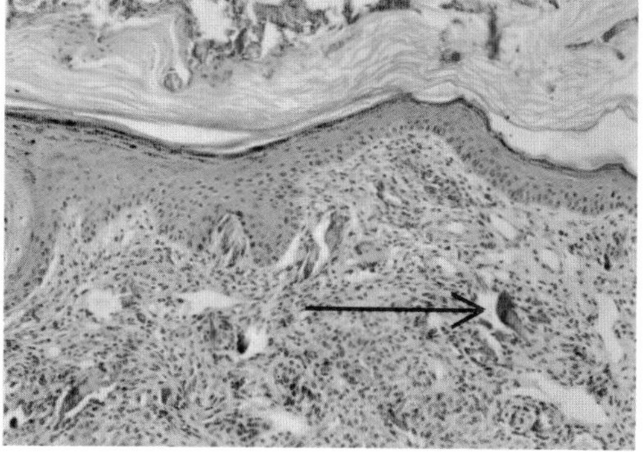

*D.* Calcinosis cutis. A calcium deposit in the upper dermis is indicated by the arrow. Several others are present in the illustration. (High power.)

by a hyperpigmented center surrounded by a rim of peeling keratin (Fig. 35:1*A*). In the presence of other characteristic lesions and symptoms, these circular areas are significant diagnostic signs. The skin is very thin and soft.

4. Other manifestations are a pendulous abdomen with large, blue veins, muscular weakness, depressive states and lethargy (Fig. 35:1*B*). There is polydipsia and polyuria. The urine specific gravity is very low (often 1.005 to 1.010). In some cases there is osteoporosis.

5. Calcinosis cutis (Fig. 35:1*C* and *D*) is seen in advanced cases and is pathognomonic of the disease when accompanied by clinical and laboratory evidence suggestive of the disease.

6. There is lymphopenia, eosinopenia and a high fasting blood sugar level.

## DIAGNOSTIC AIDS

1. There is increased urinary output of 17-ketogenic steroids.
2. Clinical and laboratory findings of polydipsia and polyuria together with hyperglycemia, lymphopenia and eosinopenia are highly suggestive.

## DIFFERENTIAL DIAGNOSIS

1. Dogs with Sertoli cell tumor have gynecomastia and other signs of feminization which are not found in hyperadrenocorticism.
2. Hypothyroidism can be differentiated by its lack of polyuria, the typical pattern of alopecia and by thyroid function tests.

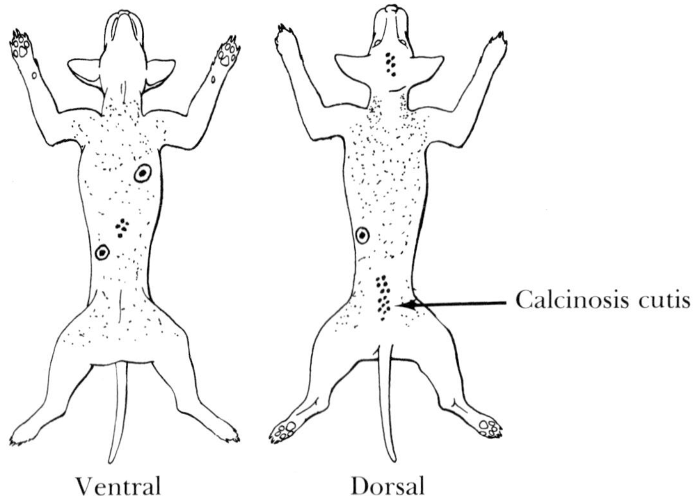


**Figure 35:2.** Hyperadrenocorticism distribution pattern.

## HISTOPATHOLOGY (FIG. 35:1*D*)

The dermis is thinner than in normal skin, accounting for the clinical impression that the skin of dogs with Cushing's syndrome feels thin. The epidermis, however, is thickened and consists of up to eight to ten layers of cells. There is a noticeable paucity of active hairs with the empty follicles filled with keratin and debris. Melanin pigment is prominent in the epidermis, especially in the basal layer. None of these changes are specific, and a diagnosis cannot be made from the histopathologic appearance alone. Calcinosis cutis, found in some advanced cases, is unique for Cushing's syndrome. Basophilic staining particles of calcium are seen within the dermis.

## CLINICAL MANAGEMENT

1. Explain the chronic nature of the disease to the owner.
2. Adrenalectomy (unilateral for adrenal tumor or bilateral for adrenal hyperplasia).
   a. Unilateral adrenalectomy is not effective in bilateral adrenal hyperplasia because hormone production of the other adrenal almost invariably increases and causes return of the same symptoms.
   b. After bilateral adrenalectomy, the animal must be kept on a lifelong maintenance therapy of mineralocorticoids as follows (Siegel, 1968):
      (1) 1 to 2 mg. of desoxycorticosterone pivalate (DOCA) injected intramuscularly daily for a 20 to 40 lb. dog.
      (2) 1 gm. of sodium chloride (table salt) daily mixed with food for a 20 to 40 lb. dog.
      (3) Long-acting DOCA can be used next. One injection of 25 mg. of DOCA (Percortin, Ciba) releases 1 mg. of DOCA per day which will maintain the dog for about three weeks.
      (4) 125 Pellets of Percortin (Ciba) can be implanted which will maintain the dog for about six months.
      (5) Potassium levels must be checked every three weeks to assure a level of 3.5 to 4.0 mEq./L.
3. Surgical removal of pituitary tumors. However, this is not feasible in the usual veterinary hospital.
4. High protein diet (P/D) because of protein catabolism.
5. Hydrochlorothiazide may be helpful in unoperated dogs to empirically reduce the polyuria and polydipsia.
6. Medicated shampoos (such as Seleen) will reduce the skin's scaliness.
7. Alpha-Keri rinses are useful for dry skin and dry hair.

### *Suggested Reading*

Bloom, F.: *Canine Medicine*. American Veterinary Publications, Santa Barbara, California, 1968.

Siegel, E. T.: Hyperadrenocorticalism. *In* Kirk, R. W. (Ed.): *Current Veterinary Therapy III*, W. B. Saunders Co., Philadelphia, 1968.

# THIRTY-SIX

# *Hypothyroidism*

Hypothyroidism is a decrease in thyroid hormone production resulting in partial alopecia, skin changes and such systemic manifestations as lethargy, gain in weight, abnormal estrus and decreased libido.

## SIGNIFICANT FACTS

1. Mild hypothyroidism is a common cause of skin and hair abnormalities.
2. Systemic manifestations are lethargy, easy fatigue, gain in weight, good appetite, constipation or diarrhea, abnormal estrus, infertility and decreased libido.
3. Hypothyroidism can be primary or secondary. The primary type results from inflammation or atrophy of the thyroid, or lack of dietary iodine. The secondary type results from pituitary insufficiency (decreased TSH output).

Not all hypothyroid patients show skin lesions and alopecia.

## LESIONS AND COURSE

1. Mild cases show a thin, dry hair coat.
2. More advanced cases start with patches of alopecia. Although a single patch is seen at first on the back or chest, the alopecia soon presents a bilaterally symmetrical distribution pattern (Fig. 36:1*B*). The head and extremities are often spared and most alopecia is on the neck and trunk.
3. Hairs are dry and brittle and they epilate easily. The coat is sparse and coarse.
4. The skin is dry, slightly scaly, superficially ridged and hyperpigmented (Fig. 36:1*C*). It is cool to the touch.
5. The condition usually progresses unless thyroid supplements are given.

**Figure 36:1.** Hypothyroidism.

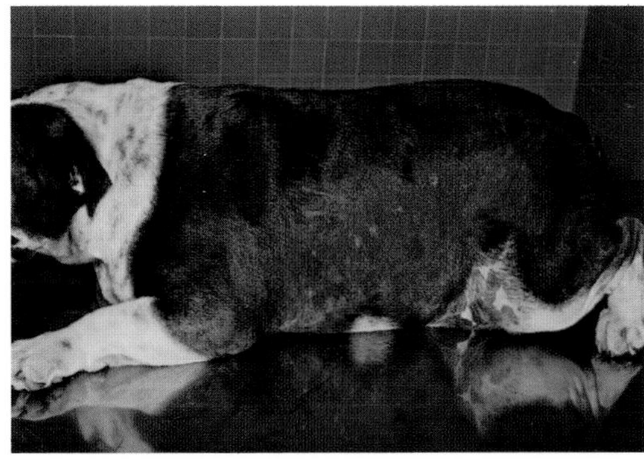

*A.* Hypothyroid patient showing obesity and patchy alopecia.

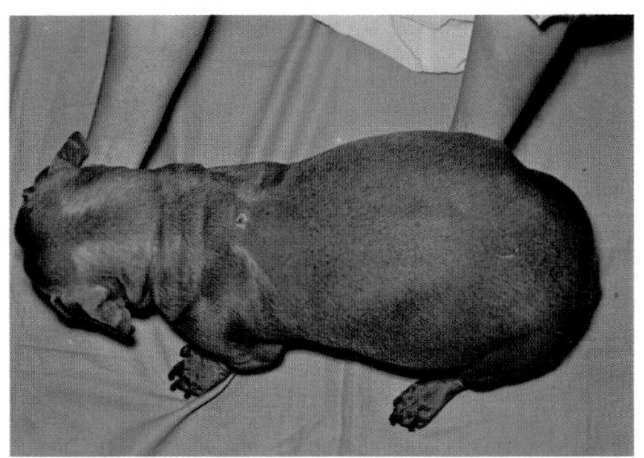

*B.* Typical bilateral distribution pattern in advanced hypothyroidism.

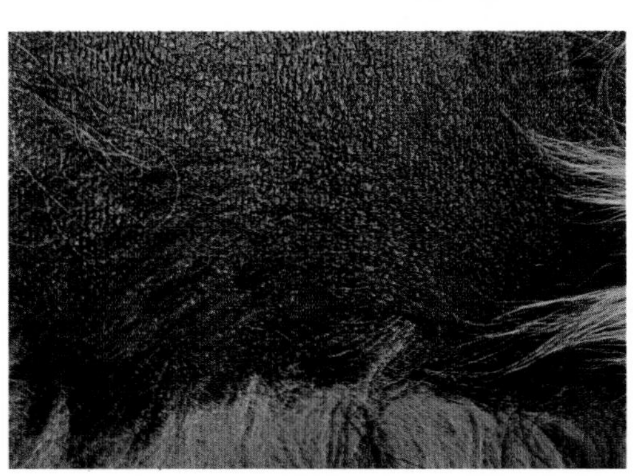

*C.* Close-up of affected area showing dry skin, ridges, hyperpigmentation and alopecia.

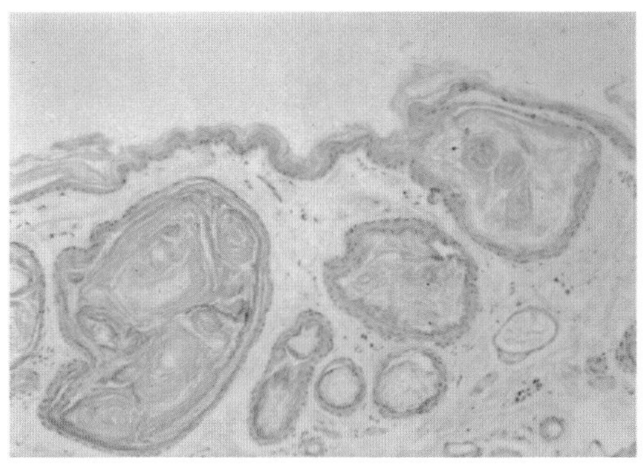

*D.* Histologic section shows "washed out" collagen, epidermal cysts and degenerating hair follicles. (Low power.)

## DIAGNOSTIC AIDS

1. There is a decreased uptake of radioactive iodine ($I^{131}$). It is below the normal of 10 to 30 per cent of the dose by 72 hours.

2. The protein-bound iodine is low. Hypothyroid dogs have a PBI of $1.0 \pm 0.5$ mcg./100 ml. whereas the euthyroid PBI is $2.4 \pm 0.6$ mcg./100 ml.

3. Total serum iodine is decreased.
   Hypothyroid dogs: $3.3 \pm 2.2$ mcg./100 ml.
   Euthyroid dogs: $7.8 \pm 3.4$ mcg./100 ml.

4. The serum cholesterol may be elevated.

5. TSH response test (see p. 175).

6. Thyroid biopsy.

7. Skin biopsy.

Normal and hypothyroid values are discussed in more detail on page 175.

## HISTOPATHOLOGY (FIG. 36:1*D*)

1. The skin of hypothyroid dogs consistently shows a thin epidermis, a "washed-out" appearance of the collagen fibers of the dermis, degenerating or absent hair follicles and tiny intradermal cysts filled with keratin and cutaneous debris.

2. Thyroid histopathology: In early cases of primary hypothyroidism there may be leukocytic infiltration and fibrosis, followed by follicular collapse and atrophy of the thyroid tissue. (Absence of thyroid histopathologic changes in conjunction with positive findings of hypothyroidism by clinical and laboratory methods suggests TSH deficiency.)

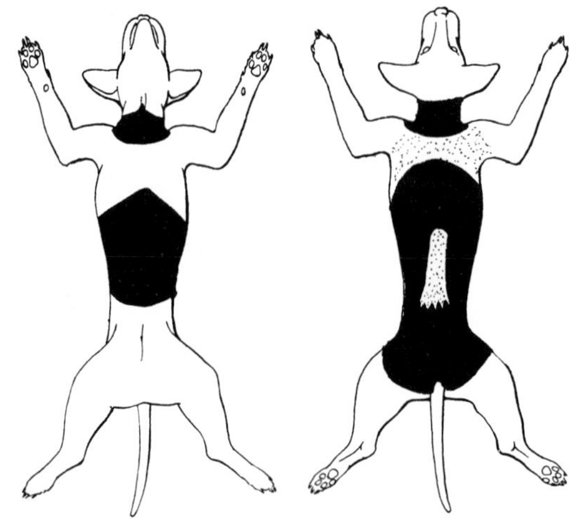


**Figure 36:2.** Hypothyroidism distribution pattern.

## DIFFERENTIAL DIAGNOSIS

1. Hyperadrenocorticism (Cushing's syndrome), in its early stage, shows a diffuse, partial alopecia similar to that of hypothyroidism. However, in the advanced stage there is more severe alopecia of the trunk and more hyperpigmentation. The skin is very thin, while hypothyroid skin is thick. Laboratory findings are helpful for differentiation.

2. Dermatomycosis shows alopecia and scaling which are not bilaterally symmetrical.

3. Seborrheic skin is greasy and more scaly than hypothyroid skin. It is warm instead of cool and there is only a minor patchy alopecia.

## CLINICAL MANAGEMENT

1. Oral administration of thyroid hormone usually reverses the symptoms and lesions in correctly diagnosed cases.

2. Desiccated USP thyroid can be used. It is important to purchase a fresh supply from reliable pharmaceutical companies. The shelf life of desiccated thyroid tablets is short (Belshaw, 1968).

3. The dose of desiccated thyroid is 3 to 6 mg./lb. of body weight daily. In the past it has been common to underdose.

4. Sodium levothyroxine (Synthroid, Flint Laboratories) is preferred to desiccated thyroid because it permits a more accurate dosage and has a longer shelf life. The dose of Synthroid for a 20 lb. dog is 0.2 mg. daily for the first four weeks. Dogs under 20 lbs. receive 0.05 to 0.1 mg. daily. Thereafter the level is reduced to the minimum amount needed to reverse the clinical manifestations. The daily maintenance dose usually varies from 0.2 to 0.5 mg. Favorable clinical improvement usually appears within four weeks.

5. Any animal receiving thyroid supplementation should be examined every three to six months, so the dose can be adjusted if necessary. Use only the minimum amount required to maintain euthyroidism.

### *Suggested Reading*

Belshaw, B. E.: Endocrinology Seminar, Proceedings of the 35th Annual Convention, American Animal Hospital Association, 1968.

Reid, Charles, F.: Hypothyroidism. *In* Kirk, R. W. (Ed.): *Current Veterinary Therapy III*. W. B. Saunders Co., Philadelphia, 1968.

Siegel, E. T., and Belshaw, B. E.: Laboratory Evaluation of Adreno-cortical and Thyroid Function in the Dog. *In* Kirk, R. W. (Ed.): *Current Veterinary Therapy III*. W. B. Saunders Co., Philadelphia, 1968.

# THIRTY-SEVEN

# *Male Feminizing Syndrome*

## *(Hypoandrogenism, Hyperestrogenism of Males)*

Male feminizing syndrome is an endocrine imbalance causing gynecomastia and lack of libido, as well as hyperkeratosis and hyperpigmentation of the flanks and genital area.

### SIGNIFICANT FACTS

1. It is a rare disorder of dogs that is a definite clinical entity and mimics the skin lesions accompanying Sertoli cell tumors.
2. There is no cryptorchidism and the gross appearance of the testicles is normal (Fig. 37-1*B*).
3. Histologic examination of the testicle fails to reveal neoplastic tissue.
4. In advanced cases the "feminizing" effect is so pronounced, the dogs become sexually attractive to other males.

### LESIONS AND COURSE

1. The lesions begin in the flanks and genital area (Fig. 37:1*A*).
2. The area of the external genital organs, posterior thighs and flanks becomes hyperpigmented, hyperkeratotic and lichenified.
3. Gynecomastia is a constant finding (Fig. 37:1*B*).
4. Ceruminous otitis externa is present.
5. A "seborrhea-like" greasiness and scaliness of the skin develop in chronic cases.

### DIFFERENTIAL DIAGNOSIS

1. Sertoli cell tumors produce similar skin lesions; however, a tumor is found in one of the testicles (which is usually retained).

**Figure 37:1.** Male feminizing syndrome.

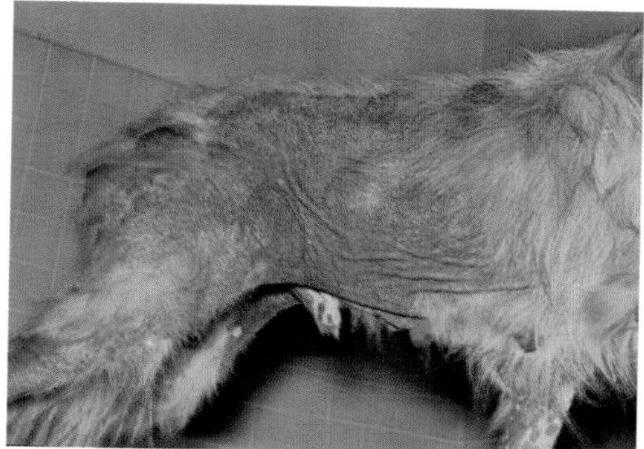

*A.* Alopecia with hyperpigmented, hyperkeratotic, lichenified skin in the flanks and thighs. The entire area is greasy and scaly.

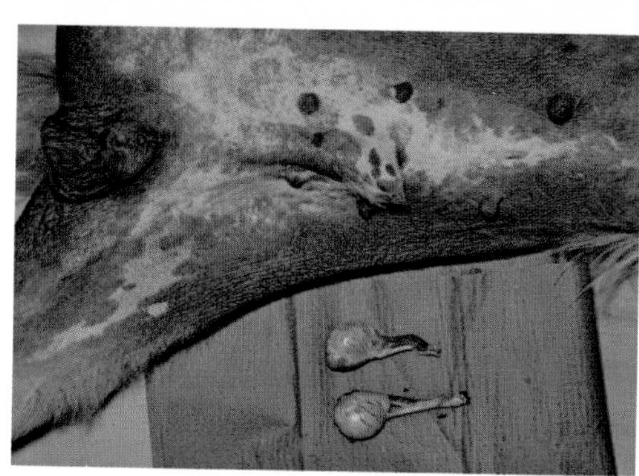

*B.* At the time of castration two small, soft testes were removed. Enlarged nipples and typical lesions of the flank and scrotum also are evident.

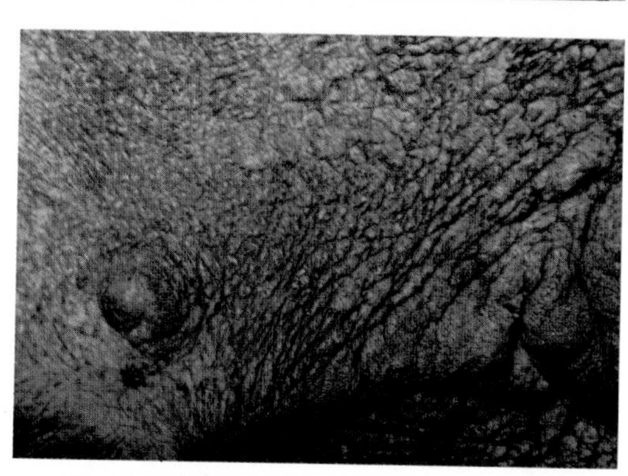

*C.* Close-up illustration of skin showing gynecomastia, hyperpigmentation, hyperkeratosis and lichenification.

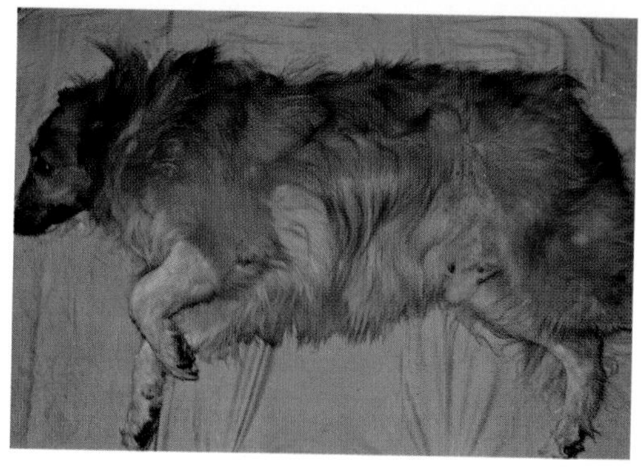

*D.* Same patient as in *A*, *B* and *C*, eight months after castration.

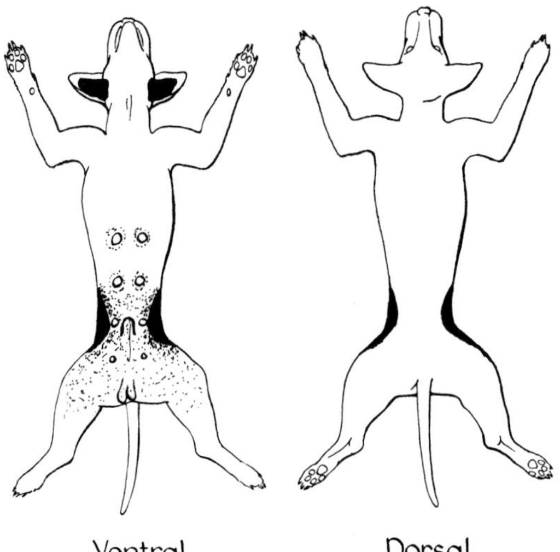


**Figure 37:2.** Distribution pattern in feminizing syndrome of male dogs (hypoandrogenism).

2. In acanthosis nigricans there is acanthosis, hyperpigmentation and keratosis too, but the lesions always start in the axillae and later spread to the ventral abdomen and hindlegs. There is no gynecomastia, and otitis may be absent.

3. Dermatomycosis is not bilaterally symmetrical.

## CLINICAL MANAGEMENT

1. Castration.
2. Administration of testosterone.
3. Administration of corticosteroids.
4. Weekly antiseborrheic shampoos.
5. Cleaning of the ears with a ceruminolytic agent.

## HISTOPATHOLOGY

1. Skin changes consist of chronic dermatitis with pronounced acanthosis, hyperkeratosis, parakeratosis and an inflammatory infiltration of the upper dermis.

### *Suggested Reading*

Muller, G. H.: Proceedings, American Animal Hospital Assn., 1964.

# THIRTY-EIGHT

## *Nail Diseases*

The nails and nail folds are subject to injury, bacterial infection (paronychia) and fungal infection (onychomycosis).

1. Paronychia (nail fold infection) is usually caused by bacteria (Fig. 38:1*A*). It may be acute or chronic, the latter being more common. Since the seat of the infection is at the base of the nail under the fold, surgical removal of the nail plate (shell) provides good drainage and is the treatment of choice. In most cases, the nail will grow back. With the animal under general anesthesia, the nail plate is grasped firmly with a strong hemostat and stripped from its attachment in one steady downward motion. Since the diseased nail usually is loose, the procedure is easily accomplished and there is little or no hemorrhage. Systemic antibiotics such as penicillin and streptomycin are effective in most cases.

2. Onychomycosis in dogs is usually caused by *Trichophyton mentagrophytes.* It frequently accompanies generalized dermatomycosis. The nail shown in Figure 38:1*B* came from a dog with a *T. mentagrophytes* infection involving over half of its skin surface. Treatment consists of permanent surgical excision of the affected nails (the entire third phalanx), followed by griseofulvin orally for several months. To prevent relapses, griseofulvin must be continued until mycotic cultures fail to grow dermatophytes.

3. Candida paronychia is rare (Fig. 38:1*C*). When *Candida albicans* becomes established in the nail fold, there is considerable pain, and some nails fall out. The remaining affected nails usually are painful and loosely attached. Nystatin or amphotericin B often is effective treatment.

4. Nails can be injured in a number of ways. Dewclaws are frequently partially avulsed so that the nail plate is loosened from its matrix. When nails are injured severely, deformities in the external plate often result, especially in cases in which the nail is split (Fig. 38:1*D*). The treatment for such severely deformed nails is surgical removal of the entire nail plate. Rarely, the entire third phalanx may need to be amputated to correct deformities.

**Figure 38:1.** Nail diseases.

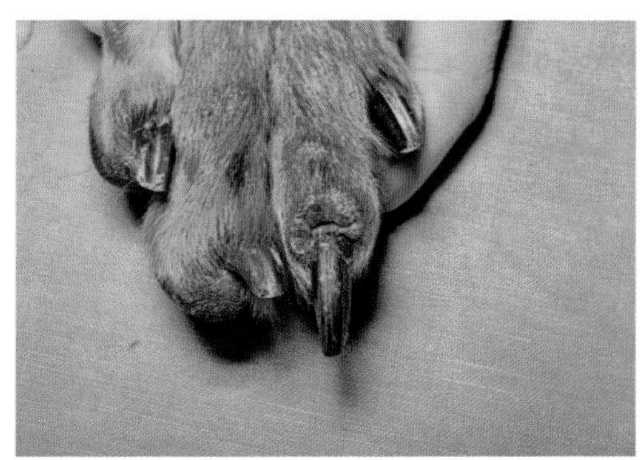

*A.* Bacterial paronychia with ulceration of the nail fold. Note the purulent exudate at the base of the nail.

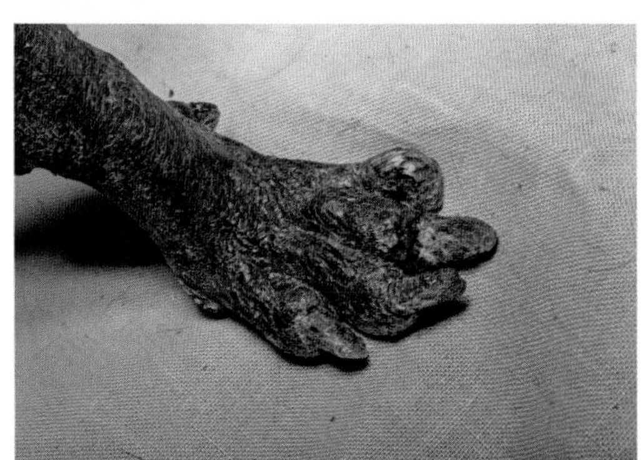

*B.* Onychomycosis in a dog caused by *Trichophyton mentagrophytes.* Nails are grossly deformed and there is secondary paronychia in the central toe.

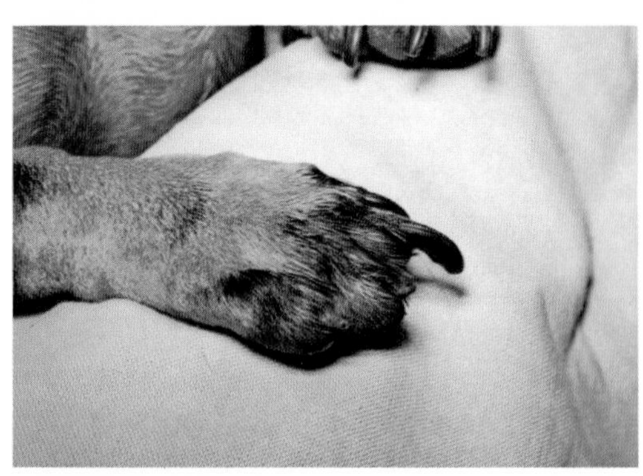

*C.* Paronychia from which *Candida albicans* was isolated. The nails fell out and the nail folds were painful.

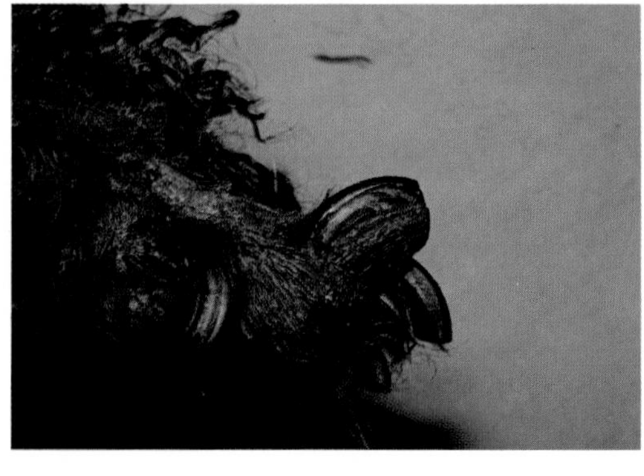

*D.* Deformed nail following an injury. Note the split and exposed matrix.

# THIRTY-NINE

# *Nasal Solar Dermatitis*
## *("Collie Nose")*

Nasal solar dermatitis is an actinic reaction upon poorly pigmented nasal and eyelid skin of collies, Shetland sheep dogs and related dogs.

## SIGNIFICANT FACTS

Nasal solar dermatitis requires a hereditary predisposition, lack of skin pigment and excessive solar radiation.

1. The specific cause of the hypersensitivity to light is unknown but there is no evidence that it results from the effect of photosensitive pigments.
2. Prior to the onset of lesions, skin in the affected areas is normal in texture. However, the disease seems predisposed to unpigmented areas of the planum nasale, nares, dorsal nasal skin, eyelids and lips.

## LESIONS AND COURSE

1. The lesions are found principally at the junction of the haired and hairless skin of the nose (Fig. 39:1*A*), but they may also appear on the lower eyelids and the lips.
2. Initially the skin becomes erythematous and alopecia develops. Exudation and crusting are common, and ulceration may appear later.
3. Progress and enlargement of the lesions are evident with the passage of each year, but are especially rapid during periods of prolonged exposure to intense sunlight. This may occur in the summer months, or during the winter as a result of reflection from snow.
4. If the patient is housed to eliminate exposure to sun, the lesions may heal by regeneration of a thin, fragile epithelium which is devoid of hair, pigment or glandular structures.

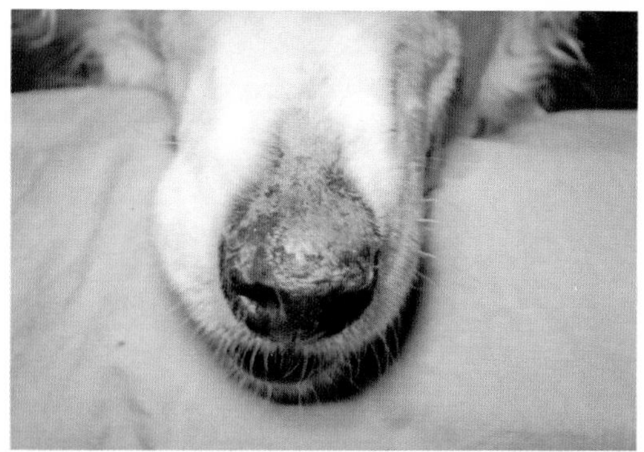

**Figure 39:1.** Nasal solar dermatitis.

*A.* Typical case showing erythema with exudation, crusting and beginning ulceration.

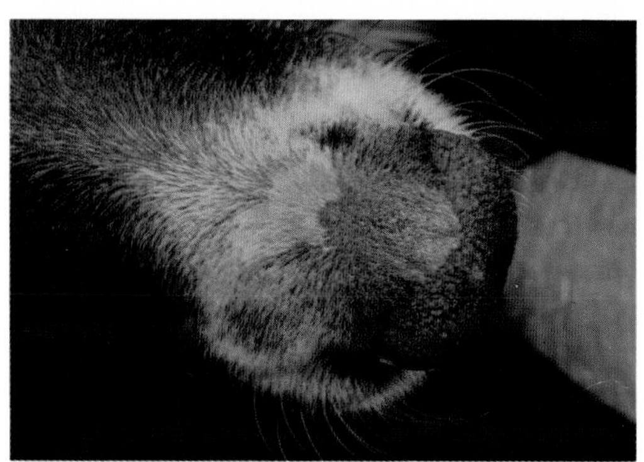

*B.* One year after completion of three tattoos, previously pink skin is now colored slate gray.

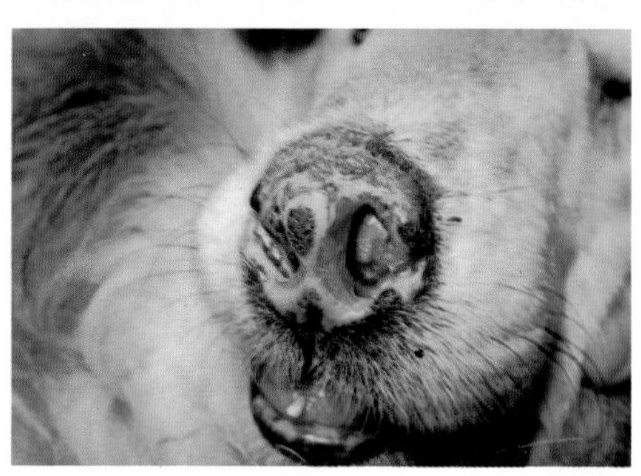

*C.* Neglected case which has progressed to a squamous cell carcinoma with erosion of nasal tissues.

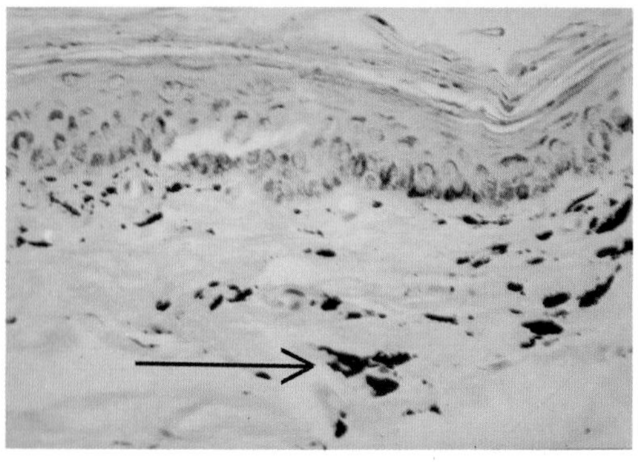

*D.* Biopsy of nose in *B* showing particles of tattoo ink within the dermis (arrow). (High power.)

5. Neglect has often allowed these irritative reactions to develop into squamous cell carcinomas (Fig. 39:1*C*). Deep ulcers form and extensive areas of the nares and nasal tip disappear, exposing unsightly nasal tissues that bleed easily.

## DIAGNOSTIC AIDS

1. The clinical appearance is typical, and the breed, history, and improvement upon removal from sunlight all give circumstantial support to the diagnosis. There are no pathognomonic tests, however.

2. Skin biopsy should be performed in advanced cases to allow pathologic examination for squamous cell carcinoma.

## HISTOPATHOLOGY

The early depigmented areas of the nose show fewer melanocytes and less melanin pigment than in normal skin. Following solar radiation there is acanthosis with intraepidermal edema. Inflammatory infiltration forms in the upper dermis, and in the lower dermis vascular dilatation is noted. Ulceration can cause disappearance of the epidermis and even the dermis and underlying cartilages. In advanced cases there is increased activity in the cells of the basal layer with the formation of large, polyhedral tumor cells which invade the dermis and subcutaneous tissue. A squamous cell carcinoma forms with cords of neoplastic cells invading to the level of the nasal cartilage.

## DIFFERENTIAL DIAGNOSIS

Nasal solar dermatitis must be differentiated from trauma (which may be asymmetrical or located in different areas), from contact dermatitis, and in advanced stages, from basal cell and squamous cell carcinomas.

## CLINICAL MANAGEMENT

1. Initial treatment should emphasize confinement of the dog indoors during the hours of sunshine, and regular systemic doses of prednisolone until the lesions are fairly well healed. Black felt marking pencils may be used to mark the lesions and help shield the skin from sunlight.

2. Systemic antibiotic therapy may be needed if there is secondary infection. Topical medications of all kinds are not effective on the nose as they are licked off promptly.

3. Tattooing with black ink is the treatment of choice for enduring protection. The ink can be applied with a Nicholsen tattoo vibrator (Fig. 39:2), or by carefully injecting the ink intradermally with a 25 gauge 5/8" needle and a tuberculin syringe. This procedure must be done under general anesthesia, and it is usually necessary to repeat the treatment at least three times at 30 to 60 day

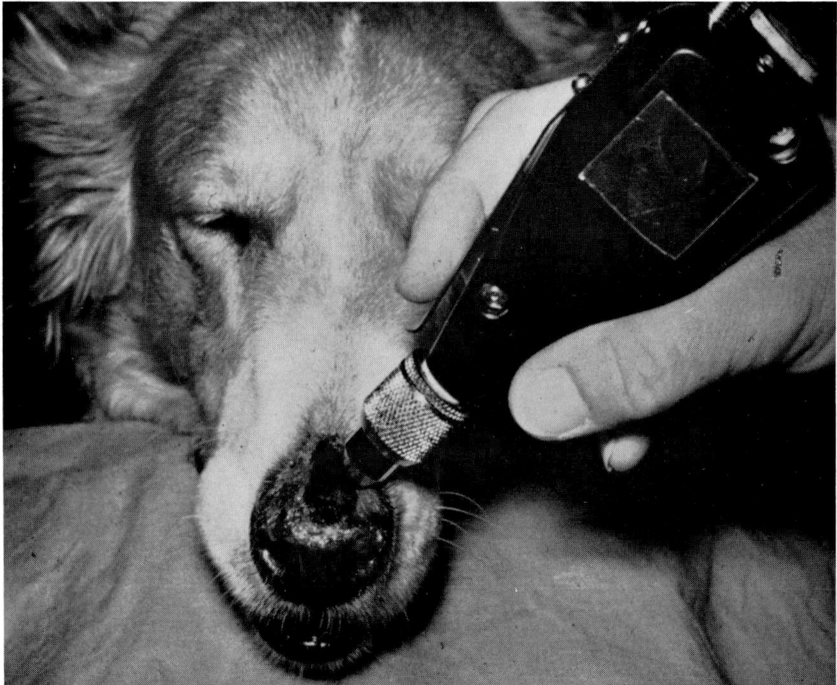

**Figure 39:2.** Preparing to use the Nicholsen tattoo vibrator. During operation the vibrator should be held perpendicular to the skin surface.

intervals. When completed satisfactorily, the tattooed skin is a slate gray color (Fig. 39:1*B*). Annual "touch-up" tattooing is necessary in many cases.

4. Ideally, the tattoo procedure should be applied to young dogs showing typical tendencies to sunlight hypersensitivity *before* the disease progresses.

5. Neglected patients which have developed squamous cell carcinoma (Fig. 39:1*C*) have no real hope for cure.

## *Suggested Reading*

Moss, L. C., and Severin, G. A.: Nasal Solar Dermatitis. *In* Kirk, R. W. (Ed.): *Current Veterinary Therapy 1966-67*, W. B. Saunders Co., Philadelphia, 1966.

# FORTY

# *Nasodigital Hyperkeratosis*

Nasodigital hyperkeratosis is marked by increased amount of horny tissue originating from and tightly adherent to the epidermis of the footpads or planum nasale.

## SIGNIFICANT FACTS

1. All photographs on the next page represent hyperkeratotic changes that occurred in adult dogs without a known history of distemper.

2. Hyperkeratosis of the footpads and nasal tip do occur in some cases of distemper; in fact, some investigators feel that "hard pad disease" is a special form of distemper, characterized by hyperkeratotic changes.

3. *Nasal hyperkeratosis* occurring without digital changes is a specific entity. Figure 40:1*A* shows such a case: a standard French poodle suddenly developed nasal hyperkeratosis at the age of five years, and his nose remained dry and horny until the end of his life at 15 years. The numerous topical medications applied did not alter the hyperkeratosis. Fissures which developed in the dry nose were treated and responded favorably to the application of Panolog ointment.

4. *Digital hyperkeratosis* occurs spontaneously in some adult dogs. The cause is not known. Figures 40:1*B* and *C* show the hard, cracked pads of a St. Bernard. The pads contained excess keratin tissue, which made walking painful for this heavy dog. Fissures and erosions added significantly to his discomfort.

5. "Corns" form in some individuals' feet as excess keratin develops in deep, circular plaques. These press into the surrounding footpad and cause pain when pressure is applied as the animal walks. Figure 40:1*D* pictures such a case in a Kerry blue terrier. The condition appeared to be hereditary, as many related animals were affected.

## LESIONS AND COURSE

1. The hyperplastic keratin which develops in this disease grows in a variety of shapes depending on its location, stage of development and the variation among individual animals.

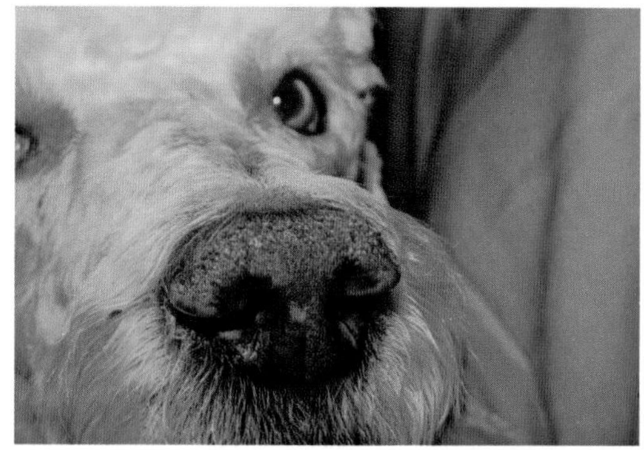

**Figure 40:1.** Nasodigital hyperkeratosis.

*A.* Nasal hyperkeratosis – horny growths of keratin adhere tightly to the epidermis of the dry planum nasale.

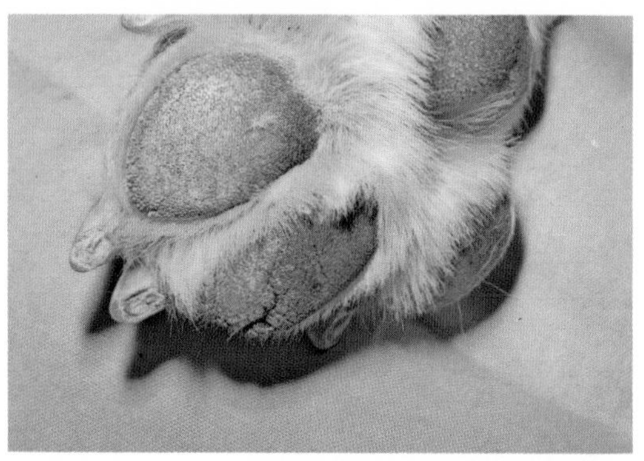

*B.* Digital hyperkeratosis – the plantar surface of the pads is thick and hard. The pad margins have a "feathered" appearance. Note the fissure on the lower pad.

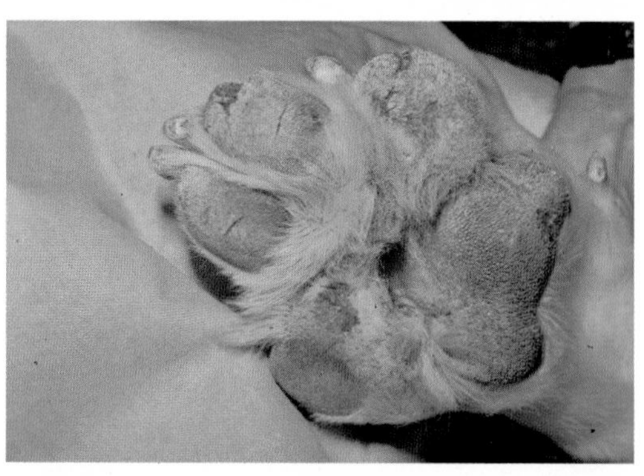

*C.* Digital hyperkeratosis and erosions of the footpads. In addition to the hyperkeratotic changes, painful erosions and fissures are seen on the foot of a St. Bernard.

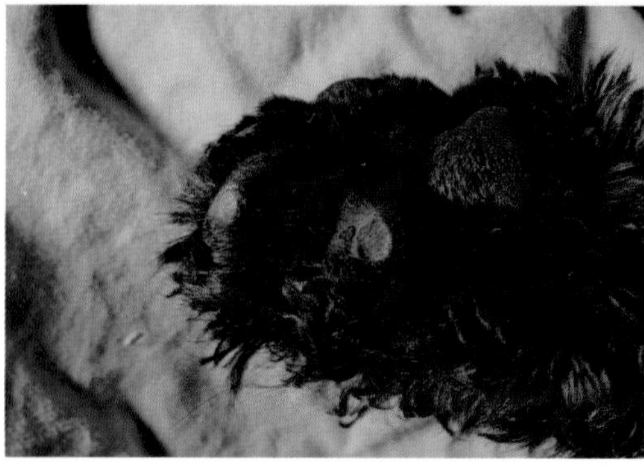

*D.* Digital hyperkeratosis – "corns" in a Kerry blue terrier. This condition is hereditary in this breed. It causes considerable disability which can be ameliorated temporarily by periodically shaving the localized hyperkeratotic plaques.

2. At times, small verrucous keratin growths appear in a regular pattern. At other times the keratin is ridged, grooved or feathered in appearance. Dryness is the common characteristic of all lesions. The planum nasale, which is moist, black, soft and shiny in normal dogs, becomes hard, dry and brittle.

3. Fissures, erosions and ulcers develop in the dry epidermal tissue.

4. When the keratin grows in circular or oval plaques on the digital pads, typical "corns" develop.

## DIFFERENTIAL DIAGNOSIS

It is necessary to distinguish between the nasodigital hyperkeratosis that accompanies certain cases of distemper (or a distemper-like disease) and those cases pictured here which arise spontaneously – of unknown cause. When distemper patients recover, those with "hard pad" changes often lose their cutaneous lesions after several months, whereas the spontaneous hyperkeratoses are chronic and often present for life.

## CLINICAL MANAGEMENT

1. Since the excess keratin formation usually cannot be stopped, treatment is directed toward relieving discomfort.

2. Excess keratin can be trimmed away with scissors when it overlaps the margins of the digital pads; and corns can be carefully pared or shaved. Care must be taken to cut only into nonviable keratin tissue.

3. Wet dressings or water soaks are useful to hydrate the keratin (which easily absorbs water). Petroleum jelly, applied immediately after the wet dressings or soaks, helps to hold moisture in the pad or basal tissues.

4. For erosions, fissures and ulcers, ointments containing antibiotics and corticosteroids (such as Panolog or Neocortef) are helpful.

5. The hyperkeratotic feet can be bandaged for short periods of time (two to five days) to protect them and to allow healing of the erosions and fissures. Furacin dressing under the bandage combats or prevents secondary bacterial infection.

6. Ichthammol ointment used once a day for two weeks exerts a beneficial keratolytic and healing effect on digital hyperkeratinized pads.

# FORTY-ONE

## *Neurodermatitis (Localized)*

Localized neurodermatitis is a chronic skin inflammation aggravated by constant licking and scratching of a local skin area.

### SIGNIFICANT FACTS

1. It is primarily a disease of cats.

2. The rough, barbed tongue of the cat is able to produce severe irritation and excoriation. A vicious lick-cyle is established as the tongue prevents healing and leaves sensitive cutaneous nerve endings exposed.

3. The primary or initiating cause may be a dermatitis with pruritus, infected ears or anal sacs, or excessive nervousness of the cat. It frequently is an anxiety neurosis caused by psychologic factors such as displacement phenomena (new pet or baby in the household, movement to new surroundings, boarding, hospitalization, loss of favorite bed or companion).

4. There is a breed predilection for the more emotional breeds such as Siamese and Abbysinian cats.

### LESIONS AND COURSE

1. Areas that the cat can lick most conveniently are the most common sites: the inside of the thigh, the lower abdomen, the lower back and tail.

2. The characteristic lesion is a bright red oval patch or red streak. Chronic cases develop lichenification.

3. The course is long and progresses slowly, sometimes remaining static for months.

### DIAGNOSTIC AIDS

The typical appearance, together with the history of constant licking, usually makes the diagnosis obvious.

Affected cats have an uncontrollable urge to lick their lesions.

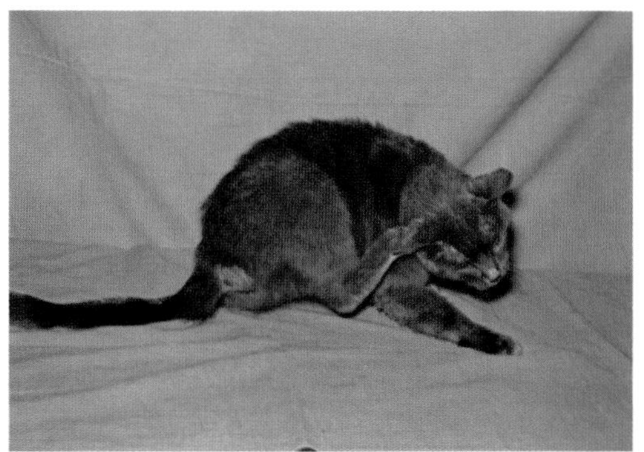

**Figure 41:1.** Localized neurodermatitis.

*A.* Constant scratching or licking is characteristic.

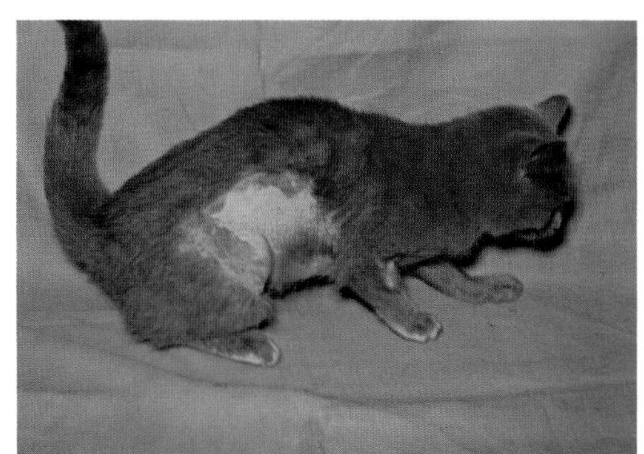

*B.* Licking removes the hair and causes a chronic inflammation of skin in the favored area.

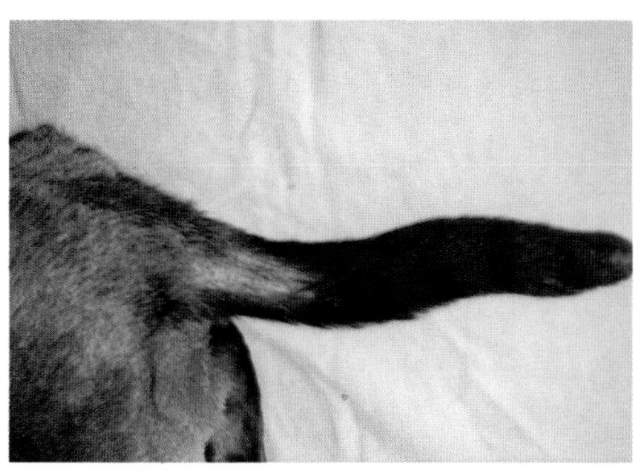

*C.* Unilateral alopecia of the tail and rump may be initiated by anogenital pain or inflammation of anal sacs.

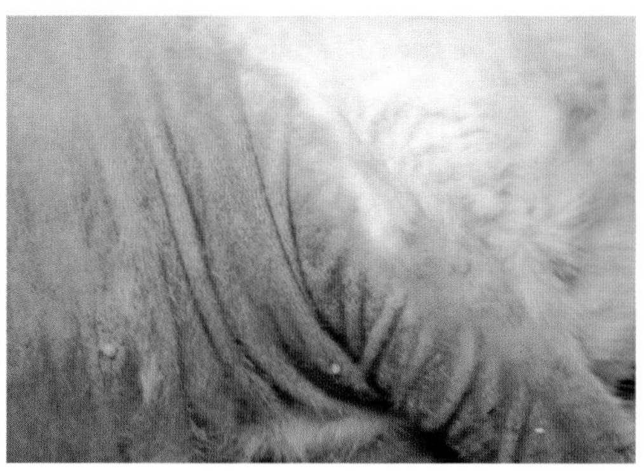

*D.* Thickened skin in the axilla, a response to the irritation of constant licking.

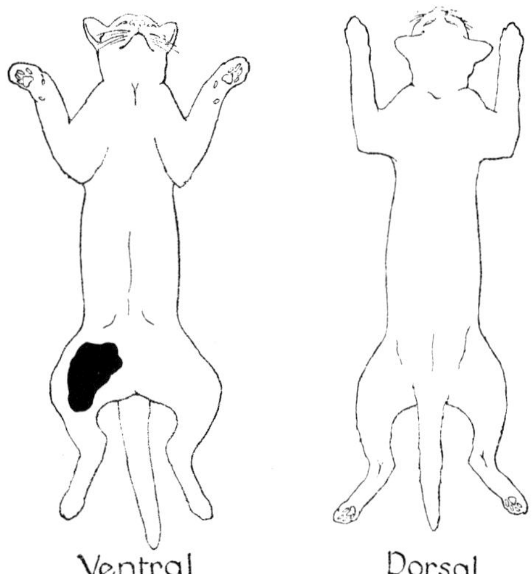


**Figure 41:2.** Localized neurodermatitis distribution pattern.

## DIFFERENTIAL DIAGNOSIS

Lesions may be confused with or develop into eosinophilic granulomas.

## CLINICAL MANAGEMENT

1. Response to treatment is poor and the condition requires much patience on the part of the owner and the veterinarian.

2. Topical medications are of little value as the cat will immediately lick them off.

3. The first systemic treatment should be corticosteroids. After an initial injection, oral medication can be used in gradually reduced dosage. Because of the severity of some cases, corticosteroids are necessary for three to four week periods. Intralesional injection of triamcinolone may be effective too.

4. Tranquilizers and sedatives can be tried alone or in combination with corticosteroids.

5. Mechanical devices (such as Elizabethan collars) are resented by cats and should be replaced by sedation if possible. In either case, reduction of medication or removal of the collar often allows a relapse to take place.

6. Once the areas are healed, occurrence can be triggered again by emotional upsets. Susceptible cats with tendencies to anxiety begin licking themselves as soon as they are boarded or psychologically stressed in other ways, and the cycle begins again.

# FORTY-TWO

## *Notoedric Mange*

Notoedric mange is a contagious parasitic disease of cats caused by *Notoedres cati.*

### SIGNIFICANT FACTS

1. Although it primarily affects cats, it can be transferred temporarily to dogs and man.
2. The mites are obligate parasites which survive off the host for only a few days.
3. It characteristically affects whole litters of kittens or older male cats and is highly contagious, spreading by direct contact.
4. Mites are more abundant and more easily demonstrated than in cases of sarcoptic mange in the dog.

Notoedric mange is highly contagious and intensely pruritic.

### LESIONS AND COURSE

1. Female mites burrow into the horny layer of the epidermis between hair follicles. These burrows appear on the surface in the center of minute papules.
2. The skin soon becomes thickened, wrinkled and folded, and later is covered with dense, tightly adhering, gray crusts (Fig. 42:1*B*). There is partial alopecia in affected areas.
3. Intense pruritus develops and the excoriations produced by scratching become secondarily infected.
4. The distribution is typical. Lesions first appear at the medial proximal edge of the pinna of the ear (Fig. 42:1*A* and *C*). They spread rapidly to the upper ear, the face, eyelids and neck. They also extend to the feet and perineum. This probably results from the cat's habits of washing, and of sleeping in a curled up position.

**Figure 42:1.** Notoedric mange.

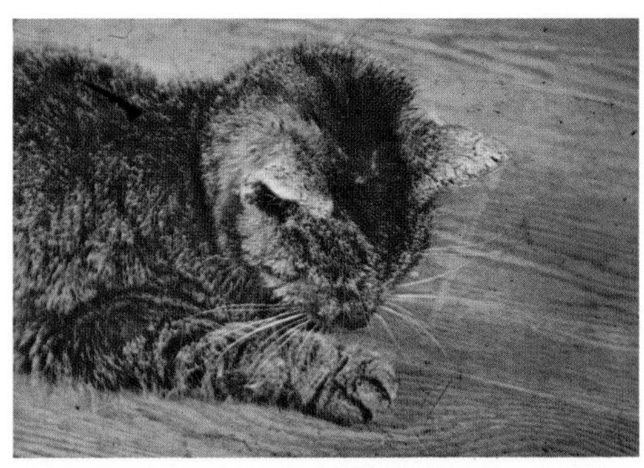

*A.* Dry crusted lesions on the edges of the ears and face are typical of notoedric mange. (Courtesy of D. W. Baker.)

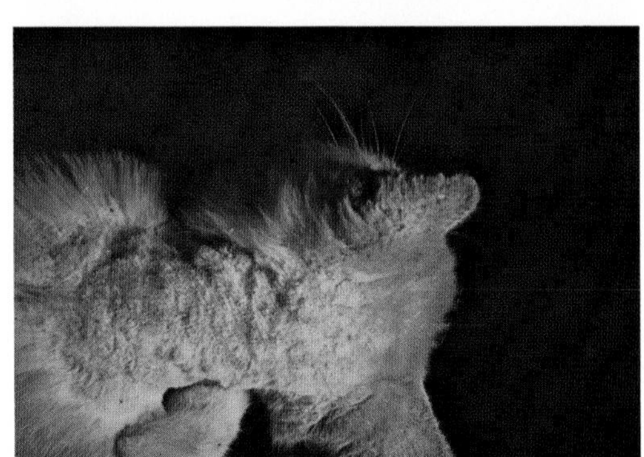

*B.* Thickened skin with dry, adherent crusts shown on an area clipped of hair for better visualization.

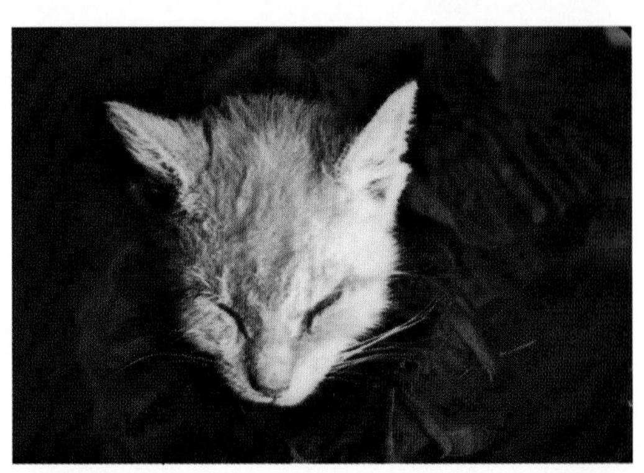

*C.* Lesions similar to *A.*

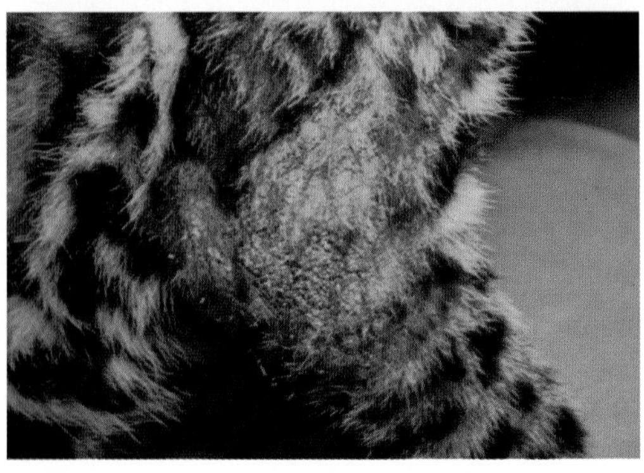

*D.* Dry, crusted gray lesions on the skin of the elbow of an ocelot.

## DIAGNOSTIC AIDS

Skin scraping of the face and ear usually produce mites.

## DIFFERENTIAL DIAGNOSIS

Lesions must be differentiated from those of dermatomycosis and fight wounds of mature male cats.

## CLINICAL MANAGEMENT

1. Most parasiticidal agents are contraindicated because of extreme toxicity to cats. Sulfur in various forms is completely safe.
2. With the cat under sedation, clip the hair from affected areas.
3. Bathe the cat in warm water and soap to loosen scales and debris.
4. Apply a 2.5 per cent warm water dilution of commercial lime sulfur solution (orchard spray). Allow to dry on.
5. Apply a commercial polysulfide solution to the affected areas every three to four days.
6. Repeat the lime sulfur dip ten days later.
7. Treat all affected cats on the premises.

### *Suggested Reading*

Holzworth, J.: Notoedric Mange of Cats. *In* Kirk, R. W. (Ed.): *Current Veterinary Therapy III*. W. B. Saunders Co., Philadelphia, 1968, p. 265.

Jubb, K. V. F., and Kennedy, P. C.: *Pathology of Domestic Animals*. Academic Press, New York, 1963.

# FORTY-THREE

## *Ovarian "Imbalance"*

Ovarian imbalance appears to produce a skin disorder of female dogs characterized by alopecia, hyperpigmentation, and lichenification of the perigenital, perineal and axillary areas.

### SIGNIFICANT FACTS

1. Until data is obtained from endocrine assays, the knowledge about this condition must come from clinical observations and the results of empirical treatments.
2. The heading "Ovarian Imbalance" probably includes several entities, but although research efforts may provide future clarification, the clinician is faced with the present need to treat his patients. For that reason, the authors include the syndrome here.
3. In many cases the skin becomes normal after spaying.
4. Anestrus or pseudocyesis is a common finding in the history.
5. Cystic ovaries are often found when the patient is spayed.

### LESIONS AND COURSE

1. Skin changes associated with ovarian imbalance are most common in bitches that are several years old.
2. The first lesions are alopecia and hyperpigmentation of the flanks, genital areas and perineum (Fig. 43:1*A*). The axillae become involved later.
3. Lichenification is a constant finding in advanced cases.
4. The vulva is often enlarged and hyperpigmented (Fig. 43:1*D*).
5. There are often crusting and enlargement of the nipples (Fig. 43:1*C*).
6. Generalized seborrhea is a common complication.

### DIFFERENTIAL DIAGNOSIS

1. Acanthosis nigricans starts in the axillae and only later involves the hindquarters.

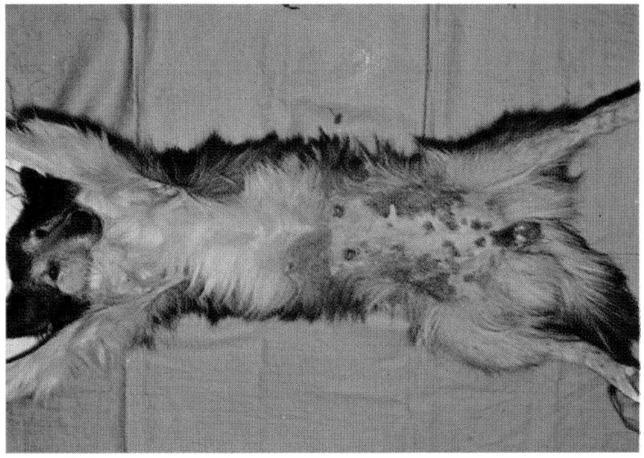

**Figure 43:1.** Ovarian "imbalance."

*A.* Bilateral lesions are restricted to the lower abdominal and pelvic areas, a reflection of the internally caused gonadal disturbance.

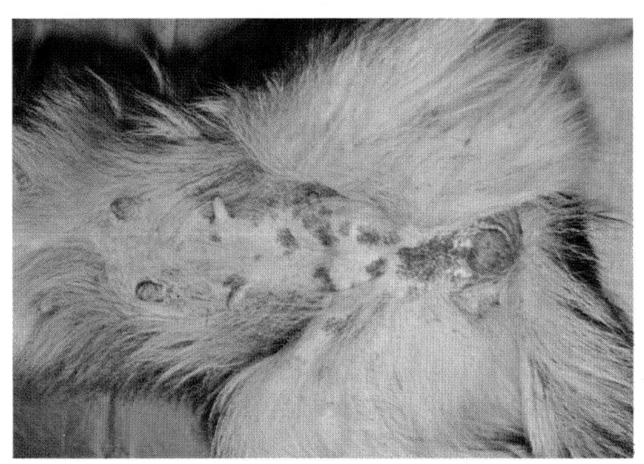

*B.* Close-up of *A* showing alopecia, hyperpigmentation and enlargement of the nipples.

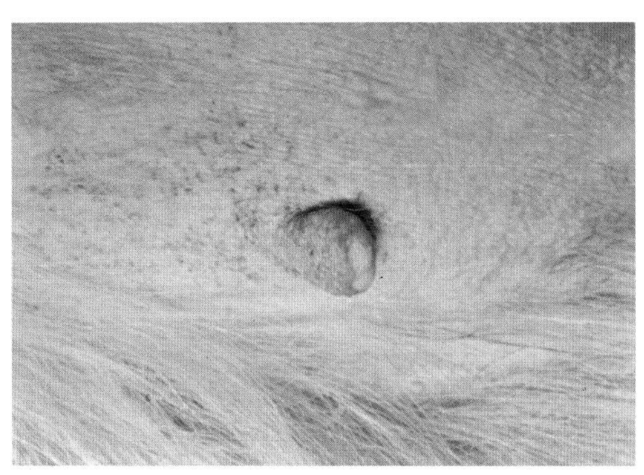

*C.* Close-up of an enlarged nipple with comedones. The nipples are as large as those of a lactating female although this bitch has never whelped.

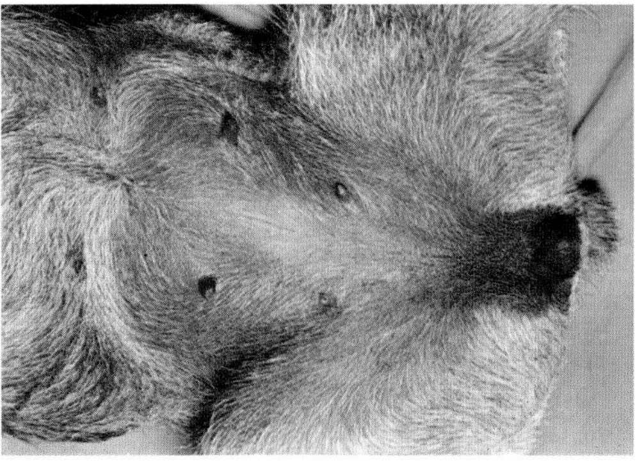

*D.* Note the hypertrophied, hyperpigmented vulva.

2. Hyperadrenocorticism is characterized by thinned instead of thickened skin.

3. Hypothyroidism is accompanied by atrophy of the external genitalia instead of hypertrophy, and distinctive laboratory tests are diagnostic.

## CLINICAL MANAGEMENT

1. Ovariectomy is effective in most cases. Unsatisfactory results can be attributed to complex adrenal-pituitary relationships.

2. Frequent antiseborrheic shampoos (once or twice weekly) are useful to help control the seborrhea.

# FORTY-FOUR

# *Pyoderma*

Pyoderma is the term applied to a pyogenic bacterial infection of the skin. It can be primary or secondary, superficial or deep, and is recognized clinically in several distinct syndromes. These will be discussed separately for the sake of clarity.

## *The Superficial Pyodermas*

*Acute moist dermatitis* ("hot spots") develops in dense-coated breeds as a result of trauma to the skin by licking or scratching at impacted anal sacs, infected ears, infestations of ectoparasites, or at minor skin irritations. The lesions have a rapid onset (hours only) and are red, moist, glistening and acutely painful (Fig. 44:2*D*). The horny layer is removed, hair is lost, and the lesion spreads rapidly. It becomes infected secondarily by a wide spectrum of organisms.

The fundamental skin reaction is similar in all types of pyoderma, varying only in severity and in location. There is acanthosis, a superficial dermal infiltrate composed of polymorphonuclear leukocytes, histiocytes, plasma cells, mast cells and numerous bacteria. This often is concentrated around the pilosebaceous units. The epidermal surface frequently is ulcerated. Epidermal edema, spongiosis and vascular dilatation is common.

Acute moist dermatitis is managed by carefully clipping the hair from the affected area. The patient may have to be anesthetized for this procedure. The skin is gently washed with pHisoHex and blotted dry. Antibiotic-corticoid sprays or lotions are applied sparingly three times daily. Systemic corticosteroids and antibiotics are sometimes used too. As the skin heals, astringent or emollient preparations are used as indicated.

Always look for the basic cause and treat this too (i.e., fleas, infected ear, impacted anal sacs or other causes); otherwise, acute moist dermatitis patches will recur.

*Skin fold pyodermas* occur in three forms: lip fold, vulvar fold and facial fold pyodermas.

Lip fold pyoderma develops in the deep folds of the lower lips of spaniels, setters and other breeds with large pendulous upper lips (Fig. 44:2*G*). This

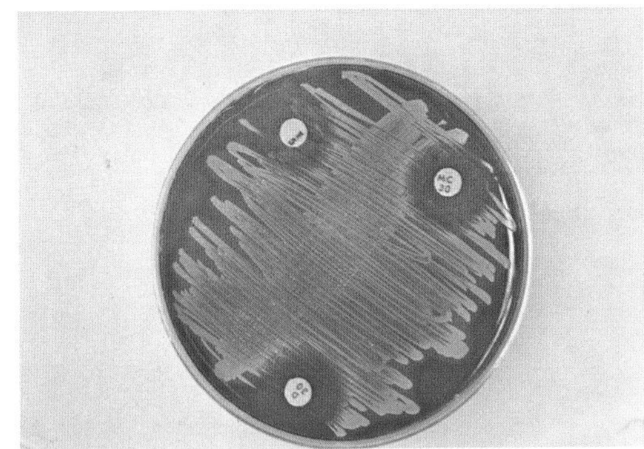

**Figure 44:1.** Gross bacteria culture characteristics.

*A. Staphylococcus aureus* grows rapidly and produces opaque, round, discrete, smooth, raised glistening colonies. Some are hemolytic (not illustrated). Antibiotic discs show good and poor inhibition of growth (blood agar).

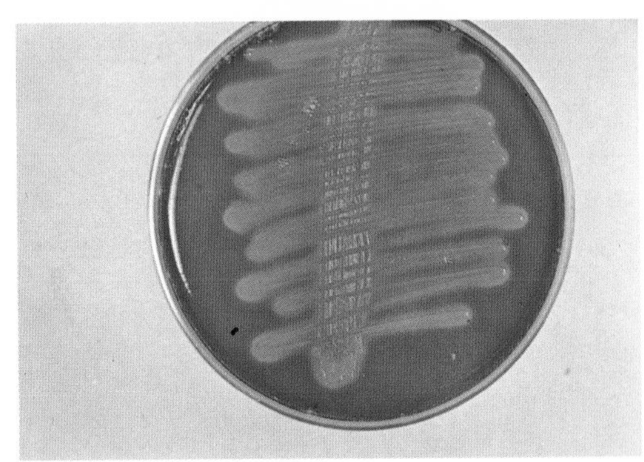

*B. Streptococcus sp.* colonies are pinpoint grayish and opalescent, resembling small drops of fluid surrounded by a clear zone of hemolysis (beta hemolysis). The size of the hemolytic zone varies (blood agar).

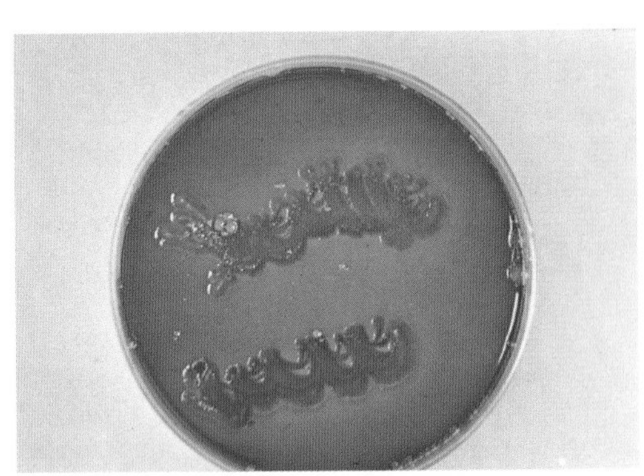

*C. Proteus mirabilis* has the ability to "swarm" on solid media as a most distinguishing characteristic. Growth often shows rippling waves or concentric rings. The color is grayish white, and the colonies produce a strong odor of decay (blood agar).

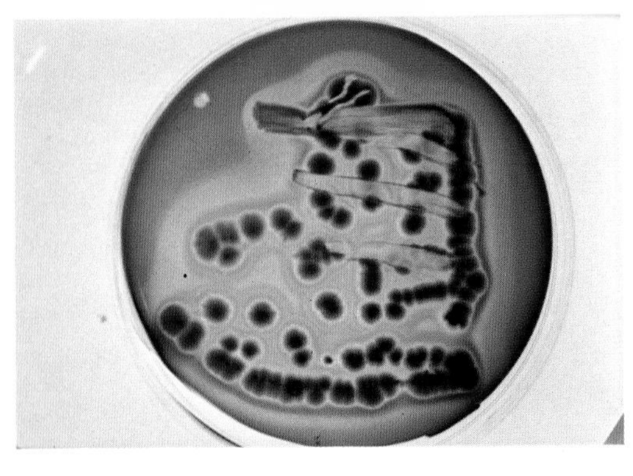

*D. Pseudomonas pyocyanea* grows dark greenish gray colonies, and their pigment production causes the agar to take on a bluish gray color (pyocyanea). It has a characteristic strong, sweet, hay-like odor (blood agar). (Additional plate on next page.)

covers the lower lip and keeps the lateral fold of the lower lip moist. The groove near the canine tooth becomes macerated, secondarily infected and is the source of a disagreeable, fetid odor. Clipping the hair, thorough cleansing of the skin, and antibacterial preparations provide only temporary improvement. Surgical extirpation of the skin fold corrects the anatomic problem, and provides an effective permanent correction. It should be done bilaterally.

Facial fold pyoderma is seen in breeds such as Pekingese which have a thick roll of skin between the nose and the eyes. Intertriginous irritation in these areas and accumulation of ocular discharges from corneal irritation establish a relatively painless but longstanding secondary pyoderma. The corneal irritation is far more important than the pyoderma, as it may result in pigmentary infiltration, ulceration and loss of sight. The best (and really only) treatment is surgical amputation of the roll of skin. However, this is a desirable beauty mark for the Pekingese breed; therefore, specific authorization from the owners should be obtained before surgery is performed. Absence of the fold is a point of severe discrimination in show animals. In some cases, temporary relief may be obtained by clipping the long hair and coating the fold with ointment.

Vulvar fold pyoderma is also an intertriginous irritation between skin folds; but in this case the folds are in the perineal region of an obese bitch that has an immature vulva. The lesions are chronic, foul smelling and unsightly (Fig. 44:2*H*). They respond poorly to medical treatment, but surgical extirpation of the folds or plastic repair to lift the recessed vulva into a more prominent position is curative. If obesity is a major cause, weight reduction results in improvement. Feeding a reducing diet (r/d) exclusively for at least three months is necessary.

*Impetigo* is a special form of superficial pyoderma which occurs as subcorneal pustules. It is a secondary infection seen in debilitating conditions such as malnutrition, severe parasitism, distemper and other systemic infections. The disease characteristically appears on the abdomen (glabrous skin) of puppies (Fig. 44:2*E*). Culture of the pus usually reveals streptococci, but staphylococci and other gram-positive bacteria are isolated occasionally. Lesions begin as multiple, discrete, erythematous macules which progress to vesicles and then to pustules. When these rupture a typical yellow exudate forms characteristic honey-colored crusts. There is no pruritus and little pain. The subcorneal pustule is covered by a parakeratotic roof and the underlying epidermal tissue is acanthotic. There is spongiosis and a superficial dermal infiltrate of inflammatory cells.

Impetigo usually responds readily to topical antiseptic and antibiotic therapy, but most cases resolve spontaneously in about one week. In extensive infections, systemic therapy with penicillin is advisable.

## *The Deep Pyodermas*

Deep pyodermas are usually associated with staphylococcal infections.

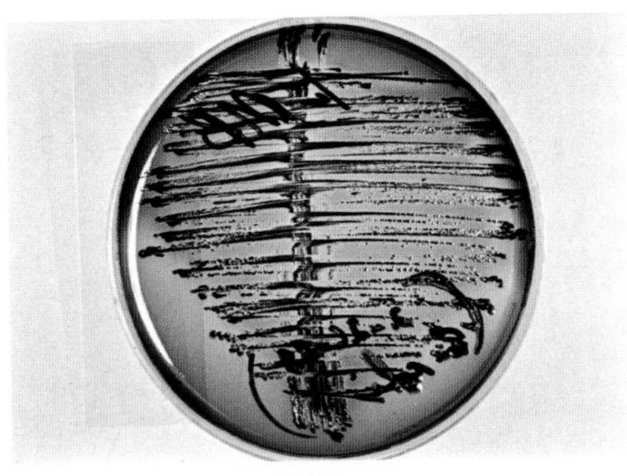

**Figure 44:2.** Pyoderma.

*A*. E. coli grows small, dry colonies which have a green metallic sheen on eosin methylene blue agar (EMB).

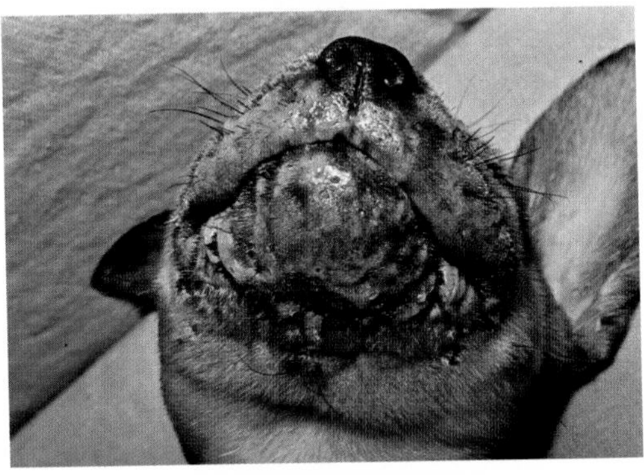

*B*. Juvenile pyoderma is characterized by swollen edematous lips with alopecia, folliculitis and pustule formation.

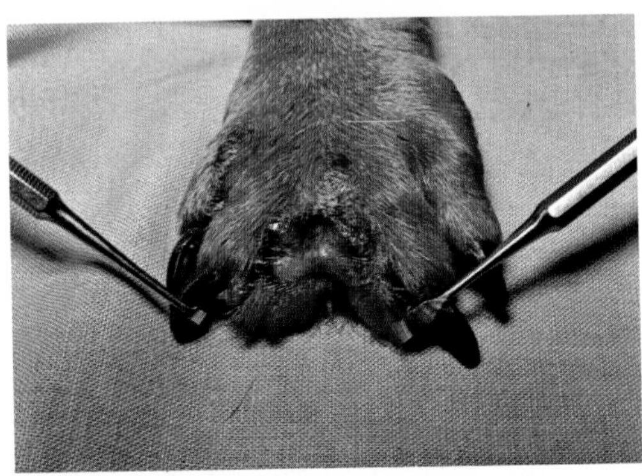

*C*. Interdigital pyoderma shows pustules and draining sinuses.

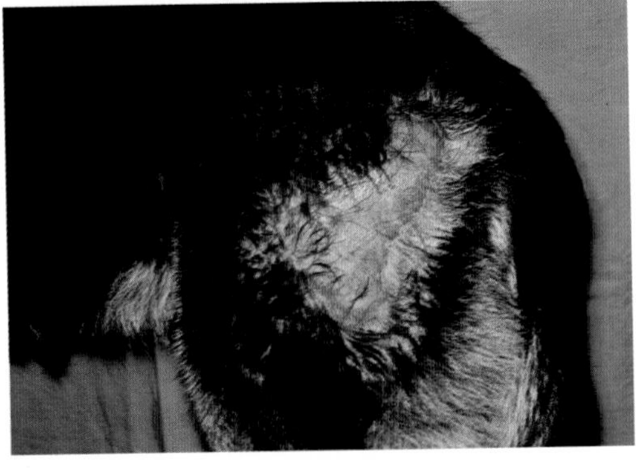

*D*. Acute moist dermatitis typically develops rapidly into a glistening, suppurative, hairless lesion bordered by a band of erythematous skin.

**Figure 44:2.** Pyoderma (continued).

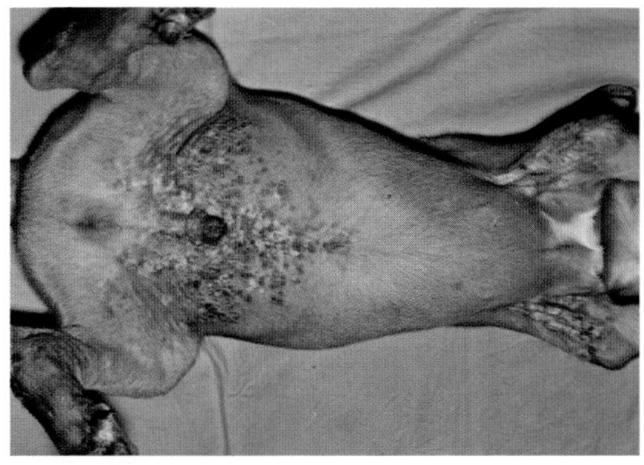

*E.* Impetigo with clusters of subcorneal pustules located on the glabrous skin of the abdomen.

*F.* Nasal pyoderma showing multiple pustules on the dorsum of the nose.

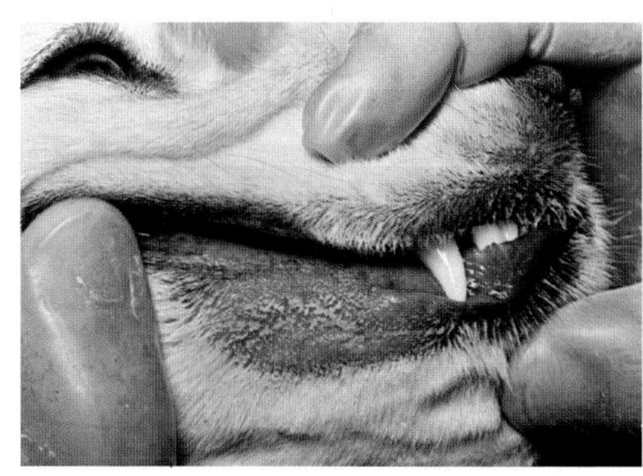

*G.* Lip fold pyoderma, characterized by erythema, exudation and a fetid odor.

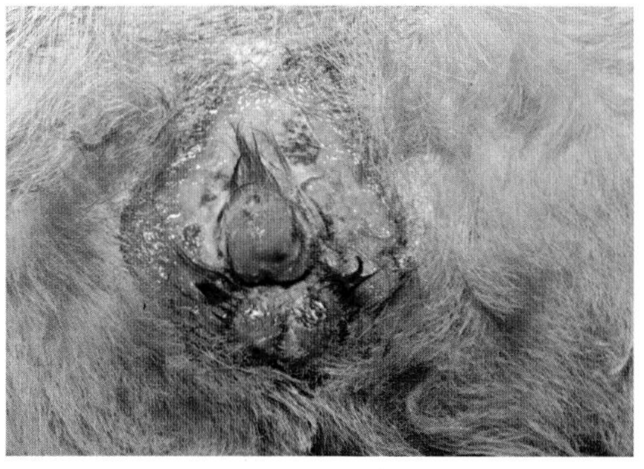

*H.* Vulvar fold pyoderma showing chronic purulent exudate.

*Folliculitis* is a more deep-seated inflammation of the skin with localization of an inflammatory infiltrate around hair follicle units. The lesions may remain as discrete papules or pustules centered around follicular openings, or they may coalesce and progress to deeper tissue and form furuncles, carbuncles and fistulas.

Deeper skin infections are commonly caused by staphylococci, but streptococci, proteus, pseudomonas, coliforms and corynebacteria are isolated occasionally (Fig. 44:1). Carefully taken cultures, and meaningful antibiotic sensitivity tests are mandatory for proper guidance of therapy in all cases of deep pyoderma.

With any deep pyoderma, a careful search should be instituted to be certain the infection is not secondary to foreign bodies such as wood slivers, awns, thorns or foxtails. However, in these cases there are usually single, localized lesions.

Microscopically, deep pyodermas differ from the superficial type by having more massive and deeper inflammatory infiltrates, more destruction of normal tissues, and by the presence of pustular and draining fistulas.

Deep pyoderma tends to localize in special areas of skin, producing specific clinical syndromes. These are called callus, nasal, juvenile, interdigital and generalized pyoderma.

*Callus pyoderma* is a secondary bacterial infection affecting the trauma-induced calluses on the elbows and hocks. The indurated skin in these areas has many folds which become macerated and infected easily. With continuing trauma the infection deepens, and ulceration and fistulas may develop. In the elbow region a chronic bursitis (hygroma) may be seen concurrently. These problems are common in large, short-coated breeds such as Great Danes, St. Bernards, boxers and English bulldogs, in which continual trauma to the points of wear produces large calluses.

Callus pyoderma may respond to intensive medical care directed at the infection. Usually, however, surgical removal of the callus is necessary. This is particularly the case if a chronic bursitis is present too. Following surgical excision it is important to prevent continuation of the trauma which initiated the callus. Soft bedding, or padding of the patient's favorite resting place will often prevent recurrence.

*Nasal pyoderma* affects the skin on the dorsal surface of the nose. It is common in German shepherds and collies (Fig. 44:2*F*), but can occur in other breeds. The infection may be irritated by the trauma of rooting along the ground, or of pawing at the area. The skin is red and swollen, and often has multiple pustules or fistulas. Permanent scars may result from destruction of the hair follicles. Although this infection usually involves mature dogs, it should be treated as juvenile pyoderma, described next. With careful treatment the prognosis is usually favorable.

*Juvenile pyoderma* affects puppies less than four months of age, and usually those of short-coated breeds such as dachshunds and pointers. This is a deep, suppurative infection caused by staphylococci which invade the skin around the puppies' lips, eyes and ears. The painful areas of skin become red, swollen and edematous (Fig. 44:2*B*). They ooze serum, and a purulent exudate forms which may become crusty. The infection is fulminating and often destroys hair follicles and causes permanent scarring. Secondary regional lymph node enlargement commonly is associated with these infections.

Juvenile and nasal pyodermas must be treated judiciously if excess destruction of hair follicles is to be avoided. Do not wash or scrub the lesions. Loose crusts can be lifted off, and topical antibiotic-cortisone medications applied with gentle patting. Aerosol sprays make excellent vehicles for such therapy. Wet dressings are also beneficial if they can be applied without patient resentment. Powders such as Furacin Soluble Powder are also useful. Because of the general infectious nature of this disease, systemic antibiotics (depending on culture results) are essential. In juvenile pyoderma, gamma globulin injections and provision of a high protein, high calorie, vitamin-supplemented diet may be beneficial ancillary measures. The course of the infection runs several weeks, but once healing begins it progresses rapidly.

*Interdigital pyoderma* is a particularly stubborn infection of the feet of short-coated breeds with a breed predilection for English bulldogs and dachshunds. It is usually associated with staphylococci, and appears as pustules and draining fistulous tracts between the toes of one or of all four feet (Fig. 44:2*C*). Trauma may be an initiating cause in some patients. (See treatment following.)

*Generalized pyoderma* is one of the most serious forms of deep skin infections. It is often associated with poor host resistance to infections, and is a secondary condition in many cases of generalized demodectic mange, as well as in malnutrition and chronic debilitating diseases. Clusters of pustules and fistulas develop in many areas, but particularly on the lateral sides of the body, legs and feet.

Hidradenitis suppurativa (apocrine gland infection) may also appear as a general pyoderma, and its treatment is quite similar. Prognosis is poor, however. It is most common in dogs of the collie type, and the ulcerative, granulating lesions are most numerous on the ventral body surface—particularly the axilla and inguinal regions.

Hidradenitis suppurativa is a troublesome infection, resistant to treatment.

Treatment of interdigital and generalized pyodermas is frustrating, as they are chronic infections which often are refractory to therapy. They need vigorous, thorough measures to obtain the best response. Pustules and fistulous tracts should be incised and curetted and followed by vigorous topical treatment. Twice daily antiseptic soaks or whirlpool baths effectively cleanse the lesions. Dilute solutions of quaternary ammonium compounds such as Nolvasan, or dilute sodium hypochlorite solutions work well for soak treatments.

Systemic antibiotics, as dictated by inhibition tests, must be used in full dosage for several weeks. Gamma globulin can be given daily for one week. An autogenous bacterin given in increasing dosage is helpful in many staphylococcus infected cases. Its use must be continued on a diminished schedule for several months for best effect. An initial subcutaneous injection of 0.1 ml. is increased every other day by 0.1 ml. until a dose of 1 ml. is reached. (However, the dosage depends on concentration of the bacterin.) The treatment is continued with a weekly injection of 1 cc. until a total of 20 cc. have been given. The

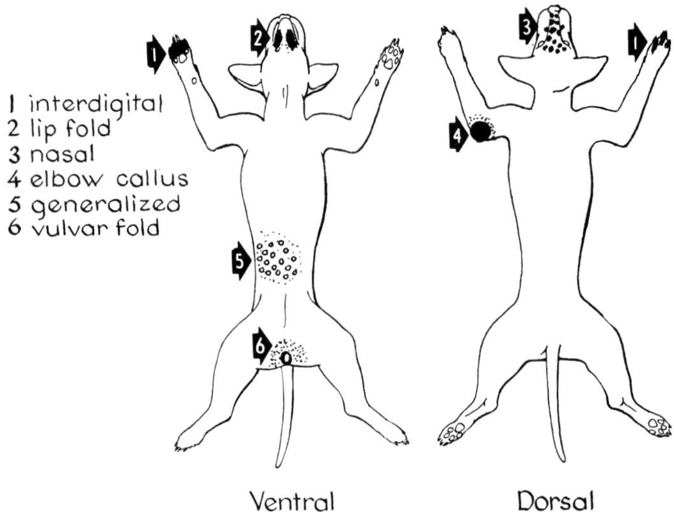


**Figure 44:3.** Pyoderma distribution pattern.

standard commercial bacterins are not particularly effective. Prognosis should always be guarded, and owners should be advised to inspect the animal frequently for signs of recurrence. Institute retreatment immediately if relapse occurs.

*Decubital ulcers* or "bedsores" are the result of prolonged local pressure in paralyzed patients. The skin over bony prominences is most frequently affected, but any area subjected to continual pressure may be involved. Although these lesions are thought to be a reflection of poor nursing care, they are almost inevitable in toxic cases. Predisposing causes are lowered nitrogen metabolism, prolonged pressure, trauma, maceration, and soiling with urine, feces or water.

Prevention should include a well-padded cage or bed (sponge or foam mats) with chamois cloth as protection over the points of wear. The patient should be rolled frequently—every two hours during the day, and several times during the night. He should be propped up in sternal recumbency much of the time. Daily, warm whirlpool baths are ideal to cleanse the skin. However, complete drying with massage and a warm air drier is mandatory following the bath. Alcohol can be gently rubbed over areas of trauma and allowed to evaporate. Powdering intertriginous areas is beneficial, too.

If ulcers develop, they should be kept scrupulously clean and dusted with antibiotic powders of B.F.I. Small foam rubber doughnuts, rolls or rings can be used to remove pressure from the ulcerated area. A high protein diet (if not contraindicated) and frequent whirlpool baths for exercise and cleanliness are also indicated. The ultimate aim is to correct the cause of the disability and get the animal ambulatory. The ulcers then heal spontaneously.

## *Suggested Reading*

Kirk, R. W.: The Pyodermas. *In* Kirk, R. W. (ed.): *Current Veterinary Therapy III*. W. B. Saunders Co., Philadelphia, 1968.

Andrews, G. C., and Domonkos, A. N.: *Diseases of the Skin*. Ed. 5. W. B. Saunders Co., Philadelphia, 1963.

# FORTY-FIVE

# *Sarcoptic Mange (Scabies)*

Sarcoptic mange is an intensely pruritic, transmissible infestation of the skin of dogs caused by the mite *Sarcoptes scabiei,* var. *canis.*

## SIGNIFICANT FACTS

1. *Sarcoptes scabiei,* the "itch mite," has an opaque, white body about 0.35 mm. long with four pairs of legs. Six-legged larvae and nymphs and oval-shaped eggs are also found in skin scrapings. The female mite forms a burrow in the epidermis into which she lays two to three eggs per day. She burrows at a rate of about 2 mm. per day and dies after two to four weeks (see p. 146).

2. Mites cannot survive longer than 48 hours off their host.

3. Sarcoptic mange affects dogs regardless of age, sex or breed.

4. The disease is highly contagious among dogs.

5. The owner and household members frequently develop visible lesions soon after the dog is affected. The mite, though host-specific, will temporarily invade the skin of man causing reddish, slightly pruritic papules (Fig. 45:1*C*). The dog mite does not form burrows in human skin and disappears from its temporary host in a few hours. The papule persists for several days. No new lesions will appear on the owner's skin after the mites are eradicated from the dog.

---

Pruritus and contagion are prominent hallmarks of sarcoptic mange.

---

## LESIONS AND COURSE

Although all cutaneous areas can be affected, the external ear is a favorite habitat of the mite (Fig. 45:1*A*). The typical distribution pattern of this dermatosis is discussed on page 90. The resulting dermatitis is characterized by erythema, papules, alopecia and the formation of small hemorrhagic crusts. Intense pruritus leads to excoriations produced by self-inflicted trauma. Secondary bacterial infection occurs in the excoriated areas.

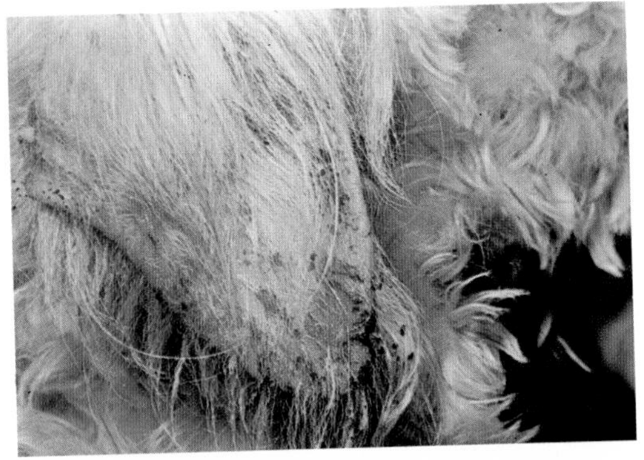

**Figure 45:1.** Sarcoptic mange.

*A.* The margin of the ear (pinna) is a characteristic site.

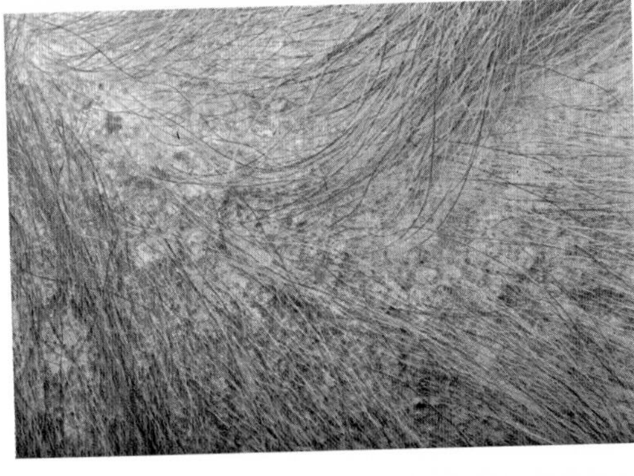

*B.* On the body, grayish crusts of sarcoptic mange mimic seborrheic dermatitis.

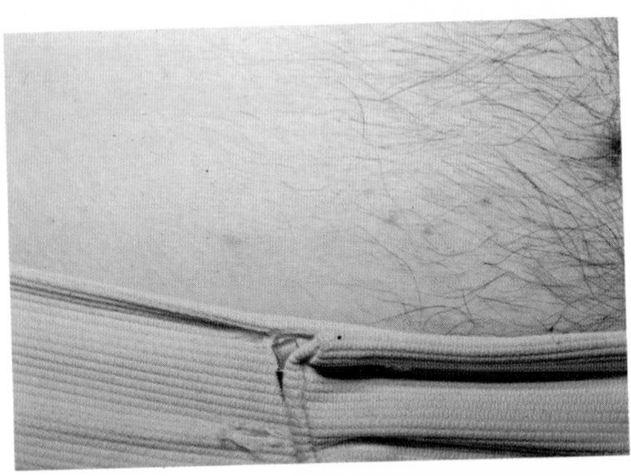

*C.* Erythematous papules above the belt line characterize the temporary invasions of human skin by *Sarcoptes scabiei*, var. *canis*.

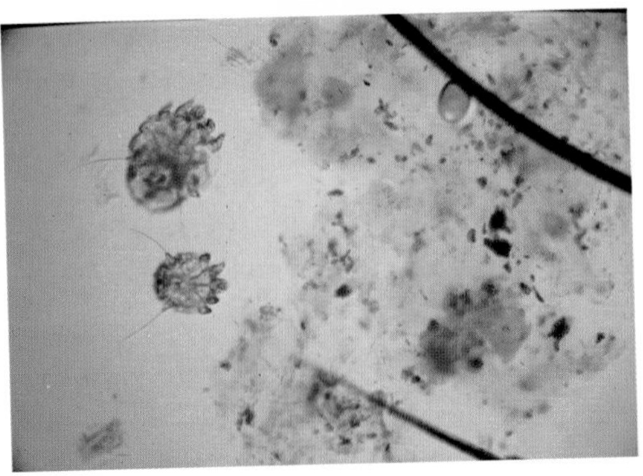

*D.* Sarcoptic mites and an egg. Small brownish pellets are the mites' fecal material.

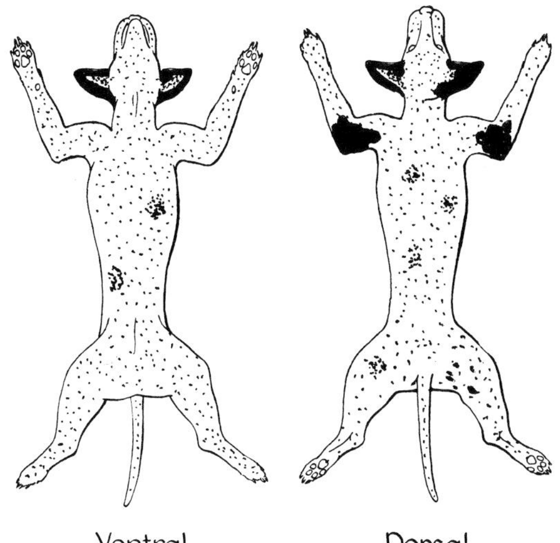


**Figure 45:2.** Sarcoptic mange distribution pattern.

The first lesions appear shortly after the mites are contracted from another dog. Unless treated, the disease becomes progressively worse—running a course of many months or even years. Without treatment, generalized involvement of the skin will occur and the dog can become emaciated and severely disabled.

## DIAGNOSTIC AIDS

Skin scraping, KOH-sugar centrifuged sedimentation, skin biopsy (see p. 93).

## HISTOPATHOLOGY

Intra-epidermal burrows contain the chitinous, basophilic-staining body of the mite. There is acanthosis with intracellular and intercellular edema in the stratum spinosum. The dermis shows an inflammatory infiltrate composed primarily of lymphocytes and eosinophils.

## DIFFERENTIAL DIAGNOSIS

In the early stages sarcoptic mange resembles allergic dermatitis; later, greasy scales form which can be mistaken for seborrheic dermatitis (Fig. 45:1*B*). Cheyletiellosis differs by its "scurfy" scales on the back, whereas scabies is especially severe on the legs and pinnas of the ears. Ringworm lesions are discrete, less pruritic and more localized.

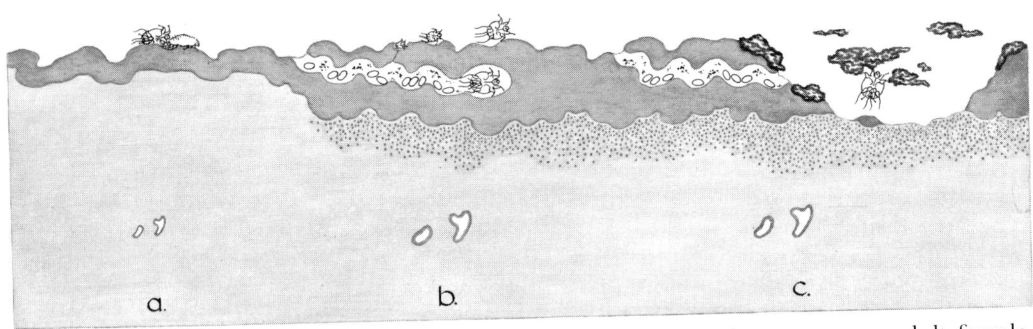


**Figure 45:3.** Sarcoptic mange dermogram. *a.* An adult male contacts an adult female *Sarcoptes scabiei* on the surface of the normal epidermis. *b.* After mating, the gravid female burrows into the epidermis and tunnels at a rate of about 2 mm. per day, leaving behind her ova and fecal pellets. As the eggs hatch, the larvae bore to the surface and form epidermal molting pockets. After molting they emerge as nymphs. The mites' activity causes the skin to react with acanthosis, hyperkeratosis, vascular dilatation and cellular infiltration of the upper dermis. *c.* Intense pruritus causes self-inflicted excoriations. The mite's burrow is opened by the trauma of scratching and the female mite is exposed and dies. Loss of mites from this process may be the reason that skin scrapings of abraded tissue fail to reveal mites. Eggs and fecal debris which remain in the burrow continue to cause pruritus, however. Oozing exudates coagulate to form crusts on the surface of the lesion.

## CLINICAL MANAGEMENT

1. Eradicate the mites! Apply one of the following acaricidal dips once a week for three weeks or until lesions disappear: Lime-sulfur, ronnel, malathion, Vapona, Kem dip. Treat all dogs on the premises to prevent reinfestation. Topical applications of benzyl benzoate, Led-O-San or USP sulfur ointment 10 per cent are useful.
2. Corticosteroids administered orally or by injection will relieve much pruritus.
3. Antiseborrheic shampoos remove scales and debris.

### Suggested Reading

Kirk, R. W.: *In* Kirk, R. W. (Ed.): *Current Veterinary Therapy III*. W. B. Saunders Co., Philadelphia, 1968.

Lapage, G.: *Veterinary Parasitology*. Charles C Thomas, Springfield, Ill., 1956.

Smith, E. B., and Claypoole, T. F.: Canine Scabies in Dogs and Humans, J.A.M.A. 199 (2), Jan. 9, 1967.

# FORTY-SIX

# *Seborrhea*

Seborrhea is a chronic skin disorder characterized by increased scale formation and abnormal sebum secretion.

## SIGNIFICANT FACTS

1. Seborrhea is arbitrarily divided into three types: seborrhea sicca (dry), seborrhea oleosa (oily) and seborrheic dermatitis (with inflammation).
2. Scale formation is the most characteristic lesion in canine seborrhea, but in man oiliness is the primary feature.
3. The cause of seborrhea is unknown; however, it secondarily accompanies such endocrine abnormalities as the male feminizing syndrome and some ovarian imbalances.
4. It is especially severe in brown and blonde cocker spaniels. A breed predilection exists for cocker spaniels and springer spaniels.

## LESIONS AND COURSE

1. There are many variations of clinical signs.
2. Seborrhea sicca (dandruff) is characterized by whitish gray or silvery dry scales, which are not oily. Scales are scattered throughout the hairs but there is little crusting of the skin (Fig. 46:1*A*).
3. Seborrhea oleosa is characterized by greasy, scaly patches. Clusters of fatty particles adhere to the hairs and resemble louse nits (Fig. 46:1*C*). In some areas the hair and skin are covered with oily masses and adherent yellowish brown greasy scales. A rancid odor, typical of seborrhea, is an unpleasant feature of these cases.
4. Seborrheic dermatitis is a variation in which scaliness and oiliness are accompanied by pruritus and erythema. Its distribution is more generalized than that of the other forms.
5. The course of seborrhea is chronic and the condition often remains with the dog for life.
6. Most cases can be satisfactorily controlled with adequate therapy, but permanent recovery or "cure" should not be expected.

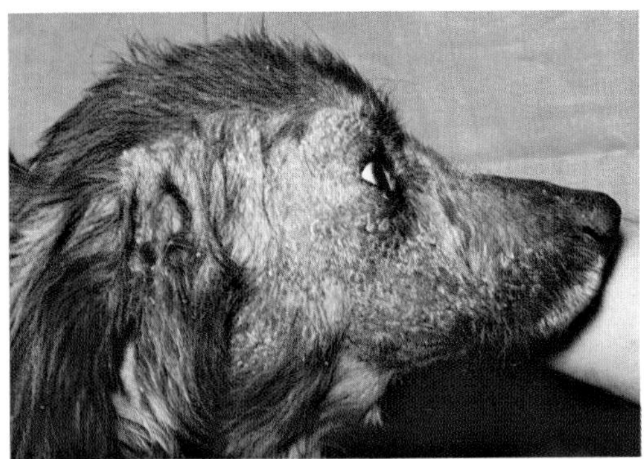

**Figure 46:1.** Seborrhea.

*A.* Head of a dog with seborrheic dermatitis of the face. Note the "dandruff" among the hairs.

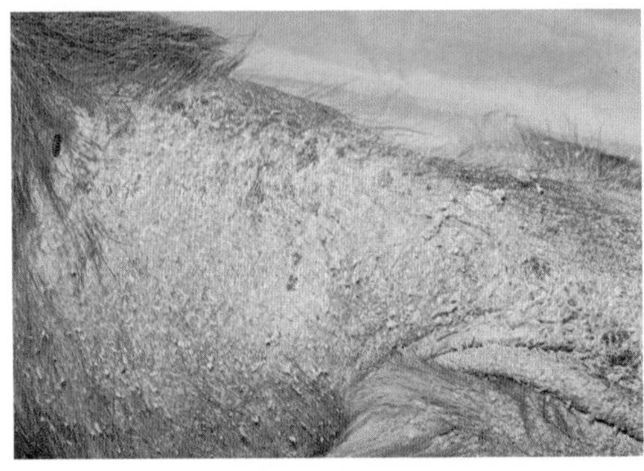

*B.* Generalized seborrhea in a dog, showing extreme scaling, flaking and partial alopecia.

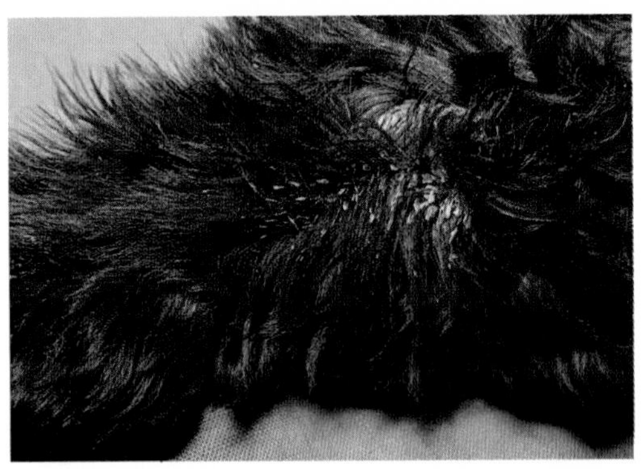

*C.* Seborrhea oleosa on the back of a cocker spaniel. Note that clusters of fatty particles adhere to the hairs and resemble louse nits.

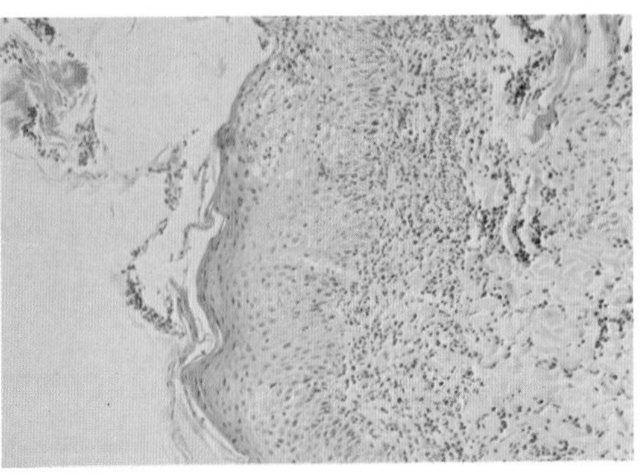

*D.* Histopathology of seborrheic dermatitis is basically that of chronic dermatitis with severe parakeratosis. Note the acanthosis and inflammatory infiltrate in the upper dermis. A seborrheic scale is in the extreme upper left. Epidermal surface at left. (Low power.)

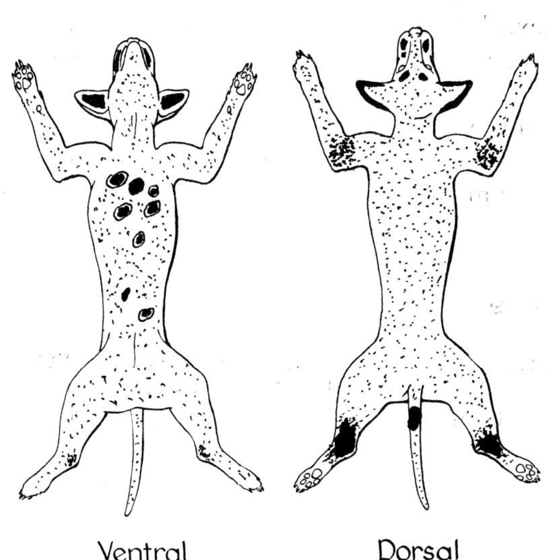


**Figure 46:2.** Seborrhea distribution pattern.

## HISTOPATHOLOGY

Microscopically, seborrhea resembles chronic dermatitis. There is papillomatosis, parakeratosis, acanthosis, intra-epidermal edema, and vascular dilatation. An inflammatory infiltrate of the upper dermis consists of plasma cells, mast cells, histiocytes and polymorphonuclear leukocytes. Follicular plugging and loss of hair are common.

## DIFFERENTIAL DIAGNOSIS

1. Dermatomycosis. The scaly, crusted, circular lesions on the chest and abdomen mimic ringworm.

2. Demodectic mange.

3. Hypoandrogenism, ovarian imbalance, and acanthosis nigricans are accompanied by secondary seborrhea. It is important to recognize the primary endocrine cause of these such cases and not to diagnose them as seborrhea.

## CLINICAL MANAGEMENT

Seborrhea is a chronic disease which can be ameliorated but not cured.

1. The objectives of treatment are to remove scales and crusts, reduce oiliness, control the seborrheic odor, relieve itching and decrease inflammation.

2. Medicated shampoos applied at intervals of three to 14 days are extremely helpful. Common ingredients of medicated shampoos are salicylic acid, sulfur, tar and hexachlorophene. Seleen, Fosteen, Sebulex and Sebutone are commercial products which are effective medicated shampoos.

3. Ointments containing tar, salicylic acid and sulfur (such as Pragmatar Ointment) are useful to reduce crusting and scaling. Sulfur reduces oiliness.

4. Corticosteroids given systemically relieve erythema and pruritus. Topical corticosteroid creams and lotions can be used for local lesions.

## *Suggested Reading*

Muller, G. H.: Canine Seborrhea. Animal Hospital *2*:228-238, 1966.

Schwartzman, R. M., and Orkin, M.: *A Comparative Study of Skin Diseases of Dog and Man.* Charles C Thomas, Springfield, Ill., 1962.

# FORTY-SEVEN

# *Thallium Poisoning*

Thallium is a cumulative, general cell poison which may produce skin lesions or systemic toxicity.

## SIGNIFICANT FACTS

1. Its common use as a rodenticide and roach poison will be terminated shortly, as over-the-counter sales have been prohibited because of its toxicity.
2. With doses over 10 to 20 mg./lb. of body weight the fatality rate is 100 per cent and the clinical signs are those of damage to central nervous system and circulatory system. Nervousness, convulsions, tremors, salivation, weakness and paralysis, together with a rapid weak pulse are seen. Reliable early signs of less acute toxicity include vomiting and profuse tarry or bile-stained diarrhea. Colic and dyspnea are often apparent. Smaller doses of thallium may be cumulative and produce the subacute or chronic syndrome described.

Thallium poisoning mimics many diseases.

3. Even with the best care, the mortality rate is extremely high (70 per cent), so that the prognosis is poor.
4. Thallium is rapidly absorbed through the oral and intestinal mucosa and through the skin. It is mainly excreted in urine but may persist in various tissues for up to three months.
5. Thallium and potassium move through cell walls together and are excreted together in the urine. Therefore, increased turnover of one increases the secretion of the other.
6. Cystine and methionine seem to protect against the alopecia and toxic effects of thallium (in rats).

## LESIONS AND COURSE

1. There are two syndromes. In acute toxicity the onset of signs is delayed 24 to 36 hours after ingestion, but the course until death is only four to five days.

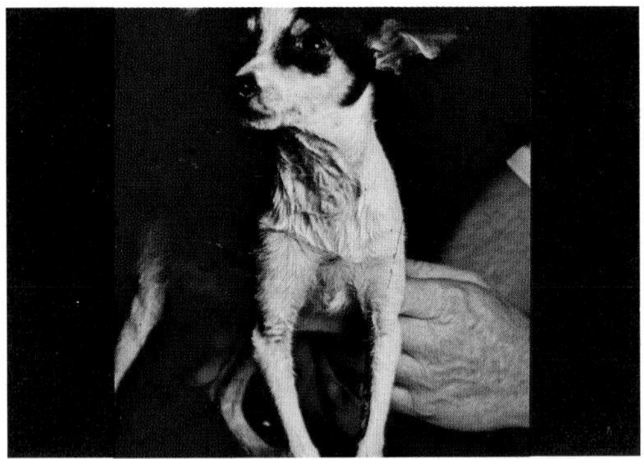

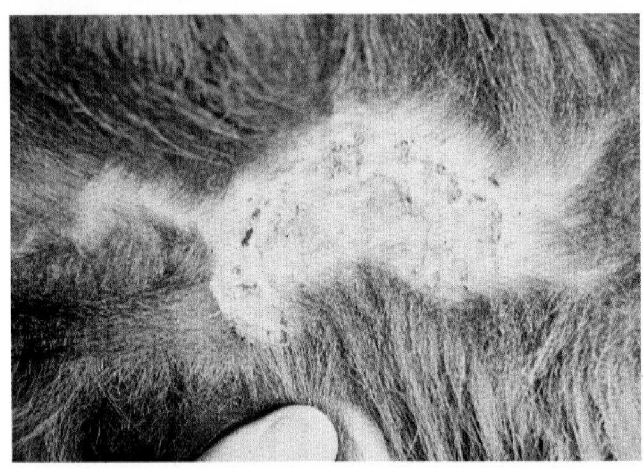

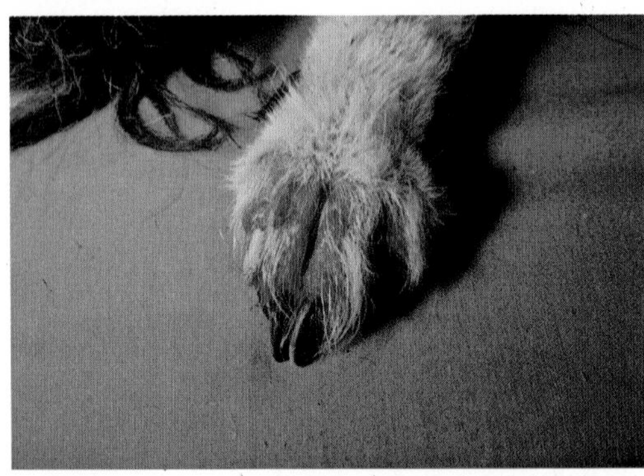

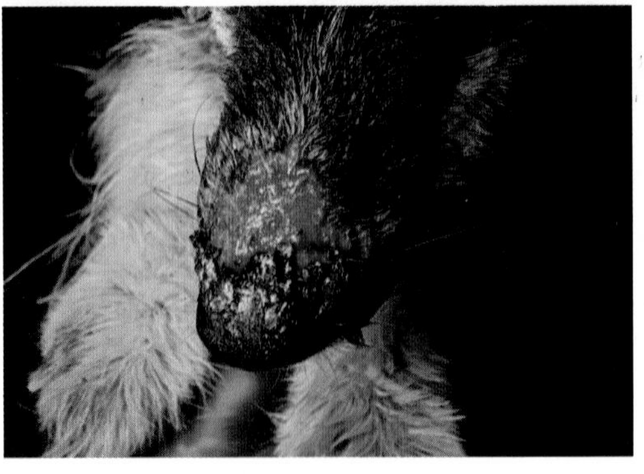

**Figure 47:1.** Thallium poisoning.

*A.* Beginning alopecia, erythema and necrosis of the skin of the neck, axilla and interdigital spaces. (Courtesy J. R. Dinsmore.)

*B.* Close-up view of skin showing alopecia, necrosis and crusting.

*C.* Erythema, alopecia and erosion of the digits and interdigital spaces.

*D.* Severe ulceration and crusting of skin of the nasal region. A purulent exudate is present.

In the chronic syndrome seven to 21 days may pass before signs appear and the course may extend to three weeks. Treatment should last seven to 21 days depending on the severity of the case.

2. Lesions of the chronic form show ulceration and hyperemia of mucous membranes and there is occasional vomiting, diarrhea and depression. Often the first sign (12 to 21 days after ingestion) is alopecia accompanied by erythema and necrosis of the skin (Fig. 47:1*A* and *B*). The skin lesions are located on the axillae, the ears, the posterior abdomen and genitalia, the interdigital frictional areas (Fig. 47:1*C*) and at mucocutaneous junctions. The lesions are slowly reversible in some cases.

## DIAGNOSTIC AIDS

1. A history showing that thallium baits were available.

2. A positive urine test for thallium. Gabriel's test with rhodamine B is simple and accurately detects thallium.

## HISTOPATHOLOGY (FIG. 47:2)

Thallium exerts a local toxic effect on epidermal cells in the process of differentiation leading to keratin formation. Degenerative changes are evident in the hair follicle and in the surface epidermis. The direct insult to the hair follicle is especially noteworthy in anagen hairs so that the hair shaft is converted to an amorphous mass, the bulb degenerates and the hair is lost. Follicular plugging is prominent.

The surface epidermis shows massive hyperkeratosis and parakeratosis with development of vacuolation of keratinocytes. Multiple spongiform abscesses are present in the upper epidermis. These areas are infiltrated with polymorphonuclear leukocytes.

A few rete ridges may be seen, and the upper dermis shows edema, extravascular hemorrhage and dilatation of vessels (hyperemia).

## DIFFERENTIAL DIAGNOSIS

Arsenic poisoning, organic phosphate poisoning, encephalitis, leptospirosis, distemper, gastroenteritis, pyoderma and pancreatitis may mimic thallium poisoning.

## CLINICAL MANAGEMENT

1. The primary objective is to remove thallium from the body. Emetics can be used early in the course. Once absorbed, thallium excretion can be promoted by oral administration of diphenylthiocarbazone (35 mg./lb. of body weight t.i.d.) and diethyldithiocarbamate (15 mg./lb. of body weight t.i.d.).

2. Potassium chloride 2 to 6 gm. orally/day may help too.

3. Peritoneal dialysis may be used in early cases.

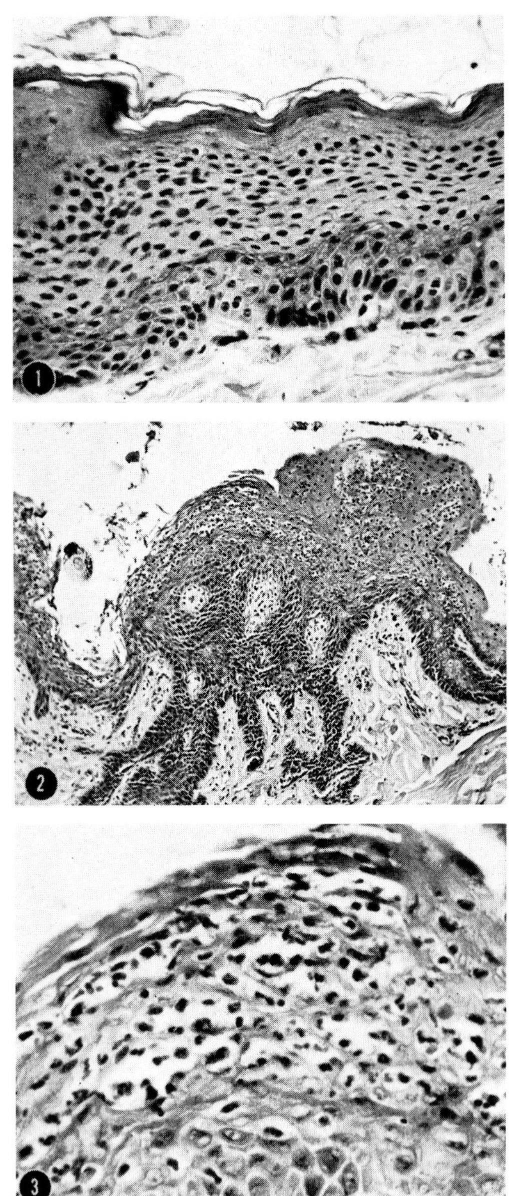

**Figure 47:2.** *1.* Canine axilla – note hyperkeratosis and massive parakeratotic scale, constituting approximately 65 per cent of epidermis. Malpighiian cells are vacuolated. H&E, × 195.

*2.* Canine axilla – multiple spongiform abscesses are present in the upper part of the epidermis. Rete ridges are elongated downward, forming a lace-like pattern. H&E, × 78.

*3.* Canine axilla – higher magnification of spongiform abscesses, showing multilocular spaces containing polymorphonuclear leukocytes. H&E, × 360. (From Jour. of Invest. Derm. Vol. 39, July, 1962.)

4. Later, the affected skin should be protected with antibiotic ointments and padded bandages.

5. Other supportive treatment may be vitally needed. Fluid injections to encourage renal function (5 per cent dextrose and water), B complex vitamins and sodium bicarbonate to combat the acidosis may all be useful.

## *Suggested Reading*

Gehring, Perry I.: Thallium Toxicity. *In* Kirk, R. W. (Ed.): *Current Veterinary Therapy III*. W. B. Saunders Co., Philadelphia, 1968.

Schwartzman, R. M., and Kirschbaum, J. O.: The Cutaneous Histopathology of Thallium Poisoning. J. Invest. Dermatology *39*:169-173, 1962.

Skelley, J. R., and Gabriel, K. L.: Thallium Intoxication in the Dog. Annals of N.Y. Academy of Sciences, Vol. III, Art. 2:612-617, 1964.

# FORTY-EIGHT

## *Callus*

A callus is a round or oval hyperkeratotic plaque that develops on the skin over bony pressure points. In dogs, the elbow and hock are the most common sites. Large breeds are especially susceptible if the dog sleeps on cement, brick or wood. The callus is hairless, gray in color, and has a wrinkled surface (Fig. 48:1). Histologically there is acanthosis, hyperkeratosis and parakeratosis. Small epidermal cysts are seen in the dermis and probably evolve from empty keratin-filled hair follicles.

Dog owners are often alarmed when they discover a callus and mistake it for ringworm, mange or some other skin disorder. Actually, most calluses are harmless and require no treatment. Only when they become extremely hyperplastic and reach unreasonable size need therapy be considered. In those cases the dogs should be discouraged from lying on hard surfaces. Foam rubber pads, carpets or blankets can make the bed or dog house a softer place. In extreme cases the callus can be removed surgically.

Callus pyoderma is a bacterial infection of a large callus with fistulization. It is discussed under the pyodermas on page 326.

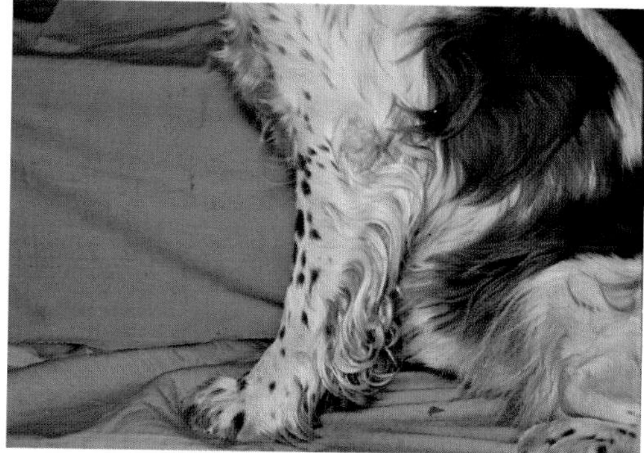

**Figure 48:1.** Callus.

Prominent elbow callus, springer spaniel.

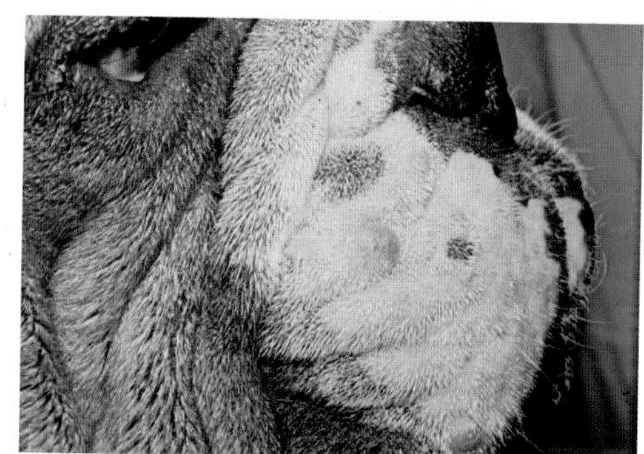

**Figure 49:1.** Canine acne.

Pustules of canis acne, lip of English bulldog. *(See page 344)*

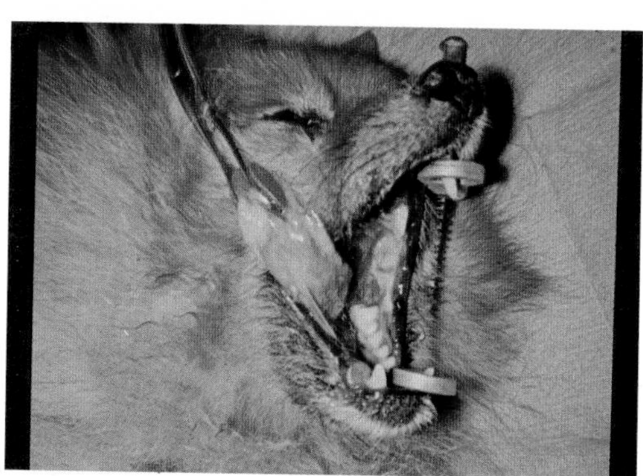

**Figure 50:1.** Candidiasis.

*A.* Oral lesions of the mucosal surface of the tongue and cheek. *(See page 345)*

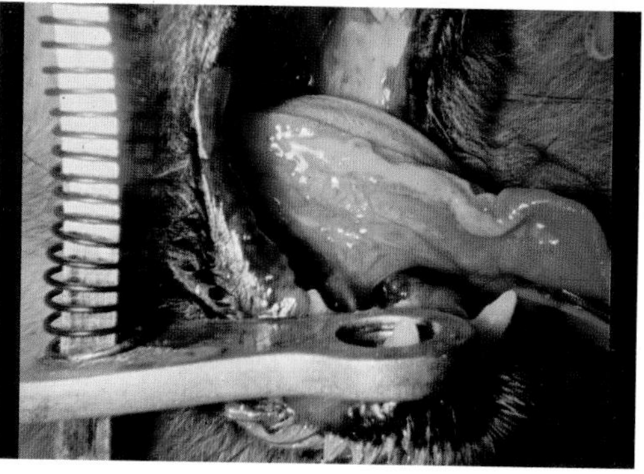

*B.* Whitish gray plaque on the cheek, and linear band of affected mucosa on the tongue. (Photos 50:1*A* and *B* courtesy of N. T. Freid.)

# FORTY-NINE

## *Canine Acne*

Canine acne affects the face in some dogs between three and 12 months of age—the time of sexual development. In certain individuals (especially boxers and English bulldogs) the disease persists into the mature years.

The primary lesion is a papule. Close examination of the face will reveal comedones that progress into erythematous papules and finally into pustules (Fig. 49:1). The chin is the most common site with upper and lower lips being next in frequency of affliction. Sometimes acne lesions are seen on the lower abdomen and medial thighs. The forehead is almost never affected.

The disease is of minor clinical importance in dogs. Their adolescent period is so short (6 to 8 months) that the pustules clear spontaneously with the onset of maturity—often without the owner really becoming aware of the condition. In dense-coated breeds, the pustules may be hidden by the hair coat.

Canine acne usually heals spontaneously when the patient matures.

In mild cases no treatment is needed. Occasionally a severely affected dog will require therapy. This is especially true of short-haired, light-colored individuals whose acne persists past sexual maturity (see Fig. 49:1). Daily shampooing of the lips and chin with pHisoHex is effective. Tetracycline should be given orally. Estrogenic hormones are helpful in resistant cases because they tend to reduce sebaceous secretion.

# FIFTY

# *Candidiasis (Moniliasis)*

Candidiasis is an infection of the mucous membrane or the skin caused by *Candida albicans.*

## SIGNIFICANT FACTS

Persisting moisture is a predisposing cause.

1. The most common and most stubborn site of infection is the oral mucosa (Fig. 50:1*A* and *B*).
2. Infection can also occur in the external ear canal, the nail folds, the anal mucosa and the vaginal mucosa.
3. Candidial skin infections are rare in dogs and cats.
4. Prolonged administration of antibiotics or persistent moisture may be predisposing factors to Candida infections.
5. The prognosis is only fair.

## LESIONS AND COURSE

1. Oral lesions consist of whitish gray plaques that tend to coalesce into linear bands surrounded by an inflammatory mucosa (Fig. 50:1*B*).
2. The lesions occur most commonly on the mucous lining of the lips, the cheeks and the ventral surface of the tongue. White papules are sometimes seen on the dorsal lingual surface.
3. A foul-smelling mucous discharge, mixed with saliva, accompanies the oral lesions.
4. In vaginal lesions there is a thin, whitish discharge.
5. Skin lesions are very rare. They consist of vesiculo-pustules covered with brownish crusts. They are usually secondary to oral, anal or vaginal moniliasis.
6. The course is chronic and some cases are refractory to treatment.

## DIAGNOSTIC AIDS

1. Smears of the exudate from typical lesions can be stained with lactophenol cotton blue and usually will reveal the yeast-like, budding cells.

2. Cultures from the affected lesions or their exudates will grow colonies of *Candida albicans* in one to three weeks. Cultures grow readily at either room temperature or at 37° C. Sabouraud's agar and special Candida agar (Pagano-Levin medium, Squibb) make good media for growth. *Candida albicans* colonies are soft, cream-colored, and have a yeasty odor.

## HISTOPATHOLOGY

The oral lesions show only chronic inflammatory changes and dermal edema. In cutaneous lesions, fungal elements consisting of small, oval, budding yeast-like organisms and hyphae are present in only the horny layer.

## DIFFERENTIAL DIAGNOSIS

Candidiasis must be distinguished from bacterial, ulcerative and gangrenous stomatitis, vulvar fold pyoderma and bacterial otitis externa.

## CLINICAL MANAGEMENT

1. Nystatin can be applied topically for Candida infections with good results. Panolog and Mycostatin are effective preparations. The affected area should be clipped if necessary, washed and dried, and Mycostatin applied topically to the skin or ear canal four times daily. Treatment should be continued after recovery to insure against relapses.

2. Oral or vulvar infections can be treated with gentian violet 1:10,000 in 10 per cent alcohol daily; or with the Mycostatin suspension four times daily.

3. In severe unresponsive cases amphotericin B may be used, but it is highly toxic (renal) systemically and should be used by that route only in desperate situations. A lotion (Fungizone) is available for safe topical use, and application three or four times daily provides effective therapy. Response may be seen in a few days in cutaneous, ear and mucocutaneous infections, but several weeks' treatment is needed for paronychia. These latter cases often relapse too.

### *Suggested Reading*

Emmons, C. W., Binford, A. B., and Utz, J. P.: *Medical Mycology*. Mycology. Lea & Febiger, Philadelphia, 1963. pp. 131-144.

Hildick-Smith, G., Blank, H., and Sarkany, I: *Fungus Diseases and Their Treatment.* Little, Brown and Co., Boston, 1964. pp. 129-205.

**Figure 51:1.** Cheyletiella yasguri.

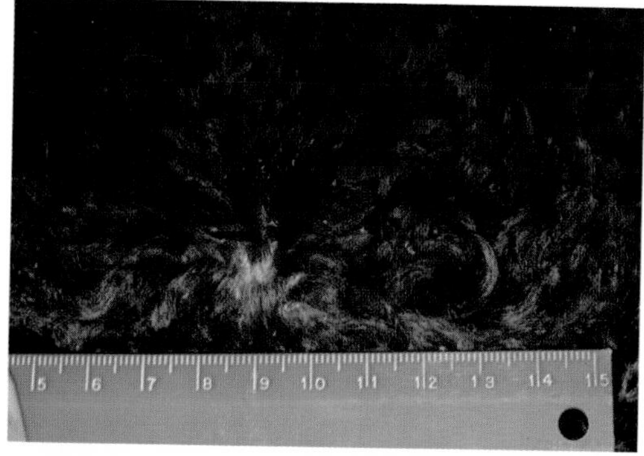


*A.* Cheyletiella adults and epidermal scales on coat and skin of puppy. Metric ruler.

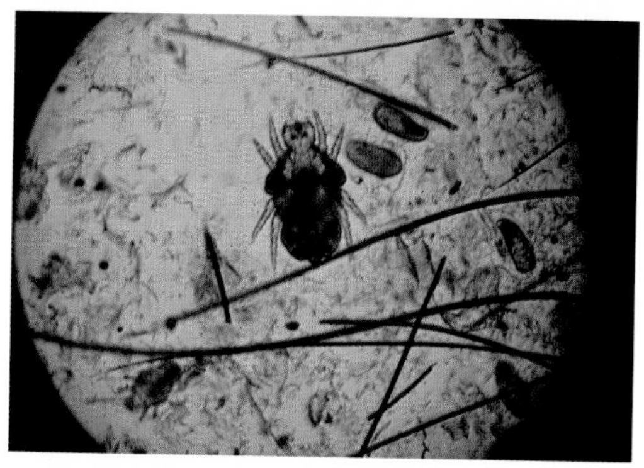

*B.* Microscopic appearance of adult, larva and egg stages of *Cheyletiella yasguri.*

**Figure 52:1.** Pediculosis. *(See page 349)*

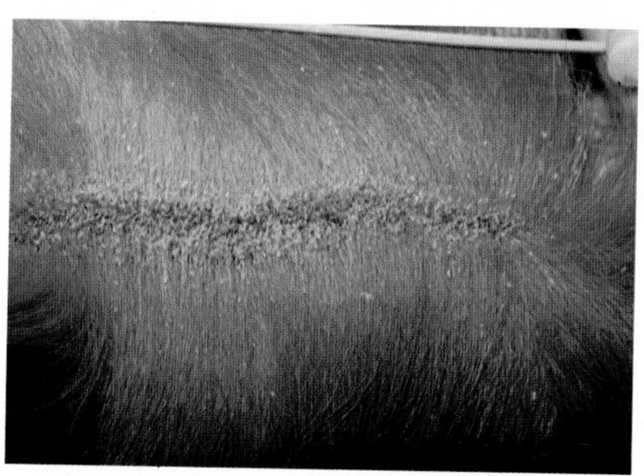

*A. Linognathus setosus* adults, (blue gray specks on the surface of the skin) and nits (white specks on the hair) illustrating severe case of pediculosis.

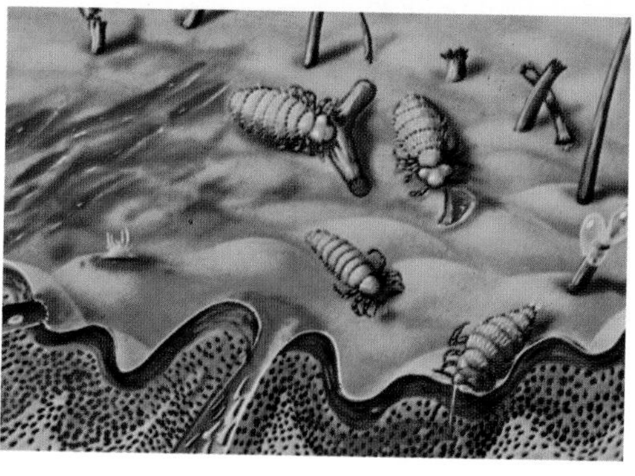

*B.* Skin diagram showing adult biting and sucking lice, a nit attached to a hair, and excoriations of the skin as a result of pruritus. (Diagram courtesy Norden Laboratories.)

# FIFTY-ONE

## *Cheyletiella Dermatitis*

*Cheyletiella yasguri* infests dogs but produces a syndrome which is often overlooked. The mites live in the keratin layer of the skin and produce a dry, scaly, gray crust in the affected areas (Fig. 51:1*A*). The appearance is suggestive of simple dandruff. Mites usually concentrate in the lumbodorsal region, but are also found along the top of the head and the nose. (See also the discussion of Cheyletiella, p. 146).

Cheyletiella dermatitis is becoming more frequent—look for it.

Pruritus and shedding of hairs are constant but not outstanding features of the disease. Cheyletiella dermatitis is primarily a kennel or pet shop problem because it spreads easily; it is particularly common in young puppies. It may also spread to man temporarily and produce a mild dermatitis. Man is not a good host, however, and repeated contact with affected dogs is necessary or spontaneous recovery occurs.

These mites are easily destroyed, and the infestation is readily controlled. The mites can live in the building for long periods; therefore, a major factor of control is proper cleansing, and treatment of the premises with insecticides. Chlordane 0.5 per cent, DDT 5 per cent, or organic phosphate products such as ronnel 1 per cent or malathion 1 per cent are effective and have residual action. All the affected or contacting animals in the area should be treated with insecticidal shampoos such as KFL, or Thionium with lindane. They may also be treated with aerosol sprays or powders (SOK). One treatment may be sufficient, but repeated treatments once weekly for three weeks ensure complete eradication.

# FIFTY-TWO

# *Pediculosis*

Pediculosis is infestation with lice.

## SIGNIFICANT FACTS

1. The common sucking louse of dogs is *Linognathus setosus*. The biting lice *Trichodectes canis* and *Heterodoxus longitarsus* are less prevalent.
2. Cats are affected by *Trichodectes felis*, a biting louse.

Lice are host-specific and spend all their lives on that host—facts which make control easier.

3. Lice are highly irritating to the host and cause intense itching. They accumulate under mats of hair, around the ears and body openings, and sucking lice produce anemia and severe debilitation.
4. Sucking lice do not move rapidly and are easily seen and caught. Biting lice may be difficult to find and capture.

## LESIONS AND COURSE

1. Lice produce few direct lesions, but excoriations and secondary dermatitis from scratching may be severe.
2. Debilitated, anemic and frustrated patients often are ill-tempered and difficult to handle.
3. The patient's coat is often dirty, matted and ill-kempt, as this is a disease of neglect. The animal often has a "mousy" odor, especially when wet.

## DIAGNOSTIC AIDS

1. Diagnosis is made by identification of the lice and their nits (see p. 154).

## DIFFERENTIAL DIAGNOSIS

Pediculosis may resemble seborrhea, Cheyletiella dermatitis, sarcoptic and notoedric mange, and *Dermanyssus gallinae* infestation.

## CLINICAL MANAGEMENT

1. All affected animals and others in close association should be treated. It is advisable to clean bedding and grooming implements too.
2. Thick mats and tags should be clipped away.
3. After a regular soap and water shampoo the animal should be soaked or sprayed thoroughly with a good insecticide.
    a. Cats: KFL shampoo. After drying they can be dusted with 2 per cent methoxychlor or 5 per cent carbaryl (Sevin) powder. Treatment should be repeated in ten to 14 days because not all the nits may be killed and any remaining will have hatched by that time.
    b. Dogs: Stronger medications with residual action can be used on dogs although lice are easily killed with the preceding preparations. Bathing in KFL or Thionium with lindane is effective. Dogs can then be dipped in 0.25 per cent DDVP. Applications of 5 per cent carbaryl (Sevin) are also useful follow-up treatments. A second treatment in ten to 14 days is recommended. These treatments are usually highly effective.
4. Severely anemic and depressed patients with extreme parasite infestations may go into shock and die following vigorous treatment. It is best to transfuse blood, give a high protein diet and reduce the number of parasites with carbaryl or other powders first. More complete treatment as previously outlined can be given several days later.

### *Suggested Reading*

Blakemore, J. C.: Macroscopic Ectoparasites. *In* Kirk, R. W. (Ed.): *Current Veterinary Therapy III*. W. B. Saunders Co., Philadelphia, 1968.

Lapage, G.: *Monnig's Veterinary Helminthology and Entomology*. Edit. 5. Williams & Wilkins Co., Baltimore, 1962.

# FIFTY-THREE

## *Feline Alopecia Universalis*

The cat pictured in Figure 53:1*A* and in Figure 69:31 has a rare case of feline generalized alopecia. A male cat was born to a normal mother which had several normal kittens in the litter.

The cat resembled a Chihuahua at first glance since it was almost hairless. Its smooth, hairless skin had a greasy feel. This resulted from the cat's reluctance to lick itself. The rough, barbed tongue is equipped for combing hair but causes pain when glabrous skin is groomed. The cat instinctively attempted to clean itself but stopped when the tongue touched the naked skin. Sebaceous glands were active, however, and a surface lipid film contributed to the oiliness of the skin and the greasy odor. It was necessary for the owner to wash the cat with soap and water twice a week. Grayish black deposits of grease which formed under the nail folds had to be removed regularly. The claws were slightly deformed.

Microscopically, the skin showed a complete absence of primary hairs (Fig. 53:1*B*). Lanugo hair follicles were found only in certain areas. The epidermis was eight to ten cells thick—much thicker than normal feline skin. Sebaceous and apocrine glands were both present but they opened directly onto the surface of the skin. The dermis appeared to be normal.

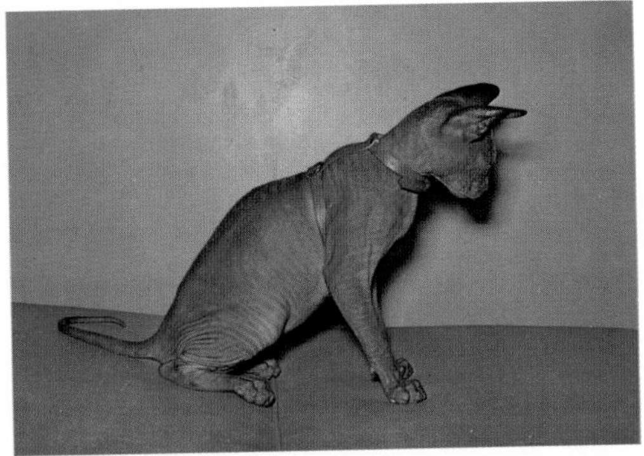

**Figure 53:1.** Alopecia universalis.

*A.* Except for a few lanugo hairs this cat has complete alopecia.

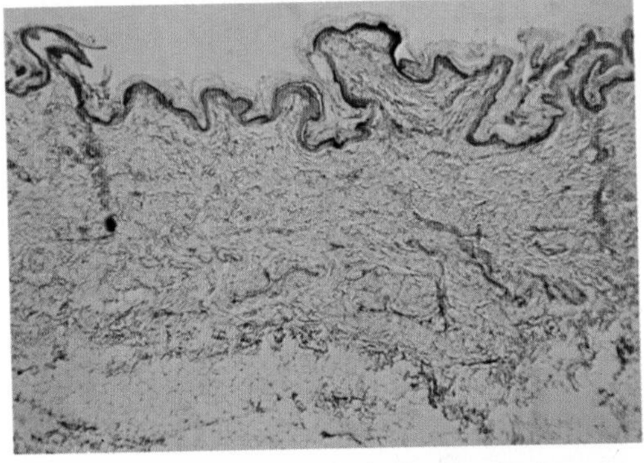

*B.* Histologic section of the skin of the cat shown in *A.* Note the hyperkeratosis, surface debris, absence of hair follicles, and relative acanthosis. (Low power.)

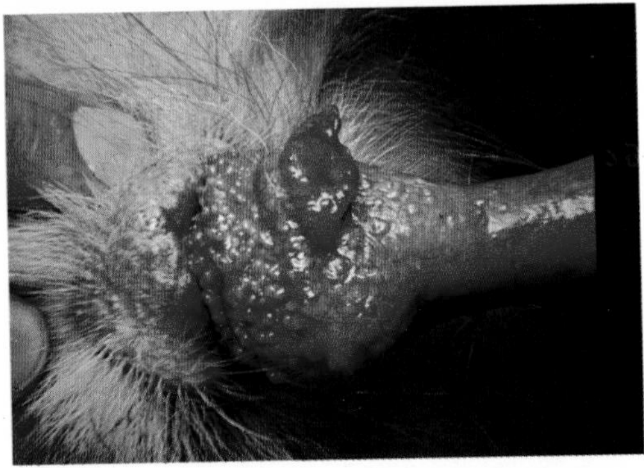

**Figure 54:1.** Transmissible venereal tumor. *(See page 353)*

*A.* The bright red nodule is a transmissible venereal tumor on the mucosa of the penis. Note the multiple lymphoid follicles, common finding in male dogs.

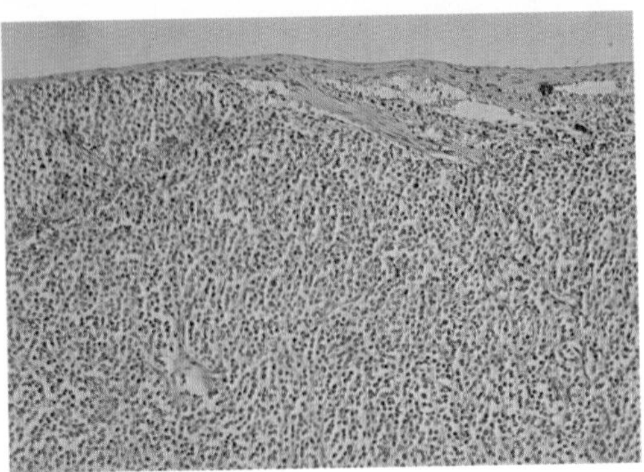

*B.* Histologic section of the tumor shown in *A.* The tumor cells are present in solid sheets with little stroma. Note the mucosal surface, and the presence of many blood vessels and hemorrhage. (Low power.)

# FIFTY-FOUR

# *Transmissible Venereal Tumor*

The transmissible venereal tumor of dogs is a disease of possible reticulo-endothelial origin which affects the genitalia of sexually mature dogs.

## SIGNIFICANT FACTS

1. There is no breed incidence, but it is slightly more prevalent in female than in male dogs.

2. The tumor is common in dogs of southern France, the Orient and Puerto Rico, but is present only sporadically in this country. It has been reported in the southeast and southwestern United States, often near military installations where imported dogs may be common.

3. Although the tumor has not been transmitted by cell free filtrates, it is readily transplanted by passage of viable tumor cells. Experimentally, it has been passed through many generations without change. Cells placed on the skin or mucosa fail to "take" unless scarification or injection enables them to penetrate this barrier. In nature, the trauma of coitus or licking causes the tumors to spread readily.

4. Spontaneous regression often develops after several months, perhaps as an immune phenomenon.

## LESIONS AND COURSE

1. The lesion usually involves the genital mucosa, and is multilobulated or nodular in shape. It is firm, friable, gray or red in color, and often ulcerated (Fig. 54:1*A*). Many grow fairly rapidly for several months and then regress and even disappear completely in six to ten months.

2. A few rare cases have spread to skin, liver and regional lymph nodes.

## DIAGNOSTIC AIDS

The clinical appearance is typical, but histologic examination is necessary for positive diagnosis.

## HISTOPATHOLOGY (Fig. 54:1*B*)

The tumor cells are uniformly round, with large hyperchromatic nuclei. The nucleoli are eccentric, and mitotic figures are common in many cases. The cells are present in solid sheets or clusters with a sparse, fibrous stroma (Fig. 54:1*B*). The tumor is vascular and may contain lymphocytes, mast cells, eosinophils and macrophages.

## DIFFERENTIAL DIAGNOSIS

Granulation tissue from wounds may resemble this tumor.

## CLINICAL MANAGEMENT

1. Surgical excision is usually successful, but the tumor is highly radiosensitive, so that this type of therapy is an excellent alternative choice.

### *Suggested Reading*

Moulton, J. E.: *Tumors in Domestic Animals.* University of California Press, Berkeley, 1961.

# FIFTY-FIVE

# *Canine Oral Papillomatosis*

Papillomatosis of dogs occurs in young animals as contagious, virus-caused, benign epithelial growths of the mouth, commonly called warts. The incubation period is approximately thirty days, and spreading occurs by implantation in scarified oral mucosa. Cats are not affected.

The lesions begin as smooth, white nodules on the lips. These soon become extremely rough and cauliflower-like, and spread to the gums, tongue and pharynx. Some animals have thousands of such nodules (Fig. 55:1). They persist for 60 to 90 days but often regress spontaneously.

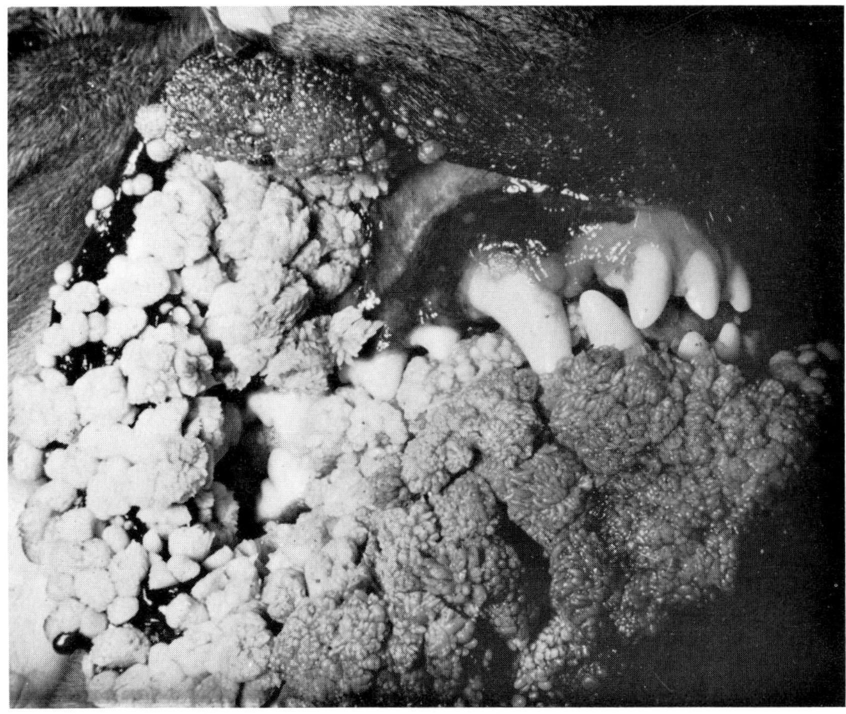

**Figure 55:1.** Severe case of oral papillomatosis.

Papillomatosis is a viral infection of young dogs.

Animals which recover from one attack are usually resistant to reinfection for life.

Histologically the lesions are papillomatous and acanthotic with thick, squamous epithelium covering thin, branching cores of dermal papillae. The inner core of normal squamous cells is surrounded by greatly enlarged vacuolated "wart cells." Acidophilic inclusions may be found in the cytoplasm and basophilic inclusions in the nuclei.

Since masses of warts make eating and mouth hygiene difficult, treatment is usually attempted to hasten resolution. Surgical removal (electro-desiccation) of the several large masses often stimulates resorption of the rest. Commercial wart vaccines are not consistently effective; however, autogenous vaccines appear to be more reliable. As with any disease which heals spontaneously, accurate evaluation of treatment is difficult. Once improvement begins, progress is remarkably rapid with complete resolution occurring in a few days.

### Suggested Reading

Bruner, D. W., and Gillespie, J. H.: *Hagan's Infectious Diseases of Domestic Animals.* Edit. 5. Cornell University Press, Ithaca, N.Y., 1965.

# FIFTY-SIX

# *Rhabditic Dermatitis*

*Rhabditis strongyloides* is the saprophytic nematode which under favorable conditions causes rhabditic dermatitis (see p. 000). It is a relatively uncommon disease which affects animals contacting infected bedding or soil. The lesions are confined to the abdomen, chest and extremities, areas which normally contact

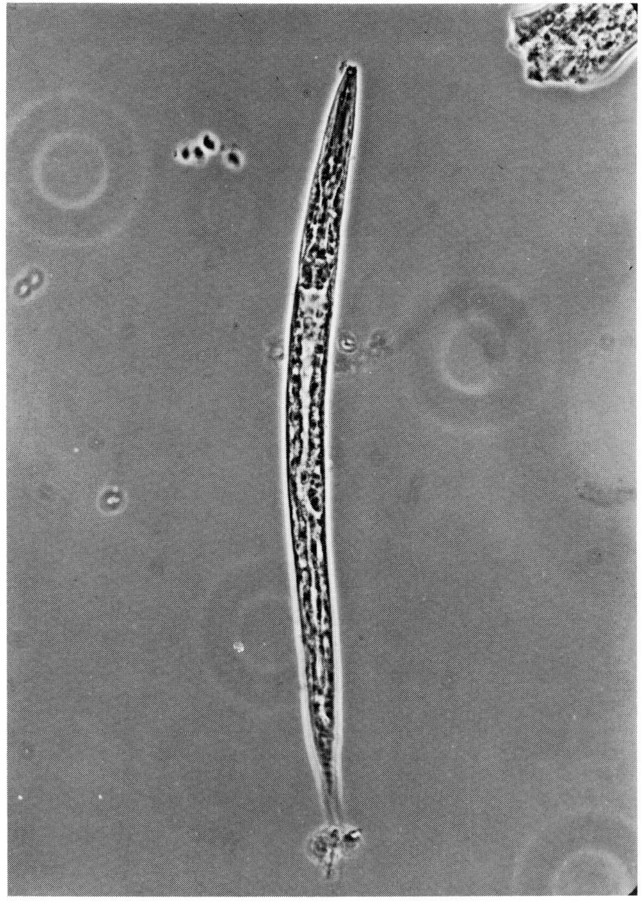

**Figure 56:1.** Larva of *Rhabditis strongyloides*.

the ground. Affected skin is hairless and erythematous, with papules, pustules and, later, scales and crusts. There is intense pruritus. Early lesions may resemble alopecic patches of dermatomycosis or demodectic mange.

Diagnosis is accomplished by observing the easily demonstrated larvae (Fig. 56:1) in skin scrapings from affected tissue. Prophylaxis depends on removal and destruction of the bedding and treatment of the premises with a residual insecticide. The patient should be treated with parasiticidal agents (see Sarcoptic Mange, p. 329). Temporary medication with prednisolone systemically (0.25 mg./lb. b.i.d.) will relieve the itching until the larvae are destroyed.

# SKIN TUMORS

*Section Six*

**Figure 57:1.** Basal cell carcinoma.

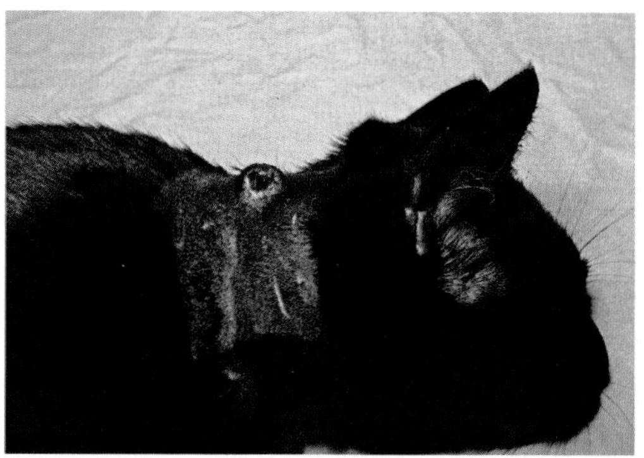

*A.* Firm rubbery nodule (BCC), that has ulcerated.

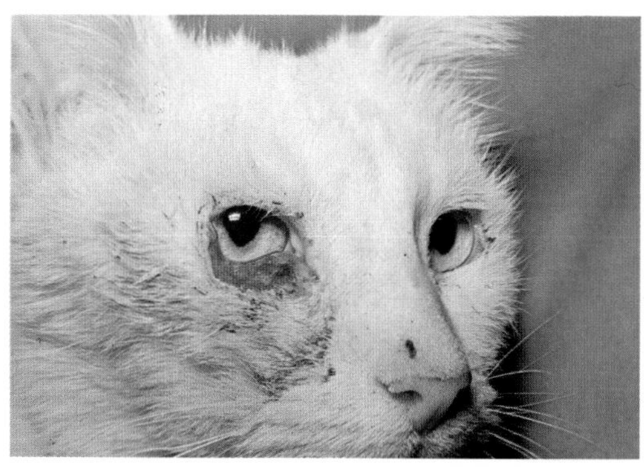

*B.* Basal cell carcinoma of the lower eyelid, a typical location.

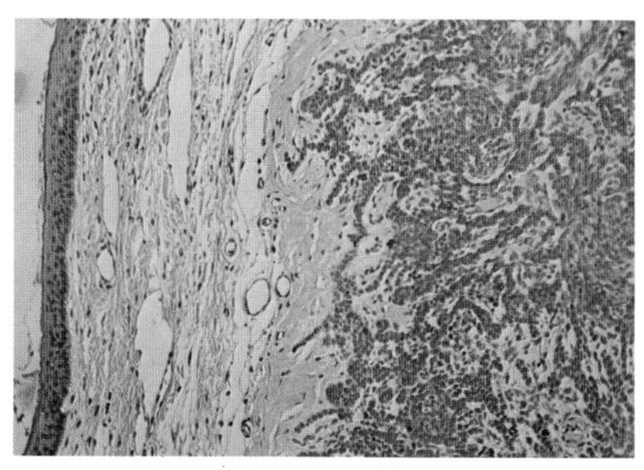

*C.* Cord-like masses of neoplastic basal cells have descended into the dermis. In an adjacent area the tumor cells are continuous with the epidermis. (Low power.)

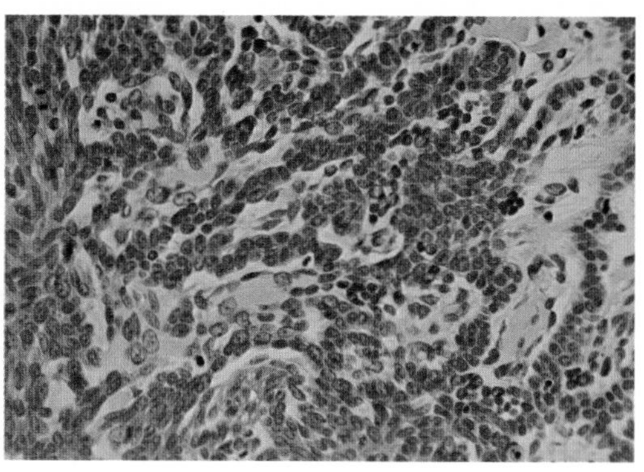

*D.* Higher magnification of *C.* Note the palisade formation of tumor cells whose long axis is at right angles to the axis of the column of cells. (High power.)

# FIFTY-SEVEN

## *Basal Cell Carcinoma*
### *(Basal Cell Tumor, Basal Cell Epithelioma)*

Basal cell carcinoma is a tumor arising from the basal cells of the epidermis, hair follicle or sebaceous gland, with a tendency for local invasion and destruction.

### SIGNIFICANT FACTS

1. This common tumor comprises 6 per cent of all canine and 27 per cent of all feline neoplasms.

2. The tumor is found in adult animals (average age six years) with no solid predilection of sex or breed, although there have been reports of an increased incidence in cocker spaniels and in male dogs.

3. In spite of its name, this tumor never exhibits metastasis.

---

Basal cell carcinomas respond well to surgical excision.

---

### LESIONS AND COURSE

1. Grossly, the tumor is a single, discrete, rounded mass which is rubbery or firm in consistency. It frequently ulcerates (Fig. 57:1*A*) and may be locally invasive into the dermis and subcutis, but it usually does not metastasize.

2. Basal cell carcinomas are most common on the head, especially around the eyes (Fig. 57:1*B*), ears and lips, but they may be found on the neck (Fig. 57:1*A*) and legs.

3. The rate of growth is slow, and they may be present for months without much change in size.

## DIAGNOSTIC AIDS

Although clinical appearance may be suggestive, biopsy or excision and histologic examination are necessary for diagnosis.

## HISTOPATHOLOGY (FIGS. 57:1*C* and *D*)

The neoplastic cells may be connected with normal basal cells of the epidermis. Long loops, festoons or cord-like masses of cells descend into the connective tissue stroma of the dermis and epidermis. The cells in these cords usually are arranged in a palisade formation with the long axis of the cells at right angles to the axis of the column of cells. The tumor cells are uniform, small in size and have ovoid hyperchromatic nuclei. Many mitotic figures are present but generally there are no signs of anaplasia.

The neoplasms arising from basal cells of the hair follicles often form masses of cells resembling hair follicles. These benign tumors are called trichoepitheliomas.

## DIFFERENTIAL DIAGNOSIS

The basal cell carcinoma may be confused with squamous cell carcinoma (which ulcerates earlier and spreads more rapidly) or with chronic ulcers. In its early stages it can be suggestive of papilloma, epidermal cyst, mastocytoma or sebaceous adenoma.

## CLINICAL MANAGEMENT

The treatment of choice is wide surgical excision. This is curative in most cases although local recurrence is possible. Radiation therapy often may be used with good results if surgical removal is impossible.

### *Suggested Reading*

Jubb, K. V. F., and Kennedy, P. C.: *Pathology of Domestic Animals.* Academic Press, New York, 1963.

Moulton, J. E.: *Tumors in Domestic Animals.* University of California Press, Berkeley, 1961.

Muller, G. H.: Basal Cell Epithelioma and Squamous Cell Carcinoma in Animals. Arch. Derm. *96*:386-389, 1967.

# FIFTY-EIGHT

# *Primary Cutaneous Lymphosarcoma*

## *(Malignant Lymphoma with Skin Manifestation)*

Primary cutaneous lymphosarcoma is a fatal malignancy characterized by severe cutaneous lesions that are closely related to lymphomas.

### SIGNIFICANT FACTS

1. This disease differs from disseminated malignant lymphoma because initially it has lesions limited to the skin. In disseminated malignant lymphoma death usually occurs within three months without associated skin lesions.

2. This disease occurs in dogs over five years of age without sex predilection.

### LESIONS AND COURSE

1. The characteristic cutaneous lesions can be present for several months (or years) before the terminal stage of lymphoid involvement begins.

2. The early stage starts with one or more bright erythematous skin patches (Fig. 58:1*B*). These enlarge to form numerous polymorphous plaques that may cover a large part of the body.

3. The skin lesions are pruritic and painful.

4. Superficial white or reddish scales cover the well-demarcated lesions, except where the surface is eroded. Brown crusts form in some areas.

5. Survival is seldom longer than three to six months from the onset of lymph node enlargement. Spontaneous temporary improvement occurs in some cases, but the disease soon continues on its relentless course. In the end there may be fever, vomiting, diarrhea, and dysphagia. Weakness, anorexia and physical collapse are followed by coma and death.

**Figure 58:1.** Primary cutaneous lymphosarcoma.

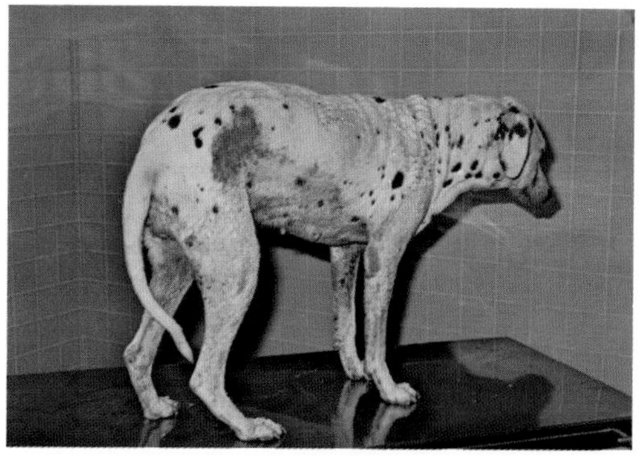

*A.* Characteristic skin lesions can be seen on this critically ill Dalmatian.

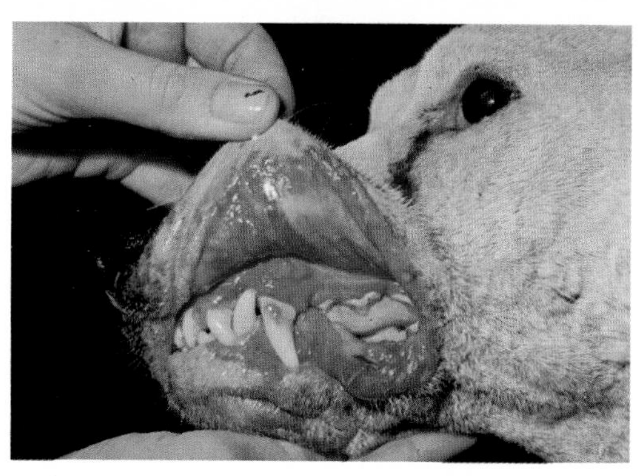

*B.* Ecchymotic hemorrhages on the oral mucosa. Note the mucous eye discharge and anguished expression.

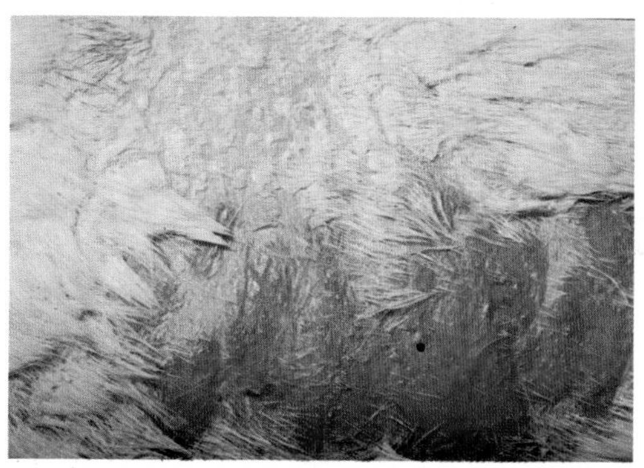

*C.* Erythematous plaque with erosions is surrounded by thin, scaly skin.

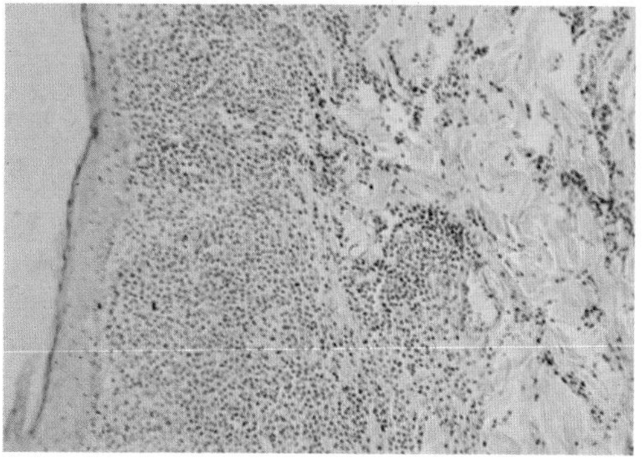

*D.* Neoplastic lymphocytes are packed tightly in the upper dermis. Epidermal surface at left side. (Low power.)

## DIAGNOSTIC AIDS

1. Skin biopsy of a plaque (see Histopathology).
2. Lymph node biopsy reveals lymphosarcoma.
3. The peripheral blood shows no abnormality in lymphocytes. A neutrophilia exists in most advanced cases and there is a normocytic anemia.

## HISTOPATHOLOGY

1. In the skin there is a sharply demarcated massive infiltrate in the upper and lower dermis. This consists of many cell types, and includes numerous histiocytes with nuclei of varying size and shapes. Immature, atypical reticulum cells are present. Mitotic figures are frequent. The infiltrate is so dense in the upper dermis that the entire area appears basophilic (Fig. 58:1*D*).
2. The enlarged lymph nodes show the typical histopathologic changes of lymphosarcoma. The entire node, especially the cortex, is filled with neoplastic lymphocytic cells that are larger than normal and have eccentrically placed prominent nuclei.

## DIFFERENTIAL DIAGNOSIS

1. Eczematous reactions to highly pruritic dermatoses (such as allergic dermatitis) may resemble cutaneous lymphosarcoma. Such reactions, however, respond favorably to corticosteroids.

## CLINICAL MANAGEMENT

This rare malignancy terminates fatally after a short course.

1. Early diagnosis, confirmed by skin and lymph node biopsies, is important so that the client realizes that improvement of the skin lesions cannot be expected and that the disease terminates fatally. Wet dressings and submerged baths will give slight relief.
2. In human patients with mycosis fungoides (a disease somewhat comparable to canine cutaneous lymphosarcoma) two treatments have been used: electron beam radiation and topical nitrogen mustard (mechlorethamine hydrochloride—Mustargen, Merck). Although at the time of this writing these treatments have not been used on canine patients, they present hope for the future.

### *References*

Arundel, F. D., and Chan, W. H.: Mycosis Fungoides—Topical Use of Nitrogen Mustard in Recurrent Cases. Calif. Med., *109*:458-461, 1968.

Haserick, J. R., and Richardson, J. H.: Remission of Lesions in Mycosis Fungoides Following Topical Application of Nitrogen Mustard. Cleveland Clinic Quarterly, Vol. 25, No. 3:144-147, 1959.

# FIFTY-NINE

## *Fibrosarcoma*

Fibrosarcoma is a malignant tumor of fibroblasts that is common in older dogs. It most often affects the mammary gland, gingiva, tongue, face (Fig. 59:1*A*) and legs. Small, firm painless nodules appear which may grow slowly for one or two years. Later they grow rapidly, and compress the surrounding tissue to form a pseudocapsule. The tumor is highly vascular and hemorrhage and ulceration is common. It is highly invasive locally, and metastasizes to the lungs.

Microscopically there are indiscriminate whorls of collagenous fibers and bundles of immature fibroblasts (Fig. 59:1*B*). The pleomorphic fusiform or polygonal tumor cells have oval hyperchromic nuclei and multiple nucleoli. Mitotic figures are common.

---

The prognosis is poor, since wide local invasion and metastasis are common.

---

The tumor is radioresistant, so *wide* surgical excision is the best treatment. If regional lymph nodes are enlarged they should be removed at the same time.

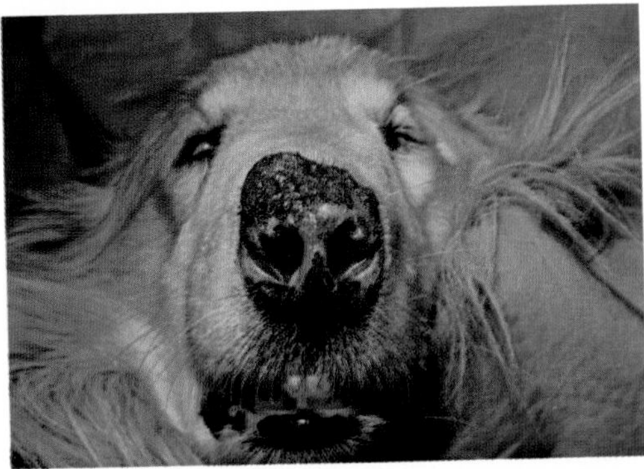

**Figure 59:1.** Fibrosarcoma.

*A.* Grossly deformed nose from fibrosarcoma. The patient also has nasal solar dermatitis.

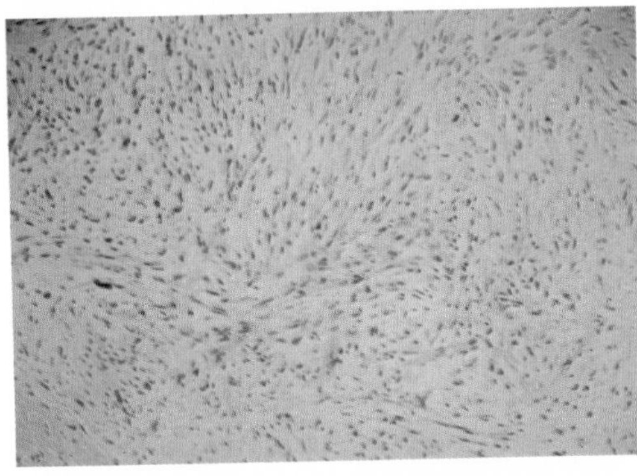

*B.* Histologic section of *A* shows swirls and an interlocking pattern of fibroblasts and fibers. (Low power.)

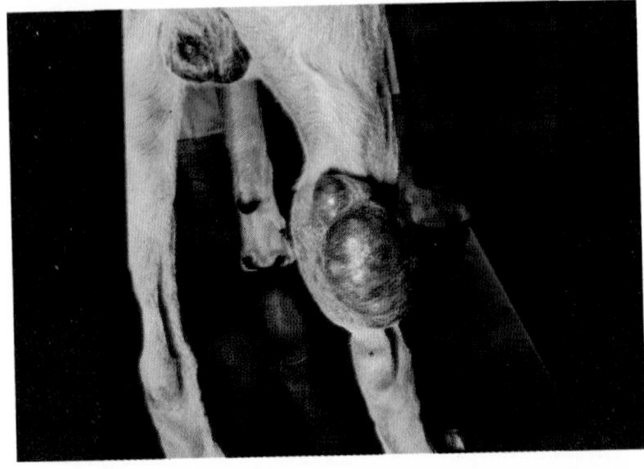

**Figure 60:1.** Neurofibroma. *(See page 369)*

*A.* This large mass recurred after two previous surgical excisions. (Courtesy G. E. Ross.)

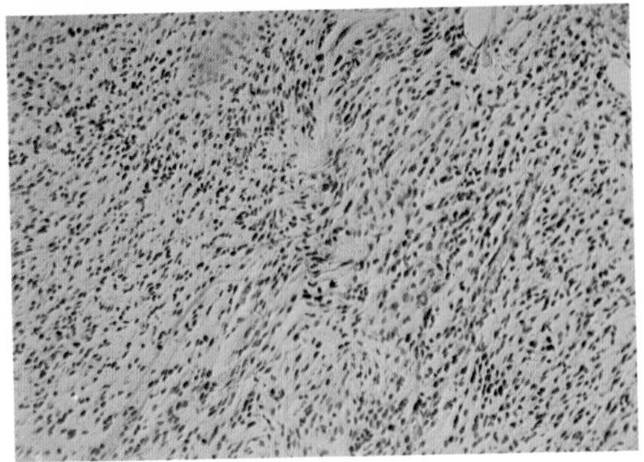

*B.* Histologic section of *A* showing interlacing bundles of cells and fibers with a palisading arrangement of nuclei. (Low power.)

# SIXTY

## *Neurofibroma*

Neurofibroma is a tumor arising from the nerve sheath cells; it may be benign, or malignant (neurofibrosarcoma). The fox terrier breed is predisposed to these tumors, which tend to occur on the skin of the back, chest and limbs. The lesions appear as firm well-defined multilobulated nodules which, in the benign form, are small and may disappear spontaneously. Although metastasis is rare, the malignant types grow rapidly and form large masses. This form of the tumor commonly recurs after surgical excision (Fig. 60:1*A*).

Microscopically, the neoplastic Schwann cells and multiple fibers form interlacing bundles and whorls (Fig. 60:1*B*). The whorls and laminations of tumor cells produce a palisading of nuclei, and this is an important point of differentiation from fibroma and hemangiopericytoma. The neurofibrosarcoma differs from the neurofibroma in that it has less fiber formation and is more cellular, with larger, more pleomorphic cells. Mitotic figures are common.

---

Neurofibromas may disappear spontaneously, or they may recur following excision.

---

Complete surgical excision is the treatment of choice.

# SIXTY-ONE

## *Histiocytoma*

### *(Transmissible Reticulum Cell Tumor, Button Tumor)*

A histiocytoma is a rapid-growing dermal tumor composed of histiocytes. It has a characteristic appearance and is found almost exclusively in young dogs.

### SIGNIFICANT FACTS

1. The histiocytoma is characterized as a neoplasm by most authorities although some believe it is an unusual inflammation.
2. It arises from histiocytes of the dermis and subcutis of young dogs, and is very rarely seen in cats.
3. There is no regrowth or metastasis and the tumor is usually classified as benign.

### LESIONS AND COURSE (FIG. 61:1*A*, *B* and *C*)

1. The gross appearance is characteristic, a small domed or button-like, circumscribed, solitary nodule. It is of firm consistency and fixed in the skin. The surface may be pink colored or ulcerated, and it usually is hairless.
2. Site predilection is not constant and they may be found on the face, lips, ears, legs, neck and abdomen.
3. This tumor grows rapidly (one to four weeks) and has been observed to regress spontaneously. Although malignancy is suggested by the rapid growth and presence of mitotic figures, it does not exhibit metastasis.

### DIAGNOSTIC AIDS

Although clinical appearance may be suggestive, biopsy or excision and histologic examination are necessary for diagnosis.

**Figure 61:1.** Histiocytoma.

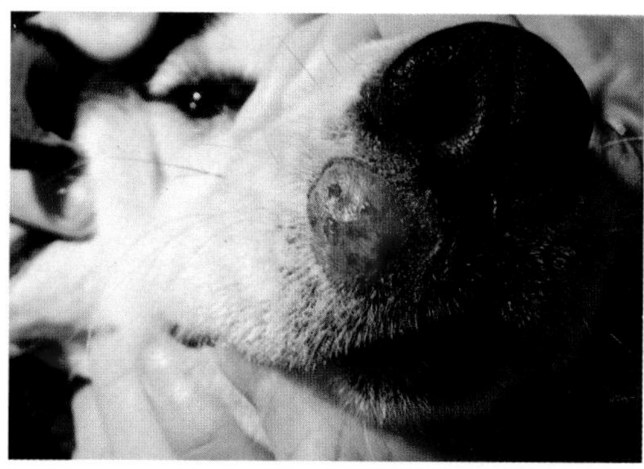

*A.* Typical location and appearance of histiocytoma. Note hairless surface with crusted exudate.

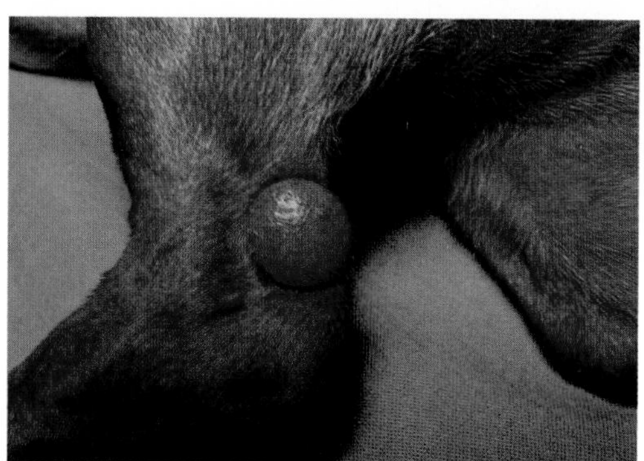

*B.* Firm, circumscribed solitary nodule in the characteristic "button" shape.

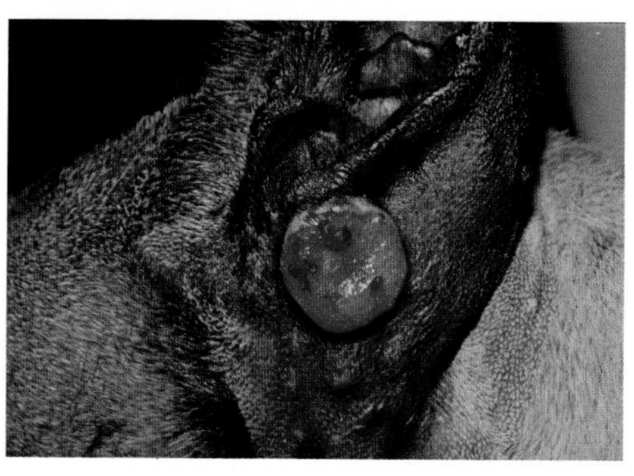

*C.* Large ulcerated histiocytoma at the base of the ear of a young Great Dane.

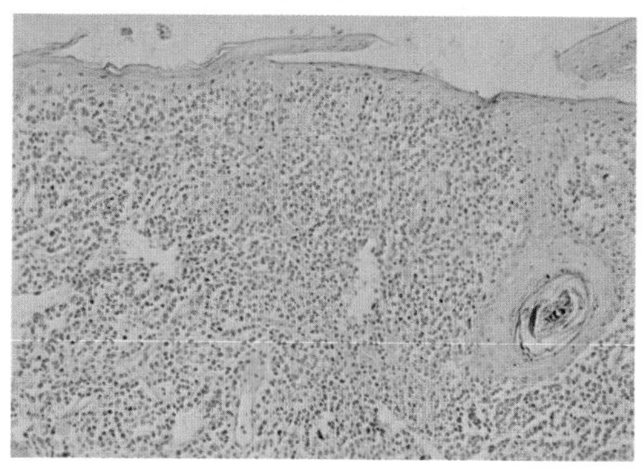

*D.* Histologic section showing normal skin, a hair follicle, blood vessels and masses of relatively uniform cellular elements which somewhat resemble inflammation. (Low power.)

## HISTOPATHOLOGY (FIG. 61:1*D*)

1. At low power the histiocytoma somewhat resembles an inflammatory exudate.

2. Under high power the neoplastic histiocytes widely infiltrate the dermis and hypodermis, clustering around the dermal adnexa and bundles of collagen fibrils. A few mast cells, plasma cells and mature neutrophils are mixed with the tumor cells and there is no definite encapsulation or line of demarcation of tumor tissue. The histiocytes have finely granular, acidophilic cytoplasm and large round nuclei with a solitary nucleolus and a uniform chromatin network. Characteristically there are many regular mitotic figures.

## DIFFERENTIAL DIAGNOSIS

There are several tumors which some authorities group together. These are mastocytoma, transmissible venereal tumor, reticulum cell sarcoma and lymphosarcoma. In most cases, history, clinical location and appearance, and histologic morphology will serve to differentiate these tumors. A circular plaque of dermatomycosis, secondarily infected, may resemble a histiocytoma.

## CLINICAL MANAGEMENT

The treatment of choice is local excision. This is simple and effective therapy.

### *Suggested Reading*

Moulton, J. E.: *Tumors in Domestic Animals.* University of California Press, Berkeley, 1961.

Mulligan, R. M.: *Neoplasms of the Dog.* Williams & Wilkins Co., Baltimore, 1949.

Ross, G. E.: Skin Tumors. *In* Kirk, R. W. (Ed.): *Current Veterinary Therapy III.* W. B. Saunders Co., Philadelphia, 1968.

# SIXTY-TWO

# *Mastocytoma*

## *(Mastocytosis, Mast Cell Tumor)*

Mastocytoma is a common dermal tumor of mesenchymal origin consisting of accumulations of mast cells.

### SIGNIFICANT FACTS

1. Mastocytoma constitutes about 13 per cent of cutaneous canine neoplasms. There is no sex predilection, but it affects older dogs (six years or more) and especially the Boston terrier and boxer breeds.

2. These tumors contain large quantities of histamine, hyaluronic acid and heparin, but there is only one report of hemorrhagic tendencies in affected animals. This involved hemorrhage following surgical excision of the tumor. The bleeding was controlled promptly by parenteral antihistamines.

3. This tumor (in the form of mast cell leukemia) has been transmitted in dogs by injections of cell free filtrates.

---

Excise mastocytomas early—they are potentially malignant.

---

### LESIONS AND COURSE

1. Lesions first appear as isolated firm nodules in the skin (Fig. 62:1*A*). They may enlarge slowly over a period of years, gradually softening and becoming poorly demarcated. The hair on the surface is sparse and may appear like "pin feathers."

2. Approximately 45 per cent of mastocytomas are found on the rear legs, perineum or external genitalia (Fig. 62:1*B*), perhaps because there are areas of normally high mast cell population.

3. After a long quiescent period some mastocytomas begin rapid growth

**Figure 62:1.** Mastocytoma.

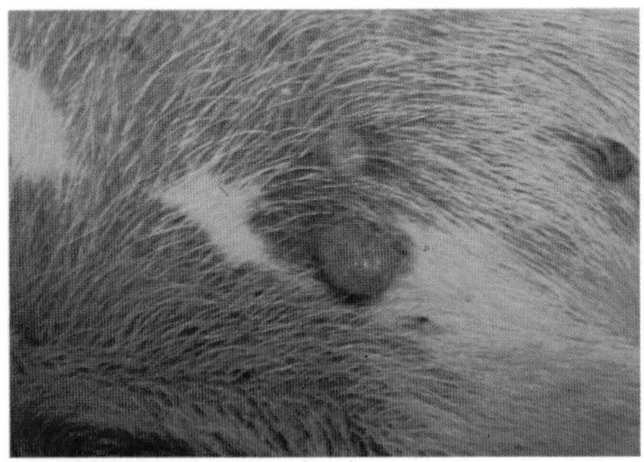

*A.* Initial mastocytoma lesion may be quiescent for many years.

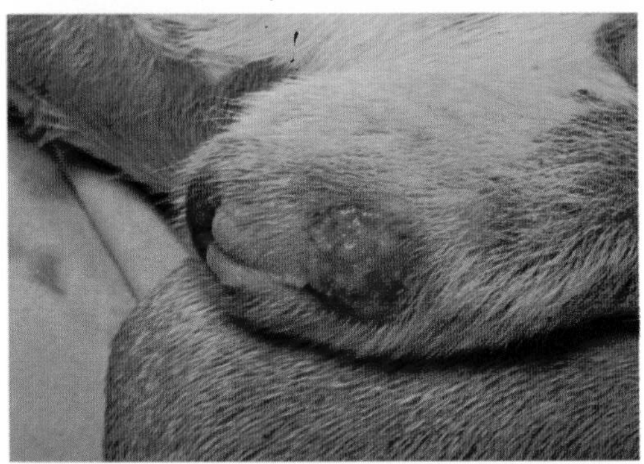

*B.* Mastocytoma on the sheath, a typical location.

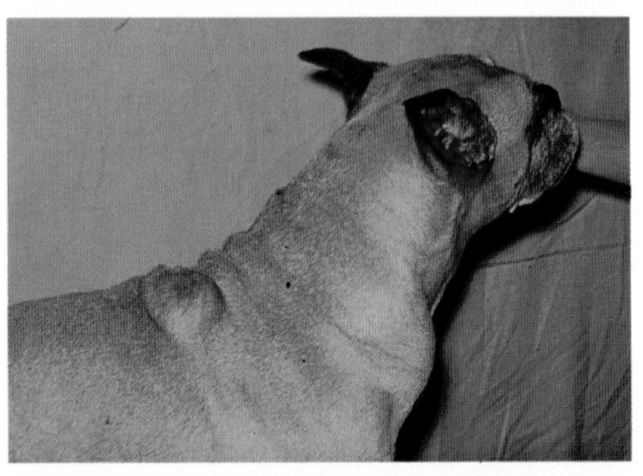

*C.* With generalized mastocytosis multiple lesions appear. They are fast-growing, firm or edematous, and spread rapidly.

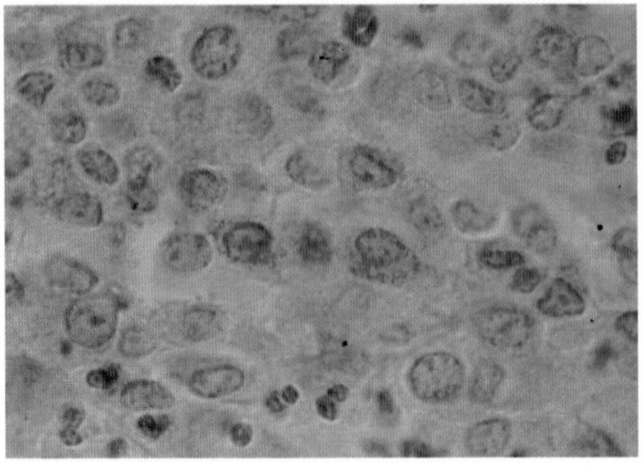

*D.* Histologic section of mastocytoma stained with toluidine blue. Note reddish purple staining cytoplasmic granules. (High power, oil immersion.)

(Fig. 62:1*C*). They become edematous, may ulcerate and spread by local infiltration; and in 10 to 20 per cent of malignant cases they may metastasize via the lymph and blood.

4. Approximately 17 per cent of these tumors recur after surgical removal, and the new growth is often more anaplastic than the original tumor.

## DIAGNOSTIC AIDS

Although clinical appearance may be suggestive, biopsy or excision and histologic examination are necessary for positive diagnosis.

## HISTOPATHOLOGY (FIG. 62:1*D*)

1. The typical mastocytoma forms sheets or cords of discrete, uniformly ovoid or polygonal cells. The infiltrate occupies the dermis and hypodermis, pushing aside connective tissue and surrounding blood vessels and epidermal appendages. Eosinophils and a few plasma cells, lymphocytes and neutrophils are mixed with tumor cells. The latter have a vesicular, central, oval nucleus and numerous cytoplasmic granules. These granules are characteristic of the mast cell and are demonstrated best with special stains. Toluidine blue stains them reddish purple (Fig. 62:1*D*); and they may be so numerous as to obscure cellular detail.

2. The atypical mastocytoma appears more malignant histologically, with anisocytosis and frequent mitotic figures. The cellular cytoplasm is reduced, and the granules are smaller, lighter staining and fewer in number. These tumors may be more malignant clinically.

## DIFFERENTIAL DIAGNOSIS

These tumors are often characteristic, but may need to be differentiated from histiocytoma, fibroma, early basal cell carcinoma and epidermal cysts.

## CLINICAL MANAGEMENT

1. Because of the malignant potentiality, this tumor should be removed by wide surgical excision at the earliest possible time. This is usually curative.

2. If the tumor recurs, or the initial surgery is performed after local invasion has started, the regional lymph nodes should be dissected and radiation therapy applied to the tumor site.

3. In inoperable mastocytomas, radiation therapy is helpful, as the tumor is radiosensitive.

4. With metastatic or advanced cases, large daily doses of systemic corticosteroids usually cause a temporary regression for several months.

### *Suggested Reading*

Moulton, J. E.: *Tumors in Domestic Animals.* University of California Press, Berkeley, 1961.

Orkin, M., and Schwartzman, R. M.: A Comparative Study of Canine and Human Dermatology: II. Cutaneous Tumors—The Mast Cell and Canine Mastocytoma. J. Invest. Derm. *32*:451-466, 1966.

# SIXTY-THREE

# *Melanoma*

A melanoma is a benign or malignant tumor composed of cells capable of forming melanosomes or premelanosomes. It may lack pigment, or have abundant uniform or mottled pigmentation.

## SIGNIFICANT FACTS

1. Conroy (1967) has divided the common benign melanomas into compound nevus, dermal nevus (Fig. 63:1*A*) and dermal melanocytoma.

The compound nevus has nests of nevus (tumor) cells in the epidermis and dermis. It is a smooth, darkly pigmented, nodular canine tumor commonly found around the eyes, although it is also present near the lips, anus and toes.

The dermal nevus' cells usually are fairly well restricted to the dermis, although some areas may show epidermal involvement.

The dermal melanocytoma (blue nevus) arises from dermal or adnexal melanocytes which have not migrated to the epidermis, but proliferate in the connective tissue.

2. Canine melanomas are most common in heavily pigmented individuals (especially Airedale, Scottish and Boston terriers, and spaniels), and predominantly in males.

3. In dogs the majority of melanomas of the mouth are malignant, but the majority of skin melanomas are benign.

## LESIONS AND COURSE

1. Benign melanomas (Fig. 63:1*A*) are small, slow-growing, well-delineated, often pedunculated hairless growths that usually are darkly pigmented. Although there are reports of malignancy developing from a benign lesion this is apparently rare. The tumors may persist for months or years without change.

2. Malignant melanomas are larger, dome-shaped, sessile growths that vary in color depending on the amount of pigment they contain. They metastasize early by way of blood or lymph channels, and are associated with high mortality. The regional lymph nodes and lungs are affected first, but widespread metastasis to other areas is common. Melanomas of the mouth (Fig. 63:1*C*) and feet are commonly malignant. The course from early diagnosis to death is often only several months.

**Figure 63:1.** Melanoma.

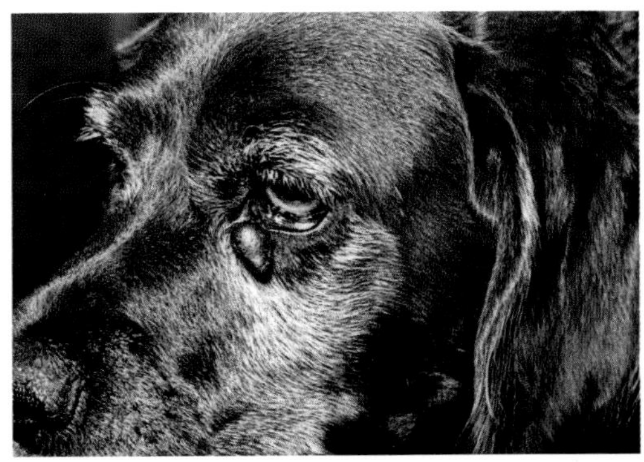

*A.* Benign melanoma (dermal nevus) in cocker spaniel.

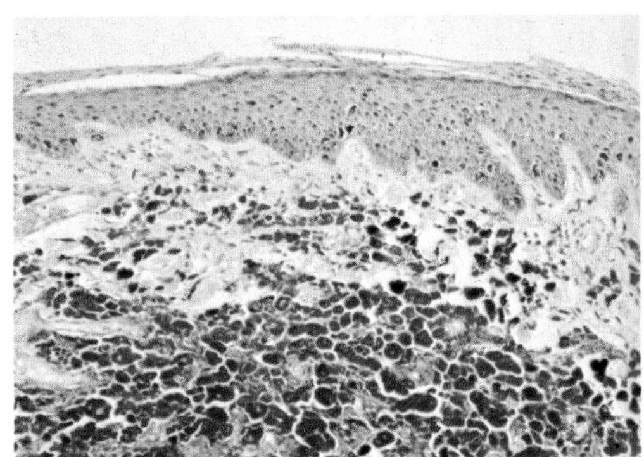

*B.* Histologic section of *A* showing acanthotic epidermis with masses of heavily pigmented benign tumor cells in the dermis. (Low power.)

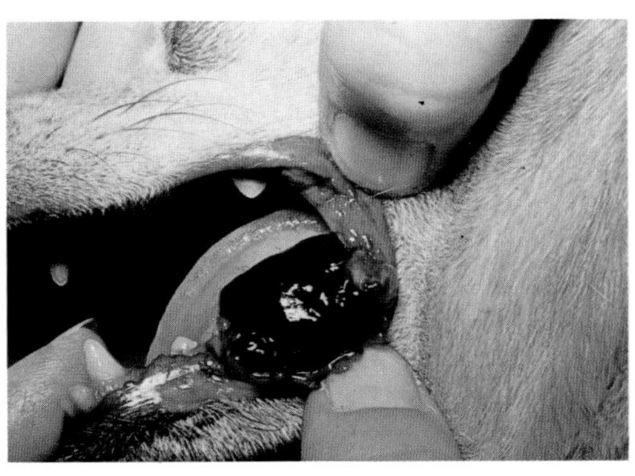

*C.* Malignant melanomas are commonly located in the oral region.

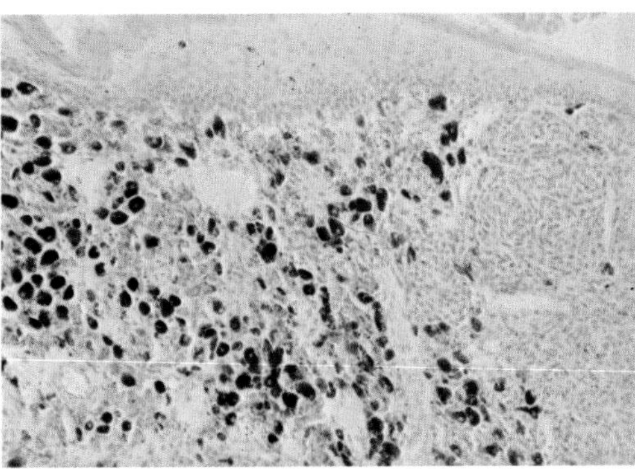

*D.* Histologic section of *C* shows mucosa of the tongue. There are many bizarre cells with variable nuclear detail and amounts of pigment. Mitotic figures are not demonstrable at this magnification. (Low power.)

## DIAGNOSTIC AIDS

Although clinical appearance may be suggestive, histologic examination of the excised tumor is necessary for diagnosis.

## HISTOPATHOLOGY

1. Benign melanomas (Fig. 63:1*B*) are covered by an acanthotic epidermis that contains more melanin than adjacent skin. The nevus cells are polyhedral, stubby or spindle-shaped, and arranged in solid masses or lobules. The cells may be compacted and overlapping or palisaded, and the nuclei are of uniform size and oval or round in shape. Dendritic cells with melanin-laden processes may intermingle with the nevus cells. If melanin pigment is abundant, bleaching may be needed to observe cellular detail.

2. Malignant melanomas (Fig. 63:1*C*) have numerous polyhedral or stubby spindle cells, but dendritic forms are rare. The cells are more loosely arranged, much larger and have only small amounts of cytoplasm. The swollen nuclei are warped and contain irregular patches of chromatin. There are often two or more prominent nucleoli and bizarre mitotic figures. Areas of necrosis and hemorrhage, and tumor invasion of adipose tissue, skeletal muscle, lymphatics and vessels all contribute to the picture of malignancy.

## DIFFERENTIAL DIAGNOSIS

1. The main diagnostic problem is to decide between malignant and nonmalignant forms. However, fibroma, lentigo, and verruca must be considered. Some highly anaplastic malignant melanomas contain little pigment and are extremely confusing at the initial examination.

## CLINICAL MANAGEMENT

Melanomas of the mouth and feet are usually malignant.

1. Small, quiescent, pigmented nodules should be widely excised and submitted for histologic diagnosis. Patients having malignant melanomas should return for regional lymph node dissection.

2. Large, growing, dome-shaped nodules should be widely excised without delay; and the regional lymph nodes should be dissected. Both tumor and nodes should be sumitted for histologic diagnosis. Chest radiographs should be obtained to check metastasis or to provide a basis for comparison with future radiographs.

### *Suggested Reading*

Conroy, J. D.: Melanocytic Tumors of Domestic Animals. Arch. Derm. *96*: 372-380, 1967.

Moulton, J. E.: *Tumors of Domestic Animals.* University of California Press, Berkeley, 1961, pp. 56-59.

Mulligan, R. M.: *Neoplasms of the Dog.* Williams & Wilkins Co., Baltimore, 1949.

# SIXTY-FOUR

## *Perianal Gland Tumors*

### *(Circumanal Gland Tumors, Adenomas or Carcinomas)*

Perianal gland tumors are common, relatively innocuous neoplasms of the specialized sebaceous glands surrounding the anus of dogs.

## SIGNIFICANT FACTS

1. These usually involve aged dogs (eight years or more) of the cocker spaniel and fox terrier breeds although any breed can be affected.
2. Only dogs are afflicted.
3. It is rare to find this tumor in females (90 per cent are males).
4. The specialized sebaceous-type cells of the perianal glands have no known function. Similar cells are found on the underside of the tail and adjacent to the prepuce, and they, too, may develop neoplasia.
5. Although adenomas and carcinomas are sometimes observed, the malignancy of the carcinoma is low.

---

Sex hormones influence perianal adenomas.

---

## LESIONS AND COURSE

1. The adenomas are small, slow-growing, single or multiple, firm nodules. They are located close to the anus, and the overlying skin is frequently ulcerated (Fig. 64:1*A*).
2. Carcinomas may appear to be similar at first, but they grow rapidly and are usually much larger when first observed, so that they may bleed or interfere with defecation.
3. The course of either type is benign, and although the carcinoma may be somewhat invasive locally, it practically never shows metastasis.

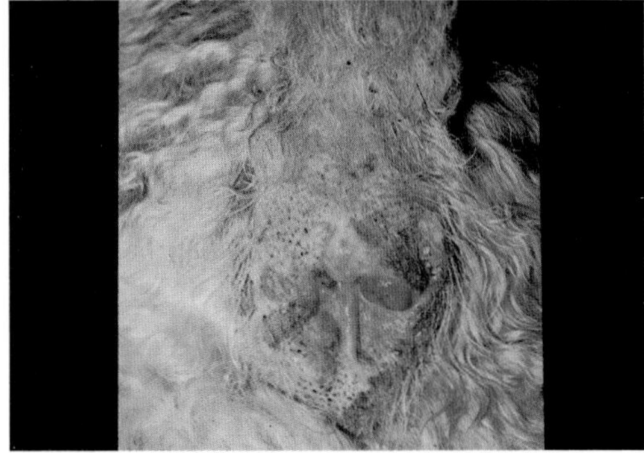

**Figure 64:1.** Perianal gland tumors.

*A.* Perianal adenoma with ulceration in an aged wire-haired fox terrier.

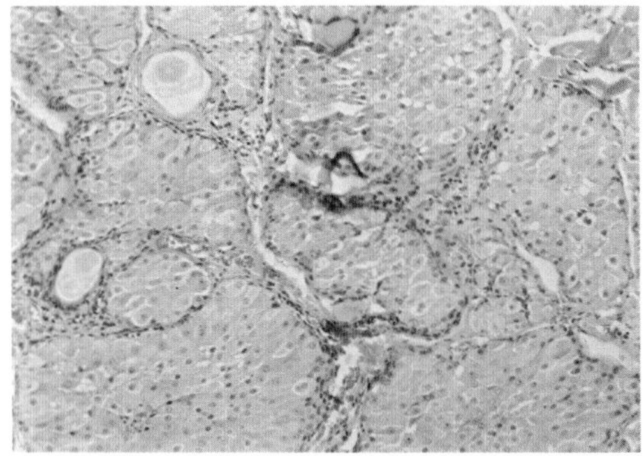

*B.* Histologic section of *A* showing polyhedral cells arranged in lobules in proximity to vessels. The lobules are surrounded by dark staining "reserve cells." (High power.)

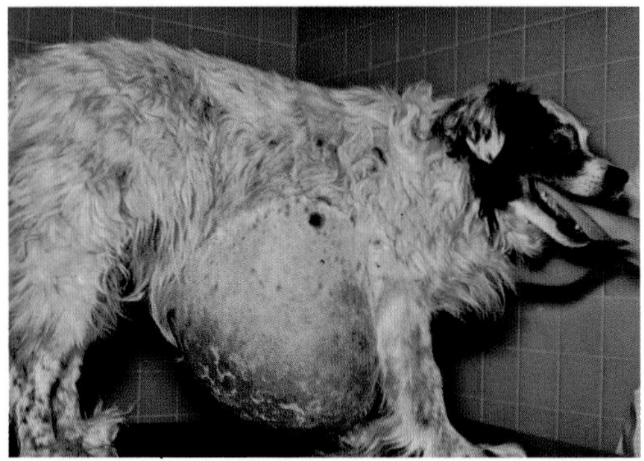

**Figure 65:1.** Lipoma. *(See page 382)*

*A.* Huge subcutaneous lipoma in an aged spaniel. Repeated trauma to the distended skin may cause secondary erythema and ulceration. Lipomas grow slowly. Surgical excision is usually easy because the tumor has a thin capsule and is relatively avascular.

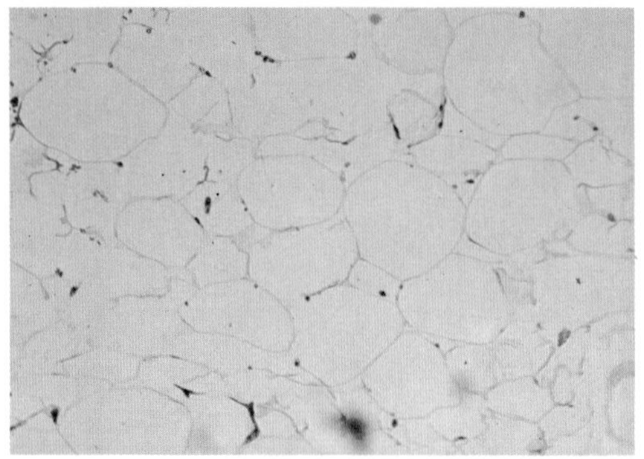

*B.* Histologic section of *A.* (High power.)

## DIAGNOSTIC AIDS

Although the clinical appearance is particularly characteristic in most cases, histologic examination is necessary for a positive diagnosis.

## HISTOPATHOLOGY (FIG. 64:1*B*)

1. The neoplastic cells of the adenoma are arranged in cords or large masses which are often aggregated into lobules. Some cells may be transformed into columnar types and arranged in duct-like structures. Others are compressed or spindle-shaped and surround laminated or hyaline bodies which resemble "pearls" of the squamous cell carcinoma. The typical tumor cells are large, polyhedral-shaped with finely granular cytoplasm and round central nuclei. "Reserve cells" are located at the periphery of the masses of tumor cells. They appear as a single row of small indistinct cells.

The stroma of the tumor is delicate connective tissue which supports many thin-walled blood vessels and lymphatics. Inflammatory cells, hemorrhage and cholesterol clefts are commonly observed.

The carcinomas are more disorderly in their growth and cell types are not well differentiated. There is invasion of vessels and lymphatics, but mitotic figures are rare. It is often difficult to distinguish between benign and malignant perianal tumors.

## DIFFERENTIAL DIAGNOSIS

This is rarely a problem, although fibromas, verrucae and mastocytomas in the region may resemble this tumor.

## CLINICAL MANAGEMENT

1. The best treatment usually is complete surgical excision.

2. Simultaneous castration is highly effective in the prevention of recurrence, or of new tumor formation.

3. The tumors are highly radiosensitive, and tumor doses of 1000 to 2000 R are adequate treatment for the benign forms. Higher doses may be necessary for the carcinoma.

4. Diethylstilbestrol or E.C.P. may cause tumor regression, but it is a temporary measure, as regrowth may appear when the therapy is withdrawn. This therapy may be useful prior to surgery to reduce the mass of the tumor, or in cases where surgery is impossible.

### *Suggested Reading*

Moulton, J. C.: *Tumors in Domestic Animals.* University of California Press, Berkeley, 1961.

Mulligan, R. M.: *Neoplasms of the Dog.* Williams & Wilkins Co., Baltimore, 1949.

# SIXTY-FIVE

## *Lipoma*

Lipoma in an aged spaniel is shown on page 380. Repeated trauma to the distended skin may cause secondary erythema and ulceration. Lipomas grow slowly and surgical excision usually presents no difficulty because the tumor has a thin capsule and is relatively avascular.

# SIXTY-SIX

# *Sertoli Cell Tumor*

Sertoli cell tumor of the testis sometimes causes marked skin changes and feminization.

## SIGNIFICANT FACTS

1. It usually occurs in retained testis, but may also occur in scrotal testes. The uninvolved testes are usually atrophied (Fig. 66:1*D*).
2. Most cases are found in dogs six years of age or older.
3. The cause of the dermatologic changes is an excess production of estrogenic hormones by the neoplastic Sertoli cells.
4. There is no consistent relationship between the size of the tumor and its ability to secrete significant amounts of estrogen.

Not all dogs with Sertoli cell tumor have alopecia and skin lesions.

## LESIONS AND COURSE

1. Hyperpigmented macules and patches of the skin are contrasted by seemingly depigmented areas in the genital area and flanks (Fig. 66:1*A*). The skin is thinner than normal in the affected areas.
2. Bilaterally symmetrical alopecia occurs in the genital area and in advanced cases in many other parts of the body (Fig. 66:2). In extremely chronic cases, almost all body hair may be lost except for a strip along the topline.
3. There is gynecomastia; in some cases the nipples resemble those of lactating females (Fig. 66:1*B*).
4. There is a lack of normal male libido, and some dogs with a Sertoli cell tumor will be attractive to other males (similar to a bitch in estrus).
5. The skin is dry, and in advanced cases the hair becomes brittle, epilates easily and is not replaced.

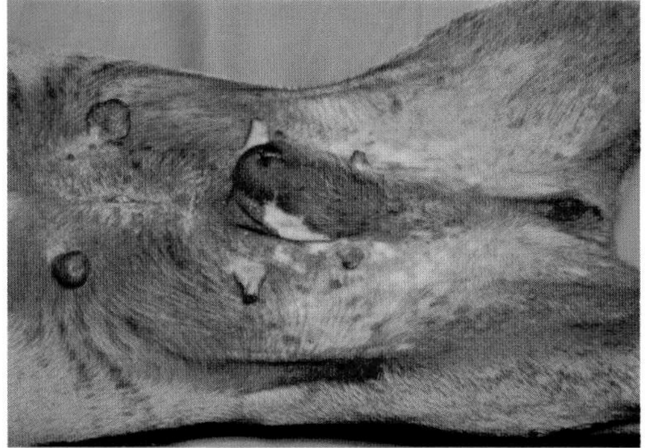

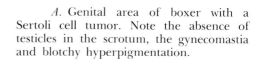

**Figure 66:1.** Sertoli cell tumor.

*A.* Genital area of boxer with a Sertoli cell tumor. Note the absence of testicles in the scrotum, the gynecomastia and blotchy hyperpigmentation.

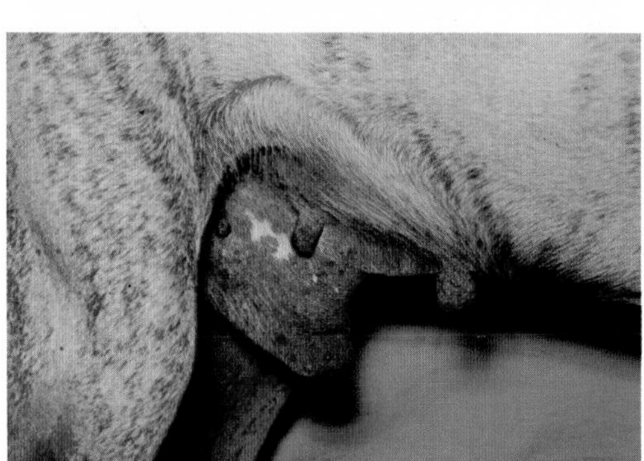

*B.* Lateral view of *A.*

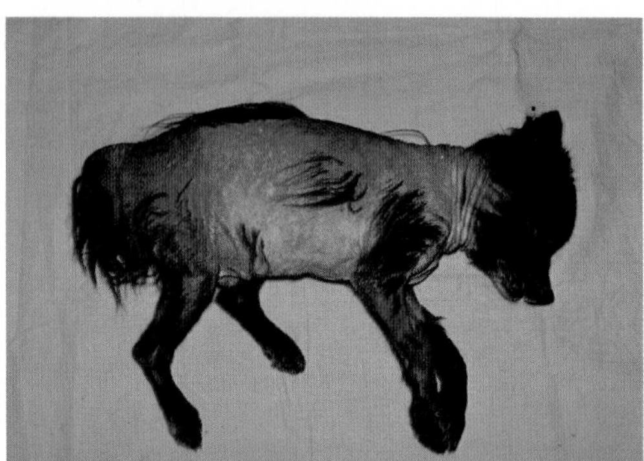

*C.* Pomeranian, whose death was caused by Sertoli cell tumor 8 cm. in diameter. Note the distribution pattern of the alopecia in this extremely advanced case.

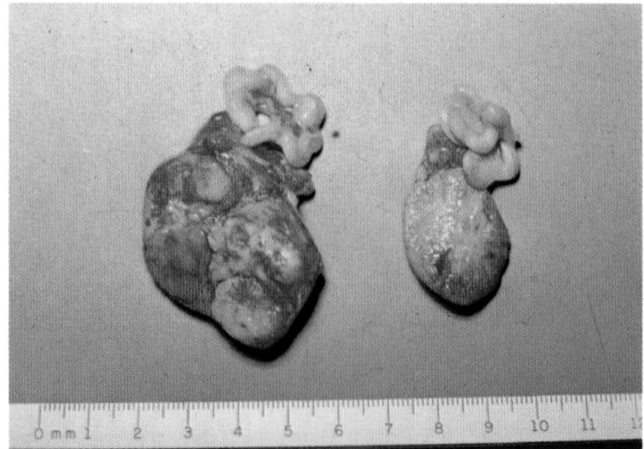


*D.* Cryptorchid testes removed surgically from dog in *A.* The left testis is neoplastic whereas the right testis is atrophied.

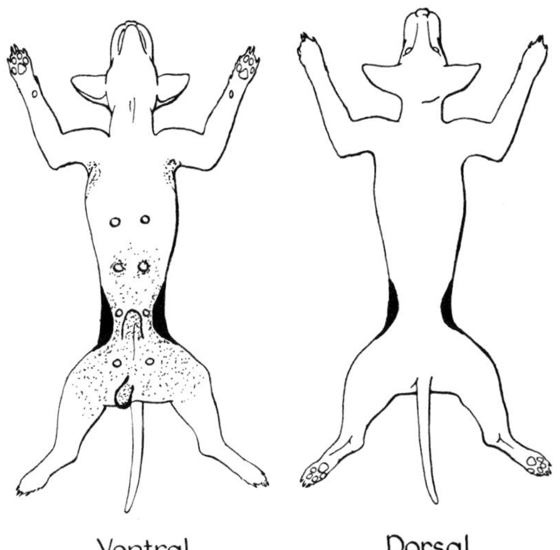


**Figure 66:2.** Sertoli cell tumor distribution pattern.

6. In early cases, skin changes are present, but there is no cachexia. As the tumor grows, the dog becomes ill and loses weight.

7. In the final stages of the disease, the dog becomes emaciated and depressed.

8. Metastasis occurs occasionally, but the primary tumor also can cause death through necrosis and toxemia.

## DIAGNOSTIC AIDS

1. Histopathologic examination of the involved testes reveals the Sertoli cell tumor.

2. Assay of the urine shows high levels of estrogen.

## HISTOPATHOLOGY

1. Skin changes consist of thinning of the epidermis, hyperkeratosis and hyperpigmentation. The surface is wavy and there are degenerative follicular changes.

2. The testicular tubules are markedly displaced and altered by masses of neoplastic tissue consisting of Sertoli cells. These cells have indistinct cytoplasmic outlines, and their small individual nuclei have a prominent basophilic chromatin pattern. Mitotic figures are frequent. Masses of necrotic cells are often found in the center of the tubules.

## DIFFERENTIAL DIAGNOSIS

1. Male feminizing syndrome (hypoandrogenism) usually occurs in male dogs with two grossly normal scrotal testes. There is more lichenification of the

flanks and more ceruminous otitis. Both testes are flaccid but contain no tumors.

2. With other endocrine imbalances, the alopecia occurs in other parts of the body in addition to the genital area. There is no gynecomastia.

## CLINICAL MANAGEMENT

1. Surgical removal of the tumorous testes.

2. Maintenance dose of testosterone (Halotestin) 0.2 mg. orally/lb. of body weight weekly until all skin changes have disappeared. Gynecomastia cannot be reversed and will remain.

## *Suggested Reading*

Moulton, J. E.: *Tumors of Domestic Animals.* University of California Press, Berkeley, 1961, pp. 153-157.

# SIXTY-SEVEN

# *Squamous Cell Carcinoma*

Squamous cell carcinoma is a malignant epidermoid tumor of squamous epithelial cells that arises from the cutaneous surface.

## SIGNIFICANT FACTS

1. This is a common neoplasm affecting older dogs.

2. It may arise spontaneously, but is often the end result of chronic irritation from coal or oil products, arsenicals, heat ionizing radiation or solar irritation. The latter results in chronic nasal solar dermatitis (p. 305) or feline solar dermatitis (p. 283), either of which may develop into squamous cell carcinoma.

## LESIONS AND COURSE

1. Lesions commonly are found on the head, ears, nose and neck of cats; and on the trunk, toes, scrotum and lips of dogs. Although older animals usually are affected, there is a wide age range. There is no sex or breed predilection.

2. This tumor appears as a raised, indurated plaque that spreads rapidly. It is firm, but ulcerates early and grows to a cauliflower or crater-like mass with a necrotic odor. Its cut surface is granular gray or yellowish white and the edge is not well demarcated.

3. Although it rapidly spreads by local invasion its metastasis is uncertain. Tumors of the feline ear tip rarely metastasize, but those of other regions may metastasize late in the course, spreading to regional lymph nodes and occasionally to the lungs.

## DIAGNOSTIC AIDS

Although clinical appearance may be suggestive, biopsy or excision and histologic examination are necessary for diagnosis.

**Figure 67:1.** Squamous cell carcinoma.

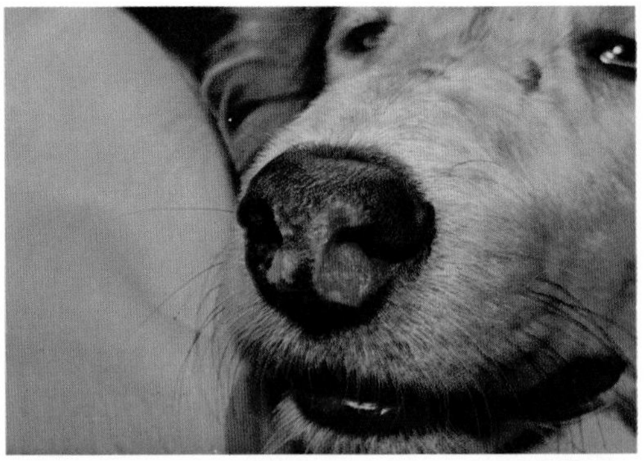

*A.* Squamous cell carcinoma inside the left nostril of a collie, with area of depigmentation of the nasal tip. Surgical removal resulted in complete recovery.

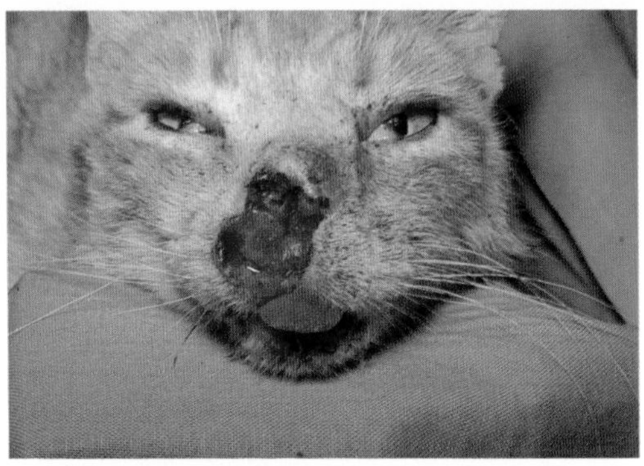

*B.* Squamous cell carcinoma that started in the nasal mucosa and became locally invasive. Highly resistant to therapy.

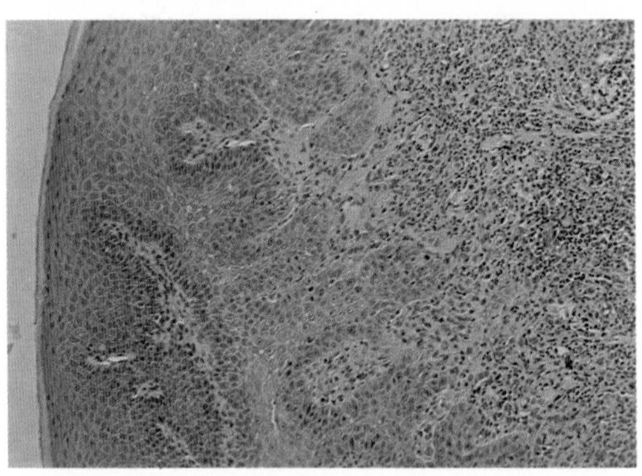

*C.* Squamous cell carcinoma. Masses of mature epidermal cells have invaded the dermis and are surrounded by a dense inflammatory infiltrate. (Low power.)

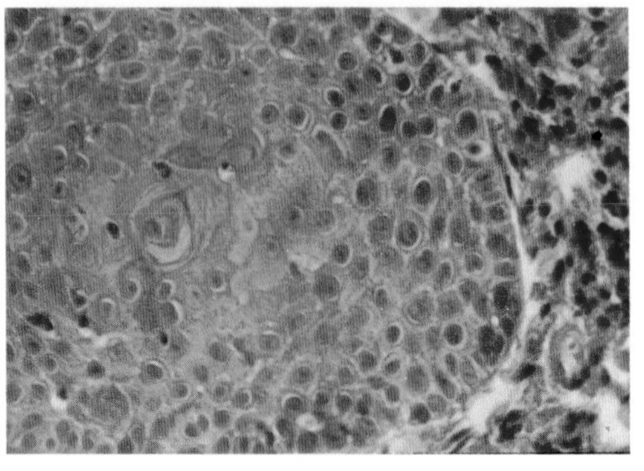

*D.* High power view of *C.* Typical large, carcinomatous squamous cells with intercellular bridges are visible in many areas. Note the numerous mitotic figures.

## HISTOPATHOLOGY (FIG. 67:1*C* and *D*)

1. Early changes are hyperactivity of basal cells of the epidermis with mononuclear cell infiltration of the dermis. Cords of epidermal cells invade the dermis and there is marked stromal fibrosis. With immature carcinomas the cells are small and hyperchromatic. In other types the cells are large and polyhedral. Usually the cells look like those of the stratum spinosum and characteristically exhibit intercellular bridges. They may form typical concentric laminations of keratin or "pearls." These cords mimic the development of the normal epidermis, with the outer layer appearing like basal cells and the central layers appearing flattened and keratinaceous.

## DIFFERENTIAL DIAGNOSIS

The squamous cell carcinoma can be confused with benign ulcers, granulomas and acute pyoderma or dermatitis. In its early stages it may be suggestive of an advanced basal cell carcinoma.

## CLINICAL MANAGEMENT

The treatment of choice is early, wide surgical excision. Regional lymph nodes should be dissected if there is a possibility of metastasis. In all cases chest radiographs should be examined carefully for evidence of tumors. Radiation therapy to inoperable tumors has not produced consistent results. However, palliation is usually the minimum result, and in some cases there is marked regression.

### *Suggested Reading*

Jubb, K. V. F., and Kennedy, P. C.: *Pathology of Domestic Animals.* Academic Press, New York, 1963.

Moulton, J. E.: *Tumors in Domestic Animals.* University of California Press, Berkeley, 1961.

Muller, G. H.: Basal Cell Epithelioma and Squamous Cell Carcinoma in Animals. Arch. Derm. *96*:383-389, 1967.

# SIXTY-EIGHT

## *Tumors of the Glands of the Skin*

### SEBACEOUS ADENOMA

This common tumor of older dogs occurs as a firm, gray, multilobulated lesion which is generally hairless and occasionally ulcerated (Fig. 68:1*A*). The tumor occurs in many breeds but is especially common in aging cocker spaniels, and it is often present in multiple foci or coexisting with other skin tumors. It may be found in skin anywhere on the body, but seems to favor the head, neck and legs.

Microscopically there are masses of relatively normal-appearing sebaceous cells which may be surrounded by one or two rows of dark-staining, palisaded reserve cells (Fig. 68:1*B*). There is a fine collagenous stroma, but no indication of invasiveness and no mitotic figures.

The treatment of choice is surgical excision, although small lesions may be removed with a scissors and the base destroyed by cauterization. There is no recurrence.

### SEBACEOUS ADENOCARCINOMA

This rare tumor differs from sebaceous adenoma in its tendency to grow to large size, its invasiveness, its anaplastic nature and cellular morphology. There are clumps of sebaceous cells, but they are highly pleomorphic with large hyperchromic nuclei (Fig. 68:1*D*). Mitotic figures are rare, and the tumor usually does not metastasize. It does ulcerate readily, however (Fig. 68:1*C*).

Treatment of choice is complete surgical excision. With adequate excision recurrence is rare.

### APOCRINE ADENOMA (SWEAT GLAND ADENOMA OR HIDRADENOMA)

These tumors are common in older dogs but rare in cats. They appear as small, slow-growing cystic nodules located about the face and head or extremities. They rarely ulcerate. Microscopically there are multiple cystic ducts and acini lined by a cuboid epithelium. The cells are often flattened by pressure from retained fluid; and papillary ingrowth of epithelium and connective tissue stroma enter the cysts. These tumors are completely benign and respond well to simple surgical excision.

## APOCRINE ADENOCARCINOMA

Fortunately this tumor is rare, as it is a rapidly invasive growth which spreads readily to regional lymph nodes and the lungs. The lesions often affect the extremities and appear as firm, fibrous nodules or plaques. Since they spread rapidly and are painful, they often give the impression of a phlegmon or cellulitis.

Microscopically there are solid cords of cells, and the glands and tubules may be partly filled with hyperchromatic neoplastic cells. There are numerous mitotic figures. Blood vessels and lymphatics are also invaded, but the tumor has a rather heavy, fibrous stroma.

Early surgical removal of tumor and regional lymph nodes offers the best hope for therapy.

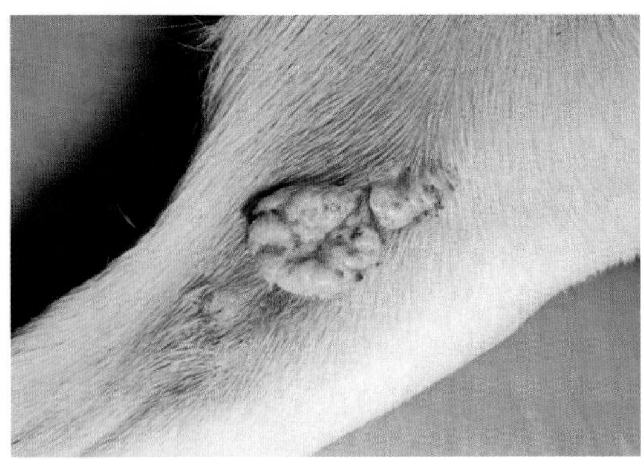

**Figure 68:1.** Tumors of glands of the skin.

Sebaceous Adenoma.

*A.* Sebaceous adenoma. Note multilobulated appearance and well demarcated borders.

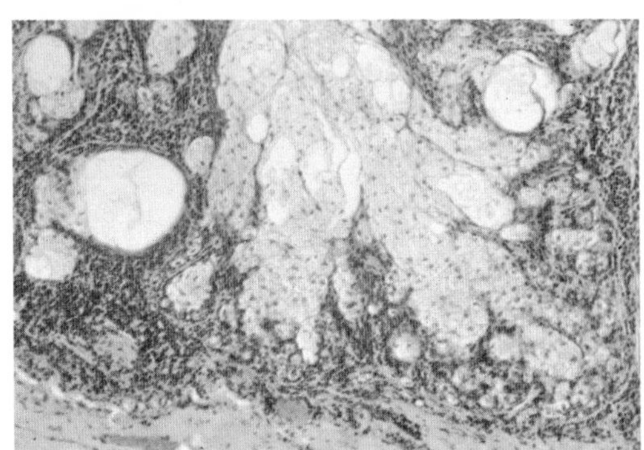

*B.* Histologic section of *A* showing clumps of sebaceous cells surrounded by dark staining "reserve cells." (Low power.)

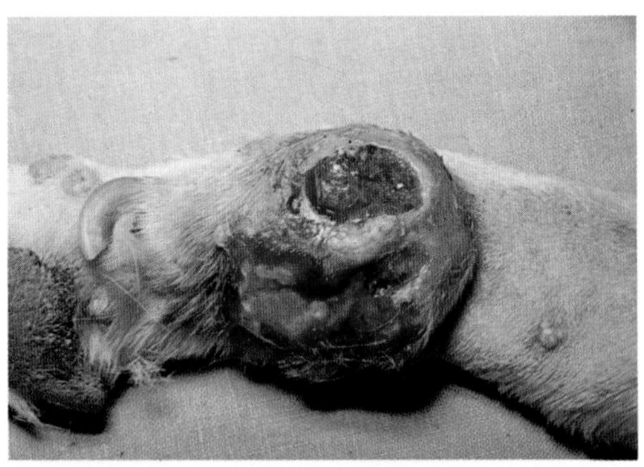

Sebaceous Adenocarcinoma.

*C.* Sebaceous adenocarcinoma that grew rapidly and is severely ulcerated.

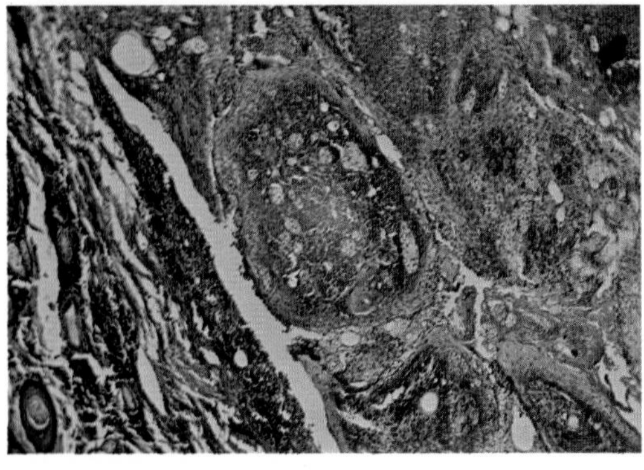

*D.* Histologic section of *C*. It is more cellular than *B* and the dark staining tumor cells are differentiated into stratum spinosum and sebaceous cells. (Low power.)

# COMPARATIVE DERMATOLOGY

*Section Seven*

# SIXTY-NINE

## *Skin Diseases, Animal and Human*

"Only a knowledge of the naturally occurring skin diseases of animals allows us to interpret experimentally produced disorders and enables us to come closer toward establishing general pathological laws."*

Julius Heller, M.D.

It is our hope that physicians and veterinarians can be encouraged to accumulate fundamental information about skin diseases – information which will be of mutual benefit. Spontaneous disease in animals offers a fruitful but incompletely exploited field of research. The conditions discussed in this section are only a few of the entities which deserve investigation.

This chapter is not intended to give detailed information about the skin of dogs and man. It is intended to survey the features which their species have in common and to point out major areas of variance and similarity. Many subjects included here are discussed elsewhere in the book in greater detail.

### ANATOMY AND PHYSIOLOGY

The major differences in human and canine skin can be attributed to the great difference in pelage. The epidermis is thin and uncomplicated in animals (dogs) with a dense hair coat (Fig. 69:1), whereas a thick epidermis protects the almost hairless human skin (Fig. 69:2). Canine epidermis is only a few cells thick and has a thin horny layer, a scanty granular layer, no stratum lucidum (except in the footpads) and very few rete ridges (except in the scrotum). The prickle cells do not have intercellular bridges except those in the footpads and the planum nasale. The epidermis of the footpads has well developed dermatoglyphics (for toughness and grip) and a thick horny layer. Interestingly, these friction areas are the only locations where mammals, such as dogs and cats, have

*Excerpt translated from the book, *Die Vergleichende Pathologie der Haut* (The Comparative Pathology of the Skin), by Dr. Julius Heller, Berlin, 1910.

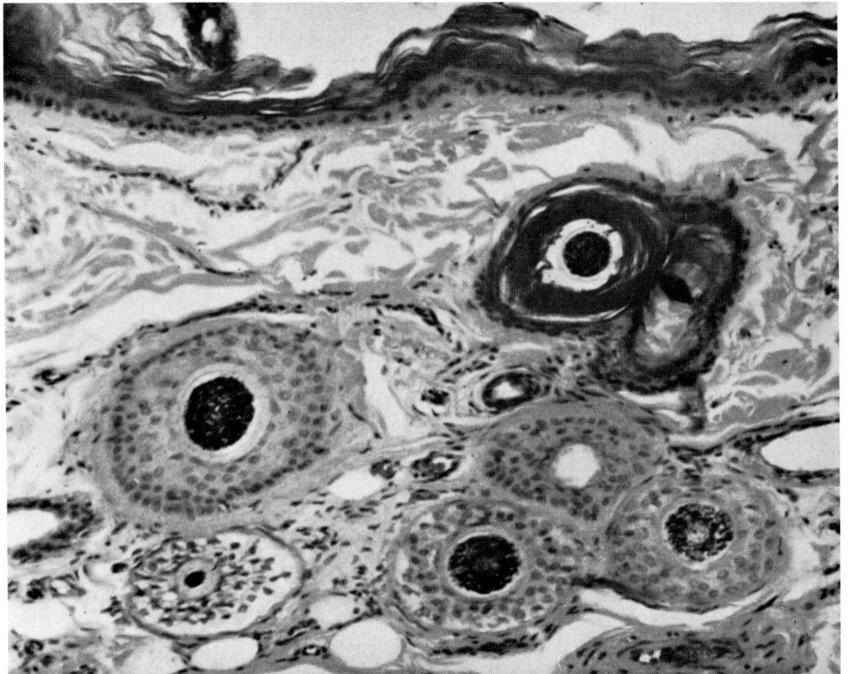

**Figure 69:1.** Normal skin, dog.

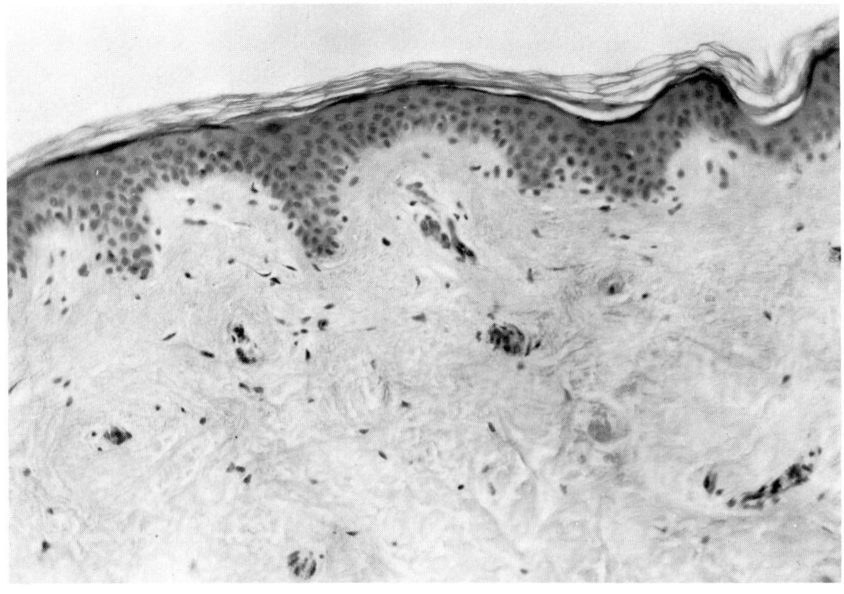

**Figure 69-2.** Normal skin, man.

eccrine sweat glands. In general, the dog's epidermal surface is more irregular than man's because of scale-like folds which form depressions from which hair follicles originate. Knob-like areas of epidermal thickening called epidermal papillae also project from canine skin (Fig. 1:14*B*).

The canine dermis is thickest where the hair is most dense (along the back) and thinnest where hair is sparse (abdomen and footpads). It is not divided into papillary and reticular layers as in man. The cellular and fibrous elements of the dermis are quite comparable, although the distribution and relative numbers of each may vary.

Sebaceous glands of both species are quite similar in histologic appearance and general function. They tend to be largest where the hairs are smallest. In dogs they are most numerous in the eyelids (meibomian glands), lips, scrotum, perineum and external ear canal. In man they are concentrated on the face, shoulders, scalp and back.

Apocrine glands have localized distribution in man—to the areolae of the nipples, axillae, and anogenital regions. In dogs they are widely distributed, one gland developing with each group of hair follicles; but they are most numerous on the face, toes and back. There are none in the nose or footpads. In both species they are modified to form mammary tissue, and the glands of Moll. They begin function with the onset of puberty in both species. All apocrine glands have a long duct which enters the animal hair follicle between the skin surface and the sebaceous duct. The gland itself is a loosely coiled structure in the dog and glomoid in the cat.

Hair is important to dogs for many functions, including insulation, protection, camouflage, ornamentation, communication and tactile sensory perception. All hairy mammals except man have sinus hair follicles with vibrissae which give them increased awareness of their surroundings.

In dogs and cats, hairs are grouped in multiple hair follicles with a large primary hair and several secondary hairs. These follicle groups are further arranged into groups of three or four. Hair growth of dogs, cats and man is basically similar in its fundamental stages. The hair cycles are similar too, as both shed in a mosaic pattern, not in waves (Fig. 1:17).

The arrector pili muscles of dogs and cats are well developed and are attached to a prominent bulge on the wall of the hair follicles (Fig. 1:1*A*).

The hair of man is largely ornamental, and is either highly prized or detested, depending on its location. Human hair is distributed widely in lanugo form, but except on the scalp and back, single hair follicles are typical of the species.

The nerve supply to canine skin is similar to man's except that the special sensory receptors are not so heavily encapsulated. The blood supply has few arteriovenous loops and this, together with the abundant pelage and lack of eccrine sweat glands, means that the dog's skin is designed for heat conservation, not for dissipation.

## TRANSMISSIBLE SKIN DISEASES

### Ringworm

Although over fifty dermatophytes are known to affect man, only twelve have involved animal species (see Table 10:1). Of these only about four are frequent causes of human ringworm (Fig. 69:5). *Microsporum canis*, found commonly on cats and dogs, and *Trichophyton verrucosum* of cattle are frequent causes of human disease. *Trichophyton mentagrophytes* also affects animals and man. The granular form is zoophilic, and the downy form is anthropophilic. *Microsporum gypseum*, a soil inhabitant, may also affect man and animals.

The zoophilic species usually produce a more acute skin reaction in man than the anthropophilic species. Veterinary dermatologists tend to classify fungus disease as dermatomycosis caused by a specific agent and avoid the titles (tinea pedis, tinea capitis and so on) used by physicians.

Certain dermatophytes are endemic in subclinical form in adult animal hosts, and in certain kennels or catteries. The overt disease (Fig. 69:3) is seen most commonly in young animals sold as pets from these establishments. They are a frequent source of exposure to children who have close contact with their pets. *M. canis* is the dermatophyte most often found.

Anthropophilic dermatophytes occasionally infect animals, but these hosts are not important in the epidemiology of the disease. Kaplan (1967) has reported cases of *M. audouinii* and *T. rubrum* in dogs. In each case the disease was transmitted to the dog by an unusual, direct and intimate contact with the human host.

Diagnosis, culture and treatment principles for ringworm are quite similar in man and animal species (see p. 251).

## Scabies

Two common species of mites from dogs and cats may produce lesions in man. *Sarcoptes scabei, var. canis*, produces sarcoptic mange in dogs—a highly contagious disease which also affects man when the mite temporarily invades the human skin. *Notoedres cati*, a related mite, affects cats, rabbits and foxes with a condition called "head mange." These mites also have been reported to temporarily affect man.

The mites are spread by direct contact and human exposure results from hugging, holding or carrying pets in the arms. Only a few minutes of contact are necessary. The mites penetrate the skin rapidly, but are thought to back out after a few hours, abandoning their unnatural host. However, they have initiated a local lesion which appears within several hours as a mildly pruritic, erythematous papule. They are small, discrete lesions which may be found on the arms, chest and abdomen. These are typically found on areas of skin above tight clothing constrictions such as belts, brassieres and girdles (Fig. 45:1*C*). Severe excoriation and secondary infections of affected areas are common.

The lesions heal spontaneously in seven to ten days if the human patient is removed from further contact with the infected animal. Most physicians use local treatment with 1 per cent gamma benzene hexachloride lotions for their patients. Veterinarians should provide whole body treatment of all affected animals once weekly for three weeks. Chlordane or ronnel dips are effective for dogs; lime sulfur dips are safe for cats (see pp. 315, 329).

## Other Mites

*Dermanyssus gallinae*, a bird mite, infests small animals and man. It is usually contracted by man when he is cleaning cages or handling infested birds,

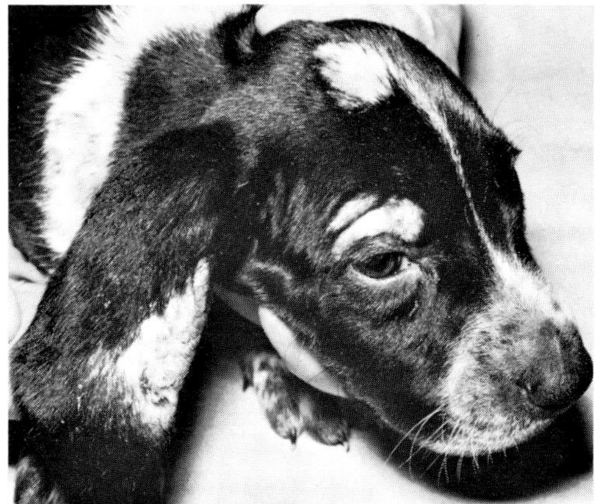

**Figure 69:3.** Ringworm, dog *(M. canis).*

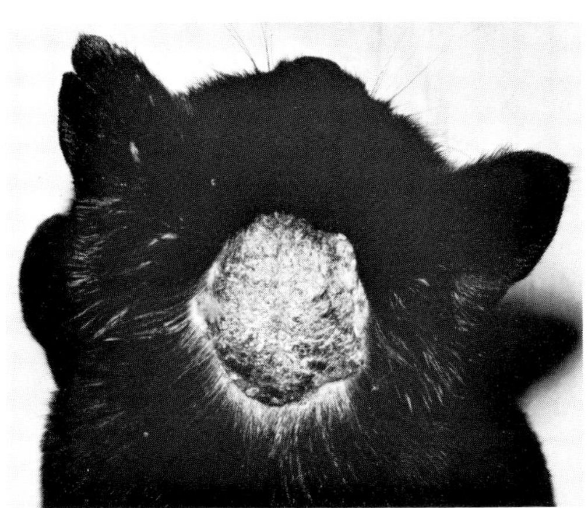

**Figure 69:4.** Ringworm, cat *(M. canis).*

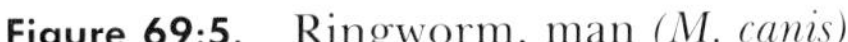

**Figure 69:5.** Ringworm, man *(M. canis).*

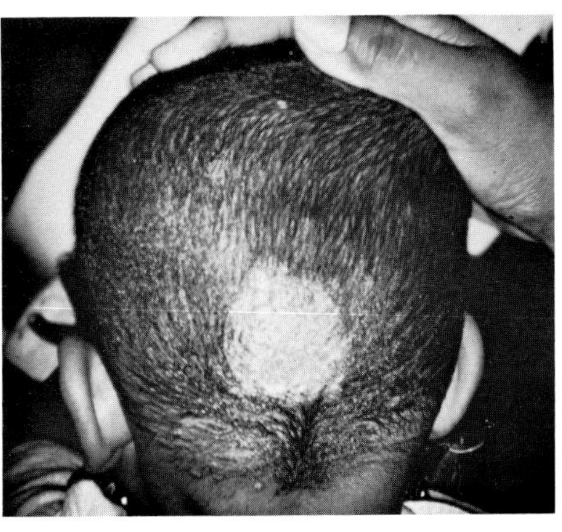

but the mites are great travelers and may move from wild bird nests or pet cages to infest other species. They may be a natural vector of eastern equine encephalomyelitis virus and so have public health significance. These mites are easily killed by insecticides, and control measures are simple and effective once the source of the infection is identified.

In man the lesions are urticarial and papulovesicular eruptions which are intensely pruritic.

### Fleas

*Ctenocephalides felis* and *C. canis* commonly affects pets and man. Certain individuals of all host species seem to be more attractive to fleas than others; and certain individuals have specific allergic reactions to their bites. The ordinary lesion is a cluster of papular wheals which in man is located on the lower extremities (Fig. 69:7), and in dogs and cats is most prominent on the dorsal lumbosacral areas (Fig. 69:6). A hemorrhagic puncture or area of petechiasis distinguishes these lesions from ordinary wheals.

Fleas are vectors of typhus, plague, tularemia and intermediate hosts of *Diplidium caninum*, therefore, their public health significance is important.

Most of the flea life cycle spent is spent off the host. The occasional feeding trips to the host cause great discomfort. This is commonly experienced by people entering flea-infested quarters which have been without a warm-blooded host for several weeks. The swarms of attacking fleas can be most distressing.

Control of fleas centers around an understanding of the life cycle and a concentration of treatment on the premises. Residual insecticides (chlordane, malathion, DDVP), or periodic treatments with other insecticides are needed. Treatment of host animals is necessary, but is only secondarily important. Complete eradication of flea infestations usually is not possible, but good control can be attained in most instances (see p. 159).

## NONTRANSMISSIBLE SKIN DISEASES

### Atopy

The term atopy (in man) is used to describe a syndrome of hay fever, asthma and eczema which is familial and in which a special antibody, called a reagin, is present. Atopic allergy presents diverse manifestations which are not pathognomonic, as they may be mimicked by nonallergic disorders (asthma, urticaria and angioneurotic edema). Specific sensitivity to atopens is not inherited, but the patient has the capacity to acquire sensitivity to them. This sensitivity is acquired by natural exposure such as by inhalation or ingestion and not by injection (Pillsbury, 1956).

Canine atopy (see p. 234) is a seasonal, familial disease which resembles its counterpart in man. Wire-haired fox terriers and the Dalmatian seem to have a special breed predilection; however, dogs of all breeds can be affected by atopy. Affected animals rub and scratch at the face and eyes and bite at the feet. There

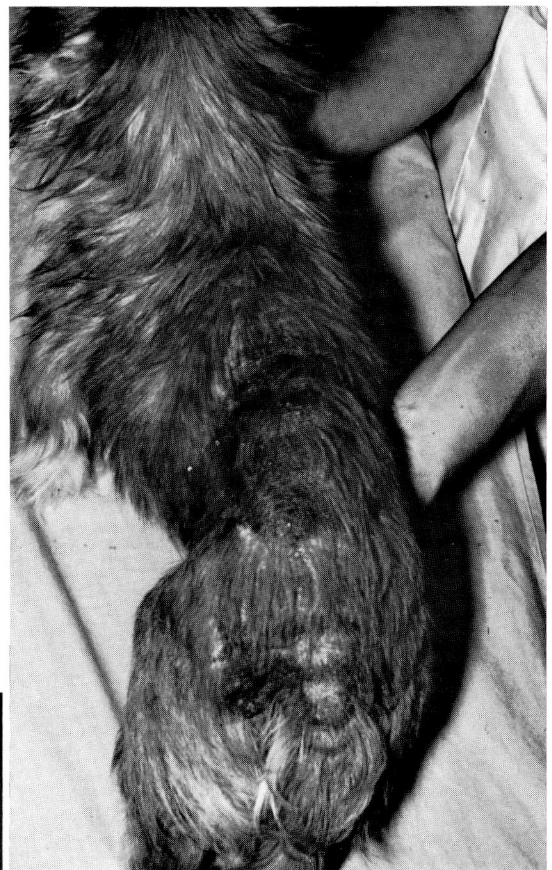

**Figure 69:6.** Flea allergy dermatitis, dog.

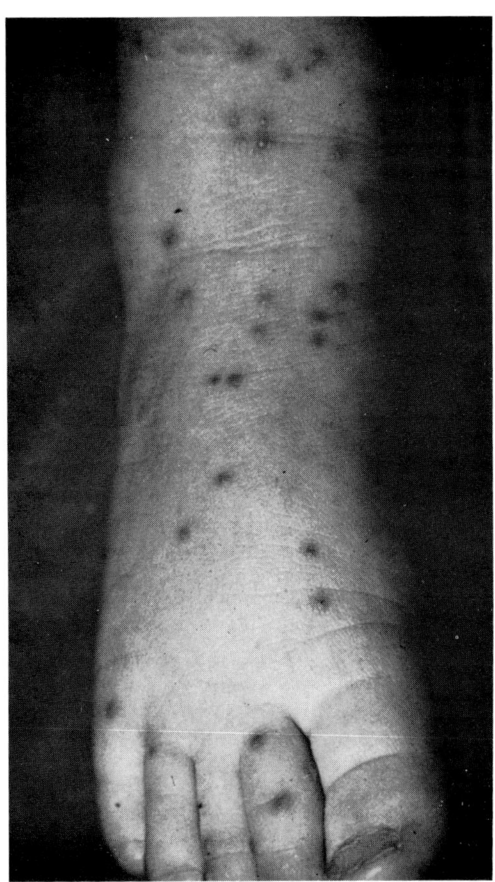

**Figure 69:7.** Fleabite lesions on the leg, man.

may be some sneezing and asthmatic or respiratory signs, and a few individuals have hyperhidrosis. As in man, affected dogs show their first signs at a young age, and a seasonal incidence may be observed. This rapidly lengthens, however, as hypersensitivity to other allergens develop.

In both dog and man, the reaginic antibody is heat labile, skin sensitizing, neutralized by antigen, and fails to develop precipitation reactions. Treatment results are somewhat comparable as antihistamine and corticosteroids both help control the signs of disease. Schwartzman (1967) reports favorable response to hyposensitization procedures in dogs, as he obtained a 75 per cent reduction of duration of signs in 22 of 25 animal patients. Pillsbury (1956) reports that temporary hyposensitization of certain human atopics provided clinical relief. However, complete desensitization rarely occurs. It is extremely doubtful if hyposensitization is of any clinical value in chronic dermatitis occurring in atopic persons.

## Contact Dermatitis

The realization that contact allergens can cause skin reactions in sensitized animals is relatively new (see p. 238).

Contact dermatitis in both man and dogs occurs in two forms, that caused by primary irritants, and that resulting from contact sensitizers which cause a delayed type of hypersensitivity. Primary irritants undoubtedly produce more animal dermatitis than sensitizers, but the latter are more troublesome to detect and manage. Primary irritants in dogs cause an acute reaction with a rapid onset, so that the history helps in diagnosis; and avoidance of re-exposure may be accomplished more easily. In dogs, irritant materials such as soaps, detergents, kerosene, insect sprays and urine may cause erythema and eczematous skin changes. The dermatologic reaction is pathologically similar to that produced by sensitizing agents.

Pruritus is often present and papules and hyperemia with excoriations may be seen early. Chronic changes include hyperkeratosis, acanthosis, fibrosis of the dermis and infiltration by mast cells and eosinophils. Similar changes are seen in human skin.

In order for allergic contact dermatitis to develop, there must be repeated, close contact between the sensitizing agent and the skin; and the skin must have the capacity to produce an allergic response. These requirements automatically limit the probability of animal cases developing. The dog's dense hair coat protects him from close contact with many agents, and the lesions that are produced appear on the abdomen, groin, axilla, perineum, muzzle and ears—places where hair is sparse (Fig. 69:8). Furthermore, repeated contacts are not so common in dogs because of differences in canine and human habits with regard to washing, use of cosmetics, clothing, jewelry and especially to contact with industrial chemicals (Fig. 69:9). Agents which have been incriminated as causing allergic contact dermatitis in dogs include chrome, nickel, leather, and wood preservatives, Vapona flea collars, detergents, bedding and carpets, medicaments, lanolin, and botanical agents such as rhus and jasmine.

Patch testing has not been used extensively in animals, but intentional exposure has been employed to give some measures of proof. There seems to be a breed predilection for dachshunds, wire-haired fox terriers and French poodles.

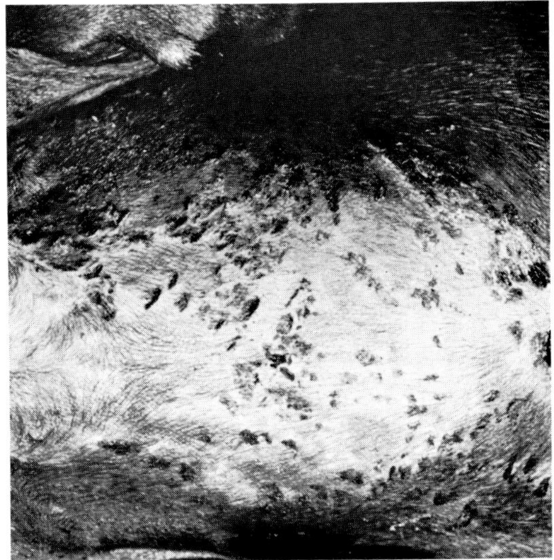

**Figure 69:8.** Contact dermatitis, dog.

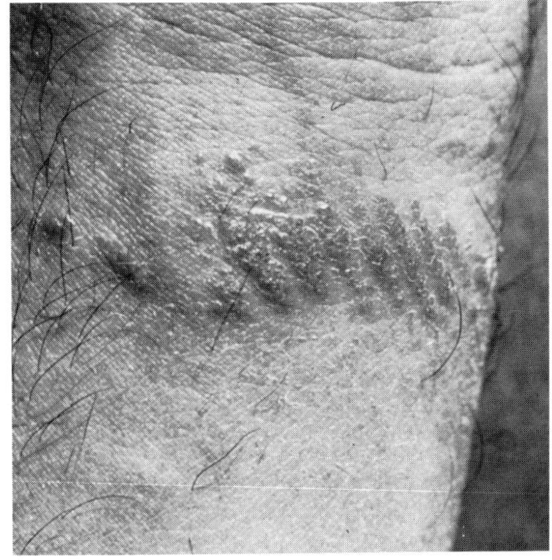

**Figure 69:9.** Contact dermatitis, man.

Clinical management in all species should emphasize finding and removing the offending agent. Corticosteroids, Burow's solution soaks, and topical emollients may be useful therapeutically.

## The Seborrheic Syndrome

The definition of seborrhea in man—a functional disturbance of the sebaceous glands with excess production of sebum and accumulation of greasy scales on the skin—may not fit dogs so well. In this species the scaliness is prominent but oiliness is less common. This clinical feature, together with the hyperkeratosis and parakeratosis seen on histologic section, suggests a defect in the process of keratinization. Even in man, although patients with seborrhea tend to have an oily skin, the relationship of the sebaceous glands to the disease is far from clear.

The disease in dogs affects all areas of skin, but is accentuated at the hocks, ears, legs and to some extent around the eyes (see p. 335). The distribution of sebaceous glands in dogs is quite uniform because of the uniform pelage, but even so, some concentration of glands is present on the tail, the anogenital region and around the eyes and lips. In man, the glands are concentrated in the scalp, face, chin and back. In both species sebaceous gland hypertrophy starts at puberty. Pillsbury (1956) reports animal experiments which show that androgens cause hypertrophy whereas estrogens cause involution. Rothman (1954) reports that androgens in the male and progesterone in the female cause sebaceous gland hyperplasia.

The cause of the seborrheic syndrome is unknown, but in dogs it is especially common in spaniel breeds (Fig. 69:10). Most cases are seen in mature dogs five to ten years old. There are three canine manifestations: a dry, scaly form (seborrhea sicca), an oily form (seborrhea oleosa) seen particularly in black cocker spaniels, and seborrheic dermatitis, with which inflammation and secondary infection are associated.

In man the disease may begin as "dandruff" of the scalp, often with increased oiliness (Fig. 69:11). The regions of the eyebrows, nasal folds, ears, and presternal and interscapular areas are affected later. The lesions are ordinarily symmetrical. As the disease progresses, erythema develops, which is sometimes diffuse but often is isolated in oval or annular patches. These lesions may be covered with adherent scales and crusts, a condition which also appears in dogs.

Treatment in both species emphasizes frequent cleansing baths to remove oil and scales and the use of tar, sulfur and salicylic acid creams topically. Systemic corticosteroid therapy is also used empirically in patients with severe seborrheic dermatitis.

Although this disease is incurable, proper management usually controls its distressing symptoms.

## Acne

In man, acne is a classic dermatologic sign of puberty. It results from an interplay of heredity and hormones, with androgens having a major effect. Estrogens tend to be inhibitory, although the importance of progesterone is uncertain and probably inconsequential.

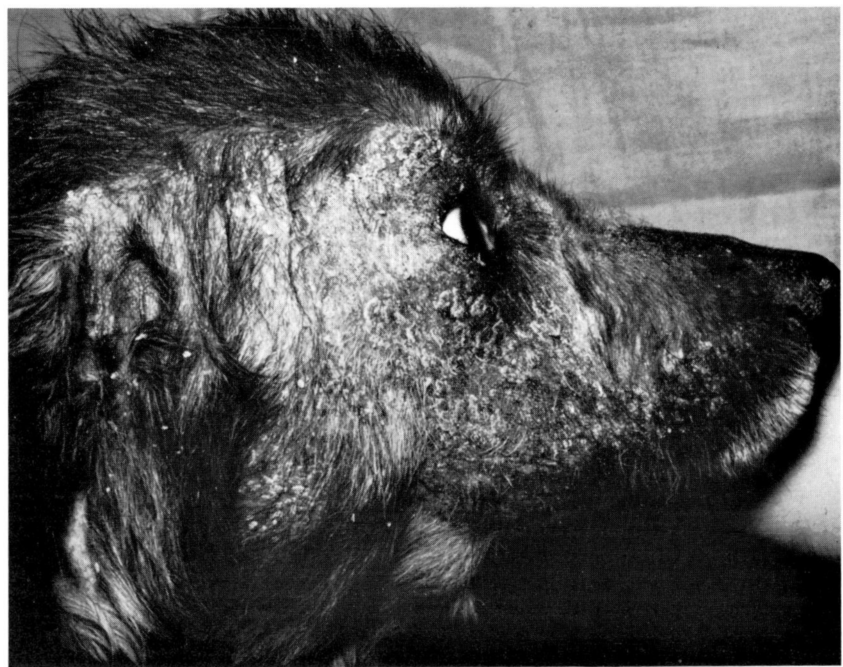

**Figure 69:10.** Seborrheic syndrome, dog.

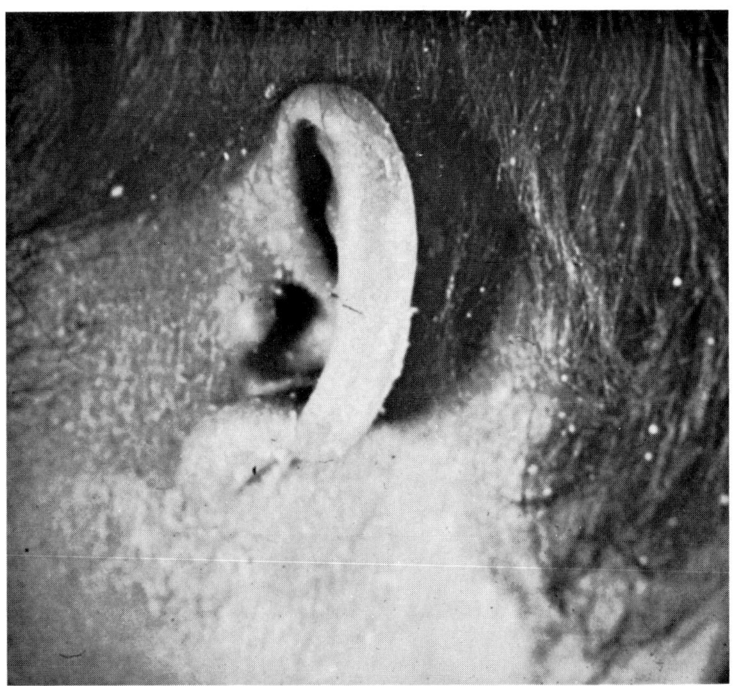

**Figure 69:11.** Seborrheic dermatitis, man.

The primary lesion of acne is the comedo or blackhead, which is a firm mass of keratin and sebum which blocks and dilates the inactive hair follicle. Comedones may be sparse or abundant in affected areas of the face and shoulders—the areas of predisposition in man. Propionibacteria are anaerobes which act on sebum in the blocked follicles to produce irritating propionic acid. This produces an inflammatory nodule. These lesions may coalesce to form sinuses and become secondarily infected. Scarring with bands, pits and hypertrophic ridges may cause permanent disfigurement (Fig. 69:13).

Feline acne is a somewhat different syndrome (see p. 000). It is localized on the chin—an area that cannot be cleaned easily by cats. Partial alopecia, comedones and pustules may form in predisposed, mature cats of either sex. A folliculitis commonly develops in the follicle under the comedo. A dense inflammatory infiltrate develops and a pustule forms. Staphylococci are often present, but the infection is rarely acute.

The feline disease does not appear to be hormonally controlled so that local treatments with antibiotics and corticosteroids, together with thorough cleansing, are usually effective treatment. In man, local cleansing and attention to diet and general hygiene are important for mild cases. However, débridement, dermabrasion and systemic antibiotic, vitamin and hormonal therapy may be needed for many cases. The severe scars and pits resulting from acne vulgaris of man are not seen in animals.

Acne-like pustules are seen in some dogs at puberty (six to 12 months), and although some lesions persist into maturity, most cases clear spontaneously by 18 months of age. The lesions consist of comedones, papules and pustules located under the chin and on the lips (Fig. 69:12). Short-haired dogs, whose skin is rich in sebaceous glands, are most commonly affected. Canine acne has a predilection for boxers, English bulldogs, Dobermans, and German shepherds (see p. 344).

## THE PYODERMAS

### Impetigo

Impetigo in man is a primary skin infection usually caused by coagulase-positive micrococci or by beta-hemolytic streptococci. It is highly contagious in young patients, but less so in adults. It begins as a thin-walled, superficial vesico-pustule which discharges a copious seropurulent exudate. This dries on the skin and forms thick, dirty crusts which are a hallmark of the disease. It is most often seen on the face and extremities (Fig. 69:15).

In dogs, impetigo is a noncontagious, secondary, pustular dermatitis usually caused by the aforementioned organisms. (See also p. 323.) It is seen in puppies in which the thin-walled pustule first appears on the abdomen or inner thighs (Fig. 69:14). Some clinicians have observed a high incidence of impetigo in puppies with distemper; however, the connection between the two diseases is not clear. Lactating bitches occasionally develop lesions on their breasts and vulva. In both species careful cleansing of the skin and topical antibiotics applied frequently cause rapid healing. In children, the severe case may require systemic antibiotic therapy.

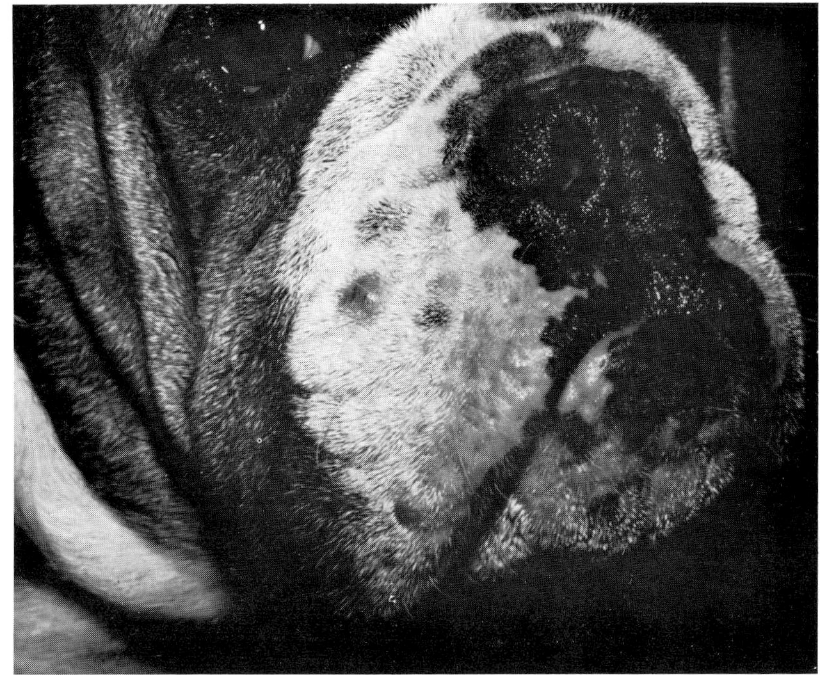

**Figure 69:12.** Acne, dog.

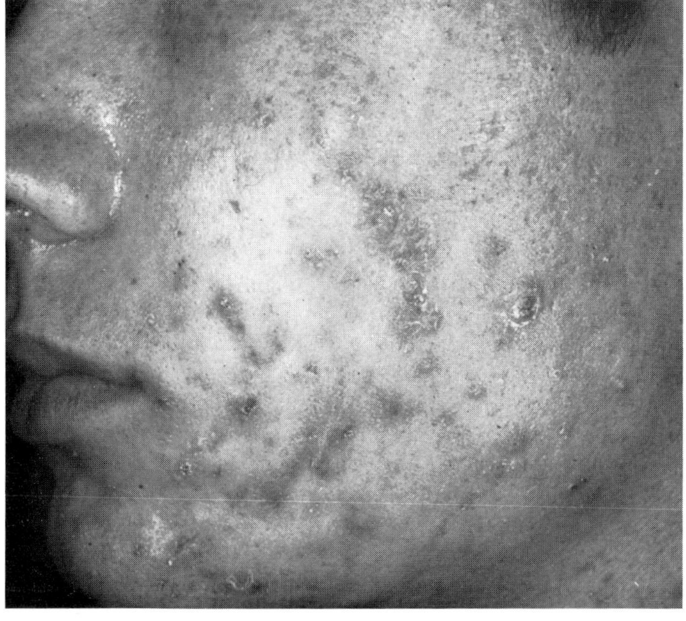

**Figure 69:13.** Acne vulgaris, man.

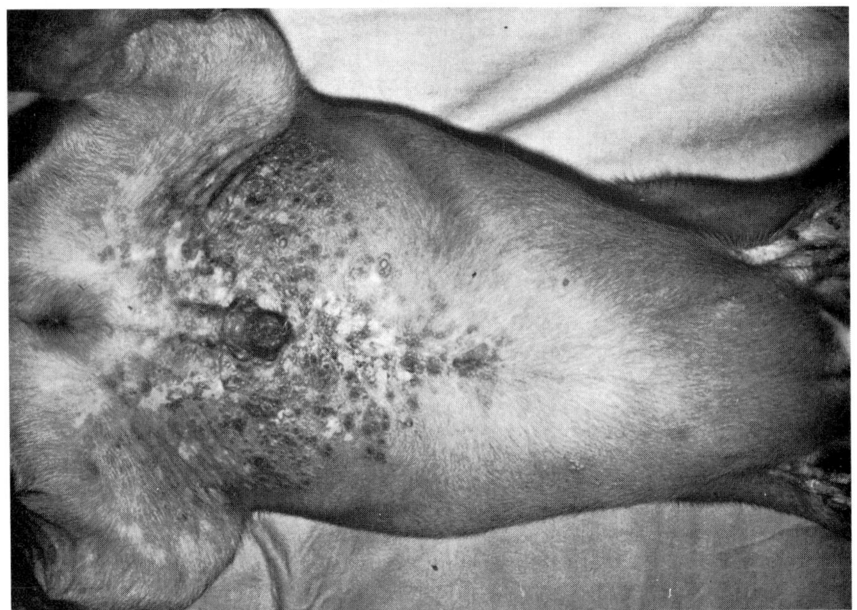

**Figure 69:14.** Impetigo, dog.

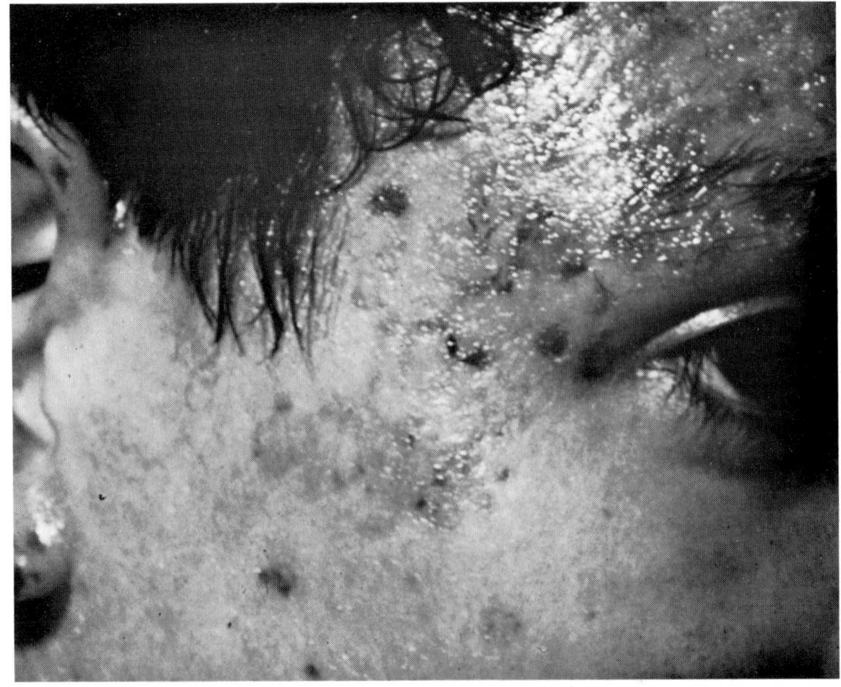

**Figure 69:15.** Impetigo, man.

### Paronychia

Paronychia is a bacterial infection (often staphylococci) of the bed of the nail or claw (see p. 303). In man it is often localized to one finger or toe and follows trauma such as a cut or scratch, or poor manicuring techniques. In animals trauma may be the inciting factor, but the condition involves multiple claws. Therapy in both species is similar, but avulsion of the claw is commonly performed for the infection in animals. The tubular shape of animal claws causes a "bottling up" of the pus and infection. Avulsion is like "pulling the cork" and establishes good drainage followed by complete healing and regrowth of the claw. (It may be deformed temporarily, however).

### Folliculitis and Furunculosis

In man folliculitis is a superficial hair follicle infection caused usually by coagulase-positive staphylococci. It is often the result of poor hygiene, friction or local irritants. Furunculosis is a deeper form of folliculitis which involves one hair follicle. Carbuncle is the term to use if several follicles are involved. They are pustules, or tender red nodules which develop a pus "point" and form a necrotic core. They are found commonly on the face, scalp, buttocks and the extremities.

Canine skin infections of this nature are usually classified as either superficial or deep pyodermas (see p. 321). Superficial pyodermas of the lip and vulvar folds or of areas easily traumatized by the dog are common and usually follow previous skin damage. The skin surface appears moist, hyperemic and swollen. There is a purulent exudate, and alopecia is complete in the center of the painful lesion. Deep pyodermas involve the entire dermis, and often subcutaneous tissues as well. Microabscesses and fistulas may be present in the deeper layers of the thickened skin. The incidence is high in short-coated breeds. The interdigital folds, lateral lower surfaces of the legs, the elbows, nose, lips and ears may be affected commonly. A coagulase-positive Staphylococcus infection is most common, but *E. coli*, Pseudomonas sp. or Proteus sp. have been found on rare occasions. Treatment of these animals is successful in about 50 per cent of the cases, but treatment requires surgical drainage, autogenous bacterins and vigorous use of properly selected systemic and topical antibiotics. Recurrence is not unusual.

Infection of the apocrine sweat glands (hidradenitis) occurs in both man and dogs. In man the condition is usually confined to the axillary area, but in dogs it can occur anywhere because of the universal distribution of apocrine glands. Canine hidradenitis requires long-term antibiotic therapy combined with surgical drainage where needed.

## DEMODECTIC MANGE

*Demodex folliculorum* is an inhabitant usually present among the normal cutaneous fauna of man. It inhabits the hair follicles and is found in areas rich in sebaceous glands, such as the face, forehead, nose and chin. It is rarely found on the extremities. There is no proof that it contributes to the pathology of any

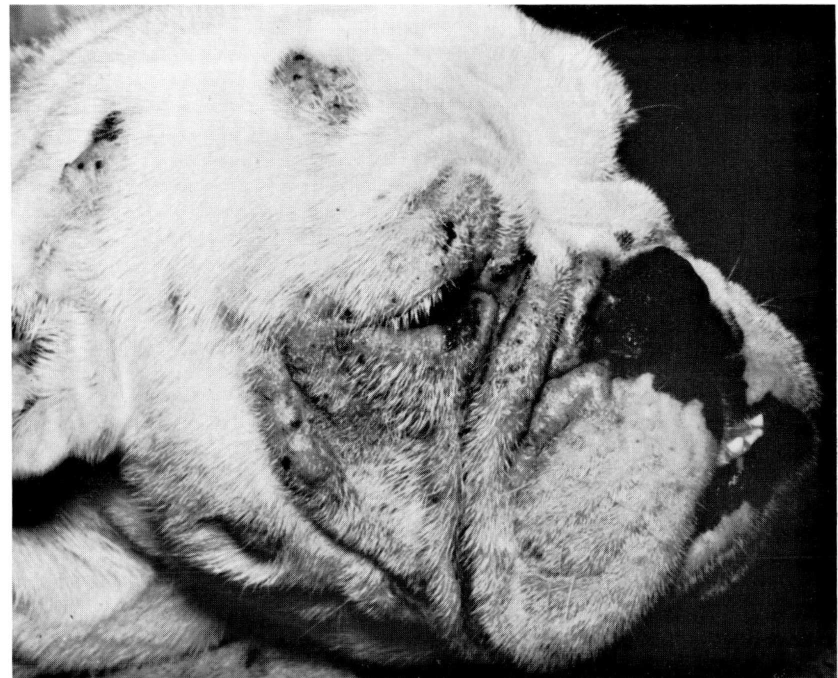

**Figure 69:16.** Demodectic mange, dog.

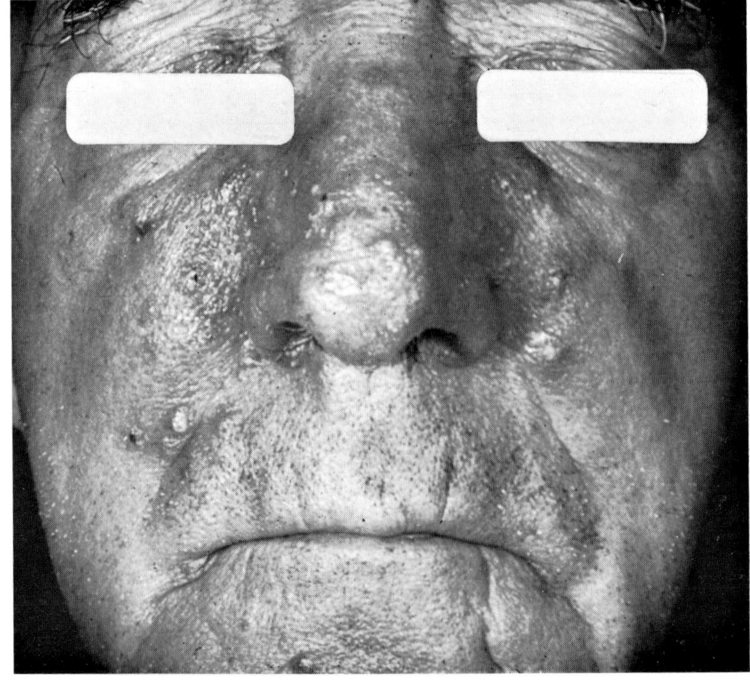

**Figure 69:17.** Acne rosacea, man.

disease in man. However, there have been reports that demodectic mites are present in large numbers in the facial skin of patients with acne rosacea (Ayres, 1932; Beerman and Stokes, 1934; Bodie, 1952) (Fig. 69:17). Demodectic mites have been reported in larger than normal numbers on the face (especially the cheeks, of middle-aged women, causing mild erythema. This condition responds favorably to application of 2 per cent sulfur ointment.

Most dogs harbor *Demodex canis* as a harmless member of the skin's fauna, but in some puppies, erythematous, alopecic patches can develop. This is called localized demodectic mange (see p. 242). It appears first on the face and extremities but the lesions may spread over most of the body (Fig. 69:16). If generalized lesions and secondary pyoderma occur, the case may become incurable. The pathogenesis of the disease in dogs is not known, but short-coated breeds have a predilection, and certain families seem to be afflicted commonly. It is rarely seen in older dogs which have not developed the disease prior to puberty. The condition may disappear at puberty, although many parasiticidal drugs have been erroneously credited with such spontaneous recoveries. Demodectic mange is a very common but poorly understood entity which should receive research attention.

## NEOPLASMS

### Verruca (Wart, Papilloma)

Warts in man are thought to be common viral infections of the skin. They are often contagious and spread to other areas, or form satellite lesions; but many times they regress spontaneously. In man, verrucae are classified by gross morphology and location. In dogs and man cutaneous verrucae appear about the head and neck as a filiform variety and the histologic appearance in both species is identical. The syndrome of oral papillomatosis of dogs (see p. 355) has not been reported in man. This viral-caused, contagious disease has an incubation period of about 35 days and is usually observed in young dogs. The pearly-white, or grayish masses may be present on the oral mucosa in huge numbers (Fig. 55:1). Usually surgical extirpation of some of the lesions causes regression of the rest, but occasional refractory cases are encountered.

The common cutaneous papilloma of older dogs is easily removed surgically. Recurrence is not common.

### Fibroma

Fibromas of dogs and dermatofibromas of man are similar entities. In both species they are slow-growing, hard cutaneous nodules that develop in the dermis or subcutis but are attached to the skin. They involve older patients and often are located on the extremities, trunk or neck. They are completely benign growths.

### Fibrosarcoma

Fibrosarcoma is the malignant tumor of fibroblasts which appears in older dogs and man. The canine tumor (see p. 367) is quite similar to the poorly differentiated (cell) variety of human fibrosarcoma. In both species this tumor arises from the subcutis as a firm nodule on the extremities. In the dog it may arise from the breasts, gingiva, trunk or neck as well as other areas. This tumor is highly invasive locally and commonly recurs after surgical excision. In the dog it ulcerates early and may metastasize to the lungs. The majority of fibrosarcomas in man are the well-differentiated type which grow slowly and do not metastasize.

## Neurofibroma (Schwannoma)

Neurofibromas are generally benign tumors, although malignant forms are observed. In dogs and man they may occur in solitary or localized forms which appear as superficial or deep, firm, round dermal tumors. The usual location in the dog is the skin of the back and legs (see p. 369). In man it is more common to find multiple neurofibromatosis (von Recklinghausen's disease), but this has not been well documented in dogs. It has been reported in other species, however, and spontaneous involution of one or more of the tumors has been noted. These tumors seldom exhibit malignant tendencies, but when they do, growth is rapid and pulmonary metastasis may occur.

## Basal Cell Carcinoma

Basal cell carcinomas in dogs and man have many similarities. They are common (dogs 7 per cent, cats 27 per cent of all tumors, and man 65 per cent of skin cancers) with a distribution predilection for the head, especially the ears, face and jaw (see p. 362). Older patients are the rule, with the tumor appearing as a solitary, discrete, round nodule of firm consistency (Fig. 69:18). They ulcerate commonly, and although they may be locally invasive, they never metastasize and are considered benign. The histologic appearance is similar in both species. In man they commonly occur on sun-exposed areas of fair-complexioned patients (Fig. 69:19), and are felt to be directly associated with photosensitivity or to x-ray exposure, burns or other irritating factors. Basal cell tumors originate from basal cells of the epidermis, and occasionally form structures resembling hair follicles. This form is found mainly in dogs and is called a trichoepithelioma. Surgical excision of basal cell carcinomas is the treatment of choice in animals, but cases in man are often treated by electrodesiccation or other modalities which minimize scarring.

## Squamous Cell Carcinoma

Squamous cell carcinoma (see p. 387) is a malignant tumor of squamous epithelium that is found most commonly on the legs, head, lips and scrotum of dogs and on the face and hands of man. It affects older patients, and in man has a high incidence in fair-skinned patients (Fig. 69:21). Sun is a major etiologic factor, but radiation, chronic heat, irritation or burns may also damage the skin and predispose to squamous cell carcinoma. The precancerous lesions of man (actinic keratosis, leukoplakia, xeroderma pigmentosum) have not been described

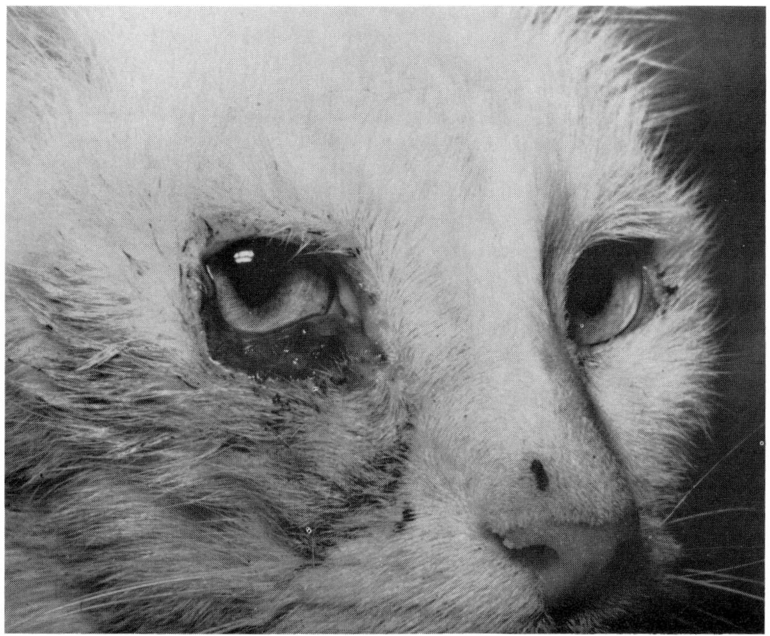

**Figure 69:18.** Basal cell carcinoma, cat.

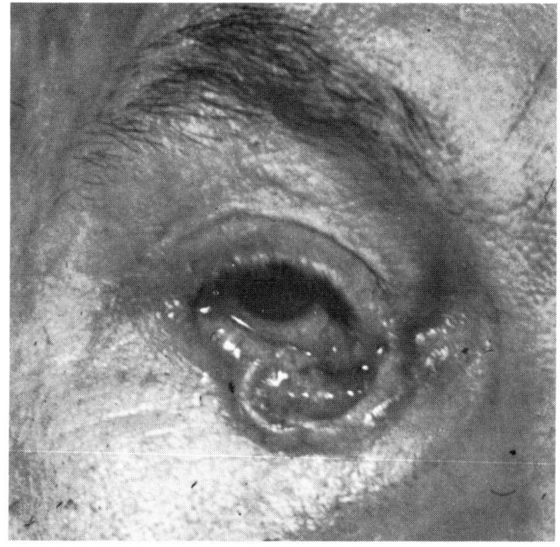

**Figure 69:19.** Basal cell carcinoma, man.

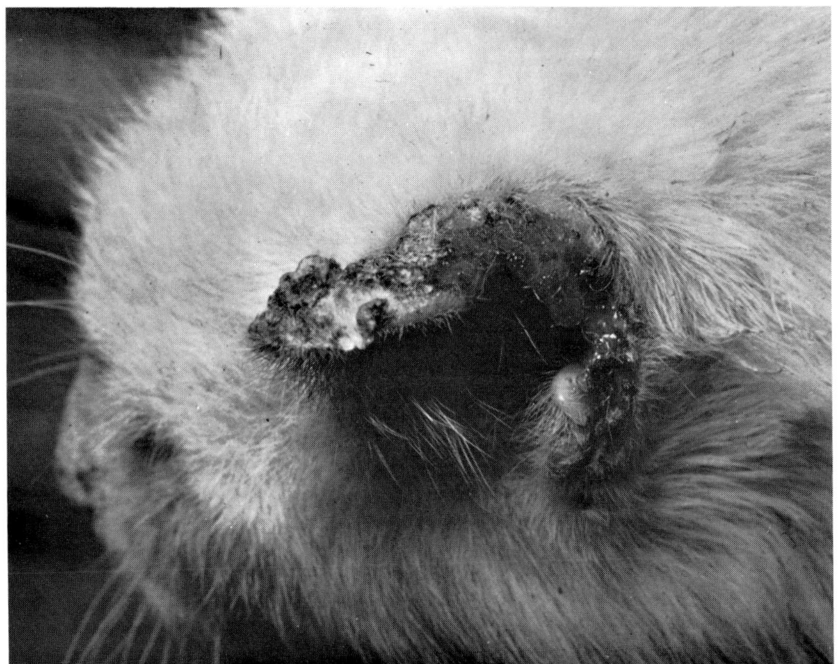

**Figure 69:20.** Squamous cell carcinoma, cat.

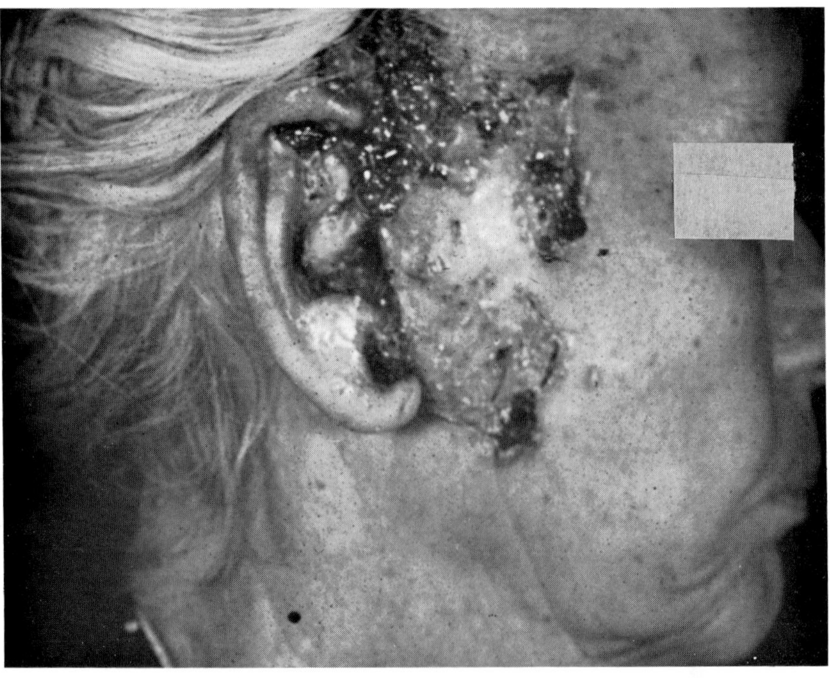

**Figure 69:21.** Squamous cell carcinoma, woman.

in dogs. The microscopic and gross characteristics of the tumor in both species, however, are similar. Clinically these tumors begin as solitary, firm nodules which ulcerate early. They are often papillary or cauliflower-like in shape. Local invasiveness and metastasis to regional lymph nodes and the lungs are common, so that the initial treatment should be vigorous. Wide-block surgical excision and dissection of lymph nodes are usually the treatment of choice.

Solar damage to hypopigmented skin which is poorly covered by hair is believed to initiate a chronic inflammation in animals. This progresses to squamous cell carcinoma in some cases. Collies and Shetland sheep dogs have a predisposition to a condition called "collie nose." The carcinomas which may result rarely metastasize (see p. 305). Cats with white ears sometimes develop squamous cell carcinoma on the exposed tips of their ears after long periods of actinic irritation (Fig. 69:20). Although these tumors are locally invasive, they rarely metastasize. Well-advanced cases require amputation of the affected pinna, and regional lymph node dissection may be necessary in lymphatic metastasis. The cosmetic affects are usually quite acceptable.

## Sebaceous Gland Tumors

Senile sebaceous hyperplasia in man is analogous to a condition in dogs described as sebaceous gland adenoma (see p. 390). Both species develop small, flat papules or cauliflower-like lesions in later life. They seem to be more common in individuals with a seborrheic tendency (i.e., cocker spaniel dogs) and in some cases their course may be modified temporarily by estrogens. Histologically, the appearance of human and canine specimens is identical.

Male dogs of certain breeds have a high incidence of tumors of the perianal gland. This gland is a modified sebaceous gland which develops multiple, benign hormonal-related tumors in older patients. These growths bear many similarities to the human senile sebaceous hyperplasia.

## Apocrine Gland Tumors

Although apocrine tumors are not uncommon in dogs or man, there are confusing reports on their incidence. Canine apocrine adenomas are usually solitary spherical tumors of the neck or extremities. These tumors may ulcerate. Schwartzman and Orkin (1962) report they have no human analogue, although they maintain that the hidradenoma papilliferum and the apocrine nevus (mixed nevus) of both species are similar.

Sweat gland adenocarcinomas are rare, but two cases seen by the authors progressed rapidly and metastasized to lymph nodes and lungs.

## Mastocytosis

Mast cell disease accounts for approximately 13 per cent of the cutaneous tumors of dogs. It has a predilection for boxers and Boston terriers in which it commonly affects the skin of the rear legs and genitalia (Fig. 69:22). Tumors begin as small, firm nodules which may remain quiescent for months. Later a

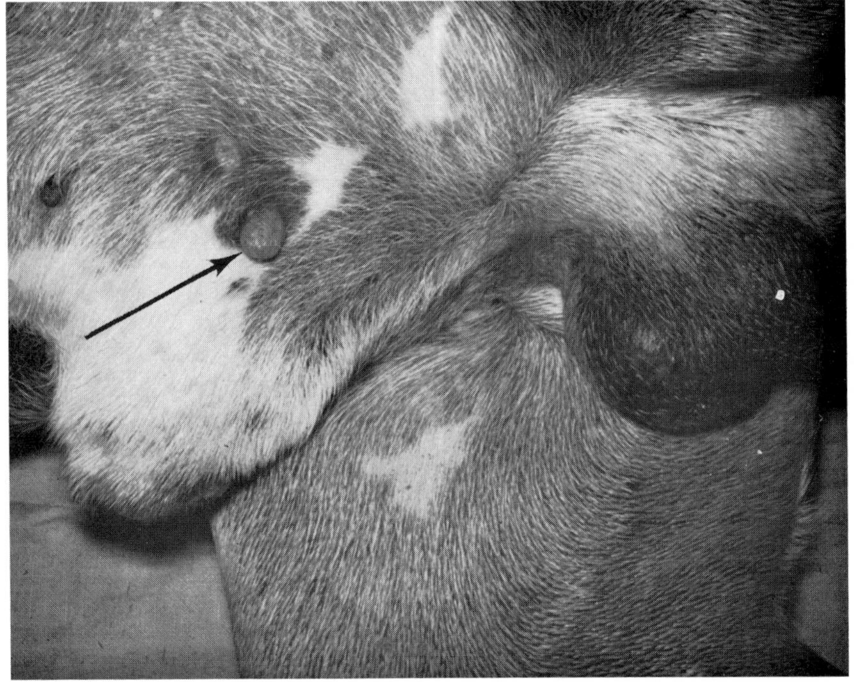

**Figure 69:22.** Mastocytoma, dog.

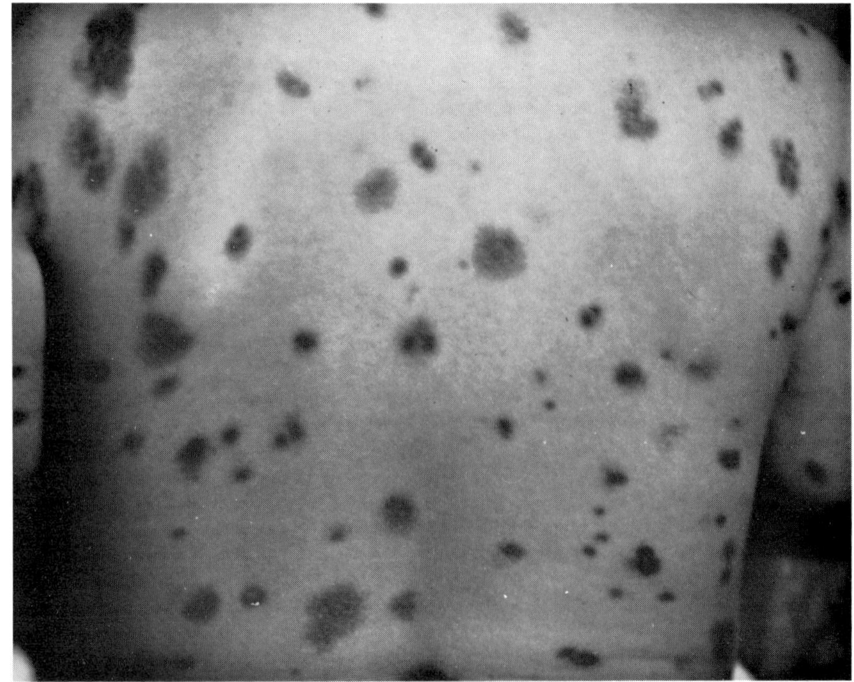

**Figure 69:23.** Urticaria pigmentosa, man.

few grow rapidly, and may become locally invasive or metastasize to lymph nodes and lungs. Following surgical excision as many as 20 per cent of the tumors may recur and the new growth is often more anaplastic than the primary tumor. Temporary (30 to 60 days) regression usually follows systemic corticosteroid therapy.

Certain cases of the disease in man have many similarities to canine mastocytosis. Urticaria pigmentosa is the traditional name for human mastocytosis. The historic type is a congenital form, characterized by multiple brown macules that urticate when rubbed briskly (Fig. 69:23). This form may disappear before puberty. Recently recognized types implicate the disease in systemic manifestations. There may be telangiectasia, visceral, bony or hematopoietic changes, and cutaneous findings may be minimal or absent. Special stains may be necessary to demonstrate the mast cells and avoid misdiagnosis.

## Melanocytic Tumors

This group of tumors has been confusing because different nomenclature was used by veterinarians and physicians. Recently, Conroy (1967) attempted to resolve this problem when he described the melanocytic tumors of dogs. Of the benign tumors, the compound nevi of man and dogs are similar, while the canine dermal melanocytoma is analogous to the blue nevus of man. The malignant melanomas of man and dogs have many disparities. In the dog they occur commonly on the feet and in the mouth and are found in older animals with heavy skin pigmentation. Cocker spaniels are commonly afflicted, and males have a higher incidence than females. In dogs over 95 per cent of oral mela-

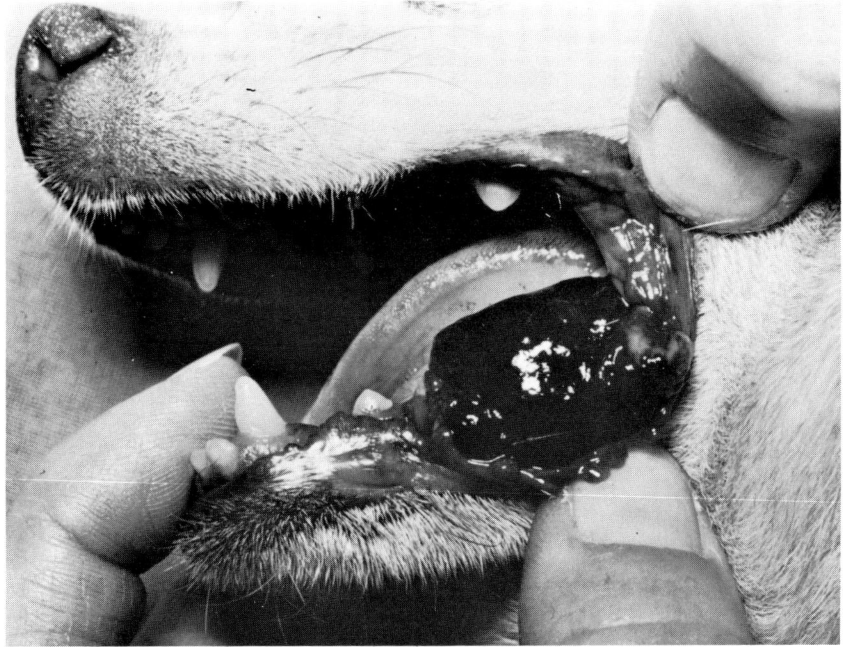

**Figure 69:24.** Malignant melanoma, dog.

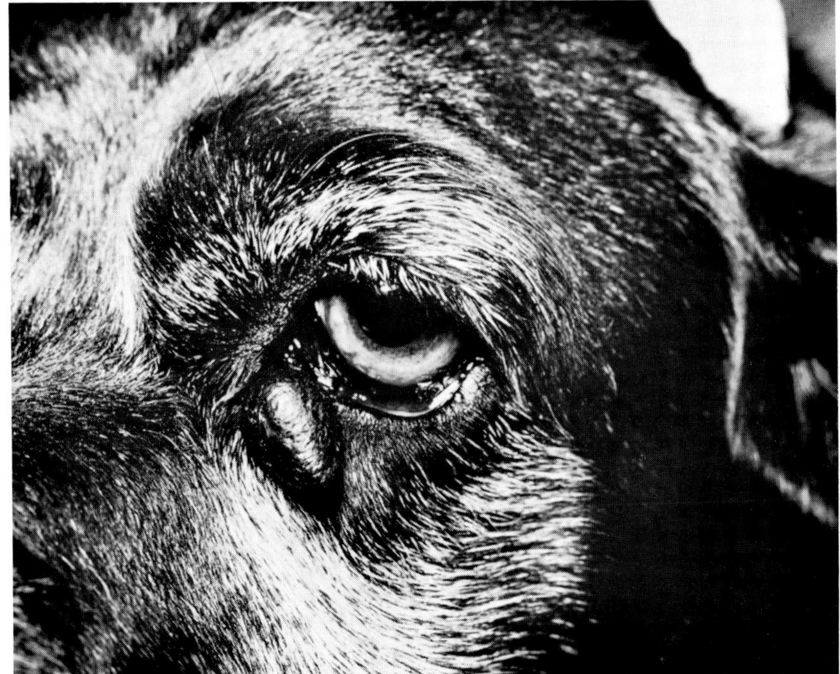

**Figure 69:25.** Benign melanoma (nevus), dog.

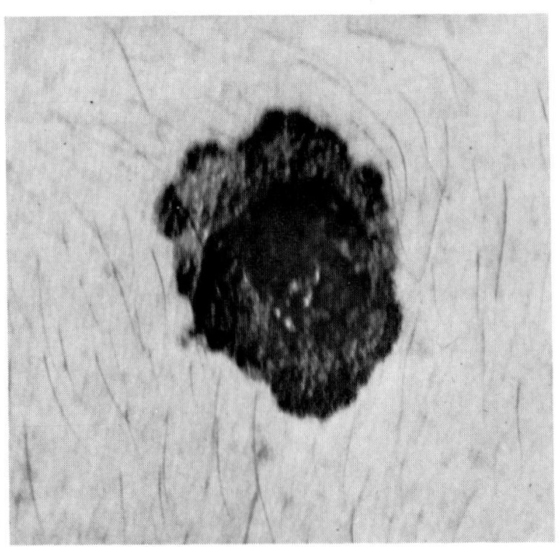

**Figure 64:26.** Melanoma (malignant), man.

nomas are malignant (Fig. 69:24) but the majority of cutaneous melanocytic tumors are benign (Fig. 69:25).

In man these tumors are most common in older, fair-skinned patients. There is no sex predilection and malignant melanomas involving mucous membranes are rare (Fig. 69:26). In both species these malignancies have similar histologic structures and in both they metastasize by lymph and blood channels at an early stage.

## Cutaneous Lymphosarcoma

A rare malignant lymphoma occurs in dogs which is characterized by severe cutaneous lesions which resemble mycosis fungoides of man. The disease begins with bright, erythematous patches on the trunk. These enlarge to form numerous polymorphous plaques that may cover a large part of the body (Fig. 69:27). Superficial white or reddish scales cover the well-demarcated lesions, except where the surface is eroded. The disease differs from malignant lymphoma (lymphosarcoma) because of its severe, irreversible skin lesions. Survival is seldom longer than three to six months from the onset of lymph node enlargement. Lymph node and skin biopsies confirm the diagnosis. For histopathology of the skin, see page 000. The human and canine skin changes are remarkably similar.

Certain phases of the disease in dogs are identical to a disease in man known as mycosis fungoides (Fig. 69:28), which is a dermatologic disease of the lymphoma type. It is also fatal but differs from the canine disease in that it remains localized in the skin for several years. In both dogs and man the disease occurs mostly in middle age: six to ten years for dogs, and 40 to 60 years for man.

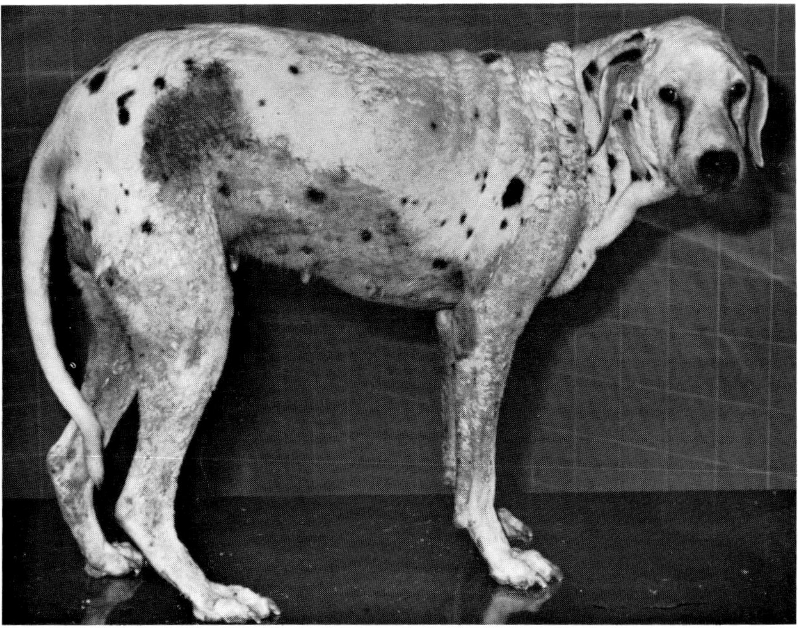

**Figure 69:27.** Primary cutaneous lymphosarcoma, dog.

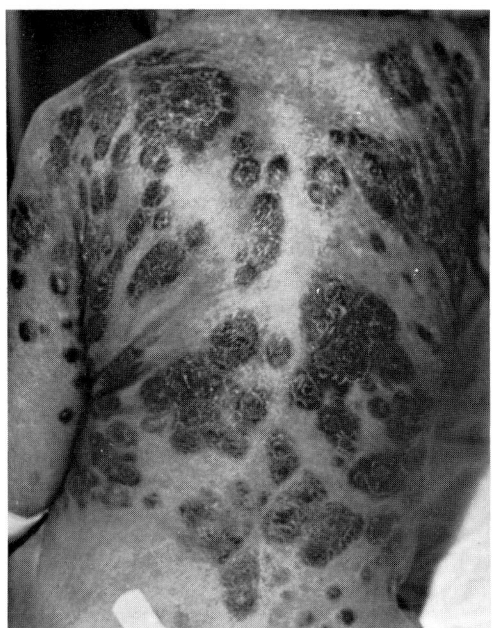

**Figure 69:28.** Mycosis fungoides, man.

## HORMONAL DERMATOSES

### Acanthosis Nigricans

Acanthosis nigricans occurs as an endocrine imbalance in dogs (see p. 225). It is especially common in the dachshund breed. The bilaterally symmetrical acanthotic lesions always start at the axilla (Fig. 69:29) and without treatment will spread to the chest, abdomen, flanks and inguinal areas. The disease is not typical hypothyroidism, but thyroid stimulating hormone and the pituitary gland may be involved. Some have called this dermatosis "frictional acanthosis" or "axillary intertrigo," but friction is not the only cause as weight reduction is not curative. In man, pseudoacanthosis nigricans is an irritative phenomenon of obese patients whose lesions mimic the real disease. The human lesions clear, however, with weight reduction.

Acanthosis nigricans in man can be benign or malignant (Fig. 69:30). The benign type may be hereditary and is seen commonly in young patients. Their lesions usually become stationary, and sometimes regress without treatments. The malignant form is found in older patients, usually associated with some fatal form of visceral cancer. The skin lesions progress as the tumor grows, but if the growth can be removed the skin lesions often regress temporarily. It is felt that the cancer is not the cause of the acanthosis nigricans since the skin lesions are often present for years before signs of the cancer appear. The skin lesions constitute grave signs which demand a thorough investigation.

## FELINE ALOPECIA UNIVERSALIS (SEE P. 277)

The photograph (Fig. 69:31) is of a black male cat born to a normal mother and the only affected kitten in a litter of five. Except for small lanugo

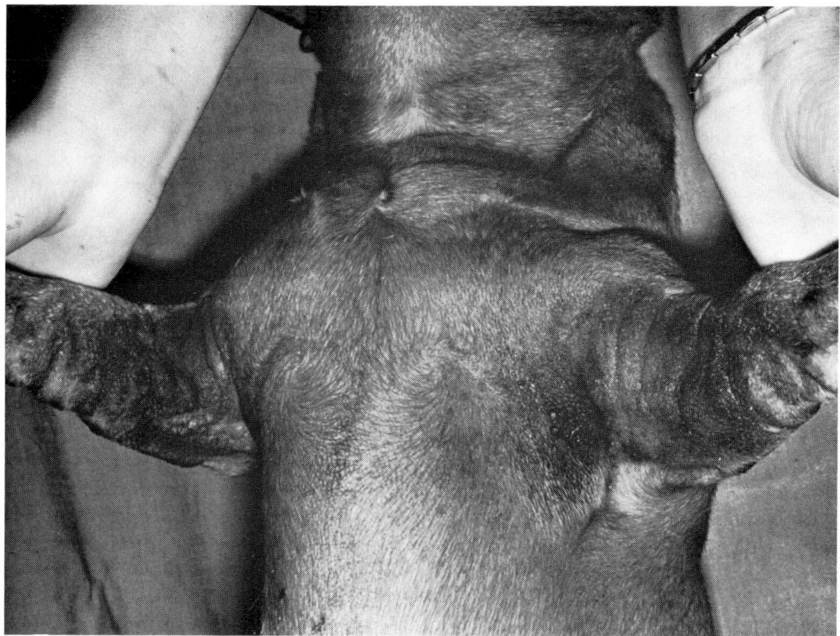

**Figure 69:29.** Acanthosis nigricans, dog.

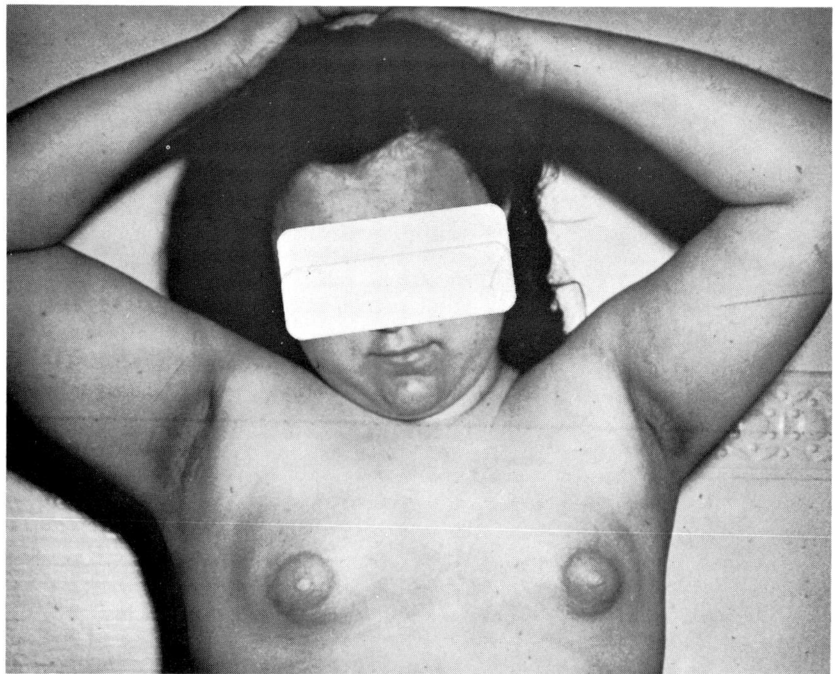

**Figure 69:30.** Acanthosis nigricans, girl.

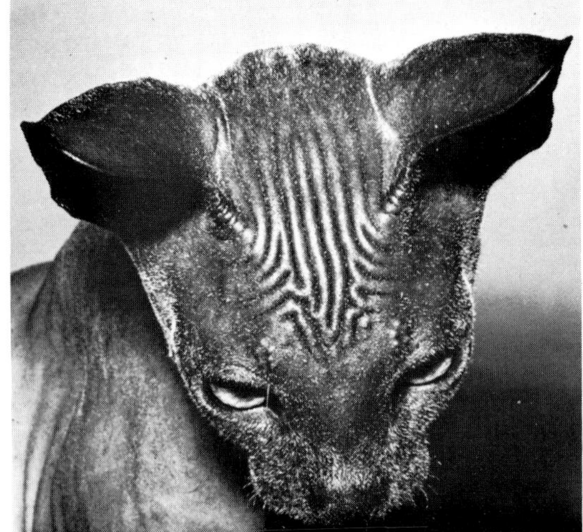

**Figure 69:31.** Feline alopecia universalis.

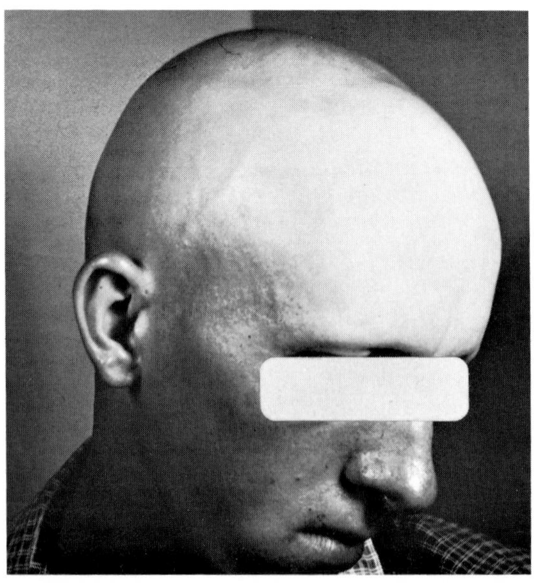

**Figure 69:32.** Alopecia universalis, man.

hairs the cat was hairless, and looked at first glance more like a Chihuahua dog than a cat (Fig. 53:1*A*). The skin of the tail was especially smooth. Since the sebaceous glands were active and the cat did not wash itself (licking the hairless skin with the rough tongue caused pain), a greasy film covered the body. Especially notable were brownish black, greasy deposits on the claws. In order to keep the cat clean and odor-free, the owner had to wash it once a week. One characteristic feature was the wrinkled forehead which is covered by hair in normal cats.

Histopathologic examination of the skin revealed a thickened epidermis and complete absence of hairs in most areas. A few scattered hair follicles were found in areas with rudimentary lanugo hairs. Sebaceous follicles opened directly onto the epidermal surface. Apocrine sweat glands were present and the dermis was normal (Fig. 53-1*B*).

Though not as completely hairless as human patients with alopecia universalis, this congenital condition of the cat resembles its counterpart in man (Fig. 69:32).

## References

Ayres, S. S., and Anderson, N. P.: Demodex Folliculorum: Its Role in the Etiology of Acne Rosacea. Arch. Derm. Syph. *25*:89-98, 1932.

Beerman, H., and Stokes, J. H.: Rosacea Complex and Demodex Folliculorum. Arch. Derm. Syph. *29*: 284-884, 1934.

Brodie, R. C. E.: Rosacea: The Role of Demodex Folliculorum. Aust. J. Derm. *3*:149, 1952.

Conroy, J. D.,: Melanocytic Tumors of Domestic Animals. Arch. Derm. *96*: 372-380, 1967.

Kaplan, W.: Epidemiology and Public Health Significance of Ringworm in Animals. Arch. Derm. *96*:404-408, 1967.

Lever, W. F.: *Histopathology of the Skin.* 4th Ed. J. B. Lippincott Co., Philadelphia, 1967.

Montagna, W.: Comparative Anatomy and Physiology of the Skin. Arch. Derm. *96*: 357-63, 1967.

Moulton, J. E.: *Tumors in Domestic Animals.* University of California Press, Berkeley, 1961.

Mulligan, R. M.: *Neoplasms of the Dog.* Williams & Wilkins Co., Baltimore, 1949.

Orkin, M.: Mastocytosis in Animals. Arch. Derm. *96*:381-385, 1967.

Pillsbury, D. M., Shelley, W. B., and Kligman, A. M.: *Dermatology.* W. B. Saunders Co., Philadelphia, 1956.

Rook, A. J., and Walton, G. S.: *Comparative Physiology and Pathology of the Skin.* F. A. Davis Co., Philadelphia, 1965.

Rothman, S.: Physiology and Biochemistry of the Skin. University of Chicago Press, Chicago, Ill. 1954.

Schwartzman, R. M.: Atopy in the Dog. Arch. Derm. *96*: 418-422, 1967.

Schwartzman, R. M., and Orkin M.: *A Comparative Study of Skin Diseases of Dog and Man.* Charles C Thomas, Springfield, Ill., 1962.

Stewart, W. D., Dante, J. L., and Maddin, S.: *Synopsis of Dermatology.* C. V. Mosby Co., St. Louis, 1966.

# A HISTORY OF VETERINARY DERMATOLOGY

*Section Eight*

# SEVENTY

# *Historical Highlights — Ancient and Modern**

By knowing the history of a specialty, we can distinguish truly new facts from those already discovered, we can prevent duplication of effort and we can avoid repeating the mistakes of others.

Almost as far back as written evidence is available, skin diseases have plagued domestic animals. Man, in turn, felt compelled to take action, often vigorous, to treat the diseased skin. Interestingly enough, a few successful remedies have survived for hundreds of years and are used today. Many others harmed more than they helped and were discontinued. Only in the last century have attempts been made to classify animal skin diseases correctly and learn about their true causes. The information in this section is from material written about veterinary dermatology in the past.

In reading ancient veterinary works it became apparent that terminology needs proper interpretation. For instance, it seems that the word "mange" was once a synonym for almost all skin diseases of animals. Although in modern times mange refers to those diseases associated with mites, many centuries ago it was a catch-all term for numerous dermatoses.†

## THE ANCIENT PERIOD

An Egyptian veterinary papyrus (Fig. 70:1) from the year 2130 B.C. contains the first written record of the treatment of animal diseases (Neffgen, 1904). The ancient hieroglyphics describe mostly eye diseases, but also mention

*Some of the historical information in this section was graciously supplied by Dr. J. F. Smithcors and important biographical information came from personal communications with Dr. Frank Kral and Prof. Dr. Otto Überreiter (Vienna).

†The word *mange* is a Middle English term (originally spelled *manjewe*) derived from the old French *mangier* (an itch) and the modern French *manger* (to eat). Originally it came from the Latin *mandere* (to chew). This condition was descriptively named from its raw, crusted, eaten-out appearance.

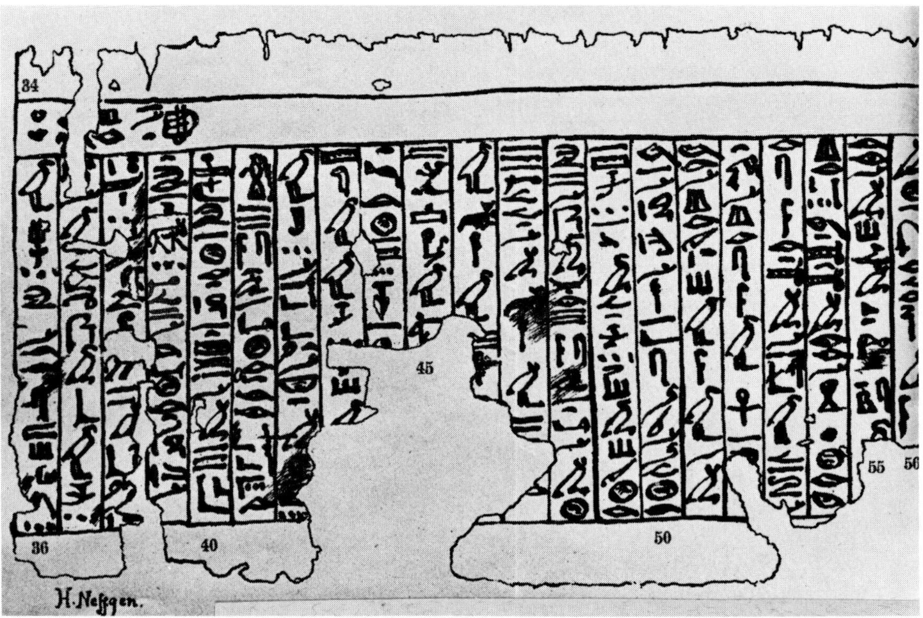

**Figure 70:1.** The veterinary papyrus of Kahun. (From Neffgen, H.: *Der Veterinär-Papyrus von Kahun.* S. Calvary & Co., Berlin, 1904.)

treatment of the skin and gums. The papyrus recommends that the body be rubbed and "fumigated" with "gourds of cucumbers." It calls for making a drying remedy for wounds. Topical medications in use at that time included the somewhat appealing beer, honey and wax, but also such repelling substances as the dung of snakes and lizards. From the earliest recorded writing to the present day, dermatologic therapy consistently included some useful remedies (e.g., wax) with others that must have been devised through ignorance and superstition.

Moses, in the 13th century B.C., gave the commandment that it was forbidden to use sheep with blemishes (Leviticus 3:1). This was interpreted by Schindelka (1908) as "sheep with mange." Another reference from the time of Moses speaks of boils breaking out in sores on both man and beast (Exodus 9:9-11). This may be considered the first reference to comparative dermatology.

The Greek physician Aesculapius (1321-1243 B.C.) was reported to have treated many animals in addition to people. Aesculapius was especially interested in skin diseases and stressed the importance of good skin care, using frequent baths, rubbing with towels and application of lotions (Postolka, 1887).

Aristotle (384 B.C.) was credited with many anatomical and physiological studies. He was said to have observed mange mites in cases of animal scabies.

The Roman scholar Pliny, the Elder (Gaius Plinius Secundus, A.D. 23-79), wrote a 37-volume *Natural History* which became one of the most widely read books of the Middle Ages (Fig. 70:2). In portions of these books the treatment of animal diseases is discussed—included many remedies for dermatoses. Pliny's treatment of skin diseases seems strictly empirical and he gives a multitude of remedies. Smithcors, in his excellent article on mange in dogs (1967), quotes Pliny as follows:

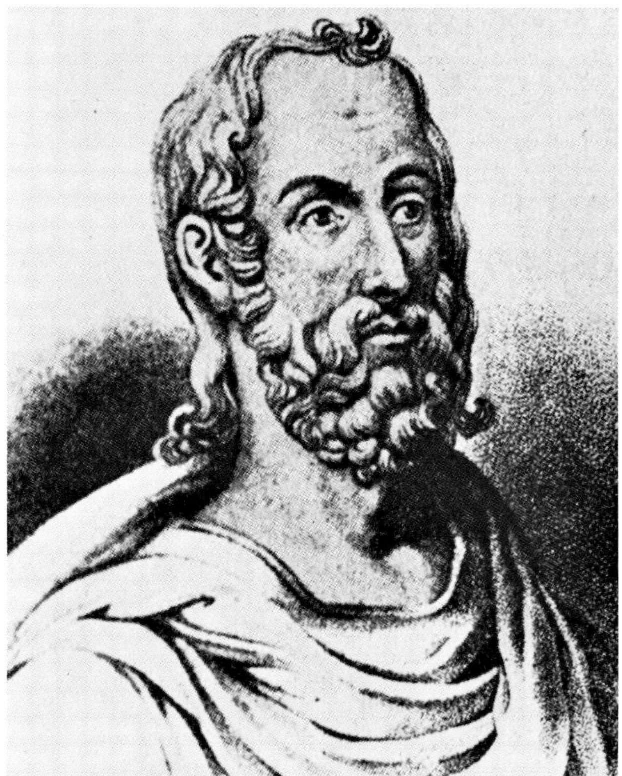

**Figure 70:2.** Pliny, the Elder, A.D. 23-79. (From Locy, W. A.: *The Growth of Biology*. Henry Holt & Co., New York, 1925. Locy borrowed this picture from Jardine: *The Naturalist's Library*.)

> The mange in dogs in healed with beasts bloud, so they be bathed therewith while it is fresh and warm, and after the same is dried upon the body, to follow it a second time the same day; and the morrow after to wash them thoroughly with lye made of strong ashes.

Then there are such unsavory remedies as skin dressings of mouse dung or urine. For mange in horses, Pliny recommends washing them in sea water in which frogs had been boiled (Postolka, 1887).

Not all of Pliny's remedies were that senseless. He recommends sulfur and tar—two remedies that have stood the test of time to this day. He also mentions the use of olive oil, fish liver oil and butter.

Pliny vindicates himself further by preferring to treat skin wounds with drying and mild remedies. However, he did not hesitate to use surgery and recommended "amputation of chronic scabies lesions." For abscesses he recomments that salt and garlic be rubbed in after lancing, following by rinsing the animal's mouth with wine (Postolka, 1887).

The Roman Vergil (Publius Vergilius Maro) lived from the year 70 to 19 B.C. and seemed especially interested in skin diseases of animals. He described mange in sheep and listed its causes as cold rain, wounds from thorns, and salty sweat after shearing. Since mange included many diseases in those days, we cannot evaluate the accuracy of the causes, but at least Vergil was one of the first to think about etiology. For treatment he recommended an ointment (of complicated and secret formula), soaks in running water, and deep cauterization of lesions. He also described anthrax and rinderpest (Postolka, 1887).

The Arabian physician Ben-Sohr, in the 12th century, discovered how mites burrow in the skin (Schindelka, 1908).

Fitzherbert states in his *Book of Husbandry* in 1523 that scabies and lice of sheep should be treated with a mixture of tar in oil or grease. The same mixture was said to be useful to repel flies and the shepherd was advised never to be without his tar box. During the same period, old German veterinary texts advised the liberal use of sulfur in goose grease for skin diseases.

George Turbervile wrote his book *The Noble Art of Venerie or Hunting* in 1576 and gave his version of the different types of mange in a chapter entitled "Of the Maunge, Tettares, Ringwormes, and Scabbes in a dogge." Here, Turbervile gave the first attempt in literature to classify skin diseases of dogs. He described the following four types of mange and gave remedies for each:

1. *Red mange* "maketh a dogges legges to swell." It is the worst type of mange and most difficult to cure. It is caused by overheating of the blood, foundering of the dog when it is hot and chafed from running over brooks and pools, or from lying in cold places. (It is difficult to determine whether he described demodectic mange with interdigital edema, cutaneous allergy or contact dermatitis.)

2. *Scaly mange* appears as patches of eroded skin the size of a man's hand. (This could be acute moist dermatitis.)

3. *Black mange* causes a black discoloration which "lyeth under the skinne" and loss of hair. (This could be hyperpigmentation and alopecia caused by endocrine imbalance.)

4. *Common mange* is caused by lack of fresh drinking water, dirty bedding, filthy kennels or foundering. It is easily cured, claims Turbervile, by applying to the skin a mixture of the following herbs: wild cress, "Enula campana," leaves and roots of wild sorrel, roots of "Roerb," roots of "Frodyles," all boiled in lye and vinegar. Use this mixture on the affected skin for four to five days.

His specific remedy for all manges is as follows:

a. Give a strong laxative.

b. Bathe the dog.

c. Draw 2 ounces of blood from the "vaine which is betwene the hough string, and the bone of his leg."

d. Apply an ointment containing:

| | |
|---|---|
| Nut oil (walnuts) | 3 lbs. |
| Oil of cade | 1½ lbs. |
| Oil of worms | 2 lbs. |
| Honey | 3 lbs. |
| Tar | 2½ lbs. |
| Vinegar | 1½ lbs. |
| Wax | ½ lb. |
| Sulfur (brimstone) | 1½ lbs. |
| Copporas | 2 lbs. |
| Verdigris | 12 oz. |

This ointment, all 18 pounds of it, is said to "kill and heale all maner of manges and itches, how strong or vehement so ever they be." Also interesting is the manner in which it is applied. The dogs are to be thoroughly washed with water, then they are dried by tying them close to a fire for one hour to make them sweat and allowing them to drink "their belly full of water." Then the ointment is applied and dogs are fed a broth of mutton boiled with brimstone and herbs to "warm them within." Continue that diet for eight days.

Turbervile described tumors, which he called "the Wolfe" and recommended surgical excision. He gave a dip for fleas, lice and ticks consisting of wild cress, sorrel leaves, mint leaves, vine leaves, "Stauesaker," saffron and salt.

Turbervile recommended the use of bichloride of mercury for ringworm. For wounds that have been sutured he applied butter as dressing so that the dog would lick it off, because its tongue's action is useful in healing the wound.

Although some of the remedies of the past seem strange and even comical to us today, we must remember to see them in the perspective of each historical period. Turbervile lived shortly after the end of the Middle Ages and in his day was probably considered a capable writer on the art of therapeutics.

## THE MODERN PERIOD

During the 17th and 18th centuries scientific progress occurred through basic investigations in anatomy, pathology and physiology.

The great social and political upheavals of the French and American revolutions at the end of the 18th and beginning of the 19th century preceded an era of medical achievements. Soon there were advances in the natural sciences, in physics and in chemistry. In 1850, Virchow founded cellular pathology, and medicine began its rapid race toward today's vast knowledge.

Many physicians consider that modern dermatology began when Dr. Robert Willan of England wrote the book *On Cutaneous Diseases* in 1808. His book greatly influenced European dermatologists such as Hebra in Germany and Rayer in France. Willan's principles laid the groundwork for most of the dermatology of the 19th century. He said that in dealing with cutaneous disease we should endeavor:

> 1. To fix the sense of the terms employed by proper definition.
> 2. To constitute general division or orders. . . .
> 3. To class and give names to such as have not been hitherto sufficiently distinguished.
> 4. To specify the mode of treatment of each disease.

These principles are as sound and applicable today as they were in Willan's time.

It was to be almost a hundred years later that the first book on veterinary dermatology was published by Schindelka (1908). In the meantime animal skin diseases were given only a chapter in general textbooks on veterinary medicine. Classification and nomenclature were vague, antiquated and confused. Some attempts were made in the middle of the 19th century to adapt human terminology to animal dermatoses. One such example is Chapter XIV in the *Handy Book of Veterinary Homoeopathy* by the English veterinarian James Moore in 1869. He bravely tried to fit animal skin diseases into human categories but failed because he was unaware of the difference in hair coat, pigmentation and epidermal thickness of animal skin. He tried to classify animal skin diseases under such headings as erythematous eruptions, vesicular eruptions, pustular eruptions and parasitic diseases. Only the last one, being etiologic, was a successful classification. Moore introduces his chapter as follows:

> Under such nondescript names as "surfeit," "mange," and so on, are conveniently clubbed together several entirely different skin diseases incidental to lower animals. These diseases can be classified, with at least some approach to diagnostic accuracy, by following the arrangement of human skin diseases into special groups.

These principles were good, but Moore got lost anyhow along the way with nonspecific terms. For instance, one of his headings is:

IV. Vesicular Eruptions
- a. Eczema
  1. Acute Mange
  2. Red Mange
  3. Foul Mange

The attempt for logic in classification, nomenclature, and diagnosis continued from 1850 to 1950. Numerous good scientific articles appeared in journals; chapters on skin diseases were included in many veterinary books. Emphasis was usually placed on diseases of large animals. It is not practical to list or discuss all the chapters. Some of them only summarized existing knowledge, but others attempted to add original observations. Two popular books containing chapters on dermatology will be discussed next.

Hutyra and Marek published the first German edition of their book *Special Pathology and Therapy of Domestic Animals* in 1905. It was revised several times and later translated into English. The last section is devoted to skin diseases of horses, cattle, sheep, swine, goats, rabbits, dogs, cats, poultry and other animals. It is well organized and much thought was given to improved nomenclature. Figure 70:4, showing demodicosis, is an example of one of the book's drawings that illustrate skin diseases.

Müller and Glass's *Diseases of the Dog and their Treatment*, appeared in its third, enlarged edition in 1911. It was based on the original German textbook by Prof. Dr. Georg Müller (Die Krankheiten des Hundes) in 1902. Although the

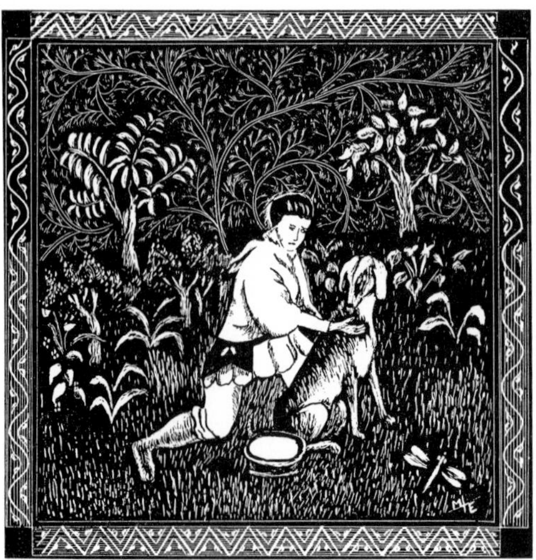

**Figure 70:3.** Dressing the skin of a dog. Detail of painting from a 16th century manuscript on the "curing of hounds." (From Smithcors, J. F.: The History of Some Current Problems in Animal Disease. *Vet. Med.* 52, 1957.)

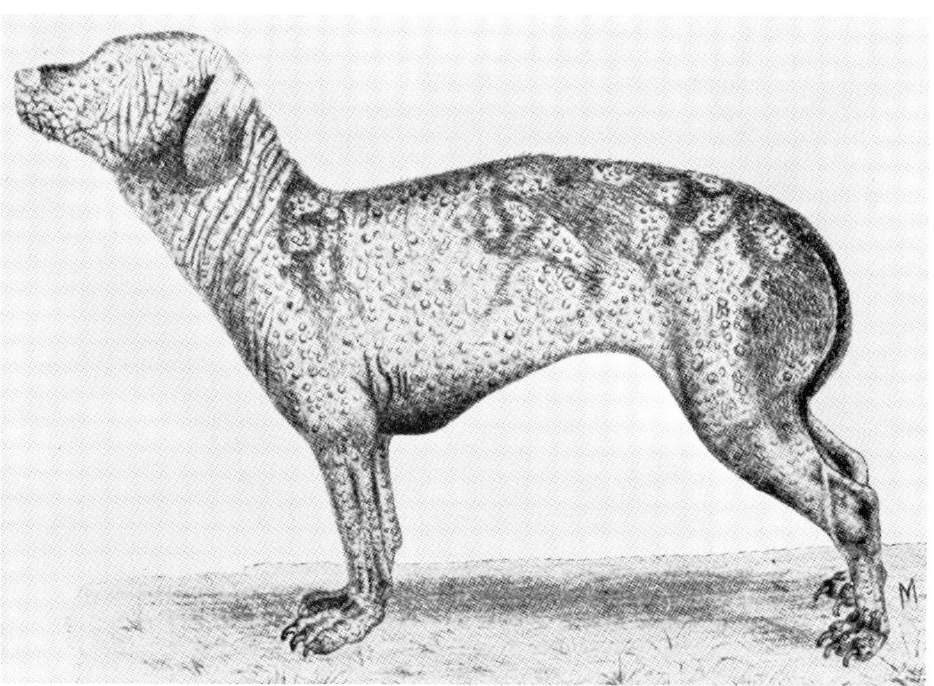

**Figure 70:4.** Demodicosis in a dog, with thickening of the skin and pustulation. (From Hutyra, F., and Marek, J.: *Spezielle Pathologie und Therapie der Haustiere.* Gustav Fischer, Jena, 1910.)

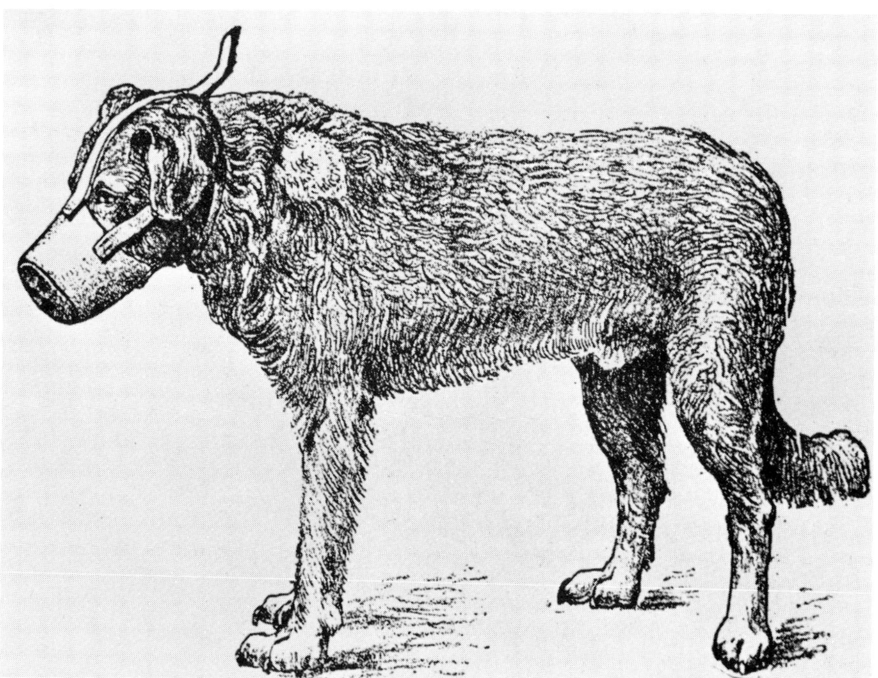

**Figure 70:5.** Moist eczema of the shoulder. Muzzle is to prevent the animal from biting it. (From Müller, G., and Glass, A.: *Diseases of the Dog and their Treatment.* The Franklin Press, Philadelphia, 1911.)

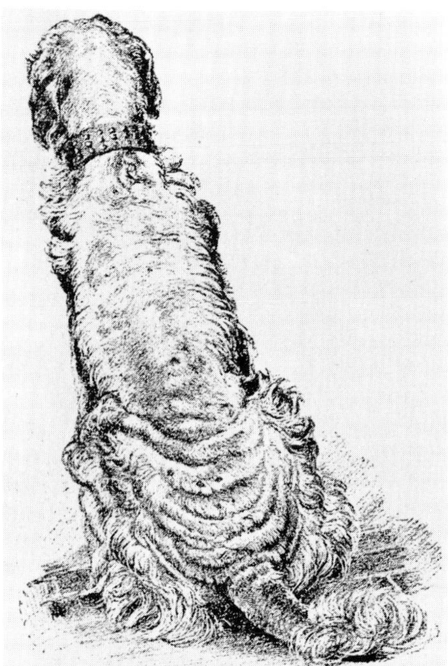

**Figure 70:6.** Chronic eczema of the back. (From Müller, G., and Glass, A.: *Diseases of the Dog and their Treatment.* The Franklin Press, Philadelphia, 1911.)

chapter on skin diseases in the Müller and Glass edition is short, it is interesting and contains several illustrations. One fourth of the chapter is devoted to "eczema," a fact which demonstrates the popularity of that term in the early twentieth century. Two drawings, showing moist eczema and chronic eczema, are included here (Figs. 70:5 and 70:6).

The main credit for progress in veterinary dermatology, however, must go to four men to whom the remainder of this section will be devoted: Schneidemühl, Schindelka, Heller and Kral.

## Schneidemühl

Georg Schneidemühl was born December 15, 1853, in Elbing, Germany. He received his doctor's degree in veterinary medicine from the School of Veterinary Medicine in Berlin. After several years as a state veterinarian and several years in private practice, he became associated with the animal clinic of Halle University in 1891. There were several further changes in his career, including one year as official veterinarian in East Africa. In 1896 he was appointed Professor of Comparative Pathology in Kiel, Germany.

Schneidemühl wrote more than 14 books, covering many diseases and branches of veterinary medicine. There is a book on each of the following: Veterinary History of Germany, Meat Inspection, Foot and Mouth Disease, Vaccination Procedures, Internal Medicine, Anatomy, Tuberculosis, Neurology, Protozoology, and Contagious Abortion.

The reason for his inclusion in this section is the outstanding chapter on skin diseases in his textbook, *The Comparative Pathology and Therapy of Man and Domestic Animals.* It was the first formal discussion of comparative dermatology and laid the groundwork for later studies by Schindelka and Heller. Each disease was described first as it occurs in man and then as it occurs in animals. His observations were clear, his organization logical, avoiding speculation when the etiology was unknown. Adapted from human dermatology are eight primary and five secondary skin lesions, and dermatoses are broadly divided into parasitic and nonparasitic diseases. Very interesting is his observation of the greater difficulty in diagnosing animal skin diseases because their bodies are covered by hair and are often heavily pigmented.

Among the diseases of comparative interest he makes the following divisions:

1. Skin diseases of man that also occur in animals: eczema, cutaneous pruritus, pemphigus, ichthyosis, hyperhidrosis, chromidrosis, acne, furunculosis, congenital alopecia, favus, impetigo, scabies, tumors and other diseases.

2. Skin diseases of man that have not yet been found in animals: erythema nodosum, psoriasis, pityriasis, lupus erythematosus, scleroderma, seborrhea, pityriasis versicolor, xanthoma, rhinoderma, xeroderma pigmentosum and other diseases.

An example of Schneidemühl's precise, clear descriptions is his discussion of eczema in dogs. It shows that he was accurately describing allergic dermatitis and contact dermatitis with acute moist dermatitis, even though the principle of hypersensitivity was unknown in his day. Here is an excerpt translated specifically for this chapter:

#### ECZEMATOUS SKIN DISEASES IN THE DOG

In the dog, eczematous skin diseases occur quite frequently. Just as with other animals, different names are in usage (eczema, summer mange, and herpes). Usually, the back, tailbase of the head and neck are the seats of the disease, rarely other parts of the body (legs). The disease has various forms and degrees of manifestation—papules, vesicles, pustules, scales and flakes—and is accompanied by more or less severe itching.

*Etiology.* Most commonly affected are young animals with fine skin or older, very well-fed dogs that are confined a lot to the room. The most manifest causes can be mechanical irritations of all kinds (chemical, heat, dust, rubbing of leather collars, repeated bathing with soaps). Aggravating factors may be predisposing causes (digestive disturbances, overly rich diet, lack of exercise). The course of the disease can be considerably complicated if the already diseased skin is infected with micro-organisms.

*Symptoms.* First there appear little light red macules which later change to papules on the back, head, neck, and the lateral surfaces of the extremities . . . . At the diseased areas the hair is bristled up, and the skin is swollen, painful and causes itching. Although in this (first) stage healing can occur, most cases progress to the formation of vesicles (eczema vesiculosum). These can then either dry up, or they burst and become covered with a serous or purulent exudate. The exudate is then likely to dry into crusts under which the skin regenerates and thus brings the process to healing. In some cases, however, the disease affects the skin very extensively. The involved and more and more enlarging areas are characterized by hair loss and oozing, and because of the continued rubbing by the animals, eventually result in suppuration and bleeding. Finally, the vesicles can also change into pustules (eczema pustulosum). The initially matted hairs fall out showing the underlying skin to be thickened, slightly bleeding, and covered with crusts. Healing can occur even at that stage, although hairless areas often remain.

In chronic cases the dog's skin is constantly reddened, thickened and painful. Also, continued scaling is noticed and in individual cases granulation tissue forms. Nevertheless, the general condition of the animals remains quite undisturbed, and only in eczematous infections of long duration are there digestive problems and weight loss.

The course varies, depending on degree and type of disorder, breed, care, and environment, and can amount to one to three weeks in acute cases, or several years in chronic cases.

## Schindelka

Although Schneidemühl and others made contributions, the real beginning of veterinary dermatology as a specialty occurred at the turn of this century when one man decided to summarize his knowledge of that subject and wrote the first book on skin diseases of domestic animals (*Hautkrankheiten bei Haustieren*). That man was Hugo Schindelka (Fig. 70:7), who completed his book in October, 1902.

Schindelka was born in the year 1853 in Znaim, a town located about 50 miles north of Vienna, Austria.* He studied both medicine and veterinary medicine. One year after receiving his medical degree from the University of Vienna in 1878, he began his studies in veterinary medicine at the Veterinary Military Institute. What caused him to abandon a career as a physician and devote the rest of his life to teaching and research in veterinary medicine is not known. In 1890 he was promoted to the rank of professor of special pathology and therapy at the University of Vienna. As a teacher he was known for his ability to organize his lectures clearly and condense extensive subject matter into a few words. Although he became most famous for his work in dermatology, he also had other interests. Surprisingly, 13 of his 42 articles dealt with ophthalmology. Together

*Znaim, Moravia (then Austria-Hungary, now Czechoslovakia).

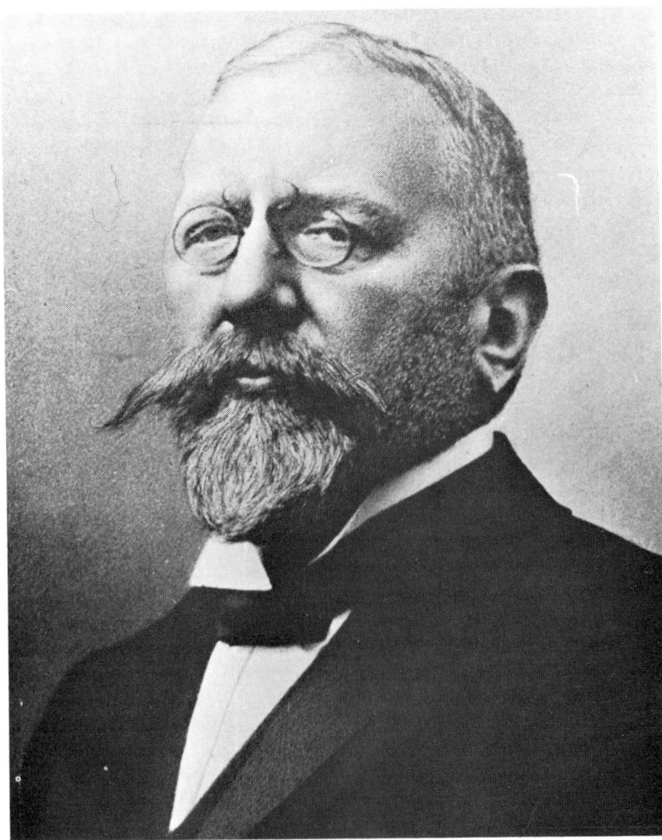

**Figure 70:7.** Hugo Schindelka, 1853-1913. (Courtesy Prof. Dr. Otto Überreiter.)

with Polansky he originated rhinolaryngoscopy of the horse. In addition to the book on skin diseases, he wrote three other books.

Schindelka's interest in dermatology was apparently stimulated by his father, who was a physician in Znaim. The senior Schindelka once wrote an article concerning work of the famous dermatologist Hebra.

One day, probably near the year 1900, Schindelka was approached by Prof. Dr. Joseph Bayer and Prof. Dr. Eugene Fröhner, the publishers of a multivolume handbook on veterinary medicine. They asked him to write a volume on skin diseases. At first Schindelka hesitated because he was aware of the lack of current knowledge of skin pathology, especially histopathology. He finally consented to write the book because of his great interest in dermatology and his access to much available clinical material.

The book is well organized and far advanced for its time. Outstanding are the detailed, lucid clinical descriptions. Schindelka had the ability to record clinical observations accurately, without adding old and inaccurate etiologic theories. It contains many excellent illustrations, e.g., Figure 70:8.

It is difficult to decide which of his disease descriptions to select for translation and inclusion in this history. Since Schindelka was the first to describe *acanthosis nigricans* in the dog, that disease is chosen. The name of the disease came from a similar disorder of man which Politzer first described and named in 1890 in the International Atlas of Rare Skin Diseases.

Following are excerpts from Schindelka's description of the disease, translated for this chapter:

> *Acanthosis Nigricans (Distrophia Papillaris et Pigmentosa)*
> Acanthosis nigricans is characterized by its typical location and by the symmetrical

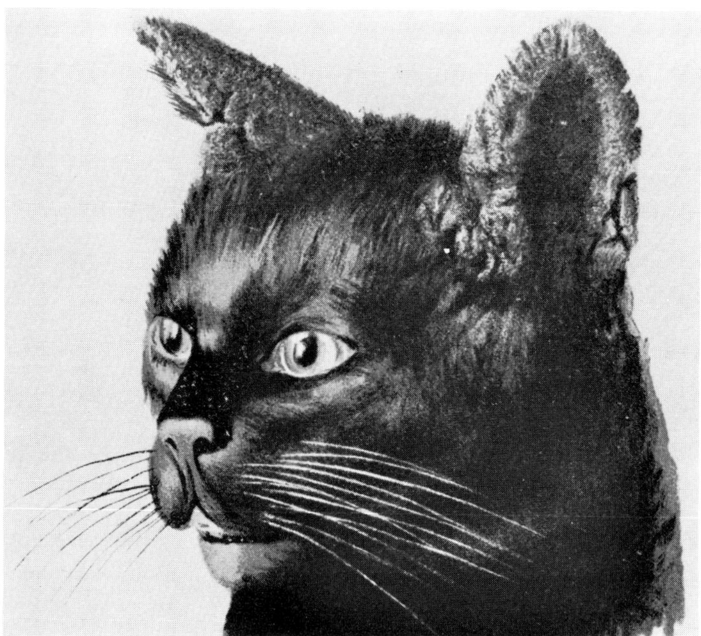

**Figure 70:8.** Notoedric mange. (From Schindelka, H.: *Hautkrankheiten bei Haustieren.* Wilhelm Braumüller, Wien, 1908.)

appearance of the skin changes which consist in hypertrophy of the papillary body, hyperpigmentation and, in most cases, hyperkeratosis.

In the dog, these skin changes occur mostly in the axillae [Fig. 70:9] and the flanks; further, in the interdigital spaces, the scrotum, the nipples, the perianal area, the ventral surface of the tail, abdomen, corners of the mouth, eyelids, and lips. Also affected can be the mucous membrane of the mouth, anus and conjunctivae. The skin lesions vary in their locations, depending on the case, and do not attain the same intensity everywhere.

Acanthosis nigricans is a skin disorder of its own kind and has no connection whatsoever with ichthyosis, as had been presumed at one time.

The changes in the skin appear gradually, without any traceable cause, and as a rule are accompanied by more or less severe itching. The causative association between this skin disorder and malignant tumors of inner organs that has been made by a number of observers in man, cannot be established in the dog. Among the seven cases that I observed, cancer was present only in one of them.

The disease is incurable and its course chronic. It progresses little by little with time intervals between the individual stages during which the skin changes regress and can almost disappear completely. In the dog, each advance is usually accompanied by pruritus.

The skin changes which develop in acanthosis nigricans are as follows:

In most cases, slight swelling and pigmentation occur in the skin of the already mentioned areas, together with hair loss. More specifically, the lesions are always symmetric, although not necessarily of the same intensity and exactly equal expansion on either side. The skin feels thickened, yet softer, more edematous, and more moist than normal skin. The borders of the affected areas are not sharply defined. Due to the fact that the normal groove pattern is more prominent, slight ridges form which are separated from each other by flat grooves, thus giving the skin a sealskin leather appearance. At the same time, pigmentary changes occur, varying between a strong gray-blue, gray-brown, or black-brown and consisting initially of irregularly defined, sporadic small macules which then enlarge peripherally and become confluent with neighboring ones until they eventually coalesce in such a manner as to give that entire skin area an almost evenly dark coloration. In its further course, the diseased skin becomes increasingly uneven. Its groove pattern gets more and more prominent with the individual ridges projecting distinctly and becoming more wart-like. In two cases I found these warts accumulated on a certain area of the skin—the axilla. They gave the appearance of several parallel curved combs. Along with these changes, the skin becomes increasingly tough and tight, and finally feels as rough as a metal "grater." In some areas, such as the extremities, the scrotum, perianal area and ventral tail, the skin thickens like that of an elephant. As a rule, no scaling is present on the affected areas with the exception of a few scanty, flaky, gray, tightly adhering scales.

The claws show striking changes in some cases. In two dogs I found them on all four paws dull, rough, dry, irregularly worn out, considerably thickened and quite feathered.

Schindelka's work had great influence on the future of veterinary dermatology—an influence still apparent today. He was the teacher, colleague and friend of Prof. Dr. D. Wirth, who wrote a special chapter on skin diseases (Wirth and Diernhofer) in 1943 and was the director of the Viennese Medical Clinic from 1920 to 1946. Schindelka was one of the teachers of Dr. Frank Kral, whose important role in dermatology will be discussed later.

Schindelka continued his work and teaching until shortly before his untimely death on April 12, 1913, at the age of 60.

## Heller

Progress in veterinary dermatology has, in the last 75 years, frequently related closely to human dermatology. Just as Schneidemühl's work was largely

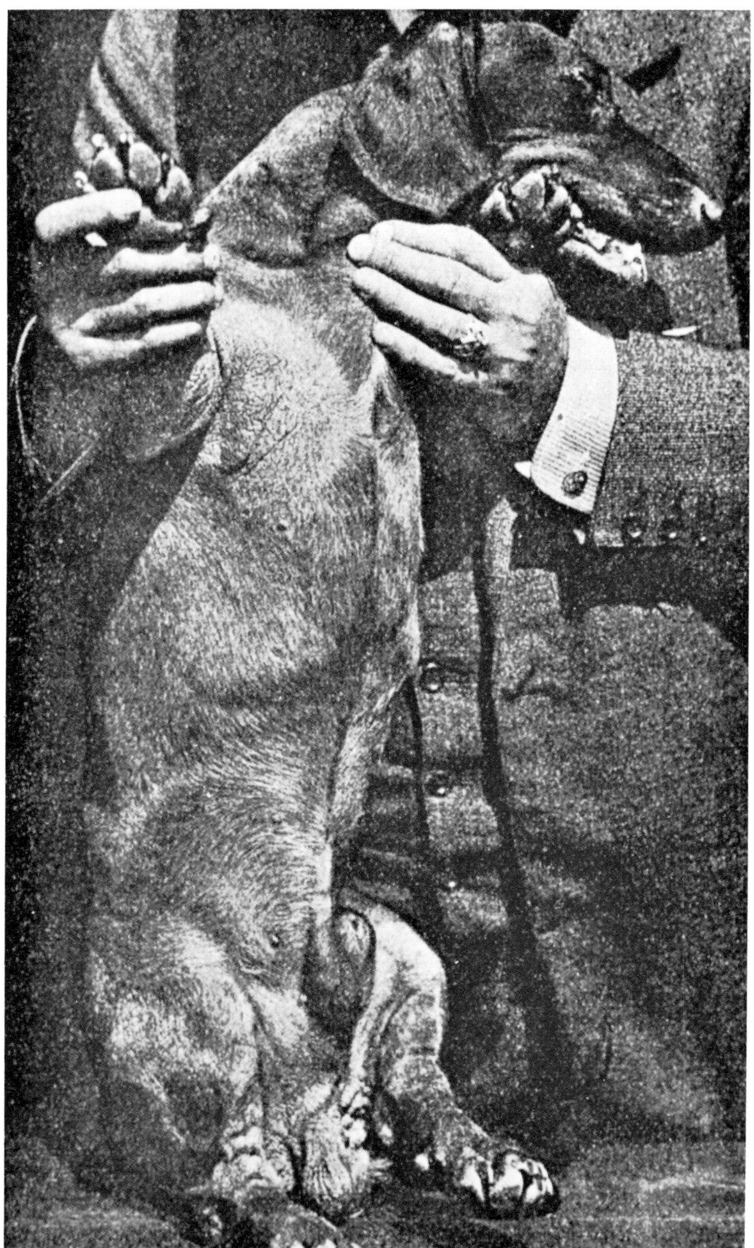

**Figure 70:9.** Acanthosis nigricans in a dachshund. (From Schindelka, H.: *Hautkrankheiten bei Haustieren.* Wilhelm Braumüller, Wien, 1908.)

in comparative medicine, Julius Heller, a German physician, had an intense interest in skin diseases of animals. His main contribution in dermatology was to write the first book devoted exclusively to comparative dermatology.

Julius Heller was born in Berlin, September 16, 1864. He studied at Heidelberg, received his degree as doctor of medicine in 1887, and specialized in dermatology and syphilology. His work covered many fields including forensic dermatology, diseases of nails, venereal diseases, histopathology of the skin, and comparative dermatology. In 1910 he was appointed Professor at the University of Berlin. The same year marked the publication of his book, *The Comparative Pathology of the Skin*. This book is unique because Heller evaluated the veterinary and zoological aspects of animal skin diseases from the point of view of the human dermatologist.

Heller began to work on this book in 1900. In 1903, when Schindelka's book was published, he realized that both would deal with a similar subject. However, he said in his foreword:

> Three years after the beginning of my studies, there appeared the first book about skin diseases of animals by Prof. Dr. Hugo Schindelka. This outstanding book was, in my opinion, written primarily for the veterinary profession. Therefore, I will continue my own book since it has a different aim from Schindelka's.

Heller's *Comparative Pathology of the Skin* is a very comprehensive work. It surveys the entire literature to that date and has many original histopathologic descriptions. These were sufficient for the range of knowledge of that time, but rather superficial in light of today's findings. This is to be expected and not to be considered criticism.

Heller wrote the following about the frequency and meaning of animal skin diseases:

> Skin diseases are comparatively more frequent in animals than in civilized man, especially in regard to the endless number of parasites that cause skin disease. Epidemics of scabies not only destroy farm animals, but also cause local extinction of wild animals (such as foxes). Fungus diseases (favus) routinely cause death in certain species (such as mice). Molluscum contagiosum is a harmless illness in man, but causes systemic illness in domestic fowl. While *Demodex folliculorum* is a harmless parasite of man, demodectic mange is often an incurable disease in animals.
>
> On the other hand, many human dermatoses are seen only seldom in animals or are seen in a different form (psoriasis, lupus erythematosus, lupus vulgaris, lichen planus, etc.).

One year before his death on December 23, 1931, Heller saw the publication of his 218-page chapter on animal dermatoses in Jadassohn's famous handbook. In this chapter Heller referred frequently to the works of Hutyra, Marek, Müller and Schindelka. The chapter preserved the knowledge that Heller had acquired since his 1910 book and filled the historical gap between 1910 and 1931. Heller had this to say:

> The pathologic anatomy of the last two decades has changed little since the appearance of my book *Comparative Pathology of the Skin* (1910). I have, therefore, concentrated on clinical aspects of animal skin diseases in this chapter.

## Kral

Modern veterinary dermatology owes a great debt to Dr. Frank Kral, whose numerous accomplishments cover many phases of large and small animal dermatology (Fig. 70:10). For half a century, since 1919, Dr. Kral has devoted his career to the study of skin diseases of animals. In 1963 he was appointed Professor Emeritus at the School of Veterinary Medicine, University of Pennsylvania.

Frank Kral was born in Albrechtice, Czechoslovakia, on August 18, 1892. He began to study medicine and later changed to veterinary medicine. Under the influence of famous teachers including Hugo Schindelka, it is not surprising that Kral's interests soon turned to veterinary dermatology. In 1919 he was appointed professor at the School of Veterinary Medicine, in Brno, Czechoslovakia, and immediately began research on skin diseases of both large and small animals. His work at the university was in close association with dermatologists of the Medical School. Under his supervision, several of his students

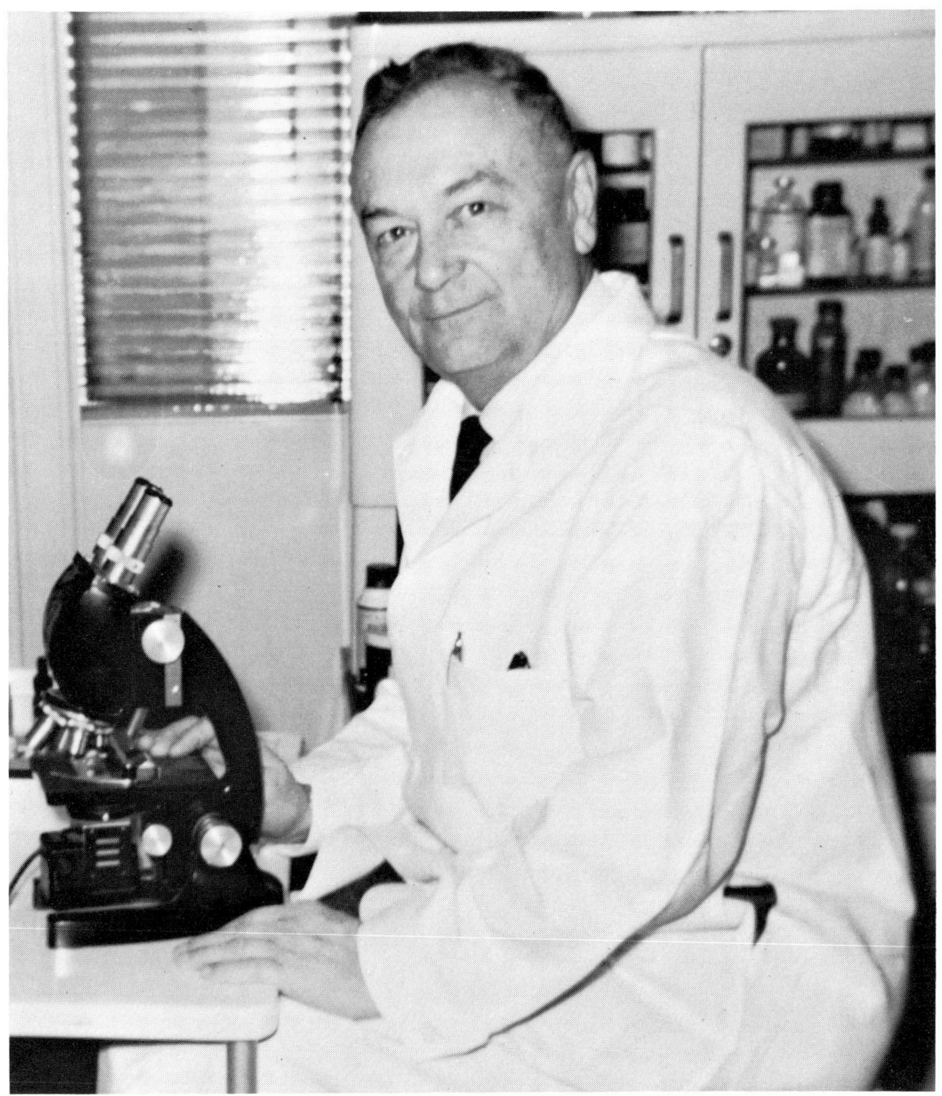

**Figure 70:10.** Dr. Frank Kral.

wrote their doctor's theses on dermatologic subjects. One of Kral's special lecture series at the Medical School dealt with infectious dermatoses transmissible from animal to man.

In 1931 he published the second book ever written on skin diseases of animals, *Veterinarni Dermatologie*.

In 1948 Kral left his native Czechoslovakia and shortly thereafter joined the staff of the School of Veterinary Medicine of the University of Pennsylvania. There he developed the famous Veterinary Dermatology Clinic and devoted himself exclusively to the treatment and investigation of large and small animal dermatoses. He was appointed to the rank of professor and wrote numerous papers on skin diseases.

His enthusiasm was contagious. Interest in veterinary dermatology soared as Kral tirelessly traveled back and forth across the United States to lecture. He spoke at meetings of medical and veterinary associations and lectured at schools of veterinary medicine as one of the most respected, most beloved, and most sought-after speakers in the veterinary field.

In 1953 he worked with Novak to revise and completely rewrite his 1931 Czechoslovakian textbook to produce *Veterinary Dermatology*, the first book on that subject in the English language. Further papers followed on fungal diseases, pyoderma, and dermatoses associated with internal disorders. As notes for a seven-city lecture tour through the United States in 1960, he produced the *Compendium of Veterinary Medicine*, a masterful summary of the subject. Two more books followed. First, with Dr. Robert M. Schwartzman, he again revised, enlarged, and completely rewrote his 1953 textbook which was published in 1964 as *Veterinary and Comparative Dermatology*. Containing over twice the number of illustrations of his 1953 book, the new work covers skin diseases of horses, cattle, swine, sheep, rabbits, poultry, dogs, cats and other animals. Finally in 1968 as a coauthor with Schwartzman he produced a color atlas of canine and feline dermatoses consisting of 100 pages of color illustrations of skin diseases.

Although Kral retired in 1963 and was appointed Emeritus Professor of Dermatology, he continued activities in his favorite specialty. Many honors have been conferred on him, including an honorary doctorate from the University of Munich (1962) and the Golden Diploma from the School of Veterinary Medicine in Vienna (1964).

## THE PRESENT PERIOD

During the last decade veterinary dermatology advanced through research, symposia and specialty organizations. Research by individuals and medical science teams resulted in a deeper understanding of animal skin disorders. Basic studies included cutaneous pathology, biochemistry, and histochemistry. Clinical dermatology and therapeutics also progressed rapidly.

Several important symposia were held which covered the subjects of clinical and comparative dermatology. These included:

The Transatlantic Conference on Canine and Feline Dermatology (Chicago and London), April, 1963.

The Symposium on Comparative Physiology and Pathology of the Skin (England), April, 1964.

Four consecutive annual symposia on Comparative Dermatology

sponsored by the American Academy of Dermatology (Chicago and Miami), 1964 through 1967.

The Symposium on Skin Diseases Common to Animals and Man, sponsored jointly by the American Medical Association and the American Animal Hospital Association (Palm Springs, California), October, 1967.

Two veterinary dermatologic organizations in America presently encourage progress and education: The Dermatology Committee of the American Animal Hospital Association (appointed in 1959) and the American Academy of Veterinary Dermatology (organized in 1964).

Further rapid advancement in veterinary dermatology is assured through such organizations and symposia. Much work lies ahead for those working in the field today, and for newcomers attracted to this specialty in the future.

## References


Fitzherbert: *Book of Husbandry*. 1523.

Heller, J.: *Die Vergleichende Pathologie der Haut*. August Hirschwald, Berlin, 1910.

Heller, J.: Die Klinik der Wichtigsten Tierdermatosen. *In* Jadassohn: *Handbuch der Haut und Geschlechtskrankheiten*. Julius Springer, Berlin, 1930.

Hutyra, F., and Marek, J.: *Spezielle Pathologie und Therapie der Haustiere*. Ed. 3. Gustav Fischer, Jena, 1910.

Moore, J.: *Handy Book of Veterinary Homoeopathy*. W. Radde, New York, 1869.

Müller, G., and Glass, A.: *Diseases of the Dog and their Treatment*. Ed. 3. The Franklin Press, Philadelphia, 1911.

Neffgen, H.: *Der Veterinar-Papyrus von Kahun*. S. Calvary & Co., Berlin, 1904.

Pliny: *Natural History of the Ubiquitous Roman of the First Century* (1600). Quotation from Smithcors, J. F.: The History of Some Current Problems in Animal Disease: V. Mange in Dogs. V. Med. *52*:127, 1967.

Postolka, A.: *Geschichte der Tierheilkunde*. Mortiz Perles, Vienna, 1887.

Schindelka, H.: *Hautkrankheiten bei Haustieren*. Wilhelm Braumüller, Vienna, 1908.

Schneidemühl, G.: *Lehrbuch der Vergleichenden Pathologie und Therapie des Menchen und der Hausthiere*. Wilhelm Engelmann, Leipzig, 1898.

Smithcors, J. F.: The History of Some Current Problems in Animal Disease: V. Mange in Dogs, Vet. Med. *52*:127-131, 1957.

Turbervile, G.: *The Noble Art of Venerie or Hunting* (1576). Facsimile edition. Clarendon Press, London, 1908.

# APPENDIX

## DERMATOLOGIC DRUGS AND EQUIPMENT

The following list of drugs and equipment is included to give brief, pertinent facts about typical dermatologic drugs which the authors have found effective. Many other excellent medications are available, but lack of space precludes their presentation here. Readers should refer to veterinary drug lists, *Current Veterinary Therapy*, *Physician's Desk Reference* and texts on pharmacology for additional, complete information.

### *Alpha-Keri*

1. Water-dispersible, antipruritic oil.
2. Contains a dewaxed, oil-soluble, keratin-moisturizing fraction of lanolin; mineral oil; nonionic emulsifiers.
3. Actions and indications:
   Deposits a thin uniform amount of oil on hair and skin to relieve itching and lubricate and soften the skin. It gives gloss to the coat. Indicated for chronic dry, pruritic skin conditions. Not for use in acute inflammations.
4. Dosage:
   Add one capful to one or two quarts of water for final rinse after bath; or spray aerosol onto wet coat and rub well.
5. Supplied:
   8 oz. bottle or 5 oz. aerosol can.
   Westwood Pharmaceuticals
   468 De Witt Street
   Buffalo, N.Y. 14213

### *Canex*

1. Acaricide for dogs.
2. Contains:
   Chloroform 7.5 per cent; rotenone 0.12 per cent; ether extracts of derris 0.38 per cent; inert 92 per cent.
3. Actions and indications:
   For demodectic, sarcoptic and otodectic mange. It is penetrating, acaricidal and safe for dogs. It may be used in the ears of cats if diluted 3:1 with mineral oil.
4. Dosage:
   Apply to affected areas topically with vigorous massage. It is best applied after clipping and bathing; application may be repeated two or three times weekly. For ear mites, apply a few drops to the ear canal and repeat three times weekly.
5. Supplied:
   Pint and gallon bottles.
   Pitman-Moore
   Indianapolis, Indiana

### *Capteen Shampoo*

1. Therapeutic shampoo.
2. Contains:
   Salicylic acid 2 per cent; captan 2 per cent; 2,2′ methylene bis (4-chlorophenol) 2 per cent; sulfur 1 per cent, in a special lathering base.
3. Actions and indications:
   Useful in the control of fungal and bacterial dermatoses of dogs and cats. It is a good cleansing agent.
4. Dosage:
   Wet coat. Work up a good lather and let remain 15 minutes. Rinse well. Repeat weekly if needed.
5. Supplied:
   6 oz. and 1 gallon plastic bottles.
   H. C. Burns
   7711 Oakport Street
   Oakland, California 94621

### *Cerumite*

1. Liquid for ear mites.
2. Contains:
   Cerumene (hexamethyltetracosane) 25.0 per cent; pyrethrin 0.05 per cent; technical piperonyl butoxide 0.5 per cent; dichlorophene 1.0 per cent; inert 73.45 per cent.
3. Actions and indications:
   Acaricidal, insecticidal and ceruminolytic qualities make it effective against otodectic infestations of the ear.
4. Dosage:
   Cleanse the ear canal and apply 5 to 10 drops to the ear canal daily. Repeat treatment in ten days.
5. Supplied:
   15 cc. plastic applicator bottles.
   EVSCO Pharmaceutical Co.
   3345 Royal Avenue
   Oceanside, L.I., N.Y. 11572

### *Colloidal Sulfur Suspension*

1. A colloidal sulfur lotion.
2. Contains:
   Colloidal sulfur 2 per cent in suspension in a pleasantly scented liquid vehicle.
3. Actions and indications:
   Sulfur is fungicidal, antiseptic and acaricidal. It is also mildly stimulating or keratolytic. The latter action is most evident with continual dosage or use of higher concentrations.
4. Dosage:
   Apply topically to affected skin twice daily.

5. Supplied:
   1 gallon bottles.
   EVSCO Pharmaceutical Co.
   3345 Royal Avenue
   Oceanside, L.I., N.Y. 11572

### *Depo-Medrol*

1. Anti-inflammatory, anti-stress agent.
2. Contains:
   Methylprednisolone acetate 20 mg./cc. for injection.
3. Actions and indications:
   Has pronounced anti-inflammatory effects and is especially helpful in various allergic dermatoses of dogs and cats.
4. Dosage:
   Single I.M. injections may last as long as one week. Dogs should receive 2 to 40 mg. per week depending on size of the patient and the severity of the condition. Cats should receive 5 to 20 mg. per week.
5. Supplied:
   5 cc. vials, 20 mg./cc.
   5 cc. vials, 40 mg./cc.
   Upjohn Company
   7171 Portage Road
   Kalamazoo, Michigan

### *Diryl Powder*

1. Insecticide, bactericide, fungicide for dogs and cats.
2. Contains:
   Malathion (0,0-dimethyl dithiophosphate of diethyl mercaptosuccinate) 4 per cent; 2,2′ methylene bis (4-chlorophenol) (Di Phenthane-70) 2 per cent; rotenone 1.25 per cent; other cube resins 2.5 per cent; inert 90.25 per cent.
3. Actions and indications:
   Insecticide, antibacterial and antifungal powder for dogs and cats.
4. Dosage:
   Sprinkle on coat; rough coat to work the powder down to the skin. Repeat two times weekly. Use on bedding or premises if needed.
5. Supplied:
   3½ oz. sprinkler top cans.
   Pitman-Moore
   Indianapolis, Indiana

### *Domeboro*

1. Tablets or powder for producing Burow's solution.
2. Contains aluminum sulfate and calcium acetate for producing Burow's solution (pH 4.2).

3. Actions and indications:
   Produces a wet dressing for anti-inflammatory cleansing, antipruritic, antiseptic and mildly astringent actions. Used for treatment of acute inflammations of the skin.
4. Dosage:
   Add one tablet or powder (1 tsp.) to 16 ounces of water. Use warm for abscesses and cellulitis; use cold for atopic dermatitis, urticaria, insect bites, acute inflammatory lesions. Apply as wet dressings, soaks, baths or irrigations for 15 minutes every 4 hours.
5. Supplied:
   Domeboro tablets, boxes of 12, 100, 500, 1000. Powder packets (½ teaspoonful) in boxes of 12, 100. Bulk powder, 4 oz. container.
   Dome Laboratories
   400 Morgan Avenue
   West Haven, Connecticut 06516

### *Fleatol*

1. Insecticidal shampoo for dogs and cats.
2. Contains:
   Ammonium lauryl sulfate 18.6 per cent; piperonyl butoxide 0.5 per cent; pyrethrine 0.05 per cent; petroleum oils 0.2 per cent; inert 80.65 per cent.
3. Action and indications:
   Kills lice and fleas, removes dirt and crusts and contains a bluing which whitens white coats.
4. Dosage:
   Wet animal, apply shampoo and work up a good lather. Allow to remain ten minutes and rinse well. Repeat once. Treatment may be repeated as often as needed.
5. Supplied:
   Pint and gallon bottles.
   Haver-Lockhart Laboratories
   Kansas City, Missouri

### *Fleavol Shampoo*

1. A mild, cleansing shampoo which leaves the hair coat soft and lustrous.
2. Contains:
   Pyrethrins 0.05 per cent; piperonyl butoxide 0.50 per cent; disopropyl cresols 0.10 per cent; inert ingredients 99.35 per cent.
3. Actions and indications:
   For cleansing skin and hair and to kill fleas, lice and other pyrethrin-susceptible ectoparasites.
4. Dosage:
   Thoroughly wet the hair. Apply shampoo and rub up a lather for five to ten minutes. Rinse thoroughly.
5. Supplied:
   6 oz., 1 gallon, 5 gallon bottles.

Norden Laboratories
Box 1227
Lincoln, Nebraska 68501

### *Fluoro-Derm*

1. Skin refrigerant for dermatologic surgery.
2. Contains:
   Dichlorotetrafluorethane in aerosol.
3. Actions and indications:
   Topical anesthesia produced by freezing. Safe, nonflammable, nonexplosive, for external use only.
4. Dosage:
   Spray on skin from distance of 4 to 6 inches for 30 seconds or until area is frosted. Blowing to enhance evaporation will hasten the process.
5. Supplied:
   8 oz. aerosol cans.
   Schucho Industries, Inc.
   250 W. 18th Street
   New York, N.Y.

### *Fostex (Fosteen) Cream*

1. An antiseborrheic skin cleanser and shampoo.
2. Contains micropulverized sulfur 2 per cent; salicylic acid 2 per cent; hexachlorophene 1 per cent; and Sebulytic surface active soapless cleansers and wetting agents.
3. Actions and indications:
   Provides maximum degreasing and degerming action and is an excellent shampoo for dandruff and oily or dry seborrhea.
4. Dosage:
   Wet the hair and skin, apply the cream and rub well to work up a lather. Rinse well. Repeat application and rinse a second time. The therapeutic shampoo may be repeated every five to ten days to manage seborrheic skin problems.

a. Supplied:
   4½ oz. jars.
   Westwood Pharmaceuticals
   468 De Witt Street
   Buffalo, N.Y. 14213

### *Fungidex Creme*

1. A fungicide, bactericide and antipruritic medication in a cream base.
2. Contains:
   Zinc undecylenate 12 per cent; undecylenic acid 5 per cent; copper undecylenate 3 per cent; dichlorophene 2 per cent in a cream base.

3. Actions and indications:
   An antimycotic and antipruritic agent for topical use.
4. Dosage:
   Clip hair from affected areas and cleanse skin. Apply cream once or twice daily with gentle massage. Continue treatment several days after lesions have healed.
5. Supplied:
   2 oz. and 1 lb. jars.
   Norden Laboratories
   Box 1227
   Lincoln, Nebraska 68501

### *Fungizone*

1. Amphotericin B lotion for topical use.
2. Contains:
   Amphotericin B 3 per cent in an aqueous vehicle with stabilizers and preservatives.
3. Actions and indications:
   Provides specific action against *C. albicans* even more effectively than nystatin. There is almost no activity against other fungi or bacteria or viruses. The vehicle and the active agent are nonirritating and can be applied safely to intertriginous skin, ear canals, perianal and vulvar areas.
4. Dosage:
   Apply liberally to affected areas three or four times daily.
5. Supplied:
   30 cc. plastic squeeze bottles.
   E. R. Squibb & Sons, Inc.
   745 Fifth Avenue
   New York, N.Y. 10022

### *Furacin*

1. Antimicrobial preparation
2. Contains:
   Nitrofurazone 0.2 per cent in a water-soluble base (dressing); or in a water-soluble solution (solution).
3. Actions and indications:
   A broad-spectrum antimicrobial agent for use in prevention and treatment of infection by organisms sensitive to its action. It is a useful agent for treating external wounds, abrasions and burns, otitis externa.
4. Dosage:
   Apply liberally to affected areas. It is best covered by a dressing to maintain contact with the tissues. Repeat dosage daily.
5. Supplied:
   Solution: 1 pint and 1 gallon jars.
   Dressing: 5 oz. and 1 lb. jars.
   Eaton Laboratories
   Norwich, N.Y.

### *Furacin Soluble Powder*

1. A water-soluble antimicrobial powder.
2. Contains 0.2 per cent nitrofurazone in a powder base composed of water-soluble polyethylene glycols.
3. Actions and indications:
   A broad-spectrum antimicrobial agent for topical application to superficial and deep pyodermas due to susceptible organisms, when the use of powder is indicated.
4. Dosage:
   Use the plastic squeeze bottle to apply the powder to the affected area one to three times daily.
5. Supplied:
   Puffer bottles of 10 gm. and 50 gm.
   Eaton Laboratories
   Norwich, New York

### *Furaspor Liquid*

1. A fungistatic and acaricidal solution.
2. Contains nitrofurfurylmethyl ether 4 per cent, in a liquid of benzyl benzoate 15 per cent, methylbenzethonium chloride 0.5 per cent and water.
3. Actions and indications:
   For the treatment of pyogenic demodectic mange and for dermatomycoses caused by fungi sensitive to nitrofurfurylmethyl ether.
4. Dosage:
   Apply topically once a day, using the sponge supplied with 60 cc. bottles. Repeat as necessary. Protect eyes. Contraindicated in cats and rabbits.
5. Supplied:
   Dauber bottles of 60 cc. and bottles of one pint.
   Eaton Laboratories
   Norwich, New York

### *Goodwinol Ointment*

1. A bland rotenone ointment.
2. Contains:
   Rotenone and orthophenylphenol in a bland cholesterol base.
3. Actions and indications:
   Acaricidal action without irritation or staining.
4. Dosage:
   Apply to affected areas once daily with massage.
5. Supplied:
   1 lb. cans.
   Goodwinol Products Corp.
   Wappingers Falls, N.Y.

### *Griseofulvin, Microsize, (Fulvicin-U/F)*

1. An orally effective, antifungal antibiotic specifically active against dermatophytes.
2. Actions and indications:
   It is absorbed after oral dosage and deposited in the basal layers of the skin, eventually coming to the keratin layers. Dermatophyte infections of the skin, hair and claws may be responsive if caused by *T. rubrum, T. mentagrophytes, T. verrucosum, M. gypseum, M. canis, M. audouini* and a few others. It is not effective against bacteria, monilia, aspergillus and most of the deep mycotic infections. It is not beneficial topically.
3. Dosage:
   10 mg./lb./day orally following a fat meal, or administration of corn oil. The same dosage can be cumulated and a total dosage given once every ten days as a massive dose. Treatment should continue until no clinical (or laboratory) evidence of infection remains. This may be six to eight weeks.
   The drug has an unpleasant taste and vomiting is a frequent complication. Dividing the dose into two or three portions often helps alleviate the nausea.
4. Supplied:
   Scored tablets 125, 250 and 500 mg. in bottles of 60 and 250.
   Schering Corporation
   60 Orange Street
   Bloomfield, N.J. 07003

### *Ichthammol, Fortified*

1. Water dispersible ointment containing ichthammol 4 per cent, salicylic acid 8 per cent, balsam of peru 4 per cent, zinc oxide ointment q.s.
2. Action and indications:
   Ichthammol penetrates the skin and stimulates peripheral circulation, salicylic acid is keratolytic and thus allows better penetration, balsam of peru is antiseptic and soothing, and zinc oxide is a mildly astringent, antiseptic base. Use for acute erythematous, pruritic and papular dermatoses, or subacute or chronic dermatitis.
3. Dosage:
   Massage well into lesions once daily until improvement occurs, then once every second or third day. Do not use on moist or pyoderma lesions.
4. Supplied:
   460 gm. plastic jars.
   Maurry Biological Co.
   Los Angeles, California

### *Lime Sulfur Solution*

1. Parasiticidal, antiseptic concentrate solution.
2. Contains:
   Calcium polysulfides 26 per cent, inert 74 per cent.

3. Actions and indications:
   The action of sulfur is applied to the skin. It is parasiticidal, antiseptic, fungicidal, stimulating and mildly keratolytic. Excellent inexpensive treatment for notoedric mange of cats and sarcoptic mange (scabies) of dogs. It is also useful as a topical fungicide in conjunction with other therapy.
4. Dosage:
   Bathe the patient with soap and warm water. Dilute the concentrate 1:40 with warm water and saturate the animal's coat and skin. Allow to dry. Repeat once every five to seven days for several treatments. Local treatment may be given with dilutions of 1:20.
5. Supplied:
   Pints, quart bottles (Orthorix Spray).
   Chevron Chemical Company
   Ortho Division
   San Francisco, California
   (Available at garden supply centers.)

### *Liquisone-F*

1. Contains prednisolone, neomycin sulfate, cerumene and tetracaine as a lotion.
2. Actions and indications:
   An antibacterial, anti-inflammatory, anesthetic lotion with good skin penetrating properties for treatment of acute otitis externa and for topical treatment of acute moist dermatitis of dogs and cats. It is effective against bacterial infections susceptible to neomycin.
3. Dosage:
   Apply topically two or three times daily. If prolonged use produces sensitivity or irritation the application should be discontinued.
4. Supplied:
   10 ml. tubes and 500 ml. bottles.
   EVSCO Pharmaceutical Company
   3345 Royal Ave.
   Oceanside, N.Y. 11572

### *Mercaptocaine Creme*

1. A soothing topical dressing with bactericidal and fungicidal action for all species.
2. Contains:
   2-mercaptobenzothiazole 2 per cent; benzocaine 5 per cent; 2-chloro-4-phenylphenol 0.2 per cent in a protecting emulsion.
3. Actions and indications:
   An antiseptic, soothing, softening cream for nonspecific dermatosis. It is mildly fungicidal and anesthetic. Benzocaine may cause sensitizing reactions in some individuals.
4. Dosage:
   Apply liberally to affected areas and repeat daily as needed.

5. Supplied:
   $2\frac{1}{2}$ oz., pint and gallon bottles.
   Pitman-Moore
   Indianapolis, Indiana

### *Mitox*

1. Ear medication effective against bacteria, fungi, ear mites and pain.
2. Contains:
   Neomycin sulfate 0.5 per cent; sulfacetamide 10.0 per cent; sodium caprylate 10.0 per cent; piperonyl butoxide 1.0 per cent; tetracaine hydrochloride 0.5 per cent, in a diffusible base.
3. Actions and indications:
   For treatment of otitis externa caused by bacteria, fungi, or ear mites.
4. Dosage:
   Cleanse ear and apply enough to fill the lower ear canal. Repeat once daily. Continue treatment at least twice weekly for two weeks to prevent reinfestation of ear mites.
5. Supplied:
   6.5 gm. and 25 gm. plastic syringes.
   Norden Laboratories
   Box 1227
   Lincoln, Nebraska 68501

### *Mulzyl Liquid*

1. Acaricidal and bactericidal lotion for dogs.
2. Contains:
   Benzyl benzoate 20 per cent; benzene hexachloride 0.9 per cent; chlorobutanol 0.5 per cent; phenylmercuric borate 0.02 per cent in a vanishing cream base 78.58 per cent.
3. Actions and indications:
   Acaricidal and antibacterial cream for topical use in localized demodectic mange and for spot treatment of sarcoptic mange.
4. Dosage:
   Apply to affected areas twice weekly with massage.
5. Supplied:
   $2\frac{1}{2}$ oz., pint and gallon bottles.
   Pitman-Moore
   Indianapolis, Indiana

### *Mycostatin*

1. Nystatin ointment and suspension.
2. Contains:
   Nystatin 100,000 units/gram in a vanishing cream base with stabilizers and

preservatives; or 100,000 units/cc. in suspension which is stable for seven days at room temperature after reconstitution.

3. Actions and indications:
   Provides specific therapy for infections caused by *C. albicans* (moniliasis).
4. Dosage:
   The ointment is useful for skin use and paronychia. The cream is preferred for intertriginous areas. The suspension is provided for oral and mucous membrane infections. Medications should be applied topically four times daily.
5. Supplied:
   Ointment: 15 and 30 gm. tubes.
   Suspension: 24 cc. bottles with each cc. = one dose (100,000 units).
   E. R. Squibb & Sons, Inc.
   745 Fifth Avenue
   New York, N.Y. 10022

### *Neo-Delta-Cortef with Tetracaine*

1. Contains prednisolone, neomycin sulfate and tetracaine as an aqueous suspension.
2. Actions and indications:
   An antibacterial, anti-inflammatory, anesthetic suspension for topical eye or ear use. It is indicated for acute inflammations and bacterial infections caused by organisms susceptible to neomycin.
3. Dosage:
   Apply topically to skin or ear infections every six hours. If sensitivity develops the application of the medication should be discontinued.
4. Supplied:
   2.5 ml. plastic dropper bottle.
   Upjohn Company
   7171 Portage Road
   Kalamazoo, Michigan

### *Neo-Polycin-HC*

1. Antibacterial, corticosteroid, topical ointment.
2. Contains:
   In each gram neomycin 3 mg.; bacitracin 400 units; polymyxin B, 8000 units; hydrocortisone acetate 10 mg. in a special base (Fuzene).
3. Actions and indications:
   It has wide-spectrum antibiotic activity and anti-inflammatory action and also helps relieve pruritus and edema. Used for secondary bacterial infections caused by organisms sensitive to its ingredients, and for seborrheic dermatitis, allergic contact and irritant dermatoses, and otitis externa.
4. Dosage:
   Apply a thin film to affected area. May be covered with a dressing if necessary. Repeat application two or three times daily.

5. Supplied:
   5 gm. tubes.
   Pitman-Moore
   Indianapolis, Indiana

### *Nivea Creme and Nivea Skin Oil*

1. Emulsions of neutral, aliphatic hydrocarbons in water with Eucerite (wool fat cholesterols). The oil is the liquid equivalent of the cream.
2. Actions and indications:
   Soothing, emollient preparations to help replenish natural lubrication and moisture to dry, rough skin. They form a nongreasy protecting film that penetrates tiny folds of skin and helps allay minor irritations.
3. Dosage:
   Apply a thin film daily as needed. Rub in well. A thin coating applied and removed acts as an effective, nonaqueous, nonirritating skin cleanser.
4. Supplied:
   Skin oil: 4 oz., 1 pint and 1 quart bottles.
   Cream: 2⅔ oz. tube and 7 oz. and 1 lb. jars.
   Duke Laboratories Inc.
   South Norwalk, Conn.

### *Nolvosan*

1. Antiseptic solution or ointment.
2. Contains:
   Chlorhexidine 2 per cent; inert 98 per cent (solution); chlorhexidine 1 per cent in cream base (ointment).
3. Actions and indications:
   Actively germicidal against gram-positive and gram-negative organisms, it is useful for sanitizing equipment, and also as a soak solution for pyodermas. Ointment form is a bland, softening and emollient preparation with antiseptic properties.
4. Dosage:
   For premises add 30 ml. to each gallon of water. For skin soaks add 15 ml. to each gallon of water. Ointment can be applied several times daily with massage.
5. Supplied:
   Gallon bottles (solution), 1 oz. tubes (ointment) and 8 oz. jars (ointment).
   Fort Dodge Laboratories
   Fort Dodge, Iowa

### *Panolog Ointment*

1. An antibiotic-corticosteroid ointment for topical use.
2. Contains:
   In each cc.: nystatin 100,000 units; neomycin sulfate 2.5 mg.; thiostreptin 2,500 units; triamcinolone acetonide 1.0 mg. in a special Plastibase.

3. Actions and indications:
   The active ingredients provide anti-inflammatory antipruritic, antimonilial and broad-spectrum antibacterial effects. It is useful against ear and skin infections caused by organisms susceptible to its ingredients, and as an adjunct to treatment of inflammatory dry or exudative dermatitis, contact and seborrheic dermatitis. It is particularly useful in otitis externa, infected anal sacs and in superficial pyoderma.
4. Dosage:
   Apply to affected areas topically once or twice daily. As the condition responds less frequent treatment is necessary.
5. Supplied:
   Tubes of 7.5 and 15 cc. and plastic bottles of 8 fluid oz.
   E. R. Squibb & Sons, Inc.
   745 Fifth Avenue
   New York, N.Y. 10022

### *Pellene Liquid*

1. Topical shake lotion.
2. Contains:
   Resorcinol 5 per cent; zinc oxide 4 per cent; calamine 2 per cent; oil of cade 1 per cent; pyroligneous acid purified 0.4 per cent; zinc hydroxide 8 per cent.
3. Actions and indications:
   A nongreasy, astringent, sedative, anodyne and absorbent lotion for nonspecific dermatoses, mild inflammations, insect bites and pruritic lesions. It may be used for otitis externa.
4. Dosage:
   Apply to affected skin once daily.
5. Supplied:
   1 oz. dropper bottles and pints.
   Pitman-Moore
   Indianapolis, Indiana

### *Petrolatum, White USP*

1. A protective ointment.
2. Contains:
   Decolorized petrolatum with not more than 10 ppm. dl-a-tocopherol as a stabilizing agent.
3. Actions and indications:
   An emollient, lubricating, hydrating and softening ointment for irritated skin, and to use as a base for compounding pharmaceuticals. Repeated heavy application may predispose to folliculitis in areas covered with hair.
4. Dosage:
   Apply a thin film daily as needed. May be covered with a dressing if desired.
5. Supplied:
   In many size jars over the counter at pharmacies.

### *pHisoHex*

1. Antibacterial, sudsing, soapless skin cleanser.
2. Contains entsufon (detergent), lanolin, cholesterols, petrolatum and 3 per cent hexachlorophene. The pH is 5.5.
3. Actions and indications:
   A bland, thorough detergent cleans the skin of dirt, scales, grease and oil and the hexachlorophene has a cumulative antibacterial action.
4. Dosage:
   Spread on the skin and gradually add water to work up a lather by rubbing. Useful as a presurgical scrub, or as an adjunct to treatment of some pyodermas, acne, impetigo, seborrheic dermatitis; and whenever a bland, thorough cleansing agent is needed.
5. Supplied:
   5 oz., 1 pint and 1 gallon plastic bottles.
   Winthrop Laboratories
   90 Park Avenue
   New York, New York 10016

### *Pragmatar Ointment*

1. A specially refined coal tar derivative in a pleasant nonstaining, washable base.
2. Contains:
   Cetyl alcohol-coal tar distillate 4 per cent; special sulfur 3 per cent; salicylic acid 3 per cent in an oil-in-water emulsion base.
3. Actions and indications:
   For subacute and chronic dermatitis and dermatoses. It is especially suggested for noninflammatory conditions for which corticosteroids are of no value. A nonstaining, pleasant ointment that produces the effects of sulfur, coal tar and salicylic acid.
4. Dosage:
   Clip the coat and apply sparingly to affected areas with massage. Apply only to affected areas once or twice daily. Avoid use in inflamed areas, near the eyes, or when it can be ingested by licking.
5. Supplied:
   1½ oz. and 1 lb. jars.
   Norden Laboratories
   Box 1227
   Lincoln, Nebraska 68501

### *Pragmatar Shampoo*

1. A medicated shampoo for treatment of a range of common skin disorders.
2. Contains:
   Cetyl alcohol-coal tar distillate 0.5 per cent; lauryl isoquinolinium bromide 0.2 per cent; hexachlorophene 2.0 per cent; isopropyl alcohol 19.0 per cent; in a special shampoo base.

3. Actions and indications:
   Useful as an aid to treatment of parasitic, hormonal and chronic dermatoses. Its shampoo action, together with the coal tar effect, benefits special cases and leaves the coat clean and soft.
4. Dosage:
   Wet coat thoroughly. Apply shampoo and rub vigorously for ten to 15 minutes. Rinse well. Repeat two times weekly or as needed.
5. Supplied:
   6 fluid oz. and 1 gallon bottles.
   Norden Laboratories
   Box 1227
   Lincoln, Nebraska 68501

***Ron - 245***

1. Ronnel concentrate for treatment of ectoparasites of dogs and cats.
2. Contains:
   Ronnel [0,0, dimethyl 0-(2,4,5-trichlorophenyl) phosphorothioate] 30 per cent; xylene 40 per cent; petroleum distillate 20 per cent; inert 10 per cent.
3. Actions and indications:
   A cholinesterase-inhibiting insecticide for use against ticks, lice and fleas of dogs. The 0.25 per cent solution can be used *with caution* on adult cats.
4. Dosage:
   1 per cent solution (30 ml. in 1000 ml. of water) can be used on premises or as a dip or sponge solution for dogs. 0.25 per cent solution (7.5 ml. in 1000 ml. of water) can be sponged onto adult cats. Treatments may be repeated at one-week intervals. (Operators should use rubber gloves to protect hands from exposure. Wash thoroughly after use.)
5. Supplied:
   Gallon bottles.
   Pitman-Moore
   Indianapolis, Indiana

***Sebutone***

1. Antiseborrheic tar shampoo.
2. Contains:
   Sebulytic, (surface-active, soapless cleansers and wetting agents); kerohydric, (dewaxed, oil-soluble, keratin-moisturizing fraction of lanolin); hexachlorophene 1 per cent; micropulverized sulfur 2 per cent; salicylic acid 2 per cent; and 0.5 per cent crude tar U.S.P.
3. Actions and indications:
   Removes oils, scales, crusts from the skin and coat and helps to relieve itching. It is helpful in seborrheic dermatitis, dry and oily seborrhea, and in cases of excess scaling.
4. Dosage:
   Wet the skin and hair, massage Sebutone into the coat for five to ten minutes,

rinse well. Repeat application and rinse again. Treatment may be repeated every five to ten days as needed. May stain white hair.

5. Supplied:
 4 oz. plastic bottle.
 Westwood Pharmaceuticals
 468 De Witt Street
 Buffalo, N.Y. 14213

### *Seleen*

1. Medicated shampoo.
2. Contains:
 Selenium disulfide 1 per cent; inert 99 per cent.
3. Actions and indications:
 A cleansing shampoo for removal of scales and debris which may be useful in seborrheic dermatitis and as an aid in the control of fleas and lice.
4. Dosage:
 Wet hair. Apply shampoo and rub up good lather. Allow to remain 15 minutes. Rinse well. Repeat at four to seven day intervals.
5. Supplied:
 $5^{1}/_{2}$ oz., pint and gallon bottles.
 Diamond Laboratories
 Des Moines, Iowa

### *Sodium Levothyroxine U.S.P. (Synthroid)*

1. Synthetic crystalline sodium levothyroxine is twice as active as the racemic (D-L) form. Synthroid 0.1 mg. is about equivalent to 65 mg. of desiccated thyroid U.S.P. However Synthroid is a uniformly potent, standardized product which simulates endogenous thyroxine in its gradual sustained effect. It has freedom from potentially allergenic protein substances.
2. Actions and indications:
 It is specific replacement therapy for absent or diminished thyroid function resulting from primary or secondary hypothyroidism.
3. Dosage:
 Individual doses must be determined for each case. Treatment can be guided by laboratory measurements and clinical judgment. Initial doses in some cases have been established at approximately 0.1 mg./20 lb./day.
4. Supplied:
 Injectable forms are available but not often needed. Tablets 0.025, 0.05, 0.1, 0.15, 0.20, 0.30 mg. are available in bottles of 100 and 500 tablets.
 Flint Laboratories
 Morton Grove, Illinois 60053

### *SOK*

1. Safe and effective insecticide for dog and cat ectoparasites (fleas, lice and ticks).

2. Contains:
   0.73 per cent Sevin [(6 and 2)-chloro-3,4-xylenol, methyl carbamate] which is a fast-acting, cholinesterase inhibitor, and a special powder vehicle.
3. Action and indications:
   Kills all stages of lice and fleas; kills ticks (even engorged females) within hours. Is safe for puppies and kittens and its base is an excellent vehicle which penetrates the hair coat to contact the skin. It is not greasy, does not stain and has no unpleasant odor.
4. Dosage:
   Apply directly to coat and ruff the hair so the powder penetrates thoroughly. Residual action lasts seven to 14 days but in severe infestations twice weekly application is desirable.
5. Supplied:
   3 oz. shaker cans.
   Upjohn Company
   7171 Portage Road
   Kalamazoo, Michigan

### *Synalar Cream 0.025 per cent*

1. Anti-inflammatory cream.
2. Contains:
   Fluocinolone acetonide 0.25 per cent in a water-washable base.
3. Actions and indications:
   Potent anti-inflammatory effect; it reduces edema, erythema, infiltration and pruritus as well as inflammation. Useful in acute and chronic superficial dermatoses in dogs, allergic dermatitis, burns and seborrheic dermatitis.
4. Dosage:
   Clip hair and apply sparingly with gentle massage to affected skin. Repeat three or four times daily.
5. Supplied:
   5 gm. tubes.
   Syntex Laboratories, Inc.
   Palo Alto, California

### *Thionium with Lindane*

1. Medicated, insecticidal shampoo.
2. Contains:
   Potassium tetrathionate 2.0 per cent; lindane 0.25 per cent; detergents 97.75 per cent.
3. Actions and indications:
   A thorough-cleansing shampoo useful in removing scales and debris in seborrhea and nonspecific dermatitis, and an aid to control of fleas, lice, sarcoptic and otodectic mites on the skin.
4. Dosage:
   Wet dog's coat, apply shampoo and work up a lather. Allow to remain at least ten minutes. Rinse. Repeat weekly if needed. Do not use on cats or pup-

pies. (Operator should wear rubber gloves and wash thoroughly after using this product.)

5. Supplied:
   6 oz. and 1 gallon bottles
   Jen-Sal Laboratories
   Kansas City, Missouri

### *Thyroid Stimulating Hormone*

1. TSH (Dermathycin) is an anterior pituitary extract free of other active constituents of the hypophysis.
2. Actions and indications:
   Stimulates thyroid activity, both growth of cellular components and synthesis of thyroxine. Used for hypothyroidism, for testing procedures, and for early treatment of acanthosis nigricans.
3. Dosage:
   1 or 2 U.S.P. units subcutaneously daily for five days. Store reconstituted drug under 40° F.
4. Supplied:
   Vials of U.S.P. units.
   Jen-Sal Laboratories
   Kansas City, Missouri

### *Tinactin (Tolnaftate)*

1. One per cent cream or solution of tolnaftate, a synthetic fungicide in propylene glycol.
2. Actions and indications:
   This nonsensitizing agent can be used on glabrous skin as a fungicide. It is reported to be useful for topical treatment of *T. rubrum, T. mentagrophytes, T. tonsurans, M. canis, and M. audouini.* Complete evaluation of its use in dermatophyte infections of dogs and cats is not yet available.
3. Dosage:
   Apply sparingly twice daily to affected skin and rub in well.
   Treatment should continue for four weeks.
4. Supplied:
   1.0 per cent cream, 15 gm. tubes; 1 per cent solution, 10 cc. plastic bottle.
   Schering Corporation
   60 Orange Street
   Bloomfield, N.J. 07003

### *Topazone*

1. An antimicrobial powder in an aerosol spray.
2. Contains furazolidone with an inert propellant.
3. Actions and indications:
   An aerosol powder for the treatment of superficial pyodermas, lacerations and infected wounds.

4. Dosage:
   Cleanse affected area. Apply Topazone once or twice daily. Hold container 6 to 12 inches from affected area and spray very lightly, applying just enough to impart a light yellow area. Repeat daily but avoid heavy application which may cause caking and retard healing.
5. Supplied:
   Aerosol containers of 85 gm. and 198 gm.
   Eaton Laboratories
   Norwich, New York

### *Vaporal*

1. Emulsifiable concentrate for resistant ticks on dogs.
2. Contains:
   Xylol 75 per cent; ronnel (0,0,-dimethyl 0 2,4,5-trichlorophenyl phosphorothioate) 5 per cent; 2,2-dichlorovinyl dimethyl phosphate (DDVP or Vapona) 4.65 per cent; related compounds 0.35 per cent; inert 15 per cent.
3. Actions and indications:
   Excellent insecticidal activity. Effective against lice, fleas and ticks on dogs. May be used to treat premises too. DDVP has a potent volatile effect. Do not use without good ventilation. Operator should use rubber gloves and wash thoroughly when through.
4. Dosage:
   Add 59 cc. to 1 gallon of water to soak or sponge dogs. Add 147 cc. to 1 gallon for treating premises. Use with good ventilation and do not contaminate food containers or food handling equipment.
5. Supplied:
   Gallon bottles.
   Florida Veterinary Laboratories
   Miami, Florida

### *Vetalog*

1. Triamcinolone acetonide aqueous suspension, tablets.
2. Contains:
   Triamcinolone acetonide 2 mg./cc. for small animal injection; tablets of 0.5 and 1.5 mg.
3. Action and indications:
   Has pronounced anti-inflammatory, antipruritic, and anti-allergic effects. There is very little mineralocorticoid activity. Particularly useful for allergic dermatoses.
4. Dosage:
   Orally: 0.05 to 0.10 mg./lb. of body weight daily initially, reduce to 0.01 to 0.02 at one week, and stop medication after two weeks if possible. Parenterally: 0.1 mg./lb. of body weight I.M. Repeat in seven to ten days if needed.
5. Supplied:
   Tablets of 0.5 and 1.5 mg. bottles of 100; parenteral: 2 mg./cc., vials of 25 and 100 cc.

E. R. Squibb & Sons, Inc.
745 Fifth Avenue
New York, N.Y. 10022

### *Vioform*

1. Three per cent iodochlorhydroxyquin in cream, ointment or lotion. Some preparations also contain 1 per cent hydrocortisone.
2. Actions and indications:
   Contains 41 per cent iodine and is thought to be a useful bactericidal and fungicidal agent.
   The lotion form is especially useful for intertriginous use; the cream is more useful for moist, acute inflammations; the ointment form is best for chronic, dry, thick and scaling lesions. These forms are used topically for dermatoses, bacterial or fungus infections for which an antibacterial, antifungal effect is desired. In some cases sensitization of the skin may occur. For this reason, and where antipruritic, anti-inflammatory action is needed, the products containing 1 per cent hydrocortisone are preferred.
3. Dosage:
   Apply topically two or three times daily and massage gently into affected area. Avoid use near eyes. Discontinue if irritation occurs. These products may cause staining.
4. Supplied:
   Cream and ointment 5 gm. and 20 gm. tubes; lotion 15 ml. plastic bottle.
   Ciba Pharmaceutical Company
   Summit, N.J. 07901

### *V-Tar Shampoo*

1. A colloidalized whole crude tar shampoo.
2. Contains:
   Colloidal, water-miscible whole crude coal tar 1 per cent; allantoin 0.2 per cent and parachlorometaxylenol 0.5 per cent in a synthetic, soap-free detergent.
3. Actions and indications:
   A medicated shampoo for the treatment of pruritus, seborrheic dermatitis, sarcoptic mange, and certain dermatomycoses in small animals.
4. Dosage:
   Shake well. Moisten coat with lukewarm water. Rub in shampoo and rinse. Repeat, massaging gently, working up a rich lather. Allow to remain in hair for 5 to 10 minutes, then rinse thoroughly. It may be used to shampoo specific areas of the animal without having to give a full shampoo.
5. Supplied:
   6 oz. bottles and 1 gallon.
   Dermavet Division
   Dermick Laboratories
   Syosset, New York 11791

### *Zinc Oxide Ointment U.S.P.*

1. A healing ointment.
2. Contains: Zinc oxide 20 per cent; liquid petrolatum 15 per cent; white ointment 65 per cent.
3. Actions and indications:
   A soothing, protective ointment which promotes healing of irritated or abraded skin.
4. Dosage:
   Apply a thin film daily.
5. Supplied:
   1 lb. jars and over the counter at pharmacies.

## SPECIAL EQUIPMENT

### *Bacterial Sensitivity Test Kits*

Media Inc.
89 Lincoln Park
Newark, New Jersey

or

Bactilab
P. O. Box 1179
Mountain View, Calif. 94040

### *Biopsy Punch*

Keyes cutaneous punch, 3½ inches long, size 2, 4, 6, 8 mm.; stainless steel.

American Hospital Supply
2020 Ridge Ave.
Evanston, Illinois 60201

### *Diagnostic Allergen Set*

EVSCO Pharmaceutical Co.
3345 Royal Ave.
Oceanside, L.I.
New York 11572

### *Fungal Culture Bottles*

Antibiotic Agar (Sabouraud's)

Derm Medical Company
P.O. Box 78595 – West Adams Station
Los Angeles 16, California 90016

or

Mycosel Agar (Mycoflask 21130)

Baltimore Biological Laboratory (BBL)
P. O. Box 175
Cockeysville, Maryland 21030

### *Head Loupe*

Opti VISOR, optical glass binocular.

Magnifier, Model No. E-5.

Donegan Optical Co., Inc.
1405 Kansas
Kansas City, Missouri 64127

MAGNI-FOCUSER
Arista Surgical Company
67 Lexington Ave.
New York, N.Y. 10010

### *Magnifying Lamp*

Model LFM-1.

Luxo Lamp Corp.
Port Chester, New York

### *Rubber Stamps*

Dog outline, cat outline, Dermatologic Case History stamp.

San Francisco Rubber Stamp Co.
94 Natoma St.
San Francisco, Calif. 94105

### *Wood's Light*

Burton's Wood's Light with 2 ultraviolet tubes and built-in magnifying glass.

Arista Surgical Company
67 Lexington Ave.
New York, N.Y. 10010

## GLOSSARY

***Abrasion***—Superficial removal of epidermis resulting in oozing and crusting.

***Abscess***—Localized collection of pus in a cavity formed by disintegration of tissue.

***Acantholysis***—Separation of the intercellular bridges in the prickle-cell layer of the epidermis.

***Acanthosis***—A diffuse hypertrophy of the prickle-cell layer of the epidermis.

***Acariasis***—An infestation caused by any mite.

***Acarus***—A mite.

***Acne***—A dermatosis characterized by a primary lesion called a comedo or blackhead. These are often inflamed or infected.

***Acral***—Pertaining to distal parts of the body, especially the extremities.

***Actinic***—Refers to the injurious effect of ultraviolet light.

***Actinodermatitis***—An inflammatory condition of the skin caused by visible or ultraviolet light.

***Adenoma***—Hypertrophy or tumefaction of a gland.

***Adnexa***—Pertaining to the skin, it means structures that are bound to it, i.e., hair, claws, and eccrine, sebaceous and apocrine glands. Extruded hair shafts and claws are more accurately called appendages.

***Allergen***—A substance that is capable of inducing an allergic state.

***Allergy***—A state in which a specific, acquired alteration in the capacity to react has developed.

***Alopecia***—Loss of hair.

***Amyloid***—A mucopolysaccharide related to chondroitin sulfuric acid which may make up the ground substance of some tissue.

***Anagen***—The phase of the hair cycle during which synthesis of hair takes place.

***Anaphylactic***—Possessing anaphylaxis.

***Anaphylaxis***—An unusual or exaggerated reaction of the organism to foreign protein or other substances.

***Annular***—Shaped like a ring.

***Anthropophilic***—Having a preference for man. Used dermatologically, pertaining to anthropophilic fungi whose primary host is man.

***Antibody***—A modified type of serum globulin synthesized by lymphoid tissue in response to antigenic stimulus, each differing haptenic structure of one antigen molecule being capable of inciting a distinct response.

***Antigen***—A substance or complex of high molecular weight, usually protein or protein-polysaccharide complex in nature, which, when foreign to the blood stream of an animal, on gaining access to the tissues of such an animal stimulates the formation of specific antibody and reacts specifically in vivo or in vitro with its homologous antibody.

***Antitoxin***—An antibody that neutralizes an antigen that is a toxin.

***Aplasia***—A condition of failure or lack of full development or growth.

***Apocrine***—Denoting that type of glandular secretion in which the secretory products become concentrated at the free end of the secreting cell and are thrown off together with the portion of the cell where they have accumulated, as in the mammary gland.

***Appendages***—Claw plates and hair shafts that hang from the skin. Adnexa is a better word for skin glands, claw matrix and the pilosebaceous apparatus.

***Arciform***—Shaped in curves (refers to the shape of lesions).

***Arthrospore***—A spore formed by septation of hyphae with subsequent separation of cells.

***Ascospore***—The sexual spore of ascomycetes, born in an ascus.

***Atopy***—A clinical hypersensitivity state which is subject to hereditary influences. Included are asthma, eczema and "hay fever." Canine atopy is characterized by sneezing, scratching, paw licking and face rubbing.

***Atrophy***—A defect or failure of nutrition manifested as a wasting away or diminution in the size of a cell, tissue, organ or part.

***Auto-immunization***—The production in an organism of reactivity to its own tissues, with appearance of certain clinical and laboratory manifestations as a result of the altered immunological response.

***Basal cell carcinoma***—A malignant neoplasm in which the proliferating cells have structural and staining characteristics of the basal cells of the epidermis and seem to stem from them positionally and developmentally.
***Benign***—Mild or not serious; not malignant.
***Biopsy***—The examination of a specimen from live tissue, usually with a microscope.
***Blister***—A thin-walled structure containing air or fluid; dermatologically, vesicles and bullae.
***Bulla***—A large vesicle or blister.
***Calcinosis***—A pathologic condition in which calcium in abnormal amounts has been abnormally deposited. The condition of calcium deposits occurring in the skin is called *calcinosis cutis*.
***Callus***—Hypertrophy of the horny layer (stratum corneum) in localized areas, especially over pressure points.
***Cancer***—A cellular tumor the natural course of which is usually fatal and often associated with formation of secondary tumors.
***Carbuncle***—A lesion consisting of multiple cutaneous abscesses that are connected by sinuses.
***Carcinoma***—A malignant new growth made up of epithelial cells tending to infiltrate the surrounding tissues and to give rise to metastases.
***Catagen***—That phase of the hair cycle in which there is transition from growth (anagen) to cessation of growth and inception of an end stage (telogen).
***Cerumen***—The wax-like secretion of the specialized apocrine glands of the ear canal.
***Chalazion***—A small tumor of the eyelid formed by a chronic inflammation of the meibomian gland.
***Chlamydospore***—A thick-walled, intercalary or terminal vegetative cell which, by thickening of the wall, has become modified into a resting spore.
***Clavate***—Club-shaped.
***Clear cell***—A kind of cell found regularly in the basal-cell layer of the epidermis (melanocyte, Langhans' cell and others).
***Collagen***—The normal fibrillar substance of the connective tissue of the dermis.
***Comedo*** (pl. ***comedones***)—A plug of keratin and dried sebum in an excretory duct (or hair follicle) of the skin.
***Confluent***—Becoming merged or running together; not discrete.
***Conidia***—Fungus spores which are abstricted in various ways from a conidiophore.
***Conidiophore***—The stalk from which conidia are abstricted.
***Contact dermatitis***—Inflammation of skin resulting from external application of a primary irritant (primary irritant contact dermatitis), or of an ordinarily harmless substance toward which a state of sensitization has been established (allergic contact dermatitis).
***Cornification***—The process of callosity or becoming horny; hyperkeratosis.
***Crust***—A dried exudate on the surface of a lesion.
***Cutaneous***—Pertaining to skin.
***Cutis***—The entire skin; frequently, the dermis.
***Cyst***—A sac, bladder or fluid-filled, circumscribed, walled process that is not inflamed.
***Dandruff***—A word used by laymen to indicate excessive scaliness of the scalp or of hairy skin.
***Degeneration***—Deterioration; change of a tissue from a higher to a lower or less active functional form.
***Demodex***—A genus of mites. ***Demodex canis*** causes demodectic mange in dogs.
***Demodicidosis***—Infestation with demodectic mites. In recent usage, abbreviated as *demodicosis*.
***Depigmentation***—The act or result of removing pigment (in skin usually implies melanin).
***Dermal***—Pertaining to the skin.
***Dermatitis*** (pl. ***dermatitides***)—Inflammation of the skin. Never a synonym for all skin disease.
***Dermatoglyphics***—Surface characteristics of the skin with respect to its folds, furrows, ridges and wrinkles.
***Dermatology***—The field of study of everything that relates to the skin in health and disease.
***Dermatomycosis***—A fungous infection of the skin.

***Dermatophyte***—A fungus living as a parasite on skin, hair or nails (claws) of man or animals.
***Dermatosis***—A pathologic condition of the skin.
***Dermis***—The corium or layer of skin between the epidermis and the subcutaneous tissue.
***Dermoid cyst***—An encapsulated mass that contains ectodermal structures such as epithelium, hair, teeth and glandular elements in disorganized arrangement and incomplete formation.
***Densensitization***—The process of reducing sensitivity. An immunologic transformation to a new state of insensitivity.
***Diffuse***—Not definitely limited or localized; widely distributed.
***Discrete***—Made up of separate parts, or characterized by lesions which do not become blended.
***Disseminated***—Disposed in separate patches.
***Districhiasis***—A double row of eyelashes.
***Dopa***—Dihydroxphenylalanine.
***Ecchymosis***—Extravasation of blood into tissue spaces.
***Eccrine***—Secreting outward (as sweat). Exocrine.
***Ectoderm***—The "external skin," the outermost of the three primary layers of the developing embryo.
***Ectothrix***—Forming a sheath of fungous spores on the outside of a hair.
***Ectropion***—Turning out of the eyelids.
***Eczema***—An inflammatory, superficial skin disease that early is erythematous, papulovesicular, oozing and crusting; and later red-purple, scaly, lichenified and possibly pigmented. Through misuse, its meaning has become vague and indefinite.
***Edema***—Swelling caused by abnormal amounts of fluid in tissues.
***Elastic fibers***—Stretchable fibers consisting of elastin fibrils held together by a cementing substance, and entwined among collagen bundles of the dermis.
***Elastin***—The normal material of elastic fibers.
***Emollient***—Softening, or a softening agent.
***Emulsion***—A preparation of one liquid distributed in small globules throughout the body of a second liquid. "A milk-like product."
***Endocrine***—Secreting within, or dispersing into the circulation; applied to organs which secrete into blood or lymph a substance, especially hormones, which has a specific effect on another organ.
***Endoderm***—The "inner skin," the innermost of the three primary layers of the developing embryo.
***Endothelium***—Layer of epithelial cells lining the cavities of heart, blood and lymph vessels and the serous body cavities.
***Endothrix***—Growing within the hair shaft without a conspicuous external sheath of spores.
***Entity***—A specific, distinct condition.
***Entropion***—Turning in of the eyelids.
***Eosinophilic***—Taking the color of eosin (pink).
***Epidermis***—The outer layer of the skin just above the dermis.
***Epidermoid cyst***—A keratinous mass in the skin enclosed by an epithelial lining. The cells of sebaceous glands seem to be the origin of these cysts.
***Epidermolysis***—Separation of dermis and epidermis (blister).
***Epilate***—To remove hair.
***Epilation***—Removal of hair.
***Epithelioma***—Neoplasia or overdevelopment of the epithelium.
***Epulis***—A growth (fibroma or sarcoma) of the gingiva or underlying bone.
***Erosion***—An eating or gnawing away, denudation or ulceration.
***Eruption***—A rapidly developing lesion of the skin due to disease and marked by redness, prominence or both.
***Erythema***—A redness of the skin produced by congestion of the capillaries.
***Erythematous***—Possessing a redness of the skin.
***Eschar***—A necrotic scab or crust usually caused by a burn.
***Excoriation***—A superficial loss of epidermis caused by scratching, biting or other physical damage.
***Exfoliation***—The shedding of leaf-like scales or layers.

***Exocrine***—Separating (or secreting) to the outside.
***Exudation***—The escape of fluid, cells and cellular debris from blood vessels and their deposition in or on the tissues. Usually the result of inflammation.
***Fibril***—A single fine thread structure (in the dermis).
***Fibroblast***—The parenchymal cells of the dermis which produce the collagen bundles.
***Fibroma***—A hard papule, nodule or tumor which histologically shows fibroblasts and their product (collagen bundles) in a dense formation.
***Fibrosis***—Formation of fibrous tissue.
***Fissure***—A splitting or discontinuity of a surface, especially one that persists.
***Fistula***—A deep, sinuous ulcer, often leading to an internal hollow organ.
***Foam cell***—A histiocyte that has imbibed lipids and has thus come to appear bubbled.
***Follicle***—A tiny, sac-like structure. In dermatology it particularly refers to the housing of the hair apparatus.
***Folliculitis***—Inflammation of a follicle or follicles.
***Fungal***—Caused by or relating to a fungus. Synonymous with the adjective *fungous.*
***Fungicidal***—An agent or procedure that kills fungi.
***Fungistatic***—An agent or process that arrests the growth of fungi.
***Fungus***—A primitive form of plant life in the subphylum of Thallophyta that is not differentiated into roots, stems and leaves, and contains no chlorophyll.
***Furuncle***—A painful, nodular abscess in the skin caused by bacteria; a boil.
***Fusiform***—Spindle-shaped; narrowing toward the ends.
***Geophilic***—Occurring naturally in the soil. Used dermatologically to refer to geophilic fungi that are found in the soil.
***Glabrous***—Smooth, referring to hairless skin.
***Gland***—An aggregation of cells specialized to secrete or excrete materials not related to their ordinary metabolic needs.
***Glands of Krause and Wolfring***—Accessory lacrimal glands located on the inner surface of the eyelids.
***Glands of Manz***—Glandular depressions at the margin of the eyelid.
***Glands of Moll***—Apocrine glands of the cilia.
***Glands of Zeis***—Sebaceous glands of the cilia.
***Glomus***—A body shaped like a ball of wool or yarn.
***Granuloma***—Tumor of granulation tissue.
***Group***—An assemblage of lesions having certain things in common, such as location or form.
***Guttate***—Characterized by lesions that are drop-shaped.
***Gynecomastia***—Enlargement of the male mammary gland.
***Hair***—A single thread of keratin.
***Haptene***—A substance that becomes antigenic when it complexes with proteins.
***Hemangioma***—A massing, overdevelopment or tumefaction of blood vessels.
***Herpetiform***—Marked by a cluster of vesicles, or having the form of herpes.
***Histiocyte***—A particular tissue cell of reticuloendothelial origin.
***Hives***—A condition characterized by wheals.
***Holocrine***—Entirely secretory. Applied to the sebaceous gland whose product is a complete shedding of cellular substance.
***Hordeolum***—An acutely painful, pyogenic infection of a sebaceous gland of the eyelid; a sty. External hordeolum involves a gland of Zeis; internal hordeolum involves a meibomian gland.
***Horn***—Hard keratin.
***Hyaline***—Colorless, transparent.
***Hyperhidrosis***—Increased sweating.
***Hyperkeratosis***—An increased thickness (cornification) of the horny layer of the skin.
***Hyperpigmentation***—Excessive coloration of the skin caused by increased deposition of pigment (especially melanin).
***Hyperplasia***—Excessive growth (of cells).
***Hypersensitivity***—A word with comparative sense meaning more sensitivity than the average. It should not be used synonymous with allergy.
***Hypertrophy***—Overdevelopment.
***Hypha***—Threadlike element of a fungal mycelium.
***Hypopigmentation***—Less than normal pigmentation.

***Hyposensitization*** — Desensitization; the procedure of decreasing or eliminating sensitivity to offending substances.
***Impetigo*** — A superficial pyogenic infection with friable, adherent crusts.
***Indurated*** — Hardened.
***Infectious*** — Caused by microbial agents; may imply it is communicable.
***Infestation*** — The state of harboring metazoal parasites on or in the body.
***Infiltrate*** — To penetrate into tissue; used especially of invasion by cells that are not normal to the location. Also, material deposited by infiltration.
***Inflammation*** — A condition of tissues reacting to injury. There are pain, heat, redness, swelling and sometimes loss of function.
***Intertrigo*** — Erythema caused by chafing of the skin between two adjacent areas, as between toes or flanks.
***Intradermal*** — Within the dermis.
***Intra-epidermal*** — Within the epidermis.
***Inunction*** — The action and result of rubbing or smearing oil or salve into the skin.
***Ischemia*** — Deficiency of blood in a part resulting from severe interference with circulation.
***Itching*** — An unpleasant cutaneous sensation which provokes the desire to scratch or rub the skin.
***Keratosis*** — A condition of excessive development of horny tissue.
***Lacuna*** — A pit, hole, hollow or cavity.
***Lanugo*** — The fine down or woolly hair.
***Lentigo*** — A lentil-shaped, pigmented spot like a freckle.
***Lesion*** — Any pathologic or traumatic deviation from normal tissue.
***Leukocytosis*** — An increased number of white blood cells.
***Leukoderma*** — A condition in which the skin is abnormally white.
***Leukoplakia*** — Flat, white patches of hyperkeratinization on mucous membranes.
***Lichenification*** — A thickening and hardening of the skin characterized by an exaggeration of the superficial skin markings and usually accompanied by hyperpigmentation.
***Liquefaction degeneration*** — Disintegration or poor delineation of the basal cell layer of the epidermis.
***Lotion*** — A liquid preparation that is applied to the skin as a paint rather than a wash.
***Lupus*** — A chronic local skin condition attended more or less with hypertrophy, absorption and ulceration. It is rarely used alone, but with a modifier, e.g., *lupus erythematosus.*
***Maceration*** — The softening and disintegration of tissue by wetting.
***Macroconidium*** — The larger of two types of conidia in fungi that bear large and small spores. See *Microconidium.*
***Macule*** — A perceptible circumscribed change in color on, in or of the skin that is not visibly raised above or depressed below the surrounding general level of the skin. Macules larger than 1 cm. in diameter are referred to as patches.
***Mange*** — A skin disease of animals caused by a mite. Sarcoptic mange (*Sarcoptes scabiei*) or demodectic mange (*Demodex canis*).
***Mast cell*** — A large cell containing metachromatically staining cytoplasmic granules and thought to contain heparin and histamine.
***Mastocytosis*** — A condition in which mast cells are abnormally abundant.
***Matrix*** — The source from which development takes place, a parental stem.
***Meibomian gland*** — A modified sebaceous gland of the eyelid not associated with cilia or hairs.
***Melanin*** — Colored protein complexes formed in many organisms by specialized cells. In shades of tan or black, the material results from a polymerization of tyrosine and desoxyphenylalanine under the influence of tyrosinase.
***Melanocyte*** — A mature cell that produces melanin.
***Melanoma*** — A neoplasm consisting of melanocytes.
***Melanophage*** — A cell that engulfs melanin.
***Merocrine*** — "Separating"; applied to apocrine glands whose product consists of some part of their cellular material which separates and is shed.
***Mesoderm*** — The "middle skin," the embryonal layer (between ectoderm and endoderm) that gives rise to connective tissue, muscle, blood, bone and other components.

***Metaplasia***—A condition in which there has been a change in cellular development.

***Metastasis***—The transfer of disease from one organ to another not directly connected with it.

***Microconidium***—The smaller of two types of conidia in fungi that bear small and large spores. See *Macroconidium.*

***Microsporum***—A genus of fungi.

***Miliary***—Resembling a millet seed.

***Multiple***—Occurring in various parts of the body at once.

***Mycelium***—Mass of hyphae making up a colony of a fungus. The fungal thallus.

***Myiasis***—Deposition of ova by flies in open wounds and development of larvae therein.

***Neurofibroma***—A tumorous lesion that is a mixture of abundant fibrous and nervous tissue.

***Nevus***—A pigmented spot on the skin. However, wide implications can be attached to the word. There are many types, such as blue nevus, compound nevus and junctional nevus.

***Nictitans gland***—Gland of the third eyelid (formerly called *Harderian gland*).

***Nigricans***—Blackening.

***Nodule***—A small node or circumscribed solid elevation that usually extends into the deeper layers of the skin.

***Nummular***—Like a little coin or round disc.

***Onychia***—Ulceration of matrix of a claw.

***Onychomalacia***—Softening of a claw.

***Onychomycosis***—A fungal infection of a claw.

***Onychorrhexis***—A breakage or brittleness of a claw.

***Oozing***—A continuing process of exudation of fluid.

***Papillomatosis***—A condition marked by tumor formation that consists of many nipple-like lesions.

***Papule***—A small, solid elevation of the skin up to 0.5 cm. in diameter. Larger, solid, elevated lesions are called nodules or tumors. Larger, *flat-topped* elevations are called plaques.

***Parakeratosis***—A condition of abnormal cornification. Clinically there is excess scaling; histologically the keratinized cells of the horny layer still possess nuclei.

***Paronychia***—Inflammation or ulceration involving the tissue fold around the claw.

***Patch***—A flat, circumscribed change in color of the skin that is larger than 1 cm. in diameter (therefore, a large macule).

***Pediculosis***—Infestation with lice.

***Petechia***—A small spot caused by minor hemorrhage.

***Photodermatitis***—Any inflammatory condition of the skin caused by the influence of light.

***Pili***—Plural of *pilus*, hair.

***Pilosebaceous***—Referring to hair and sebaceous gland as an organized apparatus.

***Pityriasis***—Conditions of the skin characterized by branny scaling.

***Plaque***—A flat-topped, solid skin elevation larger than 0.5 cm. in diameter.

***Polycyclic***—Consisting of several circular lesions.

***Polymorphous***—Referring to the simultaneous presence of several different types of primary and secondary lesions, as opposed to *monomorphous* in which all lesions of the dermatosis are the same.

***Porphyria***—Any condition resulting from abnormalities of porphyrin metabolism.

***Prickle-cell***—An epidermal cell of the Malpighian layer. ***Prickles*** are the intercellular bridges visible in this layer of the epidermis.

***Pruritus***—Intense and persistent itching.

***Pustule***—A small, circumscribed elevation of the skin filled with pus.

***Pyoderma***—A skin disease characterized by purulence.

***Pyogenic***—Producing pus or purulence.

***Reticulum fibers***—Fine thready structures thought to be young collagen fibers.

***Rhus***—A botanical genus including species such as poison ivy (*Rhus toxicodendron*) and poison oak (*Rhus diversiloba*).

***Ringworm***—Ring-shaped patches of cutaneous disease caused by dermatophytes. A synonym for fungous infection that is becoming outmoded as a medical term.

***Rodent ulcer***—Basal cell epithelioma; also, a synonym for eosinophilic granuloma (especially in cats).

***Rugose*** – Full of wrinkles.
***Saprophyte*** – Any plant organism that obtains its nourishment from dead organic matter.
***Sarcoma*** – Malignancy that develops from tissues of mesodermal origin.
***Sarcoptes*** – A genus of mites.
***Scab*** – A hard concretion on superficial wounds. It is composed of clotted blood and tissue debris. Scab is a lay term for which *crust* is medically more acceptable.
***Scabies*** – Infestation with *Sarcoptes scabiei.*
***Scale*** – An accumulation of fragments of the horny layer.
***Scar*** – A hard plaque of dense fibrous tissue that has replaced damaged dermis. It is often covered by atrophic epidermis.
***Sclerosis*** – Hardening.
***Scratch test*** – A procedure of depositing allergenic material within the epidermis after severing its continuity by a light stroke of a needle.
***Scurf*** – Obsolete word for scales and crusts.
***Sebaceous*** – Adjective from *sebum*; pertaining to sebaceous gland or its product.
***Seborrhea*** – An increase in scaling of the skin with or without increase in sebum production.
***Seborrheic dermatitis*** – An inflammatory type of seborrhea.
***Sebum*** – The waxy, oily product of the sebaceous gland.
***Septate*** – Having cross walls.
***Serpiginous*** – Creeping; referring to lesions that slowly enlarge in the shape of a crawling snake.
***Shampoo*** – Massaging and washing the hair with soap and water. Also, a preparation used for washing hair.
***Slough*** – Separation of a membrane or necrotic debris en masse.
***Solar*** – Pertaining to the sun.
***Spiral hyphae*** – Hyphae ending in flat or helical coils as in Trichophyton.
***Spongiosis*** – Intercellular edema within the epidermis having a spongy appearance.
***Spore*** – Characteristically formed cells or groups of cells which separate from the mother plant and are capable of developing into new individuals.
***Squamous*** – Full of scales.
***Steatoma*** – A cyst arising from a sebaceous gland.
***Stratum*** – A layer, especially of the epidermis.
***Stria*** (pl. ***Striae***) – A rather shallow linear depression; a furrow or channel.
***Subcorneal*** – Just under the stratum corneum.
***Subcutis*** – Tissue directly beneath the skin.
***Suspension*** – A pharmaceutical preparation in which ingredients are dispersed as visible particles and which is consequently turbid.
***Tattoo*** – Permanent coloration of the skin with pigments driven into the skin by puncture. It usually refers to a planned procedure, but the term also describes accidental introduction of pigments.
***Telogen*** – The resting or final phase of a hair cycle. That long period before a hair is shed or falls.
***Tinea*** – Superficial fungous infection of human skin.
***Tricho-*** – A prefix denoting hair.
***Trichophyton*** – A genus of fungi.
***Trombicula*** – A genus of mites.
***Tubercle*** – A compact collection of epithelioid cells admixed and surrounded by small round cells.
***Tumor*** – A swelling or enlargement of varying size that may involve any structure of the skin. Usually, but not always, neoplastic.
***Ulcer*** – A break in continuity of the epidermis with loss of substance and exposure of underlying tissue. It is slow to heal or tends not to heal at all.
***Urticaria*** – A condition characterized by wheals.
***Vacuolization*** – The process of development of small empty spaces in cells or tissues.
***Vasculitis*** – Inflammation of small blood vessels.
***Vellus*** – Fine hair that succeeds the lanugo hair.
***Verruca*** – A warty growth, often caused by a virus.
***Vesicle*** – A blister, or small sharply circumscribed elevation of the skin filled with clear fluid. Lesions larger than 0.5 cm. in diameter are called bullae. Rarely seen in dogs.

***Vibrissae*** – Long coarse hairs growing about the nose or muzzle.
***Vitiligo*** – A characteristic leukoderma of man.
***Wart*** – A small callous growth. May be caused by a virus.
***Weeping*** – A superficial inflammatory process in which there is considerable exudation of clear serum from rupture of vesicles or discontinuity of the epidermis.
***Wheal*** – A sharply circumscribed raised lesion caused by dermal edema. Many wheals produce a condition known as urticaria or hives.
***Wood's light*** – Electromagnetic energy with a wavelength of about 3650 Å; an apparatus equipped with a nickel oxide filter that produces ultraviolet light of that quality.
***Xanthoma*** – A yellow tumefaction.
***Xerosis*** – A condition of the skin of abnormal dryness.
***X-rays*** – Electromagnetic energy of wavelengths between 0.5 and 2 Å; roentgen rays.
***Zoonosis*** – A disease of animals which may be communicated to man.
***Zoophilic*** – Having a preference for animals. Used dermatologically to refer to zoophilic fungi whose primary host is an animal.

# INDEX

Page numbers in *italic* type refer to illustrations.